BINOCULAR ANOMALIES

Diagnosis and Vision Therapy

BINOCULAR ANOMALIES
Diagnosis and Vision Therapy

Third Edition

John R. Griffin
M.Opt., O.D., M.S.Ed.
Professor
Southern California College of Optometry
Fullerton

J. David Grisham
O.D., M.S.
Senior Lecturer and Associate Clinical Professor
School of Optometry
University of California, Berkeley
Berkeley

With a Foreword by

Kenneth J. Ciuffreda
O.D., Ph.D.
Distinguished Teaching Professor and Chairman
Department of Vision Sciences
State College of Optometry
State University of New York
New York

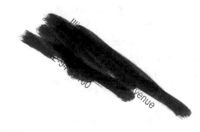

Butterworth-Heinemann
Boston Oxford Melbourne Singapore Toronto Munich New Delhi Tokyo

Every effort has been made to ensure that the drug dosage schedules within
this text are accurate and conform to standards accepted at time of
publication. However, as treatment recommendations vary in the light of
continuing research and clinical experience, the reader is advised to verify
drug dosage schedules herein with information found on product
information sheets. This is especially true in cases of new or infrequently
used drugs.

∞ Recognizing the importance of preserving what has been written,
Butterworth–Heinemann prints its books on acid-free paper whenever
possible.

Library of Congress Cataloging-in-Publication Data

Griffin, John R., 1934–
    Binocular anomalies : diagnosis and vision therapy / John R.
  Griffin, J. David Grisham ; with a foreword by Kenneth J. Ciuffreda.
  —3rd ed.
      p. cm.
    Includes bibliographical references and index.
    1. Binocular vision disorders. I. Grisham, J. David. II. Title.
    [DNLM: 1. Vision Disorders—diagnosis. 2. Vision Disorders—
  therapy. 3. Vision, Binocular. WW 140 G851b 1995]
  RE735.G74 1995
  617.7'62—dc20
  DNLM/DLC
  for Library of Congress   95–11233
                                                                  CIP

British Library Cataloguing-in-Publication Data
A catalogue record for this book is available from the British Library.

The publisher offers discounts on bulk orders of this book.

For information, please write:
Manager of Special Sales
Butterworth–Heinemann
313 Washington Street
Newton, MA 02158–1626

10 9 8 7 6 5 4 3 2 1

Printed in the United States of America

To our children
Angela, Dorothy, Katie, Kimmie, Lisa, and Scott
and
to students and practitioners of binocular vision

Table of Contents

Foreword | XI
Preface | XIII

Part One – Diagnosis

1 Normal Binocular Vision | 3
Value of Normal Binocular Vision | 3
Anatomy of the Extraocular Muscles | 5
Neurology of Eye Movements | 6
Sensory Aspects of Binocular Vision | 9

2 Vision Efficiency Skills | 17
Saccadic Eye Movements | 18
Pursuit Eye Movements | 29
Fixation | 33
Accommodation | 34
Sensory Fusion | 52

3 Heterophoria Case Analysis | 63
Tonic Convergence and AC/A | 64
Zone of Clear Single Binocular Vision | 67
Morgan's Normative Analysis | 70
Criteria for Lens and Prism Prescription | 71
Fixation Disparity Analysis | 73
Validity of Diagnostic Criteria | 81
Recommendations for Prism Prescription | 86
Vergence Anomalies | 87
Convergence Insufficiency | 88
Bioengineering Model | 92

4 Strabismus Testing | 97
History | 97
Measurement of Strabismus | 101
Comitancy | 107
Frequency of the Deviation | 121
Direction of the Deviation | 123
Magnitude of the Deviation | 125
AC/A | 128
Eye Laterality | 128
Eye Dominancy | 129
Variability of the Deviation | 129
Cosmesis | 130

5   Sensory Adaptations to Strabismus | 131
   Suppression | 131
   Amblyopia | 138
   Anomalous Correspondence | 163

6   Diagnosis and Prognosis | 185
   Establishing a Diagnosis | 185
   Prognosis | 186
   Modes of Vision Therapy | 196
   Case Examples | 202

7   Types of Strabismus | 211
   Accommodative Esotropia | 211
   Infantile Esotropia | 216
   Primary Comitant Esotropia | 220
   Primary Comitant Exotropia | 221
   A and V Patterns | 224
   Microtropia | 226
   Cyclovertical Deviations | 228
   Sensory Strabismus | 230
   Consecutive Strabismus | 230

8   Other Oculomotor Disorders | 233
   Neurogenic Palsies | 233
   Myogenic Palsies | 238
   Mechanical Restrictions of Ocular Movement | 241
   Internuclear and Supranuclear Disorders | 244
   Nystagmus | 248

Part Two – Treatment

9   Philosophies and Principles of Binocular Vision Therapy | 261
   Philosophies | 261
   Principles | 265

10   Therapy for Amblyopia | 278
   Management of Refractive Error | 278
   Occlusion Procedures | 280
   Monocular Fixation Training | 292
   Foveal Tag Techniques | 300
   Pleoptics | 305
   Binocular Therapy for Amblyopia | 309
   Progress in Amblyopia Therapy | 313
   Case Examples | 314

11 Anomalous Correspondence Therapy | 323
    Therapy Precautions | 323
    Sensory and Motor Therapy Approaches | 324
    Occlusion Procedures | 325
    Optical Procedures | 327
    Major Amblyoscope | 328
    Training in the Open Environment | 337
    Exotropia and ARC | 341
    Surgical Results in Cases of ARC | 343
    Case Management | 343
    Case Examples | 344

12 Antisuppression Therapy | 349
    Occlusion Antisuppression Therapy | 350
    General Approach to Active Antisuppression Training | 350
    Specific Antisuppression Techniques | 356
    Management Considerations | 366
    Case Example | 367

13 Vision Therapy for Eso Deviations | 371
    Diagnostic Variables | 372
    Vision Therapy Sequence for Comitant Esotropia | 372
    Vision Therapy Sequence for Esophoria | 377
    Specific Training Techniques | 378
    Case Management and Examples | 396

14 Vision Therapy for Exo Deviations | 405
    Diagnostic Considerations | 406
    Vision Therapy Sequence for Comitant Exotropia | 406
    Vision Therapy Sequence for Exophoria | 412
    Specific Training Techniques | 413
    Case Management and Examples | 427

15 Management of Noncomitant Deviations, Intractable Diplopia, and Nystagmus | 437
    Infantile Noncomitant Deviations | 437
    Acquired Noncomitant Deviations | 438
    Intractable Diplopia | 443
    Congenital Nystagmus | 447
    Acquired Nystagmus | 453
    Case Examples | 454

16 Therapy for Vision Efficiency Skills | 461
    Visual Comfort and Performance | 462
    Aniseikonia | 462
    Monovision | 465

Saccadic Eye Movements | 466
Pursuit Eye Movements | 470
Accommodation | 475
Vergences | 479
Stereopsis | 481
Case Examples | 482
Future Directions in Binocular Vision Therapy | 485

Appendixes | 387
Conversions of Prism Diopters and Degrees | 491
Visual Acuity and Visual Efficiency | 491
Stereoacuity Calculations | 442
Visual Skills Efficiency Evaluation (Testing Outline) | 493
Strabismus Examination Record | 494
Suppliers and Equipment | 496

Glossary | 499

Index | 503

Foreword

Binocular vision, ranging from optimally efficient to grossly abnormal function, represents an area in which optometry is uniquely qualified. The profession has a long history of interest, innovation, and achievement in dealing with both the diagnosis and treatment of the abnormal sensory, motor, and perceptual characteristics found in patients. The same can be said for optometry's supportive role in basic and applied research in binocular vision conducted at the various optometric academic centers. The expanding role in the area of ocular disease—as well as in the vision rehabilitation of patients with neurological dysfunction, assessment, and treatment of their relatively common binocular vision problems—has made optometry increasingly more important to the total care and functional recovery process.

I believe this third edition, now entitled *Binocular Anomalies: Diagnosis and Vision Therapy*, will continue its tradition of being the standard against which all other textbooks in this field are compared. It has been revised, expanded, and now has a co-author, J. David Grisham. Drs. Griffin and Grisham are optometric leaders in the area of binocular vision disorders. Together they selflessly share with us more than half a century of their invaluable knowledge, experience, and insight.

This textbook has several attributes that I find most appealing. First, each chapter is preceded by a detailed outline that serves to guide both the student and practitioner through the basic information and key topics. Second, numerous summary tables and figures promote more focused learning. Third, the authors provide a thorough and comprehensive approach to each topic, with straightforward discussion of the "pros and cons" of each diagnostic and therapeutic component. Fourth, they attempt to quantify their clinical observations and outcomes rather than be satisfied with more common but less useful qualitative descriptions. Finally, their respect for both basic and clinical research in the area is clearly evident. In fact, over the past two decades, both have been involved in a variety of clinical research projects and scholarly activities in binocular vision and related areas such as reading and learning disabilities.

With the above in mind, it is no surprise that Drs. Griffin and Grisham have produced a textbook of considerable merit. As optometric vision therapy continues to flourish and expand into many new, exciting, and challenging areas, it is comforting to know that such a wonderful textbook is available to provide the initial foundation for and subsequent guidance into these frontiers.

Kenneth J. Ciuffreda, O.D., Ph.D.
Distinguished Teaching Professor and Chairman
Department of Vision Sciences
State College of Optometry
State University of New York
New York

Preface

There is an increasing emphasis on primary health care in optometry and ophthalmology. As health professionals, vision care practitioners screen for general health conditions and diseases that require referral and management by allied professionals. It is no longer adequate for the clinician merely to identify eye diseases; diagnosis is the standard of care. Consequently, we include *diagnosis* in the title of the third edition. When the exact diagnosis and prognosis are known, exact and efficacious vision therapy can be prescribed and applied. The major additions to this new edition involve diagnostic categories and procedures, but important new vision therapy procedures and discussions have also been added.

We take the accepted view that *vision therapy* includes all modes of treatment of binocular vision problems, including extraocular muscle surgery when necessary and expedient. Vision training is that portion of vision therapy that encompasses orthoptics for strabismus and heterophoria, pleoptics in certain cases of amblyopia, and visual perception therapy involving learning difficulties that are visually related. This latter type of vision therapy, however, is not covered in this text on binocular anomalies. Orthoptics and pleoptics, however, are extensively discussed, as are other modes of therapy including lenses, prisms, occlusion, pharmaceutical treatment, and motivational methods for successful results. As in the previous editions, Part One covers testing, diagnosis, and prognosis, and provides an overview of management of various types of amblyopic, strabismic, and heterophoric problems. Part Two, which has been extensively updated and rewritten, deals with treatment of amblyopia, strabismus, heterophoria, and inefficient visual skills; the emphasis, however, is on vision training regimens and procedures. Each *active vision training technique* is identified by a "T" number for easy identification and referencing. Case examples are included to illustrate the implementation of vision therapy. The sampling of cases is not exhaustive but only representative to help the clinician connect the theoretical principles with the specific practical procedures in vision therapy.

We thank the following individuals for their help in making this publication possible: Drs. Morris Berman, Kenneth Brookman, Garth Christenson, Merton Flom, Richard Hemenger, Richard Hopping, Arthur Jampolsky, Janice Scharre, Clifton Schor, James Sheedy, and Bruce Wick. We also thank Richard Bertelson, Albert Garcia, Kirsten Griffin, Judith Higgins, Helen Lee, Lois Keup, Geraldine McGowan, Barbara Murphy, Diana Nguyen, Kim Nguyen, Karen Oberheim, and personnel of suppliers of equipment used in photographs, and to many other individuals whom we, apologetically, may have failed to acknowledge.

John R. Griffin
Fullerton

J. David Grisham
Berkeley

PART ONE

DIAGNOSIS

Chapter 1 / Normal Binocular Vision

Value of Normal Binocular Vision   3
Anatomy of the Extraocular Muscles   5
Neurology of Eye Movements   6
   Accommodation   6
   Conjugate Gaze Movements   7
     Saccades   7
     Vestibular Ocular Eye Movements   7
     Pursuits   7
   Vergences   8
Sensory Aspects of Binocular Vision   9
   Monocular Considerations   9

Retinal Correspondence   9
   Panum's Fusional Areas   9
   Singleness Horopter   10
Physiological Diplopia   10
Pathological Diplopia   12
Types of Sensory Fusion   12
   Color Fusion   12
   Form Fusion   12
Theories of Sensory Fusion   14
Binocularly Driven Cells and Ocular
   Dominance   15

Binocular vision pertains to the motor coordination of the eyes and the sensory unification of their respective views of the world. This is a unitary process, but for the sake of analysis it can be broken into sensory and motor components.

The sensory component starts with light emitted from or reflected off of physical objects in the external environment that is brought into focus on the retina by each eye's optics. This pattern of light energy is transformed by retinal photoreceptors into neuroelectrical impulses and is transmitted to the visual perceptual areas of the cerebral cortex and certain subcortical areas. The result of complex neural processing, which is only partially understood, is the sensation of object attributes (i.e., form, color, intensity, and position in space) that, in turn, culminates in an immediate, vivid perception of object identity and of the relations of objects in the external environment.

The motor positioning and alignment of the eyes completely subserves the primary sensory function of image unification and allows visual perception to proceed efficiently. The task of the motor system is to bring both foveas onto the object of attention within the visual field and keep them there as long as the individual requires. The motor system also holds the eyes in alignment and clear focus, thereby ensuring the maintenance of binocular vision. Frequently, however, the complete remediation of binocular vision anomalies requires attention to both sensory and motor aspects.

VALUE OF NORMAL BINOCULAR VISION

One distinctive perceptual attribute of humans, besides all other primates, is a high degree of stereoscopic binocular vision. Our skills in hunting, food gathering, and toolmaking have helped direct our evolution. In the competition for food, shelter, and safety, *stereopsis* is one of several attributes that evidently provided important advantages to those who had it. In the modern age, stereoscopic vision continues to provide individuals with important information about their environment. Whether at school, the workplace, or on the sports field, stereopsis significantly aids in making judgments about depth. It also helps stablize both sensory and motor fusion and can be considered a "barometer" of the status of binocular vision.

Besides stereopsis, there are other benefits of normal binocular vision. The most obvious benefit of having two eyes is that, in case of injury to one, there is an *eye in reserve*. This might be called the "spare tire" concept. Even though the loss of sight in one eye may cause some significant problems for an individual, losing sight in both eyes can be devastating.

The binocular individual also has the advantage of a large *field of vision* (Figure 1-1): The binocular field of vision is usually at least 30 degrees larger than the monocular field.

Binocular *visual acuity* is normally better by approximately a half-line of letters on a Snellen chart, compared with either eye alone.[1,2] The

difference is even greater when there is uncorrected ametropia in each eye.

Binocular vision often minimizes the effects of ocular disease, relative to monocular vision. Binocular summation of ocular images significantly heightens *contrast sensitivity*, by about 40%.[3] Practically speaking, this is helpful for driving at night and working under low-illumination conditions. Individuals with certain ocular diseases (e.g., optic nerve demylination in multiple sclerosis) may have profound differences in contrast sensitivity between binocular and monocular sight.

There are several vocational and avocational performance benefits in having good binocularity. Sheedy et al.[4] described superior *task performance* under binocular versus monocular viewing conditions (Table 1-1). Differences favoring binocular viewing were notable in such tasks as card filing, needle threading, and, surprisingly, word decoding. There was no significant difference, however, in letter counting on a video display terminal (VDT) and throwing beanbags accurately. These investigators concluded that stereopsis provides a performance advantage for

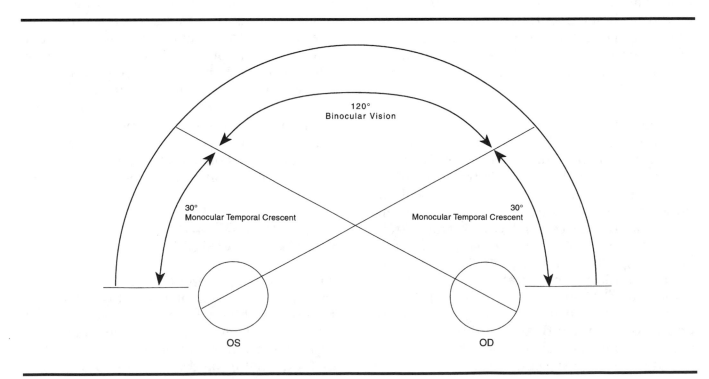

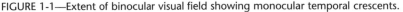
FIGURE 1-1—Extent of binocular visual field showing monocular temporal crescents.

TABLE 1-1. *Superiority of Binocular Compared with Monocular Performance.*[4]

Task	Percent	Significance (t test)
Putting sticks in holes	30%	0.001
Needle threading	20%	0.001
Card filing	9%	0.001
Placing pegs in grooves	4%	0.001
Reading (word decoding)	4%	0.05
VDT letter counting	2%	N.S.
Beanbag tossing	−1%	N.S.

many different jobs, particularly those requiring nearpoint eye-hand coordination. Several occupations (e.g., pilots, microsurgeons, and cartographers) require good binocular vision to perform their tasks safely and accurately.

Strabismus affects only a small percentage of the population, ranging from 1.3% to 5.4%,[5] but other deficiencies of binocular vision, such as convergence insufficiency and accommodative infacility, are much more prevalent and may result in bothersome symptoms and inefficient performance. Except for those individuals who have acquired strabismus and experience persistent double vision, most constant strabismics report few extraordinary visual symptoms. On the other hand, many nonstrabismics with binocular vision dysfunctions have a variety of complaints that are visual in origin, such as intermittent blur at distance or near, tired eyes after reading or viewing a computer monitor, "eyestrain" at the end of the day, print that appears to jump or move, visually related headaches, reduced depth perception, mild photophobia, and other disagreeable visual sensations. Many of these symptomatic individuals suffer from "binocular efficiency dysfunction" (see Chapter 2).

ANATOMY OF THE EXTRAOCULAR MUSCLES

Three pairs of extraocular muscles control the movements of each eye: a pair of horizontal rectus muscles, a pair of vertical rectus muscles, and a pair of oblique muscles. The rectus muscles, the superior oblique muscle, and the levator muscle (controlling the upper lid) are attached to the bones at the back of the orbit by a tendinous ring (the annulus of Zinn) that surrounds the optic foramen and part of the superior orbital fissure (Figure 1-2). The four rectus muscles, optic nerve, ophthalmic artery, N VI and two branches of N III form a *muscle cone*. The insertions of the rectus muscles are not equidistant from the corneal limbus but form a spiral, known as the spiral of Tillaux, with the superior rectus inserting the farthest away from the limbus (7.7 mm) and the medial rectus inserting the nearest (5.5 mm) (Figure 1-3). The more advanced the insertion, the greater the mechanical advantage of the muscle, e.g., the medial rectus compared with the superior rectus.

As with the rectus muscles, the superior oblique originates from the annulus of Zinn, but it courses along the superior medial wall of the orbit to the trochlea, a U-shaped fibro-

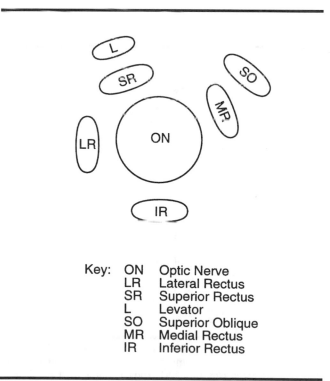

Key:
	ON	Optic Nerve
	LR	Lateral Rectus
	SR	Superior Rectus
	L	Levator
	SO	Superior Oblique
	MR	Medial Rectus
	IR	Inferior Rectus

FIGURE 1-2—Annulus of Zinn illustrating origins of the four rectus muscles and the superior oblique muscle of the right eye, inferior oblique having origin anteriorly.

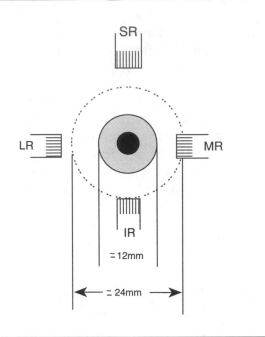

FIGURE 1-3—Spiral of Tillaux showing insertions of rectus muscles of the right eye. Starting clockwise with the medial rectus, the insertions become farther from the limbus.

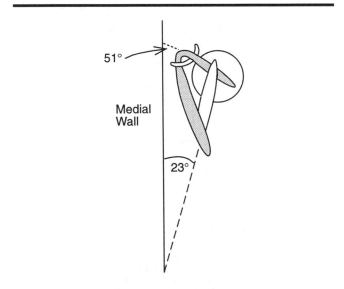

FIGURE 1-4—Diagram of relation between the superior oblique muscle and the superior rectus muscle. (Note: Both the inferior and superior oblique muscles form a 51° angle with the medial wall, and both the inferior and superior rectus form a 23° angle with the medial wall. The action fields for clinical purposes are approximately 50° and 25° for the oblique and vertical recti, respectively.)

cartilage, that acts as a pulley. Near the trochlea, the muscle tissue becomes a tendon as it passes through the trochlea and then reflects back normally at an angle of approximately 51° to the medial wall. The muscle then crosses the globe superiorly, passing under the superior rectus, to insert in the posterior, superior quadrant near the vortex veins. The trochlea, therefore, becomes the effective mechanical origin for the action of the superior oblique (Figure 1-4). The inferior oblique is the only extraocular muscle that does not originate in the orbital apex; it arises from a small fossa in the anterior, inferior, orbital wall (the maxilla bone). This muscle's course parallels the reflective portion of the superior oblique forming again a 51° angle as it courses inferiorly and laterally across the globe, over the inferior rectus, to insert in the inferior, posterior quadrant.

NEUROLOGY OF EYE MOVEMENTS

The neurology of the following systems are briefly discussed: accommodation, conjugate gaze movements, and vergence.

Accommodation

Accommodation is one member of the oculomotor triad that also includes pupil constriction and accommodative convergence, all mediated by the third nerve nucleus in the midbrain. Accommodation is a reflex initiated by retinal blur; it can, however, be under conscious control. The afferent pathway is from the retina to the visual cortex and projects from area 19 to the pretectum and superior colliculus before entering the Edinger-Westphal nucleus of the third nerve complex. Projections from the frontal eye fields (traditionally referred to as Brodmann's area 8) also enter the third nerve complex that, in part, mediates conscious control of accommodation. The efferent component of the reflex arc from the third nerve complex synapses in the ciliary ganglion and again in the ciliary muscle that, in turn, effectuates the change of lens power (Figure 1-5).

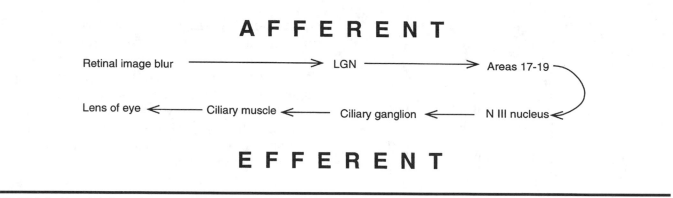

AFFERENT

Retinal image blur ──────────→ LGN ──────────→ Areas 17-19

Lens of eye ←──── Ciliary muscle ←──── Ciliary ganglion ←──── N III nucleus

EFFERENT

FIGURE 1-5—Neural pathway for accommodation.

Conjugate Gaze Movements

Conjugate eye movements are tandem movements of the two eyes, referred to as versions. These are either saccades, vestibular ocular movements, or pursuits. These three eye-movement systems share a common final pathway to the extraocular muscles, but they are neurologically distinct with different central pathways and dynamic properties.

Saccades

Saccadic eye movements refer to ballistic-type eye movements that carry the eye quickly from one target in space to another (i.e., a change in fixation). There are several types of saccades: (1) the fast phases of either vestibular or optokinetic nystagmus, (2) spontaneous saccades occurring about 20 times per minute and used to scan the environment, (3) reflexive (nonvolitional) saccades that occur in response to any new environmental stimulus, and (4) intentional saccades that carry the eyes from one target to another predetermined target.[6] The anatomy subserving voluntary saccades has been partly established by monkey studies and clinical observation in humans. For example, if there is an intention for a dextroversion (eyes that move to the right), stimulation occurs in Brodmann's area 8 (frontal eye field) in the frontal lobe of the left hemisphere. Impulses then travel to the right pontine gaze center and are forwarded to the ipsilateral nucleus of N VI. Subsequently the lateral rectus of the right eye contracts. Simultaneously, impulses travel from the ipsilateral pontine gaze center up through the medial longitudinal fasciculus that decussates to the left N III nucleus. That results in contraction of the medial rectus of the left eye. Because yoked muscles have equal innervation (Hering's Law),[7] the two eyes move in tandem. Versions are not restricted because of the simultaneous relaxation of the antagonistic yoked muscles (Sherrington's law of reciprocal innervation)[7] (Figure 1-6).

Vestibular Ocular Eye Movements

The reflexive vestibular ocular system stabilizes the eyes on a target during head movements and can be tested with the "doll's head" maneuvre. The dynamics of vestibular eye movements are relatively fast, having a latency of only 16 milliseconds compared with the pursuit system of 75 msec.[8] As the head turns, vestibular ocular reflexes (VOR) are initiated by the movement of fluid in the semicircular canals of the inner ear. For example, stimulation of the left vestibular nucleus causes impulses to travel to the right pontine gaze center. From there, the pathway to the extraocular muscles is the same as described above for saccadic eye movements. Stimulation from the left vestibular nucleus by a left head turn causes compensatory dextroversion.

Pursuits

The pursuit system mediates constant tracking of a moving target. This system is the slowest of the three. Pursuit eye movements are

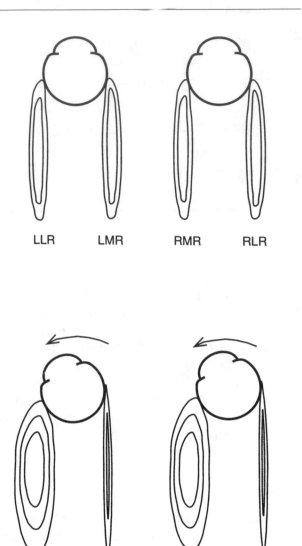

LLR   LMR   RMR   RLR

FIGURE 1-6—Hering's law and Sherrington's law evident during levoversion. The right medial rectus and the left lateral rectus (yoked muscles) contract in accord with Hering's laws. The left medial rectus is the antagonist of the left lateral rectus, and it relaxes, as does the right lateral rectus (antagonist of the right medial rectus) in accord with Sherrington's law.

mediated via the occipitomesencephalic pathway. Impulses travel from the occipital lobes (presumably from area 19) to the midbrain and pontine gaze centers, and on to the nuclei of the third, fourth, and sixth cranial nerves to innervate the extraocular muscles. Each occipital lobe is involved in the pursuit of a target, in both directions, horizontally or vertically.[9] The assumption is that the right and left oc-

cipital area is connected to each right and left pontine gaze center so that stimulation from one occipital lobe may stimulate both the left and right pontine gaze centers, for left or right pursuit movements. Because of this double coverage, pursuits may sometimes be intact despite an extensive lesion in one hemisphere of the brain that could also cause a homonymous hemianoptic visual field loss.

Vergences

Vergence refers to disjunctive eye movements, or rotation of the eyes in opposite directions. The two main types of vergence movements are *accommodative* vergence, stimulated by blur, and *fusional* vergence, stimulated by retinal image disparity. Vergences are under a degree of conscious control, but they usually are involuntary psycho-optic reflexes.[10] Vergence movements are slow and show a negative exponential waveform (velocity going from fast to slow). For most visual tasks, both vergence and saccadic eye movements are used in combination to place objects on the foveas.

Little is known about the supranuclear pathways subserving vergence eye movements, even though convergence in the monkey was produced as early as 1890 by electrical stimulation of sites in the cortex.[11] Vergence eye movements are probably synthesized bilaterally in the cerebral cortex.[12] Impulses travel from the cortex to the pretectum and rostral mesencephalic reticular formation. Innervation is integrated from several sites including the cerebellum. In the midbrain, convergence is mediated by the bilateral nuclei of the oculomotor nuclear complex (N III) that sends efferent signals to both medial rectus muscles. There is probably no single convergence center, as was once thought to be the case (e.g., "Nucleus of Perlia").

Divergence was once accepted as merely the relaxation of convergence innervation. Divergence usually is an active neurophysiologic process, as indicated by electromyographic recordings from the lateral rectus muscles.[13] The pathway centers that subserve divergence, however, are still essentially unknown.

SENSORY ASPECTS OF BINOCULAR VISION

The ability to integrate information from the two eyes into one fused image and extract depth information is dependent on the primary visual cortex (mainly in the calcarine fissure) located bilaterally on the medial aspect of each occipital lobe. Other functions of the primary visual cortex (Brodmann's area 17) include detecting spatial organization of the visual scene, brightness, shading, and rudimentary form organization. Specific points of the retina connect with specific points of the visual cortex (e.g., the homonymous right halves of the two respective retinas connect with the right visual cortex). In other words, the primary visual cortex is organized like a map of the retina. Because the eyes are separated by a distance of approximately 60 mm in humans, each eye's view of the environment is from a slightly different perspective. The sole basis for stereopsis is the horizontal disparity between the two retinal images. A little-understood neural mechanism, which is located presumably within the visual cortex, compares the retinal images from each eye for disparity information. Further neural processing in this visual pathway (also not fully understood) gives almost all people with normal binocular vision a vivid sense of three dimensionality—volume—in their visual perception of the external world.

Binocular vision seems so natural to most people that they are hardly aware that their perception of the world arises from the unification of two separate and slightly different images. They are surprised if diplopia occurs. What is truly remarkable, however, is that we usually do see images as single; this fact requires an explanation. Fusion of two ocular images requires adequate functioning of each eye and sufficient stimulation of corresponding retinal points in the two eyes to produce single binocular vision.

Monocular Considerations

For normal binocular vision, the best possible visual acuity of each eye should be attained, whether by means of spectacle lenses, contact lenses, surgical intervention (e.g., in the case of a cataract), or other possible procedures (e.g., vision therapy for amblyopia). Poor acuity of either or both eyes is a deterrent to sensory fusion. This is particularly true when the vision of one eye is much poorer than that of the other eye. The discrepancy may be due to functional reasons, such as anisometropic amblyopia and strabismic amblyopia, or it may be due to organic causes, such as macular degeneration, cataract, and optic nerve atrophy. Any organic disease must be ruled out or managed correctly before functional testing is continued and vision training procedures are begun.

Retinal Correspondence

Retinal correspondence refers to the subjective visual direction and the spatial location of objects in the binocular visual field. An individual is said to have normal "retinal" correspondence (NRC) when the stimulation of both foveas (and geometrically paired retinal areas) gives rise to a unitary percept. (The correspondence actually occurs in the cortex.) The existence of corresponding retinal elements with their common subjective visual direction is fundamental to binocular vision. Stimulation of corresponding retinal points results in haplopia (singleness of vision) even if there is normal correspondence or anomalous correspondence. (Anomalous "retinal" correspondence, conventionally abbreviated as ARC, is discussed in Chapter 5.) Conversely, double vision results when noncorresponding retinal points are sufficiently stimulated.

Panum's Fusional Areas

Rather than a point-to-point correspondence between the two eyes, there exists a point-to-area relationship subserving binocular fusion. This was first described by Panum, a Danish physiologist, in the middle of the 19th century.[14] Panum's area is "an area in the retina of one eye, any point of which, when stimulated simultaneously with a single specific point in the retina of the other eye, will give rise to a

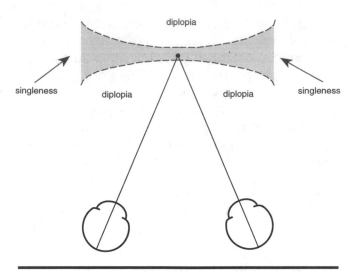

FIGURE1-7—Singleness (haplopia) horopter. Diplopia can occur for an object that is not within the horopter.

single fused percept."[7] Panum's areas are oval in shape and larger horizontally than vertically. Foveal Panum's areas are very small, only a few minutes of arc, compared with peripheral Panum's areas that may be several prism diopters in extent. The increasing size of these areas in the periphery may be related to anatomic and physiologic differences known to exist between central and peripheral retina, receptors being densely packed at the fovea but widely separated in the peripheral retina. Panum's areas parallel the increase in size of the *retinal* receptive fields, but they are functionally part of the *visual cortex* where binocular information comes together.

Singleness Horopter

Sensory fusion can also be described in terms of the location of stimuli in the visual environment. The horopter is defined as the locus of all object points that are imaged on corresponding retinal elements at a given fixation distance.[15] The *identical visual direction (IVD) horopter* is a locus of object points in which images on the two retinas provide a common visual direction. The IVD horopter is usually represented as a single horizontal line passing through the fixation point, having no thickness. The concept of Panum's fusional areas is easily visualized by reference to the IVD horop-

ter that is enveloped by the *haplopic (singleness) horopter*. This horopter is "an empirical horopter represented as having thickness corresponding to Panum's areas expressed by the anteroposterior limits through which a nonfixated test object may be displaced and still be seen as single"[7] (Figure 1-7). Note that the horopter is thicker in the periphery, corresponding to the increasing size of Panum's fusional areas. The significance of the singleness horopter, which involves the IVD horopter and Panum's areas, is that any object seen outside the horopter necessarily falls on diplopia-producing noncorresponding points. In other words, the visual world outside the singleness horopter should theoretically appear as double when retinal stimulation is sufficient. Fortunately, nature is grand; *physiological suppression* usually eliminates physiological diplopia so that most people can go about living normal lives, at least visually. Similarly, nature provides sensory antidiplopic mechanisms for the strabismic individual in the forms of ARC and pathological suppression (discussed in Chapter 5).

Physiological Diplopia

The doubling of a *nonfixated* object is referred to as physiological diplopia, because there is nothing abnormal about this phenomenon. With normal binocular vision all objects falling outside the singleness horopter can be seen as double, if sufficient attention is paid to the stimulus object. Homonymous physiological diplopia occurs when objects are beyond the point of bifixation. This is also referred to as "uncrossed" diplopia. Conversely, heteronymous ("crossed") diplopia occurs when a farther object is bifixated with a nearer object in view (Figures 1-8 and 1-9). Because of physiological suppression, these physiological diplopic images are usually unnoticed under ordinary viewing conditions.

Most patients consider seeing double to be abnormal and seek help from an eye doctor. If the examination does not reveal a paretic muscle or a motor fusion problem and physiological diplopia seems the most likely explanation, then the doctor must explain that it is a feature

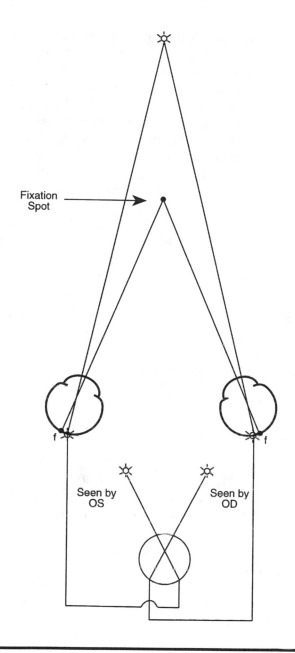

FIGURE 1-8—Homonymous ("uncrossed") physiological diplopia.

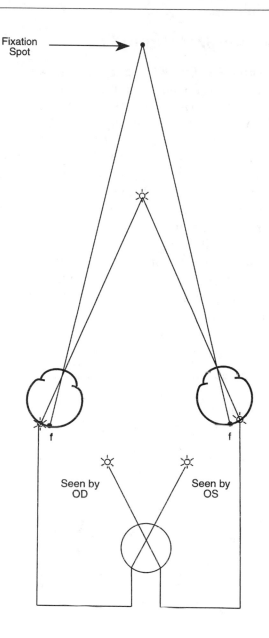

FIGURE 1-9—Heteronymous ("crossed") physiological diplopia.

of normal binocular vision that is normally unnoticed. Sometimes patients are not easily convinced of this physiological fact about binocular vision because the phenomenon seems counterintuitive. On the other hand, physiological diplopia is easy to demonstrate to a patient with normal binocular vision and can be used as a binocular vision screening technique. As the patient fixates on a pencil at 40 cm, for example, the clinician asks the patient to hold

up an index finger halfway between the fixation object and the nose. If the patient's attention is drawn to the nonfixated finger, then the finger usually appears double, like two ghost images. Patients who have active suppression of one eye due to a binocular vision disorder often cannot easily see the diplopic image. Physiological diplopia is also an important tool in vision training to help remediate binocular vision in both strabismic and nonstrabismic cases.

Pathological Diplopia

Diplopia of a *fixated* target is considered abnormal and is referred to as pathological. This occurs in cases of strabismus in which there is little or no suppression. Figure 1-10 shows one eye (left) fixating the target of regard while the esotropic (right) eye is not fixating the target. The image, rather than falling on the fovea of the right eye, is nasal relative to its fovea. This produces homonymous diplopia ("uncrossed") where the diplopic image is seen on the same side as the strabismic eye. On the other hand, in cases of exotropia, pathological diplopia is heteronymous ("crossed"), in which the diplopic image is seen on the opposite side of the strabismic eye.

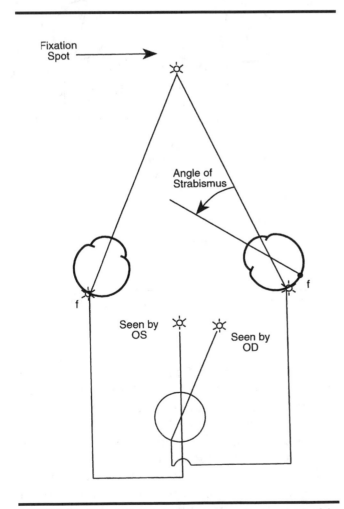

FIGURE 1-10—Pathological diplopia in an example of esotropia of the right eye. The diplopia is homonymous (uncrossed).

Cyclopean projection depicts the manner in which the visual cortex mediates subjective directionalization of the ocular images. If the cyclopean eye is compared with a clock's face, the principal visual direction would occur at the fovea (assuming normal fixation and correspondence). In Figure 1-10, assume that the nasally stimulated portion of the right eye is at the 7 o'clock position. The directional projection is, therefore, at the 7 o'clock position in the cyclopean eye. The difference of "one hour" would normally cause noticeable diplopia (assuming one image is not suppressed). When, however, the difference is only a very small fraction of an "hour," diplopia may not be obvious, as in fixation disparity. (Fixation disparity measurement is discussed in Chapter 3.)

Types of Sensory Fusion

Sensory fusion may be that of color and form.

Color Fusion

Color fusion is "a type of sensory fusion wherein spectral stimulation which differs for the two eyes is combined or integrated into a unitary percept unlike either of the stimulating fields."[7] Color fusion is independent of the singleness horopter. It is the lowest level of sensory fusion and is of relatively little importance, except that many vision testing and training procedures use color fusion (e.g., Worth dot test and anaglyphic targets).

Form Fusion

Binocular fusion of forms occurs within the singleness horopter; diplopia occurs outside the horopter. Fused binocular vision is precious, but it is possible only in a relatively small band of visual space—analogous to a vein of gold in the side of a granite mountain.

Form fusion is the driving force behind good binocularity. This is the blending of form information from the two eyes. Simultaneous perception, superimposition, flat fusion, and stereopsis are discussed.

Diplopia is the *simultaneous perception* of two ocular images of a single object. This is an important sensory phenomenon in clinical assessment and vision therapy. As discussed previously, physiological diplopia testing refers to the perception of diplopic images that lie outside the singleness horopter. Physiological diplopia training is frequently useful in vision therapy to break pathological suppression and to increase vergence ranges.

Clinicians use many tests involving pathological diplopia, particularly as part of strabismus evaluations. In cases of noncomitant strabismus, for example, pathological diplopia testing is very important to determine the severity of under- and over-actions of extraocular muscles in various positions of gaze.

Whereas diplopia results from noncorresponding retinal points being stimulated, *superimposition* of two ocular images (e.g., a bird in the cage) requires stimulation of retinal areas having common visual directions. Worth[16] classified superimposition as "first degree fusion." The importance of superimposition testing is in measuring the subjective angle of directionalization (angle S) and also assessing the degree of suppression, particularly in strabismic patients.

Worth[16] classified *flat fusion* as "second degree fusion." This is true fusion but without stereopsis. Flat fusion is defined as, "Sensory fusion in which the resultant percept is two-dimensional, that is, occupying a single plane, as may be induced by viewing a stereogram in a stereoscope in which the separation of all homologous points is identical."[7] The most important reason to consider flat fusion is for vision testing and training purposes, as in phorometry measurements, fixation disparity testing, and in amblyoscopic assessment and treatment (i.e., major amblyoscope instrumentation).

Worth[16] classified *stereopsis* as third-degree fusion. Stereopsis is defined as follows: "Binocular visual perception of three dimensional space based on retinal disparity."[7]

Figure 1-11 illustrates *central* stereopsis; the fused, small vertical line is perceived as closer than the star. Although there is lateral displacement of the vertical line, as to each eye, there will be fusion of the two lines into one vertical line, which appears centered (but closer) in respect to the star. Lateral displacement of such

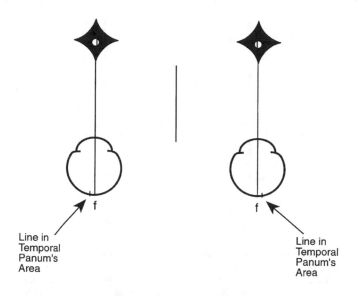

FIGURE 1-11—Stereogram for central stereopsis, induced by laterally displaced vertical lines. The fused vertical line appears closer than the star because the temporal (to the fovea) Panum's area is stimulated in each eye.

stimuli to produce stereoscopic depth is a feature of many vision therapy targets, such as vectographic slides (Vectograms®), anaglyphs, and stereograms (as in this example).

When the laterally displaced stimuli are located beyond 5° from the center of the fovea, *peripheral* stereopsis is being evaluated. In Figure 1-12 the "Y" appears to be closer to the patient and the "X" farther away in relation to the star. Clinicians also speak of stereopsis as

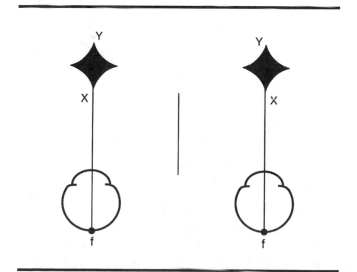

FIGURE 1-12—Example of target for peripheral stereopsis.

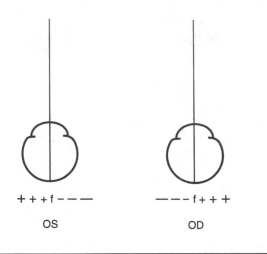

$$+++f---$$ $$---f+++$$

OS   OD

FIGURE 1-13—Stereopsis values for nearness and farness perception. Plus signs indicate nearness, also referred to as "cross disparity." Minus signs indicate distance, "uncrossed disparity." The greater the temporal Panum's area (larger plus signs) the greater the stereopsis effect, and also for the nasal Panum's area (minus signs).

"gross" or "fine." Peripheral stereopsis is necessarily classified as being "gross." Central stereopsis, on the other hand, is considered "fine" if it is 200 seconds of arc or better.

Stereoscopically fused images appear nearer to a bifixated reference point if Panum's areas are stimulated temporally from the center of the foveas. Conversely, if Panum's areas are stimulated nasally from the center of the foveas, the image seems farther from the bifixated reference point. If the temporal retina can be thought of as having positive values for nearness and the nasal retina having negative values, the concept of stereopsis related to lateral displacement is easy to understand. The greater the distance from the center of the fovea, the greater the value—either positive or negative—for the nearness and distance perceptions, respectively. This is illustrated in Figure 1-13 by the increasing sizes of the plus and minus signs toward the periphery of the retina.

Generally speaking, the finer the degree of stereoscopic discrimination, the higher the quality of binocular vision. Conversely, suppression and excessive fixation disparity may decrease stereoacuity; these anomalies often predispose a patient to asthenopic symptoms and reduced visual performance. The main value of stereopsis is that of being a clue to depth at close viewing distances. Its value to the individual is hardly significant at far distances.[17] A surgeon is more likely to need stereo depth perception than an airline pilot. Monocular clues to depth (e.g., size, linear perspective, texture gradient, and overlap) tend to predominate at far distances. Nevertheless, most passenger airlines require their pilots to have superior stereopsis since safety and prudence demand that every possible perceptual clue to making accurate depth judgments be available. That stringent criterion probably relates to stereopsis being the "barometer of binocular vision.")

Theories of Sensory Fusion

The salient features accounting for sensory fusion are retinal correspondence, retinal image disparity detection, and neural summation of information from the two eyes. A system of correspondence provides feedback whether or not the motor alignment of the eyes is in registry. Retinal image disparity detection is the stimulus to the vergence system to make correctional vergence eye movements. Also, retinal image disparities, within certain limits, are necessary for stereopsis. Research has indicated that certain striate cells in areas 17 and 18 are sensitive to horizontal disparity for the perception of stereopsis.[18,19]

Studies of higher mammals have shown that about 80% of cells in the striate cortex can be binocularly stimulated.[20] Neural summation of these binocular cells has been demonstrated by single-cell neurophysiological investigations.[18] The corresponding areas, however, must be in proper registry for maximum responsiveness. When these fields are out of alignment, they mutually inhibit one another.[21] These physiological features are the basis of the perceptual unification of the two ocular images and some of the advantages of normal binocular vision. As discussed previously, contrast sensitivity and visual acuity are enhanced by binocular neural summation.

One of the more popular older theories of binocular vision, the *alternation theory*, held that unification of the two ocular images does not, in fact, take place. The theory claimed that

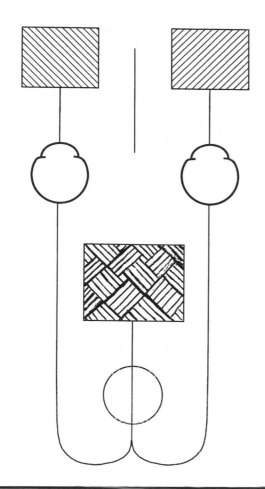

FIGURE 1-14—Cyclopean projection showing perception of retinal rivalry.

the retinal rivalry phenomenon gave evidence that the binocular field was composed of a mosaic of monocularly perceived patches. No true fusion occurred; the input for one eye would inhibit the input from the other. *Retinal rivalry* of dissimilar forms, a common clinical observation, is the primary evidence supporting the alternation theory. The mosaic pattern of the "fused" image is ever changing with certain portions at times being dominated by the left eye's responses and at other times by the responses of the right eye (Figure 1-14). This theory left many features of binocular perception unexplained, such as contrast sensitivity enhancement. Moreover, single cell electrophysiological evidence has conclusively shown this notion of binocular vision to be essentially incorrect. The more modern theory of *neural summation* is fundamental to binocular perception.

Binocularly Driven Cells and Ocular Dominance

Ocular dominance is another important physiological feature of binocularly driven cells. Only about one-fourth of these cells respond equally to input from the right and left eye; the others respond more vigorously to the input from either one eye or the other.[20] Ocular dominance of binocular cortical cells is particularly sensitive to the amount of binocular stimulation during development in infancy. Even minor obstacles to sensory fusion can have long-term consequences. Obstacles to sensory fusion, such as anisometropia, strabismus, and form deprivation (e.g., cataract), can result in a rapid shift in striate-cell ocular dominance. When most cortical cells are controlled exclusively by one eye during the sensitive period, the natural consequences are binocular anomalies. These include suppression, amblyopia, ARC, loss of stereopsis, and deficient fusional vergences. These binocular anomalies may become permanent unless timely and appropriate vision therapy takes place.

REFERENCES

1. Bárány E. A theory of binocular visual acuity and an analysis of the variability of visual acuity. *Acta Ophthalmologica.* 1946;24:63.
2. Horowity MW. An analysis of the superiority of binocular over monocular visual acuity. *J Exp Psychol.* 1949;39:581.
3. Campbell FW, Green DG. Monocular vs. binocular visual acuity. *Nature.* 1965;200:191–192.
4. Sheedy JE, Bailey IL, Muri M, Bass E. Binocular vs. monocular task performance. *Am J Optom Physiol Opt.* 1989;63:839–846.
5. Michaels DD. *Visual Optics and Refraction.* St. Louis: CV Mosby, 1980.677.
6. Glaser JS. *Neuro-ophthalmology.* Philadelphia: Lippincott; 1990:300.
7. Cline D, Hofstetter H, Griffin J. *Dictionary of Visual Science,* 4th ed. Radnor, PA: Chilton; 1989.
8. Maas EF, Huebner WP, Seidman SH, Leigh RJ. Behavior of human horizontal vestibulo-ocular reflex in response to high-acceleration stimuli. *Brain Res.* 1989;499:153–156.
9. Bajandas FJ, Kline, LB. *Neuro-Ophthalmology Review Manual.* 2nd. ed. Thorofare, NJ: Slack Inc, 1987:51–54.
10. Hoffman FB, Bielshowsky A. Über die der Wilkur entzogenen Fusionsbewegungen der Augen. *Arch Ges Physiol.* 1900;80:1.

11. Mukuno K. Electron microscopic studies on the human extraocular muscles under pathologic conditions. *Jpn J Ophthalmol.* 1969;13:35.

12. Dale RT. *Fundamentals of Ocular Motility and Strabismus.* New York: Grune & Stratton; 1982:105.

13. Tamler E, Jampolsky A. Is divergence active?: An electromyographic study. *Am J Ophthalmol.* 1967;63:452.

14. Panum PL. Physiologische Untersuchungen über das Sehen mit zwei Augen. *Kiel Schwerssche Buchandlung.* 1858:52.

15. Von Noorden GK. *Binocular Vision and Ocular Motility: Theory and Management of Strabismus,* 4th ed. St. Louis: CV Mosby; 1990:17.

16. Worth C. *Squint: Its Causes, Pathology, and Treatment.* Philadelphia: P Blakiston's; 1921.

17. Schor C, Flom MC. The relative value of stereopsis as a function of viewing distance. *Am J Optom and Physiol Opt.* 1969;46:805–809.

18. Hubel DH, Wiesel TN. Steroscopic vision in macaque monkey: Cells sensitive to binocular depth in area 18 of the macaque monkey cortex. *Nature.* 1970;225:41.

19. Poggio GF, Poggio T. The analysis of stereopsis. *Ann Rev Neurosci.* 1984;7:379.

20. Hubel DH, Wiesel TN. Receptive fields, binocular interaction and functional architecture in the cat's visual cortex. *J Physiol.* (London). 1962;160:106.

21. Nikara T, Bishop PO, Pettigrew JD. Analysis of retinal correspondence by studying receptive fields of binocular single units in cat striate cortex. *Exp Brain Res.* 1968;6:353.

Chapter 2 / Vision Efficiency Skills

Saccadic Eye Movements   18
  Objective Testing   19
    SCCO System   19
    Heinsen-Schrock System   20
    Ophthalmography   21
    Sequential Fixation Tests   22
  Subjective Testing   24
    Pierce Test   24
    King-Devick Test   25
    DEM Test   26
  Standard Scoring System   27
  Recommended Tests   28
  Summary of Saccade Testing   28
Pursuit Eye Movements   29
  Characteristics   29
  Testing of Pursuit Skills   29
    Direct Observation   30
    H-S Scale   30
    Afterimages   31
  Signs and Symptoms   31
  Summary and Recommended Tests   33
Fixation   33
  SCCO 4+ System   33
  Summary of Fixation Testing   34
Accommodation   34
  Insufficiency of Accommodation   35
    Absolute Accommodation   35
    Relative Accommodation   36
    Lag of Accommodation   37
    Nott Method   37
    MEM Retinoscopy   37
  Excess of Accommodation   38

Infacility of Accommodation   40
Ill-Sustained Accommodation   42
Summary of Accommodation
  Testing   43
Vergences   44
  Absolute Convergence   44
    Testing Techniques   44
    Functions and Norms for Absolute
      Convergence   45
    Developmental Considerations   46
  Relative Convergence Testing and
    Norms   46
    Fusional Vergences at Far   47
    Fusional Vergences at Near   49
  Vergence Facility   49
  Reflex Fusion Test   49
  Reflex Fusion Stress Test   50
  Vergence Stamina   52
  Summary of Vergence Testing   52
Sensory Fusion   52
  Simultaneous Perception   53
  Superimposition   53
  Flat Fusion   54
  Stereopsis   54
    Vectographic Methods   55
    Percentage of Stereopsis   56
    Screening for Binocular Problems with
      Stereopsis   56
    Norms for Stereoacuity   58
  Summary of Sensory Fusion Testing   58
  Recommendations from Results of
    Testing   58

For any patient being treated for binocular anomalies, the ultimate goal is the achievement of clear, single, comfortable, and *efficient* binocular vision. Vision efficiency skills refer to how various ocular systems operate over time and under various viewing conditions. Clinical evaluation of vision efficiency necessitates the assessment of sufficiency (amplitude), facility (flexibility), accuracy, and stamina of each ocular function.

Practitioners in the nineteenth century were concerned almost exclusively with clearness of eyesight and with lenses that would optimally reduce or eliminate blurred vision. Clearness and singleness of binocular vision became the issue with the advent of orthoptics. Effective therapeutic regimens for strabismus were introduced by Javal and later by others.[1]

Astute clinicians in the first half of the twentieth century became aware of the relationship between accommodation and vergence. Knowledge of the zone of clear, single, *comfortable*, binocular vision was gained through various models of vision, such as the graphical analysis approach, and through an understanding of fixation disparity (see Chapter 3).

More and more emphasis has been placed on *efficiency* of vision in the latter half of the twentieth century. This implies that efficient visual skills are related to good scholastic abilities (school) and occupational production (work), and to achievement in sports and hobbies (play). As a result, lenses and/or functional training procedures are frequently applied in clinical practice to help patients attain efficient binocular vision in these activities. (Surgery, drugs, and occlusion are not modes of therapy commonly associated with vision efficiency therapy.)

Before evaluating the efficiency of any ocular system, the prerequisite is the optimum correction of any significant ametropia. Clinicians have frequently found that correcting even small errors of refraction can result in large changes in comfort and efficiency. Furthermore, baseline data collection requires correction of ametropia.

SACCADIC EYE MOVEMENTS

There are four separate eye movement systems from a neurological point of view. These include the saccadic, pursuit, nonoptic (e.g., vestibular ocular reflexes), and vergence eye movement systems. The saccadic eye movements are abrupt shifts in fixation and are classified as *fast*, compared with pursuit and vergence eye movements.[2] A good clinical average velocity to consider would be about 300 degrees per second, which is approximately 10 times greater than the velocity of pursuit and vergence movements of about 30 degrees per second.[3] Saccadic eye movements are mainly voluntary, with the others mainly involuntary. The duration and velocity of a saccade are proportional to the magnitude of the eye movement. A 40 degree sweep would have a greater velocity and a longer duration than would a 5 degree sweep. The velocity of a saccade changes during its course, being faster at the beginning and slower toward the end of the sweep. Although this may be shown in the laboratory, it is difficult to observe clinically, even with recording instruments such as the Eye-Trac or Visagraph .

Javal may have been among the first to note that vision turns off during saccadic eye movements. This makes sense; otherwise, the world would appear to be a swimming, blurry mess as we scan our environment. This perceptual inhibition has been referred to as saccadic "blindness." It is more appropriate, however, to refer to that phenomenon as saccadic *suppression*. According to Solomons,[4] each saccadic eye movement is preceded by a latent period of about 120 to 180 milliseconds before the eye movement actually begins, and saccadic suppression begins about 40 milliseconds before the movement commences. The inhibition increases until vision perception is almost zero during the first part of the movement. It is probably not until after the saccadic movement has ended that the saccadic suppression completely ceases.

The first differential diagnostic issue is whether there is pathological etiology when deficient saccadic eye movements are found.

If voluntary versions are severely restricted, the clinician should suspect neurological problems affecting the saccadic pathway, such as myasthenia, vascular disease, or tumors that may affect supranuclear control. Other signs of neurological dysfunctioning would likely be evident in such cases. Many times, however, there may be only subclinical "soft" signs, with the patient appearing normal in all other respects. Many patients have *functional* saccadic problems, such as those from poor attention, hyperkinesis, poor visual acuity because of uncorrected refractive errors, and possibly because saccadic skills were never learned adequately.

What are the symptoms of either organic soft-sign or functional saccadic dysfunctioning? There may be several performance problems if saccadic eye movements are poor, even though the patient is otherwise considered neurologically normal. Inefficiency in reading is a major problem and a frequent complaint in such cases. Words may be omitted, lines may be skipped, or a frequent loss of place may occur when reading. "Finger reading" may indicate the need for hand support due to poor eye movement. Head movement when reading is also a common sign of poor saccades. The patient may present with a history of "having trouble hitting a ball" or "doing poorly in many athletic events." Job peformance may be affected adversely if eye-hand coordination is exceptionally poor due to saccadic eye movement problems.

Objective Testing

Clinicians should evaluate saccadic eye movements using both gross and fine targets. Fine saccades are those involved in reading (approximately 7 degrees or less). Larger saccades than these are considered gross. A patient's saccadic eye movement skills can be evaluated either on an objective or subjective basis.

Any target, such as small letters on two pencils, can be used to test for gross saccadic ability. Have the patient voluntarily look from one target to the other. That is usually done in right- and left-gaze orientations, but vertical as well as oblique orientations can be tested. If one of the patient's eyes is occluded, testing is for saccadic ductions. If both eyes are open, testing is for saccadic versions. It should be noted that even behind the occluder, the covered eye moves conjugately with the uncovered, fixating eye. There may be a difference, however, in the performance of one eye from the other during duction testing. That is an important consideration in therapy, in that the patient should have (if possible) equal saccadic skills with each eye.

SCCO System

A quick and simple routine used at the Southern California College of Optometry (SCCO) for testing horizontal saccadic eye movements is as follows. A target with a letter printed on it that is approximately equivalent to 20/80 (6/24) acuity demand is placed to the patient's right. A similar target is placed on the left. The targets are separated approximately 25 cm and held at a distance of 40 cm from the patient. The patient is asked to move his eyes alternately to each target approximately 10 times. The practitioner should look for inaccuracies i.e., either undershooting or overshooting. Scoring the results of observation is on a 4+ basis as follows: 4+ if movements are accurate, 3+ indicates some undershooting, 2+ indicates gross undershooting or any overshooting, and 1+ either the inability to do the task or an increased latency. A score of 2+ or less is considered failing, as would be any uncontrolled head movement. Hoffman and Rouse[5] considered a failure on this basis as a need for referral for vision therapy for saccadic dysfunctioning. Whether or not referral is actually made, failure should alert the practitioner at least to consider the possibility of advising vision therapy when such tests show poor saccadic skills. In other words, clinical judgment is required and referrals for vision therapy are not automatic merely because of a single poor test result.

Two alphabetical pencils may be used in the manner described above (Figure 2-1). Do not expect the young child to go all the way

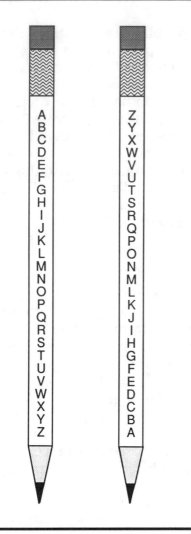

FIGURE 2-1—Alphabet pencils.

cades are automated (that is, occurring normally and simultaneously with relatively simple cognitive demands), 2 points if eye movements are stable for 20 seconds of time, and 1 point if there is adequate stamina when the test is continued for 1 minute. Thus, 10 possible points can be given using this procedure.

With regard to automated saccades, ask a simple question that is appropriate to the patient's cognitive abilities under such circumstances. For example, ask a 5-year-old patient his or her name as the patient is looking from one target to the other. A 7-year-old patient could be expected to count from 1 to 10 while maintaining accurate saccades. A 9-year-old patient should be able to count backward from 10 to 1. An 11-year-old patient should be able to count backward from 100 on down. A 13-year-old patient can normally be expected to count backward from 100 in intervals of 3. This is what we believe is meant by *automated*. Unless a reader can automatically make accurate saccades, he is unlikely to visualize and concentrate on the contents of the reading material. Frequently, when testing patients who have saccadic eye movement problems, a cognitive demand will cause patients to look in the wrong direction of the test target and

through the alphabet, but merely let the patient read the "A" on each pencil. For an adult, one pencil can be turned to expose the Z, Y, X . . . sequence. A task of A-Z, B-Y, C-X, and so on, is demanding and checks for false reporting as the patient looks from one alphabet pencil to the other. That is because it is difficult to verbalize the alphabet in the reversed sequence without seeing the letters (see Figure 2-1.)

Heinsen-Schrock System

A 10-point scale is another system recommended by Heinsen and Schrock (Table 2-1).[6] It can be performed with alphabetical pencils as previously described. For example, the patient can get 3 points if there is no head movement, 2 points if saccades are accurate, 2 points if sac-

TABLE 2-1. *Heinsen-Schrock System for Testing and Rating Saccadic Eye Movements*[6]

A	B	C
No head movement (3)	All accuracies (2)	Automated saccades (2)
Head movement, but can inhibit (2)	Slight inaccuracies (1)	Reduced automation (1)
Slight head movement persists (1)		

D	E
Stable saccades for 20 seconds (2)	Adequate stamina (1)
Stable saccades for 10 seconds (1)	

fail to make an accurate saccade. In other words, the cognitive demand can make the saccadic movements poor (and poor saccades even poorer) unless automation is achieved. It is conversely presumed that poor saccadic eye movements have an adverse effect on reading (cognitive) skills.

Ophthalmography

A good clinical ophthalmographic test for recording reading saccades is the Eye-Trac (Figure 2-2). An ideal target is a five-dot card (Figure 2-3) designed by Walton and tested by Griffin et al.[7] Griffin et al. analyzed the eye movements of 25 subjects during reading and fixation tasks

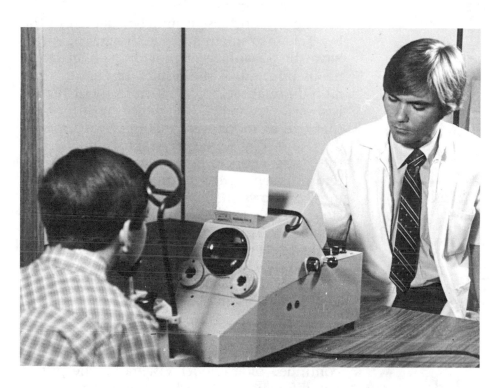

FIGURE 2-2—Eye-Trac® instrument.

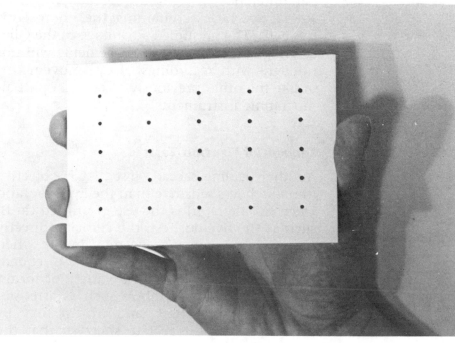

FIGURE 2-3—Five-dot card designed to test fine saccades as in the act of reading.

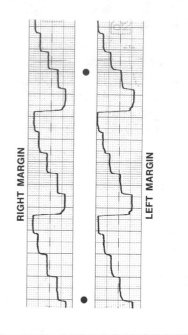

FIGURE 2-4—Good saccadic eye movements on the five-dot test.

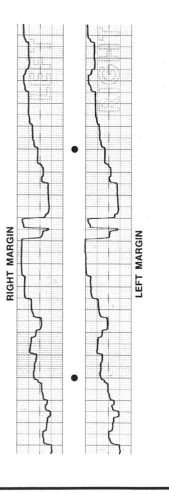

Figure 2-5—Poor saccadic eye movements on the five-dot test.

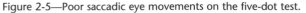

using the Reading Eye Camera™. The previously selected subjects included 12 adequate readers and 13 inadequate ones. Griffin et al. concluded that "Inadequate readers seem to have less efficient saccadic eye movements regardless of the type of material used." Besides using words as fixation targets, rows of dots were also used so that comprehension would not be an intervening factor.

The five-dot design may be adapted to the Eye-Trac instrument and the Visagraph, which have the advantage of providing an instantaneous printout of the results. In Figure 2-4, a fairly normal saccadic pattern in 5-dot testing is shown on the Eye-Trac recording strip. Note that five fixations were made for each row of dots, and they were spaced fairly equally, but there was a very slight undershooting on the return sweeps (gross saccades to the left). Figure 2-5 shows many inaccuracies and regressions on this test. This type of analysis is also possible with the Visagraph. The Visagraph is comparable to the Eye-Trac, except the individual looks at stimuli on a computer screen. Although the Eye-Trac is widely used, manufacture has been discontinued. The Ober 2: Visagraph (Figure 2-6) instrument for recording saccadic eye movements was recently introduced by the manufacturers of the discontinued older-model Visagraph, the principal difference being that the patient wears special spectacles containing the photosensitive cells. The presumed advantage of the Ober 2: Visagraph is that head movements will not interfere with recordings of eye movements, unlike the other previously discussed ophthalmographic instruments.

Sequential Fixation Tests

Another reading saccade test that is objective (but much less sensitive than the Eye-Trac and Ober 2: Visagraph) is the use of printed cards, such as the five-dot test; the clinician directly observes the patient's eye movements when evaluating dot to dot saccades. These sequential fixation tests come in a variety of forms. The dots (or other symbols such as asterisks, stars, numbers, letters, and words) may be printed on a clear acetate sheet so that the

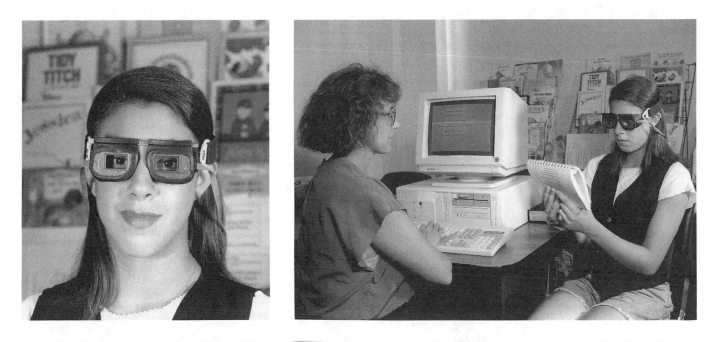

Figure 2-6—Ober 2: Visagraph™. (a) Sensors mounted in spectacle frame; (b) patient reading during computerized testing (Courtesy of Taylor Associates).

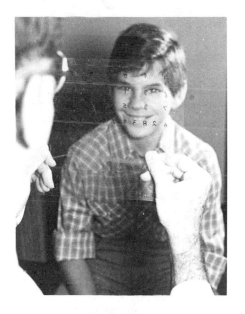

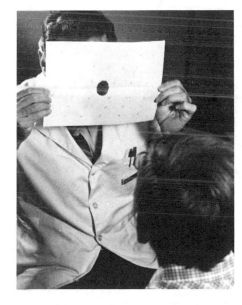

Figure 2-7—Sequential fixation test using clear sheet with printed symbols.

Figure 2-8—Sequential fixation test using an opaque card with a viewing hole.

clinician can look directly at the patient's eyes through the printed sheet to observe inaccuracies and head movements (Figure 2-7). Another variation is an opaque card on which the symbols are printed; there is a hole in the card's center for the clinician to look through to observe the patient's eye movements (Figure 2-8). Obviously, assessment of saccadic ability must be made quickly as there is no permanent printout for later analysis. Judgments are strictly qualitative and lack precision. Notwithstanding these drawbacks, experience goes a long way in making this procedure useful in the event either the Eye-Trac or Ober 2: Visagraph is not available at the time of testing. Sequential fixation tests are colloquially called a "poor person's ophthalmograph." The practitioner can increase clinical acumen with this

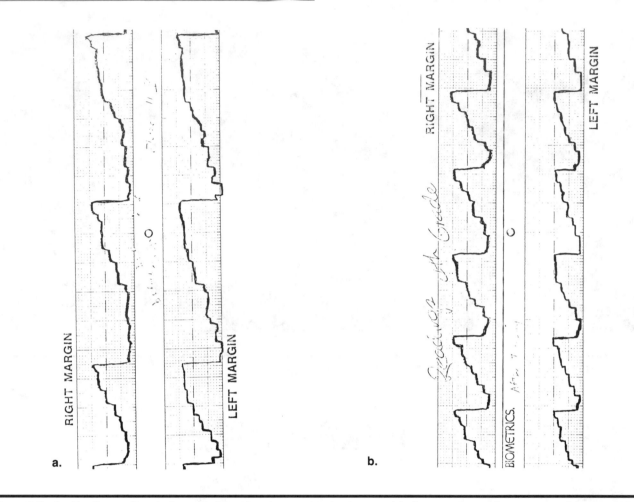

Figure 2-9—Eye-Trac® recordings before and after vision therapy showing improved performance for reading a paragraph.

simple testing procedure by comparing results of ophthalmographic recording instruments.

Whether or not the Eye-Trac or Ober 2: Visagraph is used, the patient should also be observed while reading sentences and paragraphs. Figure 2-9 shows relatively poor and good reading saccades. This patient was more efficient in reading after saccadic vision training. By testing with cognitive (paragraph) and noncognitive (five-dot) visual stimuli, a differential diagnosis can be suggested between purely saccadic problems and cognitive problems (e.g., dyslexia, poor comprehension, or unfamiliarity with certain words).

Subjective Testing

Saccades may also be evaluated indirectly by subjective means rather than directly by objec-

tive observations. The following tests are examples of subjective methods.

Pierce Test

The Pierce Saccade Test[8] is designed to evaluate the patient's gross saccadic eye movements according to age expectancies. It consists of three subtests, each of which is a series of two laterally displaced numbers. The patient is asked to hold the demonstration card (Figure 2-10) at his habitual reading distance and read each number aloud, from side to side. Holding the card too closely invalidates the test, as very large saccades would be demanded. The patient should hold the card at a distance of approximately 40 cm. A demonstration is given initially so the patient can start with the number at the top-left corner of the page and follow the arrow to the number on the top-right corner, then follow the arrow for the return sweep to the number on the left-hand side of the page, and so forth. The room should be well illuminated for testing purposes.

Once the demonstration is completed, the first subtest is begun. The three subtests become progressively more difficult since arrowed lines are missing and spacings between lines are reduced in size. The patient should read the numbers aloud as quickly as possible, but with accuracy, as in the demonstration test. This is a timed test intended for determining saccadic efficiency. Each of the three subtests is timed independently and errors are recorded. Calculate the corrected score using the following formula for each subtest:

Corrected time score =

$$\frac{30}{30-\text{errors}} \text{ X Time in seconds}$$

For example, suppose the patient takes 45 seconds to complete the first subtest, but there were no errors. The corrected score for this subtest would be 45 seconds. If there had been 10 errors, the corrected score would be 67 seconds. The total of the three corrected scores is determined and compared with the norms for the Pierce Saccade Test to judge the patient's chronological age equivalence (Table 2-2). In using the Pierce Saccade Test, the doctor has an idea if the patient's saccadic ability is above, below, or normal for his age. The Pierce test is designed for evaluating gross saccades.

King-Devick Test

The King-Devick Test was devised with fine saccades in mind. It contains five numbers per line. The numbers are randomly spaced, supposedly simulating saccades that occur when reading. Scores are evaluated in terms of errors and time; they are then compared with normed scores according to chronological age in a manner similar to that in the Pierce Saccade Test. The authors of the King-Devick Test concluded that poor saccadic ability contributes to poor reading ability.[9]

Samples of approximate norms determined by Cohen and Lieberman (in a study in coop-

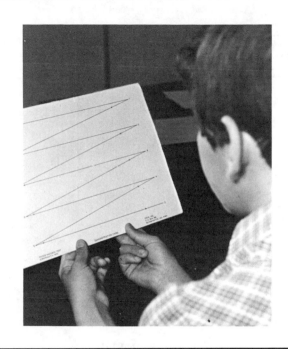

Figure 2-10—Demonstration card of the Pierce Saccade test.

TABLE 2-2. *Sample of Normative Values for the Pierce Saccade Test*

Chronological Age (Years)	Corrected Time Scores Expected (seconds)
6	150
7	125
8	100
9	82
10	70
11	65
12	59
13	55

eration with a New York Optometric Association team)[10] are given in Table 2-3. Subjects consisted of 1,202 students in regular public schools. Cohen and Lieberman found that subtests II and III were too difficult for many 6-year-old children; only subtest I is recommended; it was found to have norms of 30.98 seconds with 1.32 errors for children aged 6. The King-Devick Test includes a demonstration card (Figure 2-11a) and three test cards

TABLE 2-3. *Samples of Norms for the King-Devick Test As Determined by Cohen and Lieberman*[10]

Age	Time in Seconds (Total of 3 Subtests)	Number of Errors (Total of 3 Subtests)
6	119	17
7	101	12
8	79	3
9	73	3
10	68	2
11	57	1
12	54	1
13	52	1
14	50	0

(Figures 2-11b through 2-11d). Each test card has eight rows of 5 numbers, for a total of 40 numbers per card (as opposed to 30 per card in the Pierce Saccade Test). The numbers are sized to approximate 20/100 (6/30) reduced Snellen acuity at a viewing distance of 40 cm. Testing is done in a manner similar to the Pierce test.

DEM Test

A possible problem with the Pierce and King-Devick tests is that some individuals are basically slow in naming digits, independent of their saccadic skills. The Developmental Eye Movement Test (DEM) by Richman and Garzia[11] further refines the indirect approach to assessment of saccadic eye movements. As in the King-Devick Test, the DEM test is designed to evaluate both accuracy and speed of fine saccades as in the act of reading. The principal difference is that a subtest of naming numbers in a vertical array is included in the DEM test, presumably to determine the patient's rapid automatized naming (RAN) ability (Figure 2-12). As to the vertical columns, the DEM test manual states: "This becomes a test more heavily dominated by the individual's visual-verbal automatic calling skills (automaticity)." As in the King-Devick test, there is a horizontal array of numbers except the horizontal dimension is slightly reduced (to simulate usual reading demands) and the quantity of numbers is increased to 80 digits. This added demand is designed to assess ability for sustained performance (stamina).

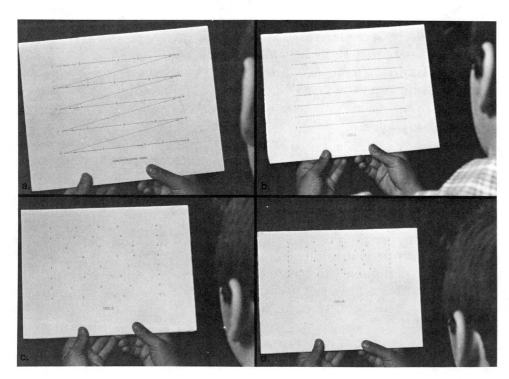

Figure 2-11—King-Devick test showing demonstration card and the three subtests. (a) Demonstration card; (b) subtest with lines; (c) subtest without lines; and (d) stimuli more crowded.

3	4
7	5
5	2
9	1
8	7
2	5
5	3
7	7
4	4
6	8
1	7
4	4
7	6
6	5
3	2
7	9
9	2
3	3
9	6
2	4

3		7	5		9		8
2	5			7	4		6
1			4	7		6	3
7		9		3	9		2
4	5			2		1	7
5			3	7	4		8
7	4		6	5			2
9		2		3		6	4
6	3	2		9			1
7			4		6	5	2
5		3	7		4		8
4			5	2		1	7
7	9	3		9			2
1			4		7	6	3
2	5			7		4	6
3	7		5		9		8

Figure 2-12—DEM Test showing: (a) vertical array of numbers, and (b) horizontal array of numbers. Similar to the Pierce test, the DEM test uses a formula to determine "adjusted" time: Adjusted time = test time X $\dfrac{80}{80-0+A}$

Key:

    Test time = Actual time for number calling on the horizontal array

    0 = Omission errors

    A = Addition errors (numbers either being repeated or added)

The essence of the DEM test is to compare the test results of vertical time with horizontal time. There are four possible outcomes:

1. Both the vertical time and the adjusted horizontal time are normal. This is considered normal performance.
2. The vertical time is normal but the adjusted horizontal time is abnormally increased. This indicates "oculomotor dysfunction" and presumably poor horizontal fine saccadic eye movements.
3. Both the vertical time and the adjusted horizontal time are abnormally increased but are approximately the same. This indicates a problem in automated number calling rather than a saccadic deficiency.
4. Both the vertical and horizontal times are abnormal but the horizontal is much worse. This indicates both a RAN problem and a saccadic eye movement deficiency.

Standard Scoring System

The aforementioned tests vary in their scoring of saccadic efficiency. A standard scoring system is desirable. Griffin[12] reported a system for saccades based on a five-point scale, in common with a five-point scale for several other visual

TABLE 2-4. *Ordinal Ranking Method for Visual Skills*

Rank	Description
5	Very strong (much above average)
4	Strong (above average)
3	Adequate (average)
2	Weak (below average)
1	Very Weak (much below average)

A ranking of less than 3 is considered failure, as referral criterion for vision therapy.

TABLE 2-5. *Ranking of Saccadic Performance on the Pierce, King-Devick, and DEM Tests.*

Rank		Results
5	Very Strong	Two or more years above average
4	Strong	One year above average
3	Adequate	Average performance for age
2	Weak	One year below average
1	Very Weak	Two or more years below average

TABLE 2-6. *Modification of the Heinsen-Schrock System for Testing and Rating Saccadic Eye Movements for a Five-Point Maximum Score*

A	B
No head movement (1.5)	All saccades accurate (1.0)
Head movement, but can inhibit (1.0)	Some slight inaccuracies (0.5)
Slight head movement persists (0.5)	Several gross inaccuracies (0.0)
Obvious persisting head movement (0.0)	

C	D
Automated saccades (1.0)	Stable saccades for 20 seconds or more (1.0)
Reduced automation (0.5)	Stable saccades for 10 seconds (0.5)
No automation (0.0)	Stable for less than 10 seconds (0.0)

E
Stamina for 1 minute (0.5)
Stamina for less than 1 minute (0.0)

Total maximum score is 5 points (i.e., no head movement, all saccades accurate, automated saccades, stable saccades for 20 seconds or more, and stamina for 1 minute).

skills. In such a scheme, each visual skill function can be ordinally ranked from 5 (best) to 1 (worst) with semantic differential descriptions (Table 2-4). An adaptation to the Pierce, King-Devick, and DEM tests is shown in Table 2-5. Such a ranking system is convenient when comparing strengths and weaknesses among various visual skills. This allows for better understanding and communication to patients and interested third parties (e.g., the patient's health insurance company). A five-point maximum ranking system which is a modification of the H-S scale is shown in Table 2-6. This is but one of the possible ways the practitioner can convert other scoring systems for saccades into a five-point scale.

Recommended Tests

A recommended sequence of saccade tests for the primary eye care practitioner is as follows: (1) SCCO 4+ system; (2) Sequential fixation testing; (3) DEM.

Summary of Saccade Testing

The clinician should attempt objective testing of saccadic eye movements even when electro-ophthalmography (Eye-Trac or Visagraph) is not available. This can be done, for example, with the SCCO 4+ system, the Heinsen-Schrock System, and sequential fixation tests.

When subjective and indirect assessment is done the Pierce Test is good for gross saccades. The DEM test accounts for deficiencies in random automatized naming (RAN) skill, important to differentiate from poor saccadic skills. Unless the RAN is known, the practitioner is unable to know whether poor horizontal saccades are due to RAN problems or actually due to saccadic deficiencies. It is desirable to convert scores into a ranking system so that there is a common denominator for each visual skill function. We propose a five-point ordinal ranking system that is easy-to-understand and convenient for patient communication purposes.

Most of the testing procedures described above are appropriate for patients 7 years and older. Some children between 5 and 6 years old can respond to some of these tests. Below age 5, however, the clinician must rely mostly on gross and objective methods, such as the SCCO 4+ system.

PURSUIT EYE MOVEMENTS

A pursuit eye movement is defined as a "movement of an eye fixating a moving object."[13]

Characteristics

According to Michaels,[14] pursuits are unlike saccades in that vision is present (without suppression as in saccades) throughout their excursions. The speed of pursuits is limited to about 30 degrees per second. They may be considerably slower, but not much faster. If the target velocity is too high, the pursuits break down into a jerky motion. The attempt to keep tracking requires the faster saccadic responses to come into play in order for the patient to regain fixation of the target.

Pursuits are a form of duction eye movements when only one eye is being tested (monocular viewing conditions); binocular viewing conditions allow for testing pursuit versions. (Versions, as with ductions, may be either saccades, pursuits, or nonoptic eye movements.) Regardless of the fact that an eye may be occluded, the covered eye moves conjugately with the fixating eye under most normal circumstances.

There may be "soft signs" neurologically in the case of jerky pursuits. Problems may be so subtle that no lesion can be found (by radiology or other means) along the occipitomesencephalic pathway. In some cases, functional training procedures may help. In many others, however, not much can be done to improve pursuits when there is a neurological organic etiology. Nevertheless, differential diagnostic testing should be considered in any event. For example, suppose a patient has voluntary saccades that are normal, but pursuit movements are significantly restricted and jerky. A supranuclear lesion affecting the occipitomesencephalic pathway would be suspected. On the other hand, if saccades are inaccurate and restricted but pursuits are normal, a frontomesencephalic pathway lesion is suspected. It is always wise to check both pursuits and saccades on a routine basis, not only to determine gross organic defects but to detect subtle problems that can also handicap individuals because of resulting inefficiencies of vision. Additionally, drugs, fatigue, emotional stress and test anxiety may adversely affect pursuit performance. For example, we have examined many children with reading difficulties in which we found a "midline hesitation" during confrontation pursuit testing using a penlight. However, no irregularity in pursuit function was found using laboratory electronic tests. On follow-up clinical testing our initial findings were repeatable. This mystery was solved when we discovered that if we moved to the patient's side, the "hesitation" also moved toward that side. The children were evidently making eye contact with the examiner, possibly because of being apprehensive under the clinical testing environment. This points out the importance of distinguishing the difference between true pursuit dysfunction and poor tracking induced by inattention, lack of cooperation, or test anxiety.

Testing of Pursuit Skills

Several objective and subjective testing procedures are discussed as examples. They are basically the same in that the tests allow for

TABLE 2-7. *Heinsen-Schrock System for Testing and Rating Pursuit Eye Movements,*[16] *Modified for Five-Point Scale*

A	10-pt. Scale	5-pt. Scale
Smooth, always on target	(3)	(1.5)
Smooth, sometimes off target	(2)	(1.0)
Jerky, generally on target	(1)	(0.5)
Jerky, generally off target	(0)	(0.0)
B		
Free of head movement	(3)	(1.5)
Head movement, but can inhibit	(2)	(1.0)
Slight head movement persists	(1)	(0.5)
Obvious persisting head movement	(0)	(0.0)
C		
Automated pursuits	(3)	(1.5)
Reduced automation	(2)	(1.0)
Much reduced automation	(1)	(0.5)
No automation	(0)	(0.0)
D		
Adequate stamina for 1 minute	(1)	(0.5)
Stamina for less than 1 minute	(0)	(0.0)

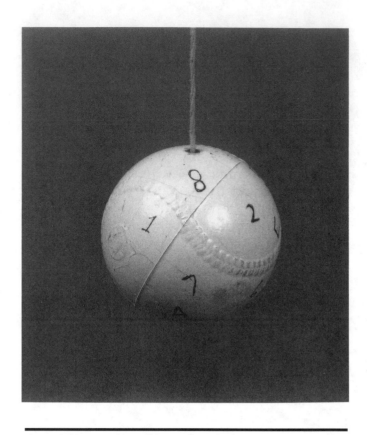

Figure 2-13—Marsden Ball for testing pursuit eye movements.

monitoring accuracy of pursuit eye movements.

Direct Observation

A quick and convenient testing and rating system for pursuits on a 4+ scale is used at the Southern California College of Optometry (SCCO).[15] A fixation target approximately the size of a 20/80 (6/24) letter is moved in front of the patient at a distance of about 40 cm. The target is moved left-right-left (one cycle), up-down-up (one cycle), and in two diagonal orientations (one cycle each) as in the lines of a British flag with the patient being instructed to track the target. A 4+ is given if pursuits are smooth and fixation is always accurate, 3+ if there is one fixation loss, 2+ if there are two fixation losses, and 1+ if there are more than two fixation losses. The patient is considered to have pursuit problems if the score is 2+ or less. If there should be any obvious head movement during testing after the patient has been instructed not to move his head, performance is considered to be inadequate. The right eye, the left eye, and then both eyes should routinely be tested by eye care practitioners, whether this or another method of testing pursuits is used. This method lends itself to testing of patients of all ages, including infants and young children.

H-S Scale

Heinsen and Schrock[6] introduced a rating system (H-S Scale) for pursuits similar to that for evaluating saccades (discussed previously). This is the 10-point scale shown in Table 2-7. Our five-point ordinal ranking system is also shown so that the very strong to very weak categories for pursuit skills can be compared with rankings of functions for other visual skills, as discussed previously for saccades. The advantage of the Heinsen-Schrock system over the SCCO 4+ system is that automation and stamina are taken into account along with head movements, smoothness, and accuracy. Either a Marsden ball (Figure 2-13) or a motorized instrument such as the Bernell Rotator (Figure 2-14) is ideal for this type of testing, although a hand-held penlight that is moved smoothly and evenly will suffice. Whatever target is used, smoothness, accuracy, head movement, automation, and stamina are to be evaluated. Using the same cognitive demands as in saccadic testing (discussed previously) and continuing the pursuits for one minute of time will allow for judgment of automation and stamina, respectively.

Afterimages

Afterimages can also be used in conjunction with a moving target to provide visual feedback for the patient to see if tracking is accurate. This is useful in both testing and training. An afterimage may be used for one eye for monocular testing, or both eyes may be stimulated simultaneously for binocular pursuit testing. The same type of afterimage generator used for testing of anomalous correspondence can be used (see Chapter 5).

Signs and Symptoms

Patients who have poor pursuit skills may also have histories of various inefficiencies. Poor readers may have poor pursuits, although the cause and effect relationship is not as great as in saccadic dysfunction and poor reading. Reading road signs from a moving vehicle would present problems in a case of poor pursuit skills. Patients with poor pursuit eye movements also tend to have significant problems in sports. It is conceivable, for example, that it would be much more difficult to track a tennis ball accurately if head movements are necessary, because the gross neck muscles are not as efficient as the finely tuned extraocular muscles. However, we saw a patient who had Duane syndrome involving each eye, which severely restricted ocular activity. This patient reported being able to play tennis "fairly well." This was in spite of head turning being necessary to see the approaching ball. Therefore, statements relating to pursuit skills and athletic skills should be made with

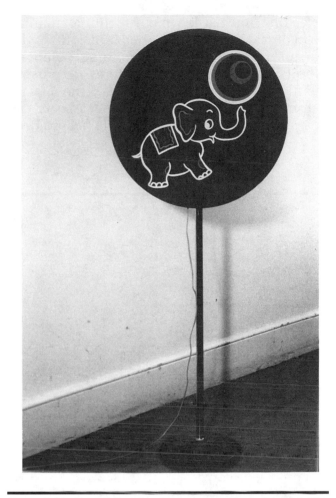

Figure 2-14—Bernell Rotation Trainer with Black Elephant Disc (photo courtesy of Bernell Corp.)

caution and with other factors (e.g., athletic prowess) kept in mind.

Supranuclear lesions restrict pursuit excursions, but also nuclear or infranuclear lesions affecting the extraocular muscles can be expected to produce many signs and symptoms. Pursuits would likely be inaccurate and jerky in the diagnostic action field of the affected muscle (see Chapter 4 regarding noncomitancy). However, these "hard" signs of neurologic impairment are relatively easy to detect, explain, and understand in contrast to "soft" signs which are possibly supranuclear. In either case, the patient with pursuit problems due to neurologic disease may have symptoms of vertigo, nausea, asthenopia, or inefficient vision for moving objects, as well as a host of other complaints.

Since pursuits are mainly involuntary and many of the neurological soft signs are incurable, one must ask what functional training procedures can do to help patients with pursuit problems. There are some voluntary aspects in the testing procedures of pursuits mentioned previously, e.g., head movement, automation, and stamina. These aspects can be improved and made more reflexive, starting from volition and progressing to automation. In many cases, accuracy and smoothness are improved as a result of functional training procedures. In cases where the pursuit problem is of functional etiology (e.g., due to inattention) the prognosis for improvement is favorable.

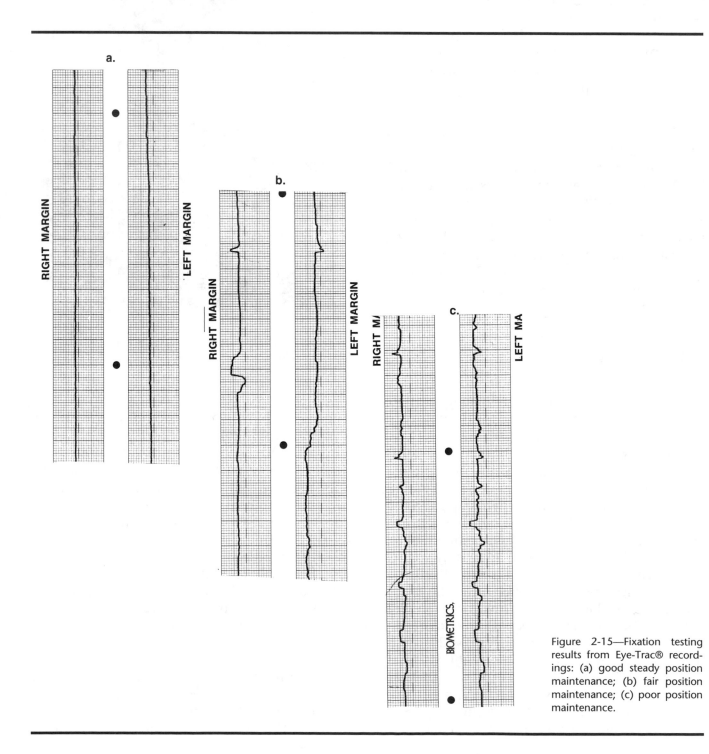

Figure 2-15—Fixation testing results from Eye-Trac® recordings: (a) good steady position maintenance; (b) fair position maintenance; (c) poor position maintenance.

Summary and Recommended Tests

Clinical assessment is important to identify neurological problems and dysfunctional visual tracking (particularly relevant to sports performance). The SCCO 4+ test is recommended for primary eye care practitioners in routine cases. Pursuit tests should usually include monocular (duction) as well as binocular (version) testing. Functional and organic causes should be differentiated. Some cases may require "diagnostic therapy" to determine if the problem is abated or not as a result of vision training.

TABLE 2-8. *System for Ranking Position Maintenance*

5	Very Strong	Steady fixation for more than 10 sec.
4	Strong	Steady fixation for at least 10 sec.
3	Adequate	Steady fixation for at least 5 sec.
2	Weak	Steady fixation for less than 5 sec. or hand support needed
1	Very Weak	Unsteady fixation almost continuously

FIXATION

Fixation is also referred to as position maintenance. Fixation is the combined involvement of all four eye movement systems, i.e., saccades, pursuits, nonoptic, (e.g., vestibular ocular reflexes), and vergences. Figure 2-15 shows Eye-Trac recordings of good versus poor position maintenance. Reading difficulties and various symptoms may occur with poor position maintenance.

True position maintenance is actually a misnomer in that there are very small movements occurring all the time during so-called steady fixation. The eyes are not motionless during fixation. According to Gay et al.,[16] the "micro" eye movements consist of rapid flicks (probably of the saccadic system) and slow drifts (probably of the pursuit system) of a very small amplitude not observable without special equipment. These small movements are thought to be useful for the purpose of correcting fixational errors to keep the fixated target precisely on the fovea, and possibly preventing retinal adaptation (fatigue).

Position maintenance can be assessed by asking the patient to fixate (monocularly) on a target. There should be no noticeable drifting or eye movement from the target of regard. If the patient cannot maintain steady fixation, have him hold his thumb at 40 cm to determine if the proprioceptive input from the "hand support" is of help in maintaining steady eye positioning. The problem may persist (e.g., due to congenital nystagmus). If the problem is psychological (e.g., lack of attention) or from other known causes (e.g., fatigue or drug effects), improvement of position maintenance is often possible through appropriate environmental changes and the efforts of functional training procedures.

SCCO 4+ System

The SCCO 4+ system is a quick and easy test for position maintenance.[5] The patient is instructed to fixate a target approximately the size of a 20/80 (6/24) letter E at a distance of 40 cm. The left eye is occluded for testing of the right eye; afterwards the left eye is tested and, then, binocular testing. Testing time is at least 10 seconds per eye. The quality of steadiness is assessed as follows: 4+ if steady for at least 10 seconds, 3+ if steady for at least 5 seconds, 2+ if steady less than 5 seconds or if hand support is needed, and 1+ if fixation is unsteady almost continuously. A 2+ or 1+ is considered failing as criteria for possible referral. Modification of the SCCO 4+ system allows for a five-point ordinal ranking system which is compatible with our recommended scale used in common for other visual skills (Table 2-8).

TABLE 2-9.   Possible Causes of a Reduction of Accommodation

1. Functional etiology:
   Binocular: deficient accommodation due to biological variation in the population, excessive nearpoint work, low illumination, low oxygen level, ocular and general fatigue or stress, vergence problems.
   Monocular: strong sighting eye dominance resulting in poor accommodation in the nondominant eye.
2. Refractive etiology:
   Binocular: manifest and latent hyperopia, myopes who do not wear spectacles at near, pseudomyopia, premature and normal presbyopia.
   Monocular: uncorrected anisometropia, poor distance refractive balance, unequal lens sclerosis.
3. Ocular disease:
   Binocular: internal ophthalmoplegia, bilateral organic amblyopia, premature cataracts, bilateral glaucoma, iridocyclitis, ciliary body aplasia, partial subluxation of lens.
   Monocular: same as above, but affecting one eye more than the other, anterior choroidal metastasis, trauma, rupture of zonular fibers.
4. Systemic diseases or conditions affecting binocular accommodation:
   Hormonal or metabolic: pregnancy, menstruation, lactation, menopause, diabetes, thyroid conditions, anemia, vascular hypertension, myotonic dystrophy.
   Neurologic: myasthenia gravis, multiple sclerosis, pineal tumor, whiplash injury, trauma to the head and neck, cerebral concussion, mesencephalic disease including vascular lesions.
   Infectious: influenza, intestinal toxemia, tuberculosis, whooping cough, measles, syphilis, tonsillar and dental infections, encephalitis, viral hepatitis, polio, amebic dysentery, malaria, herpes zoster, many acute infections.
5. Drugs, medications and toxic conditions affecting binocular accommodation:
   residual effects of cycloplegic drops, alcohol neuropathy, marijuana, heavy metal poisoning, carbon monoxide, botulism, antihistamines, CNS stimulants, large doses of tranquilizing drugs (phenothiazine derivatives), Parkinsonism drugs, many other systemic medications.
6. Emotional: Usually binocular: stress reactions, malingering, hysteria.

Summary of Fixation Testing

An ophthalmographic instrument such as the Eye-Trac is desirable for assessment of position maintenance. When this is not practical, as in very young children, a quick objective test, such as the five-point system for direct observation, is recommended. Therapy to improve position maintenance is discussed in Chapter 16.

ACCOMMODATION

Functional disorders of accommodation can be separated into four types of problems: (1) insufficiency, (2) excess, (3) infacility, and (4) ill-sustained accommodation (poor stamina). Patients can present with an accommodative dysfunction that falls into any one or all of these categories; the categories are not mutually exclusive. In fact, many patients who can be described as having an accommodative insufficiency also show signs of infacility and poor stamina. Two additional categories of accommodative dysfunction are: (5) unequal accommodation and (6) paresis/paralysis of accommodation. The etiology of these last two disorders is not functional. The first four categories do not imply an organic etiology since they often arise from functional causes, e.g., deficient physiology, overwork, or inattention. Besides describing the characteristics of an accommodative dysfunction, the clinician needs to determine, if possible, the specific etiology and seriously consider the many nonfunctional factors (Table 2-9) before the condition is assumed to be functional in origin. A review of accommodative conditions and appropriate testing follows.

Insufficiency of Accommodation

This is defined by Cline et al.[13] as "insufficient amplitude of accommodation to afford clear imagery of a stimulus object at a specified distance, usually the normal or desired reading distance. This is sometimes a problem in prepresbyopic and very often in presbyopic patients, but not too frequent in younger patients. However, pathological conditions affecting the third cranial nerve, the ciliary muscle, or the crystalline lens itself can result in paresis or paralysis of accommodation for all age groups. The use of sympathomimetic (adrenergic) or parasympatholytic (anticholinergic) drugs also result in symptom-producing lowered amplitudes of accommodation. Although isolated accommodative insufficiency in young patients is relatively rare, we saw three young male adults with isolated accommodative insufficiency within a 1-month period. All had a history of tropical illnesses of some kind. They had to wear bifocals in order to read clearly and we happened to see them after they had been to other practitioners who insisted they did not need to wear bifocals because of their youth. The accommodative amplitude in each of the three patients was practically zero, but we doubt if that had ever been tested. The resumption of wearing plus-addition bifocals solved their problems, and no further treatment was necessary. We saw another patient who was a 21-year-old college student. She had only 1 diopter of accommodative amplitude but had no other physical signs or symptoms. She had contracted influenza 3 months previously but maintained a 4-hour daily swimming schedule on a swim team. Bifocals were prescribed to relieve her nearpoint vision problems, and a subsequent neurological evaluation revealed a low-grade viral encephalitis.

The most prevalent cause of accommodative insufficiency is functional, i.e., a mismatch between a patient's physiologic accommodative capability and his/her work requirements. Chrousos et al.[16] described ten detailed cases of healthy young people who complained of intermittent blur at near. They demonstrated amplitudes of accommodation considerably below

TABLE 2-10. Donders' Table of Amplitude of Accommodation.[19]

Age (years)	Amplitude (diopters)
10	14
20	10
30	7
40	4.5
50	2.5

those expected for their respective ages (an average reduction of 6 diopters). No organic etiology for the diminished accommodation was suggested by history or could be identified by careful examination. All patients were successfully managed optically with bifocals or reading glasses, although three required the addition of base-in prisms because of exophoria at rest.

Convergence insufficiency is commonly associated with accommodative insufficiency as is accommodative infacility. Other symptoms besides nearpoint blur that are frequently reported by these patients include headaches, eyestrain, diplopia, and reading problems.[18]

Absolute Accommodation

The amplitude of accommodation is measured monocularly using the pushup method for one eye and then the other. This is *absolute* accommodation. The print size should be equivalent to 20/20 (6/6) at 40 cm, or smaller or larger depending upon the patient's maximum visual acuity. The maximum farpoint visual acuity lenses with the most plus power (also called CAMP lenses, which stands for Corrected Ametropia Most Plus) should be worn for testing. If the patient does not give reliable responses, move the target from near to far by starting at the spectacle plane and pushing it away until the designated line of print is read aloud correctly. Then go to the pushup method until first blur is reported. This is the method-of-adjustment (method-of-limits) research technique, referred to as bracketing in clinical parlance.

TABLE 2-11. *Ranking of Accommodative Amplitude*

Rank		Amplitude
5	Very Strong	1.00 D or more above average
4	Strong	0.50 D above average
3	Adequate	Average for age
2	Weak	2.00 D below average
1	Very Weak	4.00 D or more below average

Table 2-10 is an abridged table of Donders giving the amplitude of accommodation according to age.[18]

A formula to calculate the minimum expected amplitude of accommodation was introduced by Hofstetter.[18] The amplitude is equal to 15 – .25 times the patient's age:

$$A = 15 - .25(x)$$

where x is the patient's age in years.

For example, if a patient is 10 years old, the amplitude expected is 15 – .25(10), or 12.5

TABLE 2-12. *Ranking of Relative Accommodation. Dioptric Powers Represent the First Sustained Blur.*

Rank		PRA(–) and NRA (+)
5	Very Strong	*2.50 D or more
4	Strong	2.25 D
3	Adequate	1.75 to 2.00 D
2	Weak	1.50 D
1	Very Weak	<1.50 D

*The clinician should be skeptical of an NRA finding exceeding +2.50 D at 40 cm testing distance. If NRA exceeds +2.50 the testing procedure is wrong. Either the patient is over-minused or there is latent hyperopia, i.e., CAMP lenses not being worn. Theoretically, 40 cm is the farpoint (optical infinity) with +2.50 D lenses. The patient's vision should be blurred when +2.50 D power is exceeded. CAMP lenses, therefore, are absolutely necessary for reliable baseline clinical data.

diopters. If the amplitude measures only 8.5 D in the right eye, that would be very weak, since this is 4 diopters below average. Table 2-11 gives accommodative ranking. The Hofstetter formula may not hold true for very young children because their amplitudes are often clinically measured lower than would be theoretically predicted. This should be considered when testing children under the age of 6.

Semantic confusion often arises over the term *accommodative insufficiency*. Some sources (inappropriately in our opinion) refer to "accommodative deficiency" or "insufficiency" when talking about *accommodative infacility*.[19] (Accommodative infacility is discussed later in this chapter.)

Relative Accommodation

Another form of accommodative insufficiency is that of poor positive relative accommodation (PRA) and poor negative relative accommodation (NRA). The PRA is tested with minus-power lenses to first sustained blur under binocular viewing conditions. The NRA is tested similarly but with plus-power lenses. These functions are traditionally tested at 40 cm, with the patient looking through CAMP lenses for baseline reference. The patient is instructed to maintain clearness and singleness while looking at a designated line of letters (20/20 [6/6] equivalent or smaller if visible) as the plus or minus lens stimulus is increased (Table 2-12). The rate of stimulus increase is approximately every 3 seconds, in 0.25 D steps. A brief momentary blur is allowed. Approximately 5 seconds should be allowed to determine if the blur is sustained. The PRA and NRA are recordings representing the first sustained blurpoints. Failure on the PRA test is a sustained blur for 5 seconds with lens powers weaker than –1.75 D (relative to CAMP lenses). In other words, passing requires clear and sustained vision with –1.50 lenses. Failure on the NRA is similarly a sustained blur with lens powers weaker than +1.75 D. Keep in mind that relative accommodation is often limited by deficient vergence ranges. For example, an esophoric patient with a high AC/A and poor fusional divergence will likely have a reduced PRA.

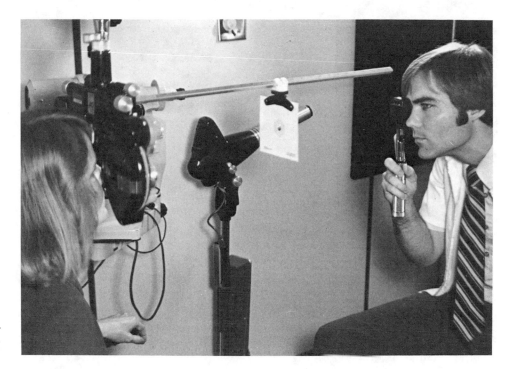

Figure 2-16—Nott method of retinoscopy to measure lag of accommodation.

Lag of Accommodation

Although lag of accommodation does not necessarily imply insufficient amplitude of accommodation, it can be thought of as a clinical form of accommodative insufficiency for a particular nearpoint target. Accommodative lag can also be thought of as *accommodative inaccuracy*, just as fixation disparity can be considered an inaccuracy in vergence. Lag of accommodation can be measured several ways, but two of the most reliable clinical methods are included here.

Nott Method

The Nott dynamic retinoscopy method is based on the linear difference between the fixation distance (usually 40 cm) and the distance of the retinoscope from the patient. This distance is converted into diopters to determine the accommodative lag.[21] The patient fixates reading material at 40 cm (2.50 D accommodative stimulus) while retinoscopy is performed through a hole in a card (Figure 2-16). The clinician physically moves toward the patient until a neutralized reflex is observed, say, at 67 cm (1.50 D accommodative response). The accommodative lag, according to the Nott method, would be 1.00 D

in this example. This test is done while the patient is behind the refractor.

With the Nott method, the accommodative stimulus does not change, because the testing distance is kept constant, and no dioptric changes are made by the intervention of additional lenses. The nearpoint rod of the refractor can be used to measure directly the dioptric distance between the fixation distance and the retinoscopic neutralization distance, i.e., the distance representing the accommodative lag.

MEM Retinoscopy

When testing is done outside the refractor, monocular estimate method (MEM) retinoscopy may be more convenient. The MEM is called "monocular" although the patient has both eyes open and testing is under binocular viewing conditions. The monocular estimate method of Haynes[21] is similar to the Nott method, except that the retinoscopic distance is kept constant. This is often at the Harmon distance (distance equal to that from one's tip of the elbow to the middle knuckle of the clenched fist measured on the outside of the arm).[13] Distances, however, may be varied, since the patient's habitual reading distance is recommended. The binocularly

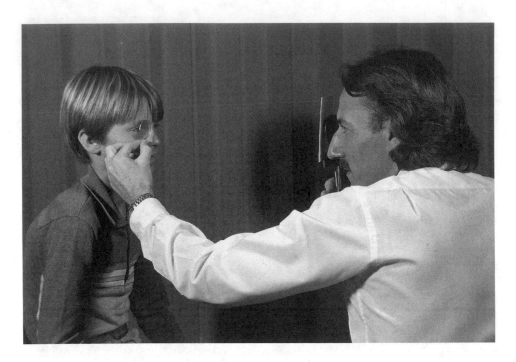

Figure 2-17—MEM retinoscopy to assess accommodative accuracy, e.g., lag of accommodation.

viewing patient is instructed to read appropriate material (for his age or cognitive level) mounted on the retinoscope. A trial lens is quickly interposed in the spectacle plane of one eye to neutralize the retinoscopic reflex (Figure 2-17). The lens is removed from the eye within a second, because latency of accommodation response is short. Tucker and Charman[22] found a mean reaction (latency) time of 0.28 second for one subject and 0.29 second for another. Therefore, the neutralizing lens must be quickly removed once it is introduced before an eye. The stimulus to accommodation possibly can be changed if the lens is before the eye for a longer duration.

The possibility of changing accommodative responses by changing accommodative stimuli must always be kept in mind when doing the MEM test.

The lens power (addition of plus) necessary to achieve retinoscopic neutralization is the estimated accommodative lag of the eye being tested at the moment. If *minus* power should be required for neutralization, accommodative excess would be indicated.

Using the Nott or MEM procedures, we believe an accommodative lag of 1.00 D or greater is cause for further investigation. This concern was shared by Bieber.[23] A high lag of accommodation suggests the possibility of the anomalies of insufficiency of accommodation, infacility of accommodation, and ill-sustained accommodation, any of which can be adverse factors in vision efficiency. Ranking of either Nott or MEM results is shown in Table 2-13. A rank of 2 or 1 is failing and referral for vision therapy may be recommended.

Excess of Accommodation

Another inaccuracy is accommodative excess. Accommodation may be excessive in focusing on a stimulus object. Accommodative excess

TABLE 2-13. *Ranking of Accommodative Lag (Insufficiency, or Inaccuracy, of Accommodation)*

Rank		NOTT or MEM Retinoscopy Lag of Accom. (either OD or OS)
5	Very Strong	+0.25D
4	Strong	+0.50D
3	Adequate	+0.75D
2	Weak	+1.00D
1	Very Weak	+1.25D

TABLE 2-14. *Ranking of Accommodative Excess Using the MEM Method of Retinoscopy.*

Rank		Lens Power Indicating Lead of Accommodation
5	Very Strong	+0.25
4	N/A	N/A
3	Adequate (borderline)	0.00
2	Weak	−0.25
1	Very Weak	−0.50 or greater

with the aid of cycloplegia can determine ametropia (i.e., farpoint). At nearpoint, however, dynamic retinoscopy is important; cycloplegia must not be used in nearpoint testing. Either Nott or MEM dynamic retinoscopy can be used to determine if there is a *lag* (i.e., insufficiency), but MEM is applicable for *lead* (i.e., excess) of accommodation. If accommodative response leads the accommodative stimulus by 0.25 D or more, we believe accommodative excess exists at that moment of testing. This observation should be verified on repeated testing. If −0.25 D is consistently required for neutralization, this is failing as to accommodative excess (Table 2-14).

Accommodative excess can also occur when excessive accommodative convergence is required to maintain fusion, as in cases of exophoria in which positive fusional convergence is insufficient. Such a patient may overaccommodate to have enough accommodative convergence to maintain single (but blurred) vision.

Although objective means for determining accommodative accuracy (with Nott or MEM

is considered to be an anomaly, sometimes referred to as spasm of accommodation, hyperaccommodation, hypertonic accommodation, or pseudomyopia. Latent hyperopia is another variation of accommodative spasm, i.e., accommodation fails to relax using noncycloplegic ("dry") refractive techniques. Cycloplegic ("wet") refraction may be indicated. Causes of spasm may be overstimulation of the accommodative system as a result of prolonged near work, emotional problems, focal infections, or unknown etiologies. Numerous symptoms may be associated with accommodative excess, such as asthenopia, blurring of distance vision, headaches, diplopia (if excessive accommodative convergence is brought into play), and inefficient performance at nearpoint (e.g., the person may hold reading material at an exceptionally close range).

Maintaining or sustaining accommodation in the absence of a dioptric stimulus is another form of accommodative excess. This form is physiological in that it is not abnormal for accommodation of approximately 1.00 D to be in play in a formless field, as in "night myopia." There is no effective therapy for this condition except the individual's becoming familiar with the set of circumstances in which it occurs and/or making appropriate adjustments to it (e.g., temporarily wearing minus overcorrections at times, if necessary, for nighttime driving).

Retinoscopy is necessary for reliable diagnosis of accommodative excess. Static retinoscopy

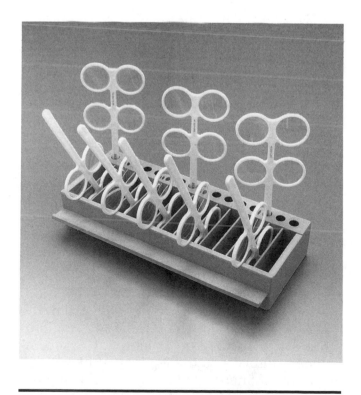

Figure 2-18—Bernell flipper devices for accommodative facility testing (photo courtesy of Bernell Corp.).

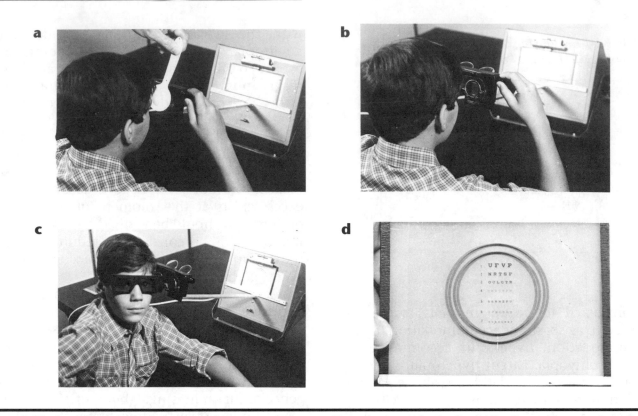

Figure 2-19—Accommodative facility testing: Trial lenses can be mounted in an attachment for the Correct-Eye-Scope. (a) monocular testing; (b) binocular testing; (c) view of polarizing filters worn by the patient; (d) vectographic target (Vectogram® #9). Line 4 is seen by the left eye, line 5 by both eyes, and line 6 by the right eye.

methods) are reliable, especially for young patients, subjective testing may also be done. This can be done with the binocular crossed-cylinder test at near. However, we do not believe this subjective method is as reliable as objective testing with Nott or MEM methods.

Infacility of Accommodation

Another aspect of accommodation is facility. An infacility of accommodation is the inability to change focus rapidly. This is also known as inertia of accommodation. Accommodative infacility can cause discomfort and reduced vision efficiency. For example, such patients typically complain of slow clearing of vision, most often blurring when looking from the "book to the board." The standard testing procedure is to use ± 2.00 D lenses. The recommended optotype is the equivalent of a 20/30 (6/9) line of Snellen letters at 40 cm while the lens power is changed from plus to minus, and so on, for 1 minute. Lenses may be mounted in a Bausch and Lomb Comparator or a similar device (Figure 2-18). Testing is done monocularly (O.D. and O.S.) and then binocularly. Suppression can be monitored with vectographic targets (Figure 2-19). Although clinicians may ask the patient to say "clear" with each stimulus change, a better technique is to instruct the patient to read each letter aloud as quickly as possible with the introduction of each lens flip. This allows monitoring of correct or incorrect responses. The number of accurate calls is recorded and converted into cycles per minute (c/m) by dividing that number by 2. For example, if the number of correct calls for an eye is 8, there are 4 c/m.

A summary of norms of facility by several investigators is included in Table 2-15. Borish stated[18] that monocular accommodative facility when tested at the patient's habitual near-point distance should have a range of lenses from +1.50 to –2.00 D with clear vision, with the normal response time being less than 5 seconds.

TABLE 2-15. *Norms for Accommodative Facility*

Investigators	Results	Comments
Alpert and Zellers[30]	±2.00 D, 11 cycles per minute monocular 8 cycles per minute, binocular, without suppression being monitored	Young adults
Burge[27]	±2.00 D, 12 cycles per minute, monocular 10 cycles per minute, binocular 7 cycles per minute, binocular, with suppression being monitored	Children and young adults
Griffin et al.[25]	±2.00 D, 17 cycles per minute, monocular	Young adults
Griffin et al.[26]	±2.00 D, 1.7 cycles per minute, monocular 13 cycles per minute, binocular 6 cycles per minute, binocular, with suppression being monitored	Young adults
Hoffman et al.[32]	±2.50 D, approximately 3 cycles per minute	Children 6 to 12 years
Liu et al.[24]	±1.50 D, 20 cycles per 64 seconds with 26 S.D.	Adults
Schlange et al.[31]	±2.00 D, 7 cycles per minute, binocular	Children
Grisham et al.[28] and Pope et al.[29]	±2.00 D, 10 cycles per 52 seconds with 24 S.D.	Children

Liu et al.[24] suggested the criterion for pass to be 20 cycles per 90 seconds, with each cycle being 4.5 seconds or each flip being 2.25 seconds.

Griffin et al.[25] studied monocular accommodative facility in 14 subjects ranging in age from 20 to 35 years. They found ±2.00 D rock to have an average value of 17 cycles per minute. The average response time to clear the minus lens was 2 seconds, and 1.4 seconds to clear the plus lens.

Griffin et al.[26] determined monocular facility compared with binocular facility. They wanted to eliminate the possibility of guessing and ensure that patients were actually seeing clearly rather than reporting "clear" with each lens flipping. Instead of manually changing targets (which were double-digit numbers), an electrical mechanism introduced random numbers (of 6-point type size at a distance of 40 cm) in synchrony with the lens-flipper mechanism. Rock of ± 2.00 D was done for 1 minute to determine the average number of cycles in a young adult population, ages 20 to 23 years. Monocular facility was approximately 17 cycles per minute. Binocular facility was approximately 13 cycles per minute, without suppression being monitored. To monitor suppression, a vectographic plate was arranged so that the leftward (first) digit was seen only by the left eye, and the right eye saw only the second digit. For example, the number "53" that appeared with the new lens change would be presented so that only the number "5" could be seen by the left eye and the number "3" by the right eye. There were only 6 cycles per minute as an average for this group of subjects when suppression was monitored. The investigators reviewed the 27 records of complete vision examinations and selected 16 subjects who showed evidence of poor visual skills and 11 who showed good visual skills. Monocular rock for the subjects with good visual skills averaged 18 cycles per minute compared with 15 cycles per minute for the subjects having poor visual skills. Binocular rock without suppression monitoring gave averages of 17 and 9 cycles per minute for the same two groups, respectively. When binocular rock was tested using suppression monitoring, there was an average of 9 cycles per minute for the subjects with good visual skills, but only 4 cycles per minute for those having poor visual skills. The authors concluded that binocular accommodative facility testing can be definitive in the assessment of a patient's binocular status.

Burge[27] used a practical clinical method to study binocular facility using suppression monitoring. He used a Spriangle Vectogram target with crossed-polarizing viewers and ±2.00 D lens flippers. The mean value results were 12 cycles per minute monocularly, 10 cycles per minute binocularly without suppression monitoring, and 7 cycles per minute with suppression monitoring. Burge's value for monocular facility was lower than those just described by Griffin et al.[26,27] He included children rather than adults only as subjects (ranging from 6 to 30 years).

Grisham et al.[28] and Pope et al.[29] established monocular accommodative facility norms for elementary school children and validated these norms by objective accommodative testing. They tested second, fourth, sixth, and eighth graders using ±2.00 D flippers at 33 cm. The target was 20/30 optotype and the child was asked to report when the print appeared to "clear" with each lens. The norms proved to be the same for all grades, except for the second graders whose responses were often inaccurate (presumably due to lapses of attention). They measured the time the subjects took to complete 10 cycles and 20 cycles on the test. Since no significant difference in c/m was found, they recommended using 10 cycles for testing children age 8 years and older. The mean time was 52 seconds with a standard deviation of 24 seconds. More than 75 seconds was considered failing. A unique feature of this study was the objective verification of the clinical procedure. The property of accommodative facility (latency, velocity, and completion time) was objectively measured using a dynamic optometer on randomly selected students. The rank correlation between the clinical and objective measurements was high (r = 0.89) indicating good concurrent validity. (Other studies are shown in Table 2-15.)

TABLE 2-16. *Ranking of Accommodative Facility with ±2.00 D*

Rank		Cycles per Minute	
		O.D. or O.S.	*Binocular
5	Very Strong	>18	>10
4	Strong	14 to 18	8 to 10
3	Adequate	10 to 13	6 to 7
2	Weak	6 to 9	4 to 5
1	Very Weak	<6	<4

*Suppression monitoring with vectographic targets.

There is no consensus on developmental norms from childhood to adulthood for accommodative facility. As to referral criteria for facility, Hoffman and Rouse[5] recommended the following: flipper test of ±2.00 D monocularly and binocularly showing less than 12 cycles per minute, with the patient viewing a 20/30 line at 40 cm, or a difference of more than 2 cycles per minute between the two eyes. In light of the results shown in Table 2-15, these referral criteria may be too stringent, especially for young children. Retesting and/or lowered initial standards should be considered during the routine testing of new patients. We recommend the cutoff criteria for pass/fail as follows: Fail if monocular facility is less than 10 cycles per minute or difference between the eyes is greater than 2 cycles per minute; fail if binocular facility with suppression monitoring is less than 6 cycles per minute. Refer to Table 2-16 for clarification and ranking of accommodative facility. These criteria do not apply to children under 7 years old. Professional judgment must be used when evaluating accommodative facility in very young children.

Ill-Sustained Accommodation

Testing for ill-sustained accommodation is similar to that for facility of accommodation except that it may show up after a period of time when accommodation is active. Speed and sufficiency may be normal in the beginning, but it may be maintained only with effort and decrease with time. The time during which the stamina decreases may be short, often within 1 minute.

Ill-sustained accommodation relates to stamina, or the power to endure fatigue.[33] It is easily detected in most routine accommodative facility testing. That is why clinicians should carry out facility testing over a period of at least 1 minute. For example, a patient with ill-sustained accommodation may begin ±2.00 D lens rock quickly and sufficiently, but the responses may become inadequate after a few flips of the lenses. If the clinician tests only one or two cycles, the patient's lack of accommodative stamina will possibly not be discovered. Ill-sustained accommodation can definitely affect performance as well as cause various visual symptoms. Individuals vary widely in their ability to meet and sustain accommodative demands for a variety of reasons, e.g., physiologic variation, medication, visual demands, and general health. Clinical experience has shown, however, that accommodative stamina can be improved in most cases when the cause is functional in nonpresbyopic patients. Therapy is the same as for accommodative facility. Monocular, bi-ocular, and binocular accommodative rock procedures are performed in the office and at home. The only difference is that sustaining ability is emphasized to a greater extent than otherwise. (Therapy is discussed in Chapter 15.)

For testing of accommodative stamina we recommend using the ranking shown in Table 2-17. These are clinical empirical observations and fully researched norms await further reports. The clinician flips the lenses at a constant rate, 6 sec/cycle. If this rate is maintained for 36 seconds under binocular conditions, the patient passes this recommended standard for accommodative stamina. Stability is emphasized as opposed to frequency of correct calls as in facility testing. It is one thing to be fast for a while, but in real life an individual will not do well if there is a lack of stamina. This is true for the accommodative system as it is for saccades,

TABLE 2-17. Ranking of Accommodative Stamina

Rank		Monocular	*Binocular
5	Very Strong	108 sec. or more	60 sec. or more
4	Strong	84 to 108 sec.	48 to 59 sec.
3	Adequate	60 to 83 sec.	36 to 47 sec.
2	Weak	36 to 59 sec.	24 to 35 sec.
1	Very Weak	<36 sec.	<24 sec.

Testing is at the rate of 6 seconds/cycle (i.e., 3 seconds per each correct response) with ±2.00 D lenses. The cut-off time isdetermined by when a response time exceeds 3 seconds on any lens flip, or whenever there is an incorrect response. *Suppression should be monitored using either anaglyphic or vectographic targets when binocular testing is done.

pursuits, and position maintenance (discussed previously).

If a patient passes the recommended criteria for accommodative facility testing with a good rate of responses consistently throughout the test, stamina testing is unnecessary.

Summary of Accommodation Testing

Accommodative insufficiency is tested in several ways. The amplitude of *absolute* accommodation is found by monocular pushups, and possibly bracketing between pushups and push-aways when necessary. PRA and NRA are binocular tests of *relative* accommodation. Dynamic retinoscopy under binocular viewing conditions, done with either the Nott or MEM method, determines an accommodative inaccuracy.

Testing for infacility introduces the element of time which relates to the efficiency of accommodative responsiveness. The standard testing procedure is to use ±2.00 D lenses, first monocularly and then binocularly. At least 10 cycles per minute are necessary for monocular adequacy, and 6 cycles per minute binocularly (with suppression monitoring). Testing for ill-sustained accommodation involves the element of time as in testing for infacility. The difference is that the quality of accurate responses as to stability and endurance is assessed, rather than mere quantity of accurate calls.

VERGENCES

Vergences are disjunctive eye movements (rather than conjugate movements, as in the three other movement systems). The occipitomesencephalic neural pathway for vergences, at least for convergence, is from area 19 to the third nerve nuclei. Vergence movements are slow (compared with saccades) and mainly involuntary. There are four components of convergence according to Maddox: tonic, accommodative, fusional (disparity), and proximal (psychic). Although authorities may disagree on this classification as being the only true one, the consensus is that the Maddox concept is useful for clinical purposes. Nevertheless, factors other than those of the Maddox classification, e.g., prism adaptation, must be taken into account in vision therapy. These are discussed in relation to case examples (along with the Maddox components) in Chapter 3 and also later in the book.

Absolute Convergence

The total amount of convergence of the visual axes from parallelism at far to a bifixated target at near is called absolute convergence, often referred to as "gross" convergence. Absolute convergence may involve all four components of Maddox, i.e., tonic, accommodative, proximal, and fusional vergence.

Testing Techniques

The clinical test for absolute convergence is performed with a small target, traditionally a pencil tip, for measuring the nearpoint of convergence (NPC). The patient views a target in the midline as it is moved closer to the spectacle plane. Any object for fixation can be used but a target requiring accurate accommodation is recommended. A small isolated letter "E" of approximately 20/30 (6/9) size at 40 cm (1.5 minutes of arc) has become a clinical standard.

TABLE 2-18. *Ranking of Results of NPC Testing.*

Rank	Description	Breakpoint (cm)	Recovery to Singleness (cm)
5	Very Strong	<5	<8
4	Strong	5 to 6	8 to 9
3	Adequate	7 to 8*	10 to 11
2	Weak	9 to 15	12 to 18
1	Very Weak	>15	>18

*A breakpoint distance more remote than 8 cm is considered failure as is a recovery more remote than 11 cm.

The examiner moves the target steadily at a rate of approximately 3 to 5 cm/sec toward the bridge of the nose of the patient. The patient is asked to look at the letter and report when it first becomes blurred and then when it appears doubled. Despite blurring, some patients may be able to maintain bifixation on the target all the way to the bridge of the nose (i.e., approximating the spectacle plane). Most patients, however, will have a breakpoint several centimeters from the spectacle plane (Table 2-18). After the blurpoint is reported (although not reported by many patients) and the breakpoint is measured, the target is withdrawn in a similar manner and at the same speed to determine the point of recovery. Supplementary testing in up-gaze and down-gaze may be included as warranted, e.g., in cases of A or V patterns. (Refer to discussion on comitancy in Chapter 4.)

These clinical measurements are usually recorded in centimeter values, although they may alternately be expressed in prism diopters units. If, for example, the breakpoint is 7 cm from the spectacle plane, the magnitude in prism diopters of absolute convergence can be calculated trigonometrically. The following formula, however, is convenient for clinical purposes:

$$\text{Prism Diopters} = \text{IPD}\left(\frac{100}{X + 2.7}\right)$$

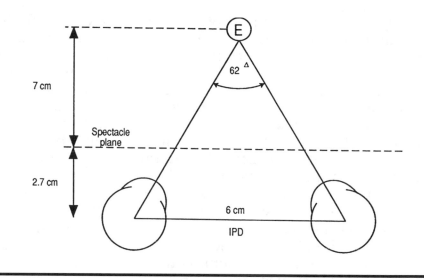

Figure 2-20—Example of NPC Conversion from centimeters to prism diopters.

If, for example, the interpupillary distance (IPD) is 60 mm (6 cm) and the NPC in breakpoint is 7 cm:

$$\Delta = 6\left(\frac{100}{7+2.7}\right)$$

$$\Delta = 62$$

Note: The 2.7 cm distance is the approximate distance from the center of rotation of the eyes to the spectacle plane (Figure 2-20).

Functions and Norms for Absolute Convergence

NPC testing allows three functions of absolute convergence to be assessed: sufficiency (amplitude), facility (flexibility), and stamina. Norms listed below are from Griffin,[34] Hoffman and Rouse,[5] and from our clinical experience.

Sufficiency of absolute convergence is determined by the usual testing method of pencil pushups, as described above; a small detailed target is recommended rather than a pencil tip. The blurpoint is so variable among the normal population that norms have not been established. Ideally, however, blurring should not occur until the target approaches a distance in the range of 10 to 15 cm. On the other hand, the breakpoint should be much less remote, normally 7 to 8 cm or closer. Either diplopia of the target reported by the patient or loss of bifixation (as observed by the examiner) at a distance exceeding 8 cm is considered "failing" which can be used as a cutoff point for referral considerations (see Table 2-18). Certainly a remote NPC greater than 10 cm is definitely failing. The reporting of diplopia is a subjective test. Subjective NPC results should be corroborated with objective testing results (observation of examiner). Ordinarily, direct observation of the patient's eyes will suffice, but greater accuracy is possible by observing the corneal reflexes from an auxiliary penlight source held a few centimeters above the letter E fixation target. This is a modified Hirschberg test. (Refer to Chapter 4 for discussion on Hirschberg testing.) Suppression may be indicated if there is no report of diplopia and the clinician observes a lack of bifixation.

Facility of absolute convergence can be assessed indirectly by the patient's ability to recover bifixation. Clearness of the target is not necessarily demanded, only singleness, for normative evaluation purposes. The patient should be expected to recover singleness (and objectively be observed by the examiner that bifixation has in fact recurred) at a distance of 10 to 11 cm or closer as the target is withdrawn. Poor vergence recovery is indicated if the distance is more remote. In other words, a recovery beyond 11 cm is considered "failing" and referral for vision therapy should be considered (see Table 2-18).

Stamina of absolute convergence is assessed by repeating the break/recovery testing four times, for a total of five routines. Poor stamina is indicated if the endpoints are more remote upon repetition. Any decrement in performance over this time period is considered failing or, at least, suggestive of a dysfunction of gross convergence. Note that the training effect of repeated NPC testing may result in prism (vergence) adaptation which theoretically should help the patient converge more sufficiently. If, however, sufficiency is reduced upon repetition because of lack of stamina, the individual most likely has significant binocular problems. Referral for vision therapy should be considered. In summary, *stamina* is an important function to evaluate, as are *facility* and *sufficiency* of absolute convergence.

Although NPC normative data are not well established for infants and preschoolers, practitioners of vision therapy are well aware of the fact that infants of 1 year of age can converge their eyes to view a target at very close distances. Wick[35] reported this in a patient not quite a year old.

Developmental Considerations

Absolute convergence, as measured during NPC testing, is composed of four components: tonic, accommodative, proximal, and fusional vergence. The developmental periods of each of the components are different and should be taken into account by clinicians examining infants and toddlers.

Schor[36] summarized that tonic vergence is stimulated by intrinsic innervation; accommodative vergence responds to blur; and psychic vergence is dependent upon perceived distance. These are "open-loop" responses and do not demand heavily on visual feedback mechanisms. For example, one eye may be occluded but convergence will occur if the unoccluded eye responds to the accommodative demand of a minus lens, which would cause accommodative convergence. Fusional (dispar-ity) vergence, on the other hand, is a "closed-loop" response requiring sensory feedback from retinal image disparity. Tonic vergence can be measured at birth, often a "low tonic" convergence resulting in an exo deviation. Accommodative vergence is evident, to some extent, within a few weeks after birth. Proximal convergence is evident in the neonate as shown by the difference between the deviation in lighted surrounds (usually exo) and the deviation of the visual axes in darkness (usually eso).

According to Schor,[37] however, "It is clear that the binocular disparity vergence system is the last of the oculomotor functions to develop. Little is known about the age at which the response is adultlike." The following section on disparity vergences, therefore, presents established norms for adults. We believe these are applicable, however, to older children and perhaps those down to age 7. Although the physiology is present in children for them to respond to testing, attentional problems may cause unreliable results in many cases. Nevertheless, our clinical impression is that a 7-year-old child should have approximately the same magnitudes of sufficiency, facility and stamina of vergence functions as older children and adults. This is assuming attention is good and optimal performance is attained during testing. In general, testing of very young children requires objective testing to a large extent.

Relative Convergence Testing and Norms

Convergence is the traditionally used term for both convergence and divergence. The general term "vergence" is probably preferable when discussing relative vergences rather than the semantically restrictive "con" prefix being included. This would avoid the necessity of awkward or superfluous denotations such as "negative fusional convergence" and "positive fusional convergence." The terms, *relative vergence, fusional vergence*, and *disparity vergence* may be used interchangeably for most clinical purposes. (Refer to Chapter 3 for further discussion on relative vergences.) The stimulus for fusional vergence eye movements is retinal disparity with other intervening variables excluded. This means that a constant testing distance is maintained during increasing prismatic stimuli. Relative vergence is conveniently measured from the ortho demand point which simplifies clinical recording. For example, a patient views a target at 40 cm while base-out demand is increasingly introduced with Risley prisms. The blur, break, and recovery points are recorded directly from the scale on the instrument as though the patient (and every patient) is orthophoric. The actual magnitude of the disparity vergence response, however, must take into account the fusion-free position of rest which involves the effects of tonic, accommodative, and proximal vergence. If, for example, a patient has exophoria of 6^Δ at 40 cm and the blurpoint with base-out demand is 10^Δ, the total fusional (disparity) vergence response would be 16^Δ. Suppose another patient has an esophoria at 40 cm of 4^Δ, the total fusional (disparity) vergence response would be only 6^Δ for the 10^Δ base-out demand. This method of measurement complicates establishment of norms for clinical usefulness. Conveniently, however, relative vergences measured from the common-denominator-ortho position allow for norms to be standardized. This is why *relative* vergence is the preferred term for clinical purposes.

Clinical testing of relative vergence should begin with divergence testing. This is because prism adaptation to base-out is relatively strong and prism demands may contaminate the base-in findings, making the fusional divergence response appear to be falsely much weaker than otherwise. According to Schor's hypothesis,[37] "the stimulus to vergence adaptation is the effort, or output, of the fast fusional vergence controller." In other words, the reflex-disparity-vergence output resulting from Risley base-out prisms can induce prism adaptation during actual clinical testing. Therefore, fusional divergence testing should precede testing of fusional convergence. By tradition in clinical practice, however, farpoint BI and BO vergence testing precedes nearpoint BI and BO vergence testing. The clinical sequence is (1) fusional divergence at far; (2) fusional convergence at far; (3) fusional divergence at near; (4) fusional convergence at near. Despite the possible contaminant of prism adaptation (especially with BO prism), clinicians find it more convenient to finish farpoint testing before going to nearpoint testing. Therefore, we recommend maintaining the traditional sequence, for sake of clinical ease and expediency.

Fusional Vergences at Far

Fusional divergence at far is also known as negative fusional vergence, negative fusional convergence (NFC), and negative disparity divergence, among the several designations for this function. For sake of consistency and historical precedence in this text, we adhere to "NRC at 6 m" as the clinical nomenclature of choice. The stimulus to fusional divergence is retinal image disparity (which is base-in demand). The responses of tonic, accommodative, and proximal vergences must be minimized, to the extent possible, so that only fusional vergence is measured. Fusional divergence can be measured by several clinical methods. The most common method to measure NRC is with the use of Risley prisms in a phoropter. From a distance of 6 m the patient is instructed to view a vertical column of letters, normally of 20/20 (6/6) subtense, but the letter size may vary depending on the best attainable acuity of the patient. If, for example, the patient's best corrected visual acuity is 20/40 (6/12), that particular minimum angle of resolution for letters should be used for testing. CAMP (corrected ametropia with most plus) lenses for maximum visual acuity at far must be used for all baseline testing. This is for reliability of all visual skills.

When vergence ranges are tested with Risley prisms, the speed of prism induction should be standardized. If the rate is too slow, the patient may have an excessive degree of prism adaptation, and falsely pass the test. If the prism demand is introduced too rapidly, the patient may falsely fail the test. Most clinicians have found that the best overall rate of introduction of Risley prism power is approximately 4 prism diopters per second. We recommend this rate for all sliding vergence testing whether with Risley prisms, Vectograms, ana-

TABLE 2-19. *Ranking of Results of NRC Testing at 6 Meters (BI).*

Rank	Description	Breakpoint (Δ)	Recovery to Singleness (D)
5	Very Strong	8	6
4	Strong	7	5
3	Adequate	6	4
2	Weak	5	3
1	Very Weak	4	2

TABLE 2-20. *Ranking of Results of PRC Testing at 6 Meters (BO)*

Rank	Description	Blurpoint (Δ)	Breakpoint (Δ)	Recovery to Singleness (Δ)
5	Very Strong	>14	>24	>15
4	Strong	11 to 14	21 to 24	12 to 15
3	Adequate	8 to 10	16 to 20	9 to 11
2	Weak	7	15	8
1	Very Weak	<7	<15	<8

glyphs, or targets in stereoscopes. As Grisham[28] pointed out, "Test results are markedly influenced by such procedural factors as speed and smoothness of prism power induction, amount of contour in the fixation target, and phrasing of instructions (i.e., "Tell me when the target doubles," as opposed to "Try to keep the target single.")

We recommend the following standard routine:

1. Have the patient view a column of 20/20 (6/6) letters (or the patient's minimum angle of resolution if acuity is worse).
2. Instruct the patient to try to keep the letters clear and report if there is any blurring. The Risley prisms are rotated symmetrically. Note: be skeptical if a blur is reported on base-in testing at far. A blurring could be due to an incorrect

refractive status, such as latent hyperopia, or else the patient is overminused. Therefore, it is vital to do vergence testing with the patient looking through CAMP lenses. The first sustained blur exceeding 2 seconds is recorded. Blurring should be that amount of degraded form acuity that would be caused by +0.25 D overcorrection at 6 m. Demonstrate this to the patient, if necessary, for reliable reporting for "blur." Again, blurring should not normally occur with BI prism testing at 6 m.

3. Instruct the patient: "Try to keep the target single but tell me when the target doubles." The first sustained diplopia is recorded. If the patient reports a momentary diplopia that does not exceed 5 seconds, that is disregarded. The amount of prism causing a "sustained" diplopia is recorded for "break."
4. After the endpoint of sustained diplopia is reached, reduce the prismatic demand (at the rate of 4^Δ/sec) until sustained singleness (but not necessarily clearness) is reported. A good instruction is: "Tell me when the double images join again into one." This endpoint is recorded for the recovery value.

Once the break and recovery values for negative relative convergence (NRC) are recorded, these findings may be evaluated as to normal versus abnormal. Table 2-19 shows a ranking system whereby ranks of 2 or less are abnormal and, thus, failing. Ranks of 3 or more are passing. This indicates 6^Δ break and 4^Δ recovery are passing. These are in accord with Morgan's norms (discussed in Chapter 3).

Positive relative convergence (PRC) at 6 m is tested in a similar manner as for NRC. The difference is that base-out prism demands are given, rather than base-in. Unlike NRC at 6 m, a blurpoint is usually expected when base-out prism demand (PRC at 6 m) is increased. Some patients, however, do not report blurring, only break and recovery. We have found that with proper instruction and demonstration, over 90% of nonpresbyopic patients are able to appreciate the blurpoint at 6 m with base-out prism demand. A blurpoint of 7^Δ is "weak" and it should be at least 8^Δ (Table 2-20). The breakpoint should be at least 16^Δ and recovery should be at least 9^Δ. Otherwise, the cutoff criteria for passing are not met for break and recovery.

Fusional Vergences at Near

The nearpoint testing procedure for fusional divergence is similar to that at farpoint, except a blurpoint is expected. It is referred to simply as negative relative convergence (NRC) with the 40 cm testing distance implied. Ranking standards are shown in Table 2-21. All nearpoint testing of fusional divergence is done at 40 cm. The base-in demand is presented to the patient in the same manner as discussed above for other fusional vergence testing. The blurpoint should be at least 12^Δ for passing. The breakpoint should be at least 20^Δ and recovery at least 11^Δ.

Fusional convergence at 40 cm is done similarly, as discussed above. Base-out prism demand is increased gradually until the endpoints of blur, break, and recovery are reached. The blurpoint is called positive relative convergence (PRC). Pass-fail criteria are shown in Table 2-22 along with rankings from very strong to very weak. A blurpoint less than 15^Δ is failing, as is a breakpoint less than 19^Δ, and a recovery less than 8^Δ. These findings are entered in the patient's record. If a blur is not reported, place an X to denote this as such, e.g., X/18/7.

Vergence Facility

Vergence facility depends on both amplitude and speed of vergence movements. The quantity and quality of disparity vergences should be evaluated. (Discussion will be limited to horizontal vergence facility of fusional divergence and convergence.) Grisham[28,38] studied the vergence tracking rate, using 2^Δ jump-vergence steps in 8 subjects, 4 of whom had "normal vergence characteristics" and 4 who had "abnormal" heterophoric or vergence characteristics, based on clinical data. He found that the normal group had an average minimum stimulus duration of 0.84 sec per step, and the

TABLE 2-21. *Ranking of Results of NRC Testing at 40 Centimeters (BI)*

Rank	Description	Blurpoint (Δ)	Breakpoint (Δ)	Recovery to Singleness (Δ)
5	Very Strong	>18	>26	>18
4	Strong	14 to 18	22 to 26	14 to 18
3	Adequate	12 to 13	20 to 21	11 to 13
2	Weak	11	19	10
1	Very Weak	<11	<19	<10

TABLE 2-22. *Ranking of Results of PRC Testing at 40 Centimeters (BO)*

Rank	Description	Blurpoint (Δ)	Breakpoint (Λ)	Recovery to Singleness (Δ)
5	Very Strong	>23	>28	>18
4	Strong	18 to 23	22 to 28	13 to 18
3	Adequate	15 to 17	19 to 21	8 to 11
2	Weak	14	18	7
1	Very Weak	<14	<18	<7

abnormal group had a significantly longer duration of 1.67 sec per step. Grisham cited the observation of Rashbass and Westheimer "that normal disparity vergence eye movements take on the order of 1 sec to complete independent of step stimulus amplitude" and said that his study "compares well with the observation of Rashbass and Westheimer." Grisham also found that the normal and abnormal groups could be differentiated according to other dynamic properties of fusional vergence response, including percentage of completion of step responses, response velocity, and divergence latency (but not convergence latency).

Reflex Fusion Text

Clinically, we recommend evaluating vergence facility by direct observation. A small-power prism, the vergence stimulus, is inserted before one eye as the patient fixates a detailed target.

The latency, velocity, accuracy, and stamina of vergence responses can be directly observed and assessed. Without eye movement recording equipment, these dynamic components cannot be quantified, but with practice the clinician can make accurate and valid judgments regarding quality of reflex vergence function by closely noting the eye movements stimulated by the prism. A virtue of this technique is that it is objective, relying only on tester observations. It can be used to confirm subjective vergence testing or with patients who have unreliable subjective responses, e.g., young children, some aged patients, and some handicapped patients.

The procedure is simple, but accurate observation and interpretation take practice. A 6^Δ prism is inserted before the sighting dominant eye as the patient fixates a target at 40 cm. In exophoric cases, convergence is evaluated first with a base-out prism, and then with base-in prism. Conversely with esophores, base-in prism is initially used, then base-out. Since the patient is viewing binocularly, the prism is a vergence stimulus. Usually, there is a mixed version and vergence response to a small-increment prism. A normal vergence response would represent little or no version movement of eye without the prism; most of the vergence movement would be by the eye with the prism. The larger the version response of the nonprismed eye, the longer is the latency of the vergence system. Velocity of the vergence component is directly observed and rated as slow, moderate, or fast based on clinical experience with this test. If there is one smooth vergence movement to the prism, the response is considered accurate, whereas, if a series of vergences are observed, inaccuracy is evident. Stamina can be noted by rapid, repeated observations of the speed and accuracy of vergence responses in a particular direction.

Reflex Fusion Stress Test

An attempt to quantify the reflex fusion test has been made by establishing norms for teenagers and adults. Ten cycles of prism rock are timed in a particular direction, base-out or base-in. The clinician inserts and removes the prism when each vergence response is completed. Direct observation of responses is the basis for reintroducing the prism, but in cases when the responses are particularly slow and the point of complete bifixation is difficult to see, then subjective responses of sensory fusion (singleness versus diplopia) by the patient may be helpful. Using 10 cycles of 6^Δ BO, the norm is 22 seconds ±3 (S.D.) and for 6^Δ BI, it is 21 seconds ±4 (S.D.). Using the standard deviation as the basis for clinical evaluation, a patient's vergence responses are considered slow if the completion time is 25 seconds or longer.

In many cases of vergence infacility, the completion time is considerably longer than 25 seconds. Prolonged latency, slow velocity, and inaccuracy can all contribute to increasing the total time. Some patients having vergence fatigue may not even complete the 10 cycles and manifest diplopia or suppression during the test. Diplopia is noted subjectively by the patient's report. Objectively, the clinician observes the patient's failure to make a correct vergence response. A suppression response is noted if there is no movement of either eye to the vergence stimulus. In this case, the patient has suppressed the eye behind the prism. In summary, a prolonged completion time, isolated version, alternate versions, or no movement to the prism are all responses considered to be abnormal and indicative of a fusional vergence dysfunction.

Kenyon et al.[39] studied "dynamic" vergence responses to stimuli at two different distances, 25 and 50 cm. They tested fusional facility of vergence since disparity vergence was being tested as in "jump" vergences as opposed to "sliding" vergences as may be tested with Risley prisms. An absence of disparity vergence was found in all strabismic individuals and in some who had amblyopia with no strabismus. Accommodative convergence, rather than fusional (disparity) vergence, was used to attempt to bifoveate the target.

From the literature and clinical experience, we believe clinical testing of vergence facility can be useful in evaluating the quality of a patient's binocular status and possibly the patient's developmental-perceptual status. Pierce[40] reported a difference in vergence facility between normal and learning-disabled children. Other studies[41,42] reported developmental differences

TABLE 2-23. *Summary of Studies on Vergence Facility*

Investigators	Fusional (Disparity) Vergence Facility (c/min. = Cycles per Minute)	Comments
Kenyon et al.[39]	None in strabismics	Also none in some amblyopic subjects without strabismus
Pierce[40]	8^Δ BI and 8^Δ BO, 10 c/min. (median); screening criterion of 7.5 c/min.	Median for children; 7.5 c/min. recommended as cutoff for "normal" versus "learning-disabled" children
Stuckle and Rouse[41]	8^Δ BI and 8^Δ BO, approx. 7 c/min.	Mean for 6th graders
	8^Δ BI and 8^Δ BO, approx. 5 c/min.	Mean for 3rd graders
Mitchell et al.[42]	8^Δ BI and 8^Δ BO, 6.53 c/min.	Mean for 6th graders
	8^Δ BI and 8^Δ BO, 5.05 c/min.	Mean for 3rd graders (cutoff criterion of 3 c/min. recommended)
Moser and Atkinson[43]	8^Δ BI and 8^Δ BO, 8.14 c/min.	Young adults
Rosner[44]	Screening: 6^Δ BI and 12^Δ BO, 3 c/0.5 min.	At farpoint
	12^Δ BI and 14^Δ BO, 3 c/0.5 min.	At nearpoint
	Goals: 6^Δ BI and 12^Δ BO, 18 c/1.5 min.	At farpoint
	12^Δ BI and 14^Δ BO, 18 c/1.5 min.	At nearpoint
Jacobson et al.[45]	5^Δ BI and 15^Δ BO in relation to the phoric position of each subject, 8.6 c/min.	Young adults with no vision problems; jump vergences with two sets of vectographic targets
Delgadillo and Griffin[46]	5^Δ BI and 15^Δ BO versus 8^Δ BI and 8^Δ BO	Approximately same results (adult subjects)

between schoolchildren in the third and sixth grades being around 5 and 7 cycles per minute, respectively, using 8^Δ BI and 8^Δ BO flippers (Table 2-23). Moser and Atkinson[43] found an average of 8.14 cycles per minute in young adults using 8^Δ BI and 8^Δ BO in vergence facility testing. Rosner[44] stated criteria for screening (for referral) and for ultimate goals as follows: 6^Δ base-in and 12^Δ base-out at farpoint and 12^Δ base-in and 14^Δ base-out at nearpoint. The goal of at least 18 cycles in 90 seconds is desired at farpoint and nearpoint using free-space orthopic and chiastopic fusion without instrumentation or filters. (These types of fusion are discussed in Chapters 13 and 14.)

Jacobson et al.[45] studied vergence facility in 41 young adults with no referable vision problems or significant binocular problems. Two sets of Quoits vectographic targets were used, the upper pair having a base-in demand, and the lower pair a base-out demand. Testing was done

at 40 cm. A 5^Δ base-in demand was presented relative to the patient's nearpoint heterophoric eye positioning. [A nearpoint phoria is also referred to as *fusional supplementary convergence (FSC) value.*] For example, if the patient had an esophoria of 4^Δ at nearpoint, only 1^Δ base-in was set in the upper Quoits slides. Similarly, a 15^Δ base-out demand relative to the near phoria was set in the lower Quoits slides, or in this example, the setting would be at 19^Δ base-out. The investigators found it necessary to make these adjustments for the heterophoria because many subjects could not perform a range of 20^Δ using absolute 5^Δ base-in and 15^Δ base-out. The principal problem for many subjects was with base-in demands, particularly if the subjects were esophoric at near. A mean of 8.6 cycles per minute was found. This would indicate a rather low recommended number for screening and referral purposes. If absolute base-in and base-out powers of 5^Δ and 15^Δ, respectively, are used,

TABLE 2-24. *Vergence Facility Tested with 8^Δ BI and 8^Δ BO at 40 cm and with 4^Δ BI and 8^Δ BO at 6 m.*

Rank		Cycle/Minute (c/m)
5	Very Strong	>15
4	Strong	11 to 15
3	Adequate	5 to 10
2	Weak	3 to 4
1	Very Weak	<3

Note: Suppression should be monitored with anaglyphic or vectographic targets with targets equivalent to "20/30" being clear and single with each prism flip. The Vectographic Slide is recommended for 6 m and Vectograms as used for accommodative facility are recommended for testing at 40 cm.

TABLE 2-25. *Vergence Stamina with 8^Δ BI and 8^Δ BO at 40 cm and with 4^Δ BI and 8^Δ BO at 6 m at the Rate of 6 Seconds per Cycle.*

Rank		Seconds
5	Very Strong	>90
4	Strong	66 to 90
3	Adequate	30 to 65
2	Weak	18 to 29
1	Very Weak	<18

Note: Suppression should be monitored as in vergence facility testing.

we believe a screening criterion of 5 cycles per minute is useful as a cutoff value when suppression is monitored. A training goal, however, would be much larger.

Delgadillo and Griffin[46] found that 5^Δ BI -15^Δ BO gave approximately the same results as 8^Δ BI and 8^Δ BO; therefore, either test can be used at nearpoint, at least in adults with normal binocular vision.

Considering the above reports and from our clinical experience we recommend evaluating vergence facility as shown in Table 2-24. For children of ages 7 to 11 a lenient cut-off crite-rion for failing is 4 or less cycles per minute; 5 c/m or more would be passing as to the question of referral for vision therapy being considered. These criteria apply at 40 cm with 8^Δ BI and 8^Δ BO as well as at 6 m with 4^Δ BI and 8^Δ BO prism demands. Although the criteria appear to be lenient, some of the earlier reports recommending greater values for cycles per minute did not include suppression monitoring. We have found that patients generally are much slower when vectographic targets and viewing filters are used, reduced perhaps as many as 3 to 5 c/m, whether in children or adults. We believe, therefore, that the criteria in Table 2-24 can apply to both children and adults for evaluation of vergence facility.

Vergence Stamina

Vergence stamina is tested when vergence facility is tested over a period of time at a constant rate of stimulus change. (Slowing of responses should be noted.) This is analogous to accommodative stamina. Vergence stamina is tested at 40 cm with 8^Δ BI and 8^Δ BO at the rate of 6 seconds per cycle (3 seconds per clear fusion response). The patient is instructed to see the target as clear and single. Testing at 6 m is done with 4^Δ BI and 8^Δ BO flip prisms every 3 seconds, so that testing is at the rate of 6 seconds per cycle. The cut-off point is 30 seconds (Table 2-25). The patient should be able to maintain clear and single vision with each flip for at least 30 seconds.

Summary of Vergence Testing

As with accommodation, vergences are classified as either absolute or relative and testing is to determine the sufficiency, facility, and stamina. Accuracy of vergence is assessed with fixation disparity testing (discussed in Chapter 3), which is analogous to accommodative accuracy assessed with dynamic retinoscopy.

SENSORY FUSION

The systems of saccades, pursuits, fixation, accommodation, and vergences are principally motoric from a clinical perspective. However, there must be sensory (and usually perceptual and often cognitive) input so visual functioning can occur. Clinical testing of sensory fusion also involves a motoric component. Nevertheless, for instructional purposes it is convenient to deal with motor fusion and sensory fusion as though they were separate keeping in mind that this distinction is artificial and that they are really indissoluble.

On a clinical basis, motor fusion can be considered as basically involving the amplitude and speed of various ranges of vergences. On the other hand, the basic clinical concern in sensory fusion is with the question of suppression. Sensory fusion is classified according to the Worth taxonomy into three categories: first-, second-, and third-degree fusion. (Refer to Chapter 1 for theoretical discussions of these degrees of sensory fusion.)

In clinical diagnosis there are four levels regarding sensorial fusion of form. This classification is a modification of the categories of fusion recommended by Worth.[47] They are as follows:

Simultaneous Perception (diplopia)

Superimposition (first-degree fusion)

Flat Fusion (second-degree fusion)

Stereopsis (third-degree fusion)

These categories of binocular sensorial status can be conveniently tested by using vectographic, colored filters, and the numerous stereoscopic methods employing septum arrangements. (Many various methods and instruments are presented in this book, particularly in case examples.)

Simultaneous Perception

Although simultaneous perception is classified as one of the levels of sensory fusion, there is actually no real fusion with this particular binocular demand. Simultaneous perception is determined to be present merely by the patient's awareness of binocular images at the same time. In clinical usage, simultaneous percep-

tion refers to the stimulation of noncorresponding retinal points which give rise to diplopia. An example is shown in Figure 1-10 where the fixated light is seen diplopically because the dioptric image is on a noncorresponding point of the deviated right eye.

The usual test applied in determining if a patient can appreciate simultaneous perception is to elicit a diplopic response when one object (e.g., penlight) is fixated. When deep suppression interferes with diplopia testing, it may be desirable to stimulate a noncorresponding point somewhere outside of the suppression zone. This is conveniently done by placing a vertically oriented loose prism before the deviating eye to elicit a diplopic response. If a sufficiently large base-down prism is placed before the right eye, the dioptric image of the light is located below the suppression zone (inferior retina) and will be perceived (in the visual field) above the fixated one. When suppression is very deep, this technique is useful in determining the horizontal subjective angle of deviation.

Simultaneous perception testing may be carried out by using two objects rather than one. These targets are usually stereograms designed for use in a stereoscope. A familiar example is the Keystone Test 1 (DB-10A). A picture of a pig is seen only by the left eye, a dog by the right eye. If the suppression zone is very large and encompasses one picture, one of the animals will appear to be missing.

Superimposition

The superimposition of two dissimilar targets is known as first-degree fusion. However, when this occurs, confusion rather than true sensory fusion exists because similar targets are not being integrated; they merely have common oculocentric directions. Since two dissimilar objects stimulate corresponding retinal points and are perceived as superimposed, the definition of superimposition is satisfied.

With the exception of the Maddox rod test, superimposition testing usually requires more instrumentation than a penlight in free space. Stereoscopes containing a different target for each eye (e.g., a fish seen only by the left eye

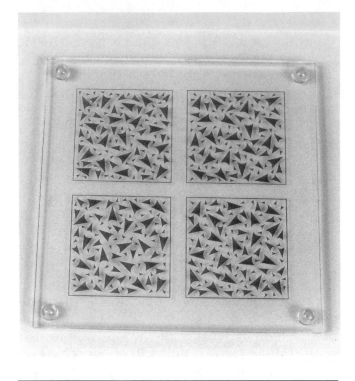

Figure 2-21—Frisby test. Random patterns are printed on each side of a transparent plate. The patient is to locate in which of four squares is the stereoscopically perceived circular target.

and a tank seen by the right eye) are usually necessary (see Figure 5-6).

Flat Fusion

This is true sensory fusion and is the integration of two similar ocular images into a single percept. There may be one target in free space, such as a page of print, or there may be two identical targets in a stereoscope. In any event, this type of target must be two-dimensional and identical in form for each eye to be classified as a flat fusion stimulus.

Such targets are the most frequently employed in testing and evaluating motor fusion (fusional divergence and convergence). Usually Snellen letters or printed words are used as targets to be fused with the incorporation of unfused suppression clues in the test-design. An example of a flat fusion target with a test-design for extrafoveal suppression is shown in Figure 5-7. If the angular separation from the center of the target to a suppression clue is greater than 5 degrees, testing for peripheral

suppression is being done. Testing for foveal suppression requires a suppression clue to be located in or near the center of the target. Therefore, the location of the clues that are suppressed determines the size of the suppression. These specifications regarding targets for determination of suppression size are listed in Table 5-1 (Chapter 5). In cases of heterophoria, however, foveal suppression is usually the concern, rather than larger suppression zones occurring in strabismus. Similarly, depth of suppression is necessarily evaluated in cases of strabismus but not too often in heterophoria. (Testing for depth of suppression is discussed in Chapter 5.)

Stereopsis

Stereopsis is the perception of three-dimensional visual space due to binocular disparity clues. These test targets are similar to those of flat fusion with one exception; there is lateral displacement in certain portions of the target. The displacement of a set of paired points (referred to as homologous points) is relative to the position of other pairs of homologous points on the stereogram. For example, in Figure 1-11 consider the star as the figure that is fixated and fused. The small vertical lines are displaced inwardly (base-out, or crossed disparity effect) relative to the fused star. Assume the patient is concentrating on the fused star. The vertical lines are imaged on each retina temporally in relation to the star. This causes the fused image of the lines to appear closer than the star. The opposite would be if the lines were disparately nasalward on each retina. The rule to remember is that if the retinal disparity is temporalward from the center of each fovea, the stereoscopic image will appear closer; if the retinal disparity is nasalward, it will appear farther. If the disparities become too far apart, the lines can no longer be fused (by remaining within Panum's areas) and are seen diplopically. They fall on points too disparate and cause diplopia in the same manner as in simultaneous perception testing. However, if the disparities are not too great, the targets are fusible even though they do not fall exactly on corresponding retinal points. This is due to the allowance in disparity afforded by Panum's area. It is this small fused disparity that is responsible for stereopsis. As in flat fusion testing, there are suppression clues in stereopsis testing, and these are those portions of the stereogram that are supposed to be seen in depth, relative to a fixated point. In the above example, the clues are the fused lines. The lack of depth may be an indication of suppression.

Vectographic Methods

Applying the principle of polarization to the testing of vision allows the use of suppression clues during fairly natural conditions of binocular viewing. For such testing, the patient wears polarizing filters in the form of spectacles. The polarizing filter for one eye must be rotated to an angle 90 degrees from the filter for the other eye. This achieves mutual exclusion of light coming to each eye. Thus, when the test targets are also polarized, one eye cannot see certain portions of the test target that are visible to the other eye. In the United States the filters in commercially available polarizing spectacles are usually oriented at 45 and 135 degrees; those manufactured in some other countries are often set at 90 and 180 degrees.

Several frequently used vectographic tests for stereoacuity are listed in Table 2-26. There are other nonvectographic tests (e.g., Frisby, Lang) that are illustrated in Figures 2-21 and 2-22.

Stereoacuity may also be evaluated by comparing the relative distance of two objects in free space, such as in the traditional Howard-Dolman peg test. This is designed for farpoint measurements. The test consists of two black movable vertical rods viewed through an aperture against a white background. The patient is seated at a distance of six meters from the rods and instructed not to move his head. Otherwise, lateral parallax will be induced, thereby invalidating testing procedures. The rods are moved by the patient, either nearer or farther from each other, by means of strings until they appear to be equally distant; i.e., in the same plane. The distance error is determined from an average of several trials. This is converted from millimeters into seconds of arc and represents

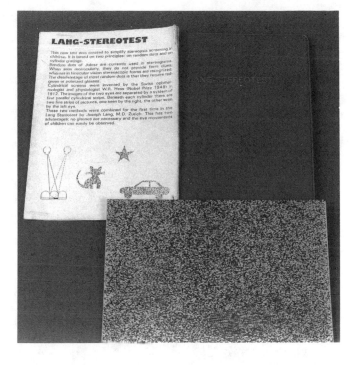

Figure 2-22—Lang test. Images for the eyes are separated by fine parallel cylindrical strips to create perception of stereopsis.

TABLE 2-26. *Frequently Used Vectographic Tests of Stereoacuity*

Contoured (local stereopsis)
    Stereo Tests (Fly) (nearpoint testing)
    Stereo Reindeer Test (nearpoint testing)
    Vectographic Slide (farpoint testing)
Non-Contoured (global stereopsis)
    Randot Stereotest (nearpoint testing)
    Random Dot E Stereotest (near to far testing)

---

the stereoacuity (Table 2-27). For example, if the error (the distance the patient misaligns the two pegs) is 60 mm, the stereoacuity is 20 seconds of arc. Because there may be a constant error due to a skewed or tilted horopter, however, testing results may be invalid. The *standard deviation* of the mean would represent a truer index of stereoacuity. This would take about 15 trials and is the reason this is seldom done on a routine clinical basis. An apparatus of the Howard-Dolman type may be custommade or obtained through commercial sources.

TABLE 2-27. *Howard-Dolman Test for Stereopsis. Performed at 6 Meters. Assume IPD of 60 mm.*

Alignment error (mm)	Stereoacuity
5	2
10	3
20	7
30	10
40	13
50	16
60	20
80	26
100	33
200	66
300	99
400	132
500	165

Stereoacuities were determined by the following formula:
Eta = IPD (x)/d^2 x 206,000.
Eta: symbol for stereoacuity in seconds of arc
IPD: interpupillary distance in mm
x: alignment error in mm
d: testing distance from patient to rods in mm

TABLE 2-28. *Approximate Corresponding Values for Stereoacuity in Seconds of Arc and Shepard Percentages*

Seconds of arc	Shepard percentage
1000	4
400	16
200	31
100	51
50	72
40	78
20	95
15	100
10	106

Shepard percentages are calculated using the following
formula of Fry: percent stereopsis $= \dfrac{10100}{eta + 81} - 5$

Percentage of Stereopsis

Occasionally practitioners are asked to report percentage values of stereopsis for patients rather than values recorded in seconds of arc. Percentage scales were empirically determined by Dr. Carl F. Shepard for such purposes. Calculations and information pertaining to this method were presented by Fry.[48] Table 2-28 gives percentage values corresponding to stereoacuity in seconds of arc.

Screening for Binocular Problems with Stereopsis

The level of stereopsis determines the level of binocular status in most cases. Stereopsis is the "barometer" of binocularity. If stereopsis is good, the binocular status is good. But the opposite cannot always be said with certainty. That is, a patient may be found to have no stereopsis but have normal sensory and motor fusion in all other respects. Some individuals may lack cortical binocular disparity cells. Hine[49] cited a study of Richards[50] that reported that 30% of subjects showed inabilities to detect disparity, comparing crossed and uncrossed disparity processing. It was implied that such stereoanomalies are genetic in origin. If lack of both types of disparity detectors (i.e., crossed and uncrossed) is inherited, an individual may lack normal binocular vision and be at risk for strabismus. Hine stated, "It is important in developing and improving motor fusion ranges." This is particularly so in small-angle strabismics, who can develop good fusional amplitudes but yet may have a poor prognosis for developing bifixation (with central, fine stereopsis).

In light of this discussion, one may wonder why random dot stereo tests, even gross ones, apparently seem to be effective in detecting sensory binocular anomalies of suppression, anomalous correspondence, and amblyopia. Conversely, the stereo tests with contoured patterns must be within relatively sensitive criteria to be effective in this regard. The difference in criteria between the two types of stereopsis tests may have something to do with "local" versus "global" stereopsis. Cline et al.[13] defined *local*

STEREOACUITY AND LEVEL OF INDUCED ANISOMETROPIA

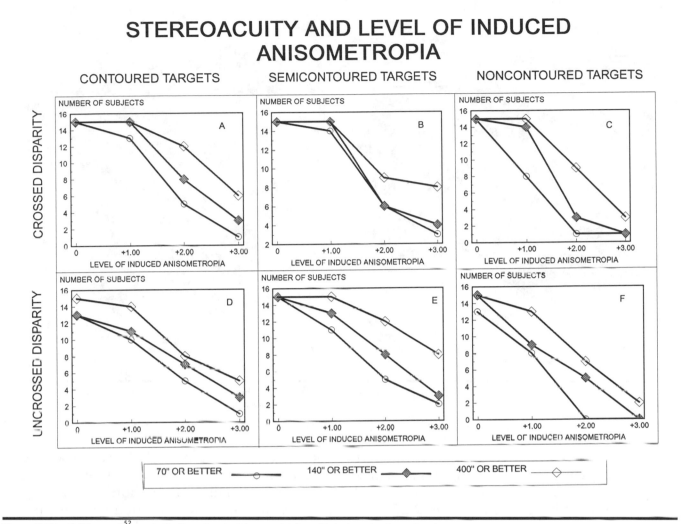

Figure 2-23—Griffin et al.[52] study finding decreased stereoacuity with induced anisometropia.

stereopsis as a "very simple disparity stimulus pattern such as, for example, a stereogram with two parallel vertical line segments seen by each eye with slightly differing lateral separations." On the other hand, they defined *global stereopsis* as that "elicited by the disparity of portions and/or clusters within relatively large stereogram patterns, involving complex textured surfaces and repetitive elements for which many disparately paired details might provide ambiguous or even conflicting stereopsis clues without destroying the overlying percept of depth, believed by Julesz to represent a perceptual interpretation process differentiable from local stereopsis."

Hamsher[51] confirmed the hypothesis that "the right hemisphere is dominant for global stereopsis but not local stereopsis. The additional mechanism(s) needed to achieve global stereopsis, while working with stereoscopic mechanisms, may not be of a strictly stereoscopic but of a more general visuoperceptive nature, perhaps those involved in utilizing subtle cues to achieve form recognition."

There may be two different types of stereopsis, global requiring more "visual perception" than local. It may be that people with poor binocularity have a lack of development in this regard. This could be the reason they do relatively poorly on random dot types of stereo tests. A study by Griffin et al.[52] corroborates this concept by showing that induced optical anisometropia degrades global stereopsis more rapidly than local stereopsis (Figure 2-23).

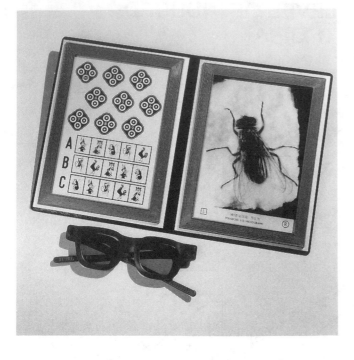

Figure 2-24—The "Fly" stereopsis test, contoured targets. (Courtesy Stereo Optical Co.)

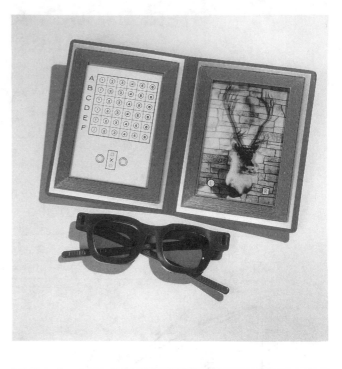

Figure 2-25—The "Reindeer" stereopsis test, contoured targets. (Courtesy Stereo Optical Co.)

Examples of stereopsis tests that are contoured (local stereopsis) are shown in Figures 2-24 and 2-25; examples of noncontoured (global stereopsis) are shown in Figures 2-26 and 2-27.

Norms for Stereoacuity

Rankings of stereoacuity scores are clinically practical for possible referrals and for assessment of stereopsis before and after vision therapy. These are listed in Table 2-29 for contoured (local) and noncontoured (global) stereopsis. Note that leniency is given for global stereopsis. These rankings apply to patients 7 years and older. Professional judgment is required when evaluating test results of children under 7 years of age.

Summary of Sensory Fusion Testing

In cases of heterophoria, flat fusion testing is done for purposes of measuring binocular accommodative facility, relative vergence ranges, and testing for fixation disparity. Stereopsis is generally an index to binocular status, although some patients are stereoblind even though other visual skills may be normal. Ranking of stereoacuity may be done in a manner similar to ranking of other visual skills.

Recommendations from Results of Testing

Referral for vision therapy is appropriate if there are symptoms of discomfort and performance problems that are related to poor visual skills, including saccades, pursuits, fixation, vergences, and sensory fusion. Referrals should take into account these considerations and not be made just because a finding (or even several) is below average. Professional judgment is called for whenever referral decisions are being made. Isolated abnormal findings may be spurious. A general pattern of binocular dysfunction provides the strongest basis for making a diagnostic statement. For example, suppose a patient is found to have asthenopic symptoms when reading, exophoria of 14^Δ, insufficient positive relative convergence, and

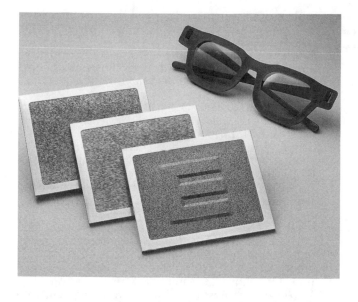

Figure 2-26—Random Dot E stereopsis test, noncontoured targets. (Courtesy Stereo Optical Co.)

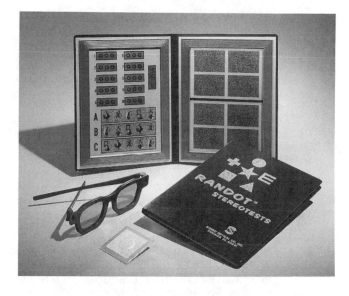

Figure 2-27—Randot stereopsis test, noncontoured and semi-contoured targets. (Courtesy Stereo Optical Co.)

vergence infacility. The doctor can be reasonably confident that there is fusional vergence dysfunction. It is important to have guidelines, however, as to what is normal and what is abnormal for each and every function. It would be ludicrous for internists who are checking cholesterol levels not to know what is considered normal. Similarly, we have given these visual skills norms as tentative guidelines for eye care practitioners to consider. We believe they are reliable and practical for clinical use. Rankings define in common terms what is strong or weak so that each visual skill function can be assessed and documented before and after vision therapy.

Referral to other professionals is indicated if the patient's complaints are not fully abated, even though there was successful completion of the vision therapy program. Therapy for vision efficiency skills is covered in Chapter 16. For example, if the patient has an attention deficit or hyperactive disorder, medical referral may be indicated. If a child, for example, has "Streff syndrome"[53,54] and continues to have psychological problems even after vision dysfunctions are abated, appropriate referral to a mental health professional is indicated. Similarly, if a patient is found to be dyslexic,[55-58] referral for educational therapy is necessary.

TABLE 2-29. *Ranking of Results of Stereopsis Testing (seconds of arc).*

Rank	Description	Contoured	Noncontoured
5	Very strong	Better than 20	Better than 30
4	Strong	20 to 30	31 to 50
3	Adequate	31 to 60	51 to 100
2	Weak	61 to 100	101 to 600
1	Very weak	Worse than 100	Worse than 600

REFERENCES

1. Revell MJ. *Strabismus: A History of Orthoptic Techniques.* London: Barrie and Jenkins, 1971.21-22.
2. Moses RA. *Adler's Physiology of the Eye,* 7th ed. St. Louis: CV Mosby; 1981:137.
3. Gay AJ, Newman NM, Keltner JL, Stroud MH. *Eye Movement Disorders.* St. Louis: C. Mosby; 1974:2-8.
4. Solomons H. *Binocular Vision: A Programmed Text.* London: William Heinemann Medical Books; 1978:151.
5. Hoffman LG, Rouse M. Referral recommendations for binocular function and/or developmental perceptual deficiencies. *J Am Optom Assoc.* 1980;51:119-125.
6. Heinson A, Schrock R. Personal communication, 1981.
7. Griffin DC, Walton HN, Ives V. Saccades as related to reading disorders. *J Learning Disabilities.* 1974;7:52-58.

8. Pierce J. Information available from Dr. John R. Pierce. Birmingham, Ala: University of Alabama, School of Optometry.

9. King AJ, Devick S. The Proposed King-Devick Saccade Test and its relation to the Pierce Saccade Test and reading levels. (Senior Research Study) Chicago: College of Optometry, 1976.

10. Cohen A, Lieberman S. Report in Manual of the NYSOA-KD Saccade Test. South Bend, Ind: Bernell Corp; 1993.

11. Garzia RP, Richman JE, Nicholson SB, Gaines CS. A new visual-verbal saccade test: the Developmental Eye Movement Test (DEM). *J Am Optom Assoc.* 1990;61:124-135.

12. Griffin.JR. Visual skills: ranking scores of clinical findings. *Optom Monthly.* 1984;75:451-454.

13. Cline D, Hofstetter H, Griffin J. *Dictionary of Visual Science,* 4th ed. Radnor, Penn: Chilton; 1989.

14. Michaels DD. *Visual Optics and Refraction: A Clinical Approach.* St. Louis: CV Mosby; 1980:417.

15. Gay AJ, Newman NM, Keltner JL, and Stroud MH. *Eye Movement Disorders,* St. Louis: CV Mosby; 1974:50-54.

16. Chrousos GA, O'Neill JF, Lueth BD, Parks MM. Accommodation Deficiency in Healthy Young Individuals. *J Ped Ophthalmol Strabismus.* 1988;25:176-178.

17. Daum KM. Accommodative Insufficiency. *Amer J Optom Physiol Opt.* 1983;60:352-359.

18. Borish IM. *Clinical Refraction,* 3rd ed. Chicago: Professional Press; 1975:169-170.

19. Day R, Miller S, Wilson R. eds. *Current Optometric Information and Terminology,* 3rd ed. St. Louis: American Optometric Association; 1980:1-2.

20. Nott IS. Dynamic skiametry: Accommodation and convergence. *Am J Physiol Opt.* 1925;6:490-503.

21. Haynes HM. Clinical observations with dynamic retinoscopy. *Optom Weekly.* 1960;51:2306-2309.

22. Tucker J, Charman WN. Reaction and response times for accommodation. *Am J Optom.* 1979;56:490-503.

23. Bieber JC. Why nearpoint retinoscopy with children? *Optom Weekly.* 1974;65:54-57.

24. Liu JS, Lee M, Jany J, Ciuffreda KJ, Wong JH, Grisham D, Stark L. Objective assessment of accommodation. Orthoptics, I: dynamic insufficiency. *Am J Optom Physiol Opt.* 1979;56:285-94.

25. Griffin JR, Britz D, Zundell M. A study of variables influencing the facility of accommodation. Ketchum Library, Southern California College of Optometry, Fullerton, 1972.

26. Griffin JR, Clausen D, Graham G. A new apparatus for accommodative rock. Ketchum Library, Southern California College of Optometry, Fullerton, 1977.

27. Burge S. Suppression during binocular accommodative rock. *Optom Monthly.* 1979;79:867-872.

28. Grisham JD. Treatment of binocular dysfunctions. In: *Vergence Eye Movements.* Schor CM, Ciuffreda KJ, eds. Boston: Butterworth-Heinemann; 1983:607-623.

29. Pope RS, Wong JD, Mah M. Accommodative facility testing in children: norms and validation. OD thesis. Berkeley, Calif: School of Optometry, University of California; 1981.

30. Alpert T, Zellers J. A normative study of accommodative facility. Ketchum Library, Southern California College of Optometry, Fullerton, 1980.

31. Schlange D, Kostelnik K, Paterson D. Accommodative facility: a normative study. Chicago: College of Optometry, 1979.

32. Rouse MW, Ryan JM. The optometric examination and management of children. In: Rosenbloom AA, Morgan MW, eds. *Pediatric Optometry.* Philadelphia: Lippincott; 1990:180.

33. Duke-Elder S, Abrams D. System of Ophthalmology, vol. 5. *Ophthalmic Optics and Refraction.* London: Henry Kimpton, 1970:463.

34. Griffin JR. Vision Efficiency Therapy Course #637A, Laboratory Syllabus. Fullerton, Calif: Southern California College of Optometry; 1995.

35. Wick B. Vision therapy for preschool children. In: Rosenbloom AA, Morgan MW, eds. *Pediatric Optometry.* Philadelphia: Lippincott; 1990:283.

36. Schor C. Visuomotor development. In: Rosenbloom AA, Morgan MW, eds. *Pediatric Optometry.* Philadelphia: Lippincott; 1990:83-85.

37. Schor CM. Fixation disparity and vergence adaptation. In: Schor CM, Ciuffreda KJ, eds. *Vergence Eye Movements.* Boston: Butterworth-Heinemann; 1983:485.

38. Grisham JD. The dynamics of fusional vergence eye movements in binocular dysfunction. *Am J Optom Physiol Opt.* 1980;57:645-655.

39. Kenyon RV, Ciuffreda KJ, Stark L. Dynamic vergence eye movements in strabismus and amblyopia: symmetric vergence. *Investigative Ophthalmol.* 1980;19:60-74.

40. Pierce JR. Lecture. Minneapolis, Minn: Northern Central States Optometric Conference; 1973.

41. Stuckle LG, Rouse M. Norms for Dynamic Vergences. Ketchum Library, Southern California College of Optometry, Fullerton, 1979.

42. Mitchell R, Stanich R, and Rouse M. Norms for Dynamic Vergences. Ketchum Library, Southern California College of Optometry, Fullerton, 1980.

43. Moser JE, Atkinson WF. Vergence Facility in a Young Adult Population. Ketchum Library, Southern California College of Optometry, Fullerton, 1980.

44. Rosner J. Lecture notes: course no. 548. Houston: University of Houston, College of Optometry; Spring 1979.

45. Jacobson M, Goldstein A, Griffin JR. The Relationship between Vergence Range and Vergence Facility.Ketchum Library, Southern California College of Optometry, Fullerton, 1979.

46. Delgadillo H, Griffin JR. Vergence facility and associated symptoms: a comparison of two prism flipper tests. *J Behavioral Optom.* 1992;3:91-94.

47. Worth C. Cited by Revell MJ. *Strabismus.* London: Barrie and Jenkins, 1971:32.

48. Fry G. Measurement of the threshold of stereopsis. *Optom Weekly.* 1942;33:1032.

49. Hine NA. Random-Dot stereogram: Survey of the clinical uses and reliability. *Aust J Optom.* 1980;63:123-129.

50. Richards W. Stereopsis and stereoblindness. *Exp Brain Res.* 1970;10:380-388.

51. Hamsher K deS. Stereopsis and unilateral brain disease. *Investigative Ophthalmol Vis Sci.* 1978;17:336-343.

52. Griffin JR, Super S, Lee RA, DeLand PN. Study conducted at the Southern California College of Op-

tometry. Presented at annual meeting American Academy of Optometry. Orlando, Fla: 1992.

53. Streff JW. Preliminary observations on a nonmalingering syndrome. *Optom Weekly.* 1962; 53:536-537.

54. Gilman GD. A case in point: optometric or psychological problem? *J Am Optom Assoc.* 1981; 52:609-610.

55. Christenson GN, Griffin JR, Wesson MD. Optometry's role in reading disabilities: resolving the controversy. *J Am Optom Assoc.* 1990;61:363-372.

56. Cardinal DN, Christenson GN, Griffin JR. Neurological-behavioral model of dyslexia. *J Behav Optom.* 1992;3:35-39.

57. Griffin JR. Office testing for dyslexia. *Current Opinion in Ophthalmol.* 1992;3:35-39.

58. Guerin DW, Griffin JR, Gottfried AW, Christenson GN. Concurrent validity and screening efficiency of the dyslexia screener. *Psychol Assessment.* 1993;5: 369-373.

Chapter 3 / Heterophoria Case Analysis

Tonic Convergence and AC/A   64
   Calculated AC/A   65
   Gradient AC/A   65
Zone of Clear Single Binocular
   Vision   67
Morgan's Normative Analysis   70
Criteria for Lens and
   Prism Prescription   71
   Morgan   71
   Clinical Wisdom   72
   Sheard   72
   Percival   73
Fixation Disparity Analysis   73
   Definition and Features   73
   Measurement   75

Prescribing Prism   81
Validity of Diagnostic Criteria   81
Recommendations for Prism
   Prescription   86
Vergence Anomalies   87
Convergence Insufficiency   88
   Basic Exophoria   89
   Divergence Excess   89
   Divergence Insufficiency   90
   Basic Esophoria   90
   Convergence Excess   91
   Basic Orthophoria with
     Restricted Zone   91
   Normal Zone with Symptoms   92
Bioengineering Model   92

Most clinical systems used in the analysis of vergence disorders are conceptually based on the interaction of the four Maddox components of vergence: tonic, accommodative, fusional and proximal. Graphical analysis, with roots extending from Donders[1] and Maddox[2] in the nineteenth century, uses a Cartesian coordinate system to illustrate relations between accommodation and vergence. To this day, clinicians may find it helpful to draw a graph of phorometry measurements (i.e., heterophoria, relative vergence, and relative accommodation) to visualize better the interactions. A graph can readily reveal various clinical syndromes and alert the clinician to inconsistencies in the data. The analysis implies relation between accommodative response and vergence eye position, in which changes in accommodation affect vergence and, conversely, changes in vergence affect accommodation.

By convention, the graph is plotted with accommodative stimulus, in diopters, on the ordinate (Y axis) and vergence stimulus, in prism diopters on the abscissa (X axis). A diagonal line (Donders' line) is drawn representing convergence for all points in space along the midsagittal plane with no prism or lens addition. This is also called the *demand line* (Figure 3-1). The exact positioning of the demand line on the graph is influenced by the interpupillary distance of the patient, but for standard diagrammatic purposes, the graph is traditionally scaled for an interpupillary distance (IPD) of 60 mm. In cases of a large IPD (e.g., 70 mm), the convergence demand for

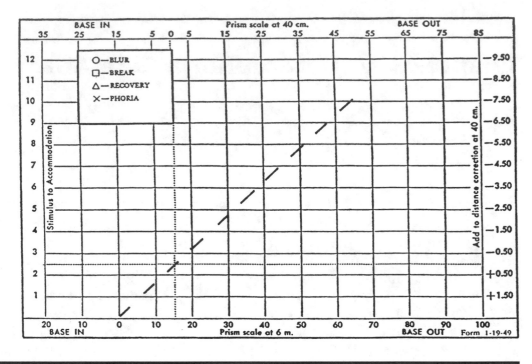

Figure 3-1—Graphical illustration of the demand line, shown as dashed.

binocular eye alignment becomes greater with increasing accommodative stimuli for near-point targets. Conversely, the convergence demand is less for a small IPD (e.g., 50 mm). For fixation distances beyond 20 cm, however, the error is small and can be ignored for clinical purposes.

TONIC CONVERGENCE AND AC/A

Tonic vergence position of the eyes is indicated by the farpoint heterophoria measurement. The alternate cover test at far (6 meters) with the corrected ametropia most plus (CAMP) lenses is the standard method of establishing this position. Unless otherwise specified, this rule of testing with CAMP lenses in place applies to all testing procedures involved in the investigation of binocular anomalies.

In some cases of excessive heterophoria or intermittent strabismus, prolonged occlusion of an eye is necessary to reveal the full magnitude of the tonic deviation. This is because the effects of fusional vergence responses do not always immediately decrease by momentarily covering one eye.

Measurement of the farpoint heterophoria position through a phoropter can introduce other sources of error through psychic and accommodative vergence effects. Nevertheless, phorometry measurements of heterophoria are usually valuable since these data are compared with other clinical data taken under similar testing conditions.

Nearpoint heterophoria is conventionally measured at 40 cm in the primary position. This is measured with either the alternate cover test (objectively) or by phorometry (subjectively). During testing it is extremely important to control the influence of accommodation. The patient should be instructed to fixate a detailed nearpoint target requiring precise focus while being reminded to keep the target perfectly clear. With small children, precise focus can be ensured by asking them to identify a small letter or figure as the measurement is taken. Proper dissociation of the eyes and relaxation of fusional vergence are necessary to measure the angle of deviation at near. When fusional vergence is completely inhibited, the near heterophoria measurement represents a combination of tonic vergence and accommodative convergence being stimulated at the near testing distance. There may also be psychic vergence effects that are stimulated by testing at a near distance, but these are usually small and essentially ignored during routine clinical evaluation.

The relation between accommodative-convergence and accommodation is referred to as the "ACA ratio," or more properly, the AC/A. The ratio means that for every diopter of accommodative response, a certain amount of accommodative-convergence (depending on the value of the AC/A) is brought into play. For instance, if the AC/A is 6^Δ per 1.00 diopter of accommodation, a patient who accommodates 2.50 diopters will have an increased convergence of the visual axes of 15^Δ.

Calculated AC/A

There are several ways to calculate the AC/A from far and near deviations. The general formula is

$$AC/A = IPD +[(Hn-Hf)/(An-Af)]$$

Where

IPD = Interpupillary distance in centimeters
An = Accommodative demand at near in diopters
Af = Accommodative demand at far in diopters
Hn = Objective angle of deviation at near (Δ)
Hf = Objective angle of deviation at far (Δ)
Note: ESO deviations have positive (+) values
EXO deviations have negative (−) values

This formula assumes that the CAMP lenses are in place and the AC/A is linear. Any two viewing distances can be used but they are customarily 6 m and 40 cm. Flom[3] offered a clinically useful form of this general formula. AC/A = IPD + M (Hn−Hf), where M is the fixation distance at near in meters. In this case, the fixation distance must be at 6 m, or farther. For example, assume that a patient with a 60 mm interpupillary distance has 15^Δ of exophoria at far and is orthophoric at the near fixation distance of 40 cm. The AC/A would be $12^\Delta/1D$. It is calculated as follows:

$$AC/A = 6 + .4 [0- (-15)]$$
$$= 6 + .4 (15)$$
$$= 12 (i.e., 12^\Delta/1D)$$

An AC/A of this magnitude is considered very high. The normal calculated AC/A range is from 4/1 to 7/1. An AC/A greater than 7/1 is high; less than 4/1 is low. If another patient has 15^Δ exophoria at near as well as at far, the AC/A is 6/1. Note that the size of the IPD directly affects the magnitude of the calculated AC/A; the larger the IPD the larger is the AC/A.

Table 3-1 gives the calculated answers for various angles of deviations at far and near. By looking at this table, two useful rules become readily apparent. First, the AC/A is equal to the patient's interpupillary distance when the deviations at far and near are the same. For instance, ortho (0) on both scales for angle H intersects at 6/1. The AC/A is 6/1 on the chart wherever the angles of deviation are equal. Also, a zero AC/A is very improbable, and a negative one is probably impossible. The table indicates those spurious combinations that could produce either a zero or negative AC/A. If these questionable combinations occur, the measured magnitudes of deviation for far and near should be rechecked. For example, if the patient has an IPD of 60 mm and a measurement of ortho at far and 15^Δ exo at near, the combination indicates an AC/A of zero, which suggests an error in clinical testing. However, this deviation of ortho at far and 15^Δ exo at near is possible if the IPD is larger. If, for instance, the IPD is 70 mm, instead of 60 mm, the AC/A would be 1/1, which is possible.

Gradient AC/A

The magnitude of the AC/A may also be arrived at by measuring the effect of spherical lenses on vergence. At far, minus lenses are used for this purpose; at near, either plus or minus lenses will give the value. Regardless of the testing distance, the AC/A should be determined with the patient wearing CAMP lenses.

The following is an example of how the gradient method may be used. The patient has exophoria of 15^Δ at far, determined by objective means such as the cover test or possibly by

TABLE 3–1. *Calculated AC/A Depending on Far and Near Magnitudes of the Angle of Deviation for an Interpupillary Distance of 60 Millimeters.*

		Angle H at Far														
		EXO								ESO							
		35	30	25	20	15	10	5	0	5	10	15	20	25	30	35
ANGLE H AT NEAR	EXO — 35	34	32	30	28	26	24	22	20	18	16	14	12	10	8	6
	30	32	30	28	26	24	22	20	18	16	14	12	10	8	6	4
	25	30	28	26	24	22	20	18	16	14	12	10	8	6	4	2
	20	28	26	24	22	20	18	16	14	12	10	8	6	4	2	0
	15	26	24	22	20	18	16	14	12	10	8	6	4	2	0	
	10	24	22	20	18	16	14	12	10	8	6	4	2	0		
	5	22	20	18	16	14	12	10	8	6	4	2	0			
	0	20	18	16	14	12	10	8	6	4	2	0				
	ESO — 5	18	16	14	12	10	8	6	4	2	0					
	10	16	14	12	10	8	6	4	2	0						
	15	14	12	10	8	6	4	2	0							
	20	12	10	8	6	4	2	0								
	25	10	8	6	4	2	0									
	30	8	6	4	2	0										
	35	6	4	2	0											

Key: H is the objective horizontal angle of deviation of the visual axes.
     EXO is either exophoria or exotropia.
     ESO is either esophoria or esotropia.

subjective diplopia testing, e.g., Maddox rod. A spherical lens of –2.00 D is placed before each eye. The patient is instructed to focus and clear the fixation target while looking through the lenses. When the patient reports that the target is clear, another measurement of the angle of deviation is made. If the lenses cause the angle to change, for example, from 15^Δ exo to 5^Δ exo, the gradient AC/A is 5/1. This is determined by dividing the change in the deviation by the change of accommodative stimulus (i.e., the power of the added lenses). Thus, 10 divided by 2.00 equals 5^Δ/1D.

Clinically, the gradient AC/A is most often determined at near by using a phoropter. The nearpoint heterophoria is measured subjectively by either the von Graefe method or Maddox rod. Spheres of +1.00 D are added and the heterophoria is remeasured. The magnitude change of the angle of deviation indicates the gradient. Greater precision is usually gained by using +1.00 D, then –1.00 D added lenses to evaluate the amount of deviation change. If there is a large depth of focus, then either +1.00 D or –1.00 D may be insufficient stimuli to elicit a sufficient accommodative response. In such cases, larger increments of lens power might be required.

Comparing the gradient with the near-far calculation method, the gradient method will usually give a lower AC/A. A gradient value of more than 5/1 is considered high. The depth of focus causes the reduced AC/A magnitude, particularly if low-powered lens additions are used. The calculation method usually yields a higher value, probably because proximal convergence is a factor when fixation is shifted from far to near. Both methods are useful, however. In general, the calculated AC/A is more reliable than the gradient method, but the gradient value

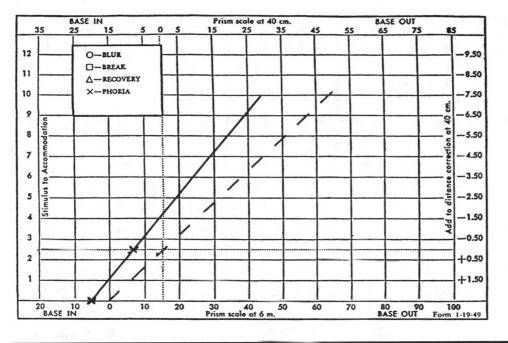

Figure 3-2—Phoria line, shown as a solid line. The X markings represent direct measurements of the phoria.

may be more useful for prognosis because it directly shows what direct effect added lenses have on the angle of deviation. Added lenses are often used in vision therapy to change the magnitude of deviation, in cases of both phoria and strabismus.

In graphical analysis, the far and near heterophoria measurements taken through a phoropter are plotted; a straight line is drawn to connect them. This is called the *phoria line*. The AC/A can be determined by direct inspection by noting the change in the deviation per unit change in accommodative stimulus. The *phoria line* is clinically useful since it predicts the magnitude of the heterophoria at various testing distances (Figure 3-2).

ZONE OF CLEAR SINGLE BINOCULAR VISION

The zone of clear single binocular vision (ZCSBV) is a graphical representation of the functional relations between accommodation and vergence. The ZCSBV is enclosed by the extremes of accommodation and vergence that can be elicited while maintaining clear, binocular fusion. The vertical limits of the zone are traditionally designated by the absolute amplitude of accommodation. (Monocular testing results are used because of well-established norms.) This is determined by the pushup amplitude of accommodation test. At each particular viewing distance, the horizontal limits of the zone represent the base-in and base-out blurpoints, usually measured with Risley prisms. Ideally, the divergence limit is measured before the convergence limit (at each viewing distance) to reduce the effect of prism adaptation. Relative vergence blurpoints are indicated by circles. They are plotted for at least two viewing distances, customarily at 6 m and 40 cm. At 40 cm they are designated by circles for NRC (negative relative convergence which is base in to blur), and PRC (positive relative convergence which is base-out to blur); at 6 m they are the base-in to break (designated by a square since blur should not normally occur) and the base-out to blur findings.

During prism vergence testing, it is customary to record the blur (and the break and recovery points) in a particular vergence direction, convergence or divergence, at each viewing distance. If there is no blurpoint reported by the patient, the breakpoint (diplopia) is charted; this is symbolized by a square. The

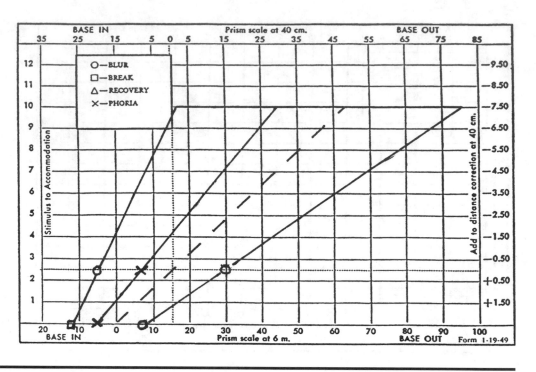

Figure 3-3—Zone of clear single binocular vision (ZCSBV). Vision is blurred outside the enclosure.

blurpoints of negative relative accommodation (NRA) and positive relative accommodation (PRA) are also designated by circles and are often added to the charting of the ZCSBV (not illustrated in Figure 3-3 but shown in Figure 3-5).

The zone of *single* binocular vision can also be plotted (Figure 3-4). This enclosure is formed by connecting the breakpoints. It is usually larger than the zone of clear single binocular vision. The area difference between these two zones represents the use of accommodative vergence to maintain a single image (at the expense of clarity). As base-out prisms are introduced, alignment of the eyes is maintained by fusional convergence. Similarly, the accommodative posture of the eyes is also stimulated through the convergence-accommodation/convergence (CA/C) reflex. A normal accommodative *lag* can often become a small *lead* of accommodation without the patient reporting accommodative blur due to the effect of an eye's depth of focus. At some point of increasing prism demand, however, fusional convergence is exhausted; the only way a patient can then maintain binocular alignment and fusion is to recruit accommodative

convergence. This results in excessive accommodation for the fixation distance. Target blur is then reported when the depth of focus is exceeded. As base-out prism induction is continued, a point is reached even where accommodative vergence is inadequate. Binocular fusion is then lost (i.e., the breakpoint) and diplopia is reported (see Figure 3-4).

There are a number of characteristics of the ZCSBV that can be useful in clinical interpretation. A plot of the zone allows the clinician to predict how a patient will respond to various prisms, lenses, and viewing distances. Some of the important attributes of charting a zone of clear single binocular vision are illustrated in Figure 3-3. These are as follows:

1. The ZCSBV approximates a parallelogram slanting toward the right due to the influence of the AC/A. The AC/A line serves as the axis of the zone. If there is a large deviation from a parallelogram, then spurious data points should be suspected and retesting is indicated.
2. The slope of the zone is influenced by the slope of the AC/A. The slope of the zone often deviates slightly from the

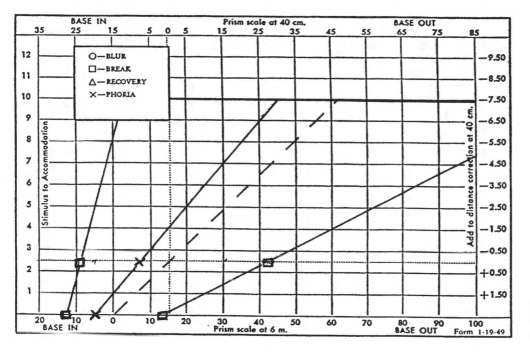

Figure 3-4—Zone of single binocular vision (ZSBV). Vision is diplopic outside the enclosure.

demand line. Large deviations, however, are probably associated with binocular anomalies (e.g., very steep slope indicating excessive esophoria at near).

3. The vertical limits of the zone represent the amplitude of accommodation. This can be judged as either sufficient or insufficient for the patient's age and work requirements.
4. The horizontal limit of the zone represents the ranges of fusional divergence and convergence. This can be judged as either sufficient or insufficient for the patient's work requirements.
5. The base-out blur limit of the zone is more steep (i.e., fans out) from the base-in to blur line and from the phoria line, primarily because of the influence of proximal (psychic) convergence for nearpoint targets, but also possibly because of convergence ("prism") adaptation with nearpoint "stress" during testing with base-out prism demands.
6. Normally, there is no blurpoint for fusional divergence at far. That limit is indicated by a break (diplopia) point. If a blurpoint is found, then the most

likely explanation is that the refractive error is not fully corrected with most plus for hyperopia or is over-corrected with minus in a case of myopia. This blurpoint usually indicates a spasm of accommodation.

The horizontal limits are the same as drawn previously in this example, but the limits of relative accommodation are added (Figure 3-5). (Refer to Chapter 2 for discussion of NRA and PRA.)

The clinically relevant features of the ZCSBV are often the relations between its constituent parts, i.e., the demand line, the phoria line, the range of fusional vergence, and the amplitude of relative accommodation. Custom dictates specific names for each of these features. Positive relative convergence (PRC) and negative relative convergence (NRC) are the ranges of fusional (disparity) vergence to the blurpoint that are measured relative to the *demand* line (see Figure 3-3). These are the values directly measured using the Risley prism vergence technique in both convergence and divergence directions. Another way to describe the horizontal extent of the ZCSBV is to refer to the vergence

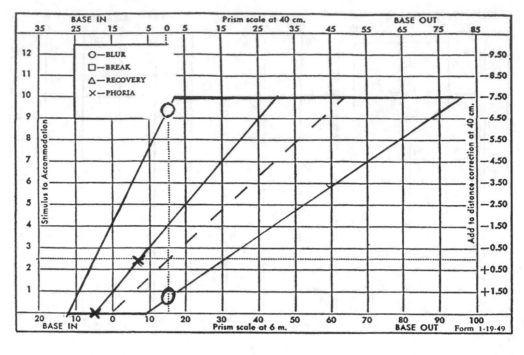

Figure 3-5—ZCSBV showing charting of the NRA (lower circle) and the PRA (upper circle).

ranges relative to the *phoria* line. Positive fusional convergence (PFC) is the amount of convergence measured between the phoria at any particular viewing distance to the base-out blurpoint (or break point if no blur point is found). Similarly, negative fusional convergence (NFC) is represented by the amplitude between the phoria line and the base-in to blur line (divergence blur limit).

Sheard[4] emphasized the relation between the phoria direction and the compensating fusional (disparity) vergence range. When discussing Sheard's concept, the term *reserve* vergence is used. It is the relation between the phoria position and the compensating vergence range that has clinical relevance according to Sheard.[4] The significance and utility of these relations will be discussed later in this chapter.

Gross convergence (NPC) is not usually charted, but may be calculated. A conversion formula (cm to Δ) for clinical use is:

$$\text{Gross convergence } (\Delta) = \text{IPDcm} \left(\frac{100}{\text{NPCcm} + 2.7} \right)$$

Note: 2.7 is a correction factor for the distance from the spectacle plane to the center of rotation of the eyes.

Example: If the IPD = 60 mm and the pushup NPC = 5 cm from the spectacle plane (bridge of the nose), then Δ = 6 x 100/5 + 2.7 = 78 prism diopters.

MORGAN'S NORMATIVE ANALYSIS

Morgan is a principal founder of binocular vision case analysis. He accumulated and analyzed clinical phorometry data on 800 nonpresbyopic adults, 20 to 40 years old.[5] Morgan established clinical norms for his patient group and suggested expected values for clinical evaluation (Table 3-2). He recommended using 1/2 of a standard deviation from the mean to represent clinically suspicious findings. (These expected values are factors in the vergence clinical ranking system recommended in Chapter 2.) Morgan also evaluated the pattern of clinical findings by determining correlation coefficients for various zone components.[6] His results are presented in Table 3-3. His important contribution demonstrated the quantitative strength of these relations. Other findings also deserve interpretation. For example, the corre-

TABLE 3–2. *Clinical Norms of Morgan*[5]

Test	Mean	1/2 SD	Acceptable Range
Phoria, far	1^Δ exo	±1	Ortho to 2^Δ exo
BO blur far	9^Δ	±2	7^Δ to 11^Δ
BO brk, far	19^Δ	±4	15^Δ to 23^Δ
BO rec, far	10^Δ	±2	8^Δ to 12^Δ
BI brk, far	7^Δ	±2	5^Δ to 9^Δ
BI rec, far	4^Δ	±1	3^Δ to 5^Δ
Phoria, near	3^Δ	±3	Ortho to 6^Δ exo
BO blur, near	17^Δ	±3	14^Δ to 20^Δ
BO brk, near	21^Δ	±3	18^Δ to 24^Δ
BO rec, near	11^Δ	±4	7^Δ to 15^Δ
BI blur, near	13^Δ	±2	11^Δ to 15^Δ
BI brk, near	21^Δ	±2	19^Δ to 23^Δ
BI rec, near	13^Δ	±3	10^Δ to 16^Δ
PRA	−2.37 D	±0.62	-1.75 D to −3.00 D
NRA	+2.00 D	±0.25	+1.75 D to +2.25 D

TABLE 3–3. *Morgan's Correlations between Selected Clinical Findings*

Functions	R
Age and Amplitude of Accommodation	− 0.80
PRA and Amplitude of Accommodation	+ 0.80
PRC blur and break	+ 0.70
NRC blur and break	+ 0.50
NRA and PRC	+ 0.50
PRA and NRC	+ 0.50
NRA and PRA	− 0.50

Key: PRA, Positive relative accommodation
      PRC, Base-out to blur at near
      NRC, Base-in to blur at near
      NRA, Negative relative accommodation

lation between PRC and NRA was +0.5, a moderate correlation. A direct association exists between these two features of the zone; the larger the PRC, the larger is the NRA. In many cases, accommodation can limit vergence; conversely, vergence can limit accommodation. This relation suggests the possibility of clinical syndromes as Morgan astutely pointed out.

Morgan demonstrated that certain features of the ZCSBV tend to be congregated. Morgan's group "A" findings are amplitude of accommodation, PRA, and NRC. Group "B" findings are NRA and PRC. (Morgan also proposed another classification, group "C," that includes the far and near phorias, the gradient AC/A, and the calculated AC/A.) When group A findings are low, group B findings tend to be high; Morgan refers to this case type as *accommodative fatigue*. The treatments of choice are often a plus add for reading or vision training that would better balance A and B findings. When group B data are low and group A high, then the case type is referred to as *convergence fatigue*. The recommended treatment would be either base-in prism to balance the two groups or fusional convergence (base-out) vision training.

CRITERIA FOR LENS AND PRISM PRESCRIPTION

Many people have contributed to graphical case analysis over the years; several researchers and clinicians have recommended various criteria for the prescription of prisms and adds to balance various elements within the ZCSBV. Unfortunately, little research has been done to check the validity or reliability of these criteria. Clinical popularity has waxed and waned over the years depending on the fashion of the time. The selection of one criterion over another is usually based on a particular clinician's training, experiences, and biases. Several criteria in use are reviewed.

Morgan

Morgan's expected ranges for near and distance heterophorias have been used as clinical values for the prescription of prism or added lens power. The idea is that if a patient has an excessive phoria falling outside the expected values, a prism or spherical lens additions are prescribed to compensate for the phoria. The lens or prism shifts the demand line relative to the phoria line so that the measured phoria then falls within expected limits as can be graphically shown.

This prism prescription criterion will be referred to as the *Morgan's Expected Criterion*. For example, if a patient suffers from eyestrain while reading and has an exophoria of 10^Δ at near, the spectacle prescription would be 4^Δ base-in to reduce the phoria to 6^Δ exo with respect to the new demand; this is a limiting expected value.

Clinical Wisdom

Another criterion based on the amount of the heterophoria is called the *Clinical Wisdom Criterion*. Its origin is obscure, but it seems to be passed on from one generation of clinicians to the next. The criterion varies with the direction of the deviation. If a patient has ocular symptoms and poor performance associated with an excessive exophoria, then clinical wisdom would recommend prescribing prism in the amount of 1/3 the angle of deviation to bring symptomatic relief. For example, if the exophoria measures 12^Δ by cover test, then 4^Δ BI would be prescribed. The prism amount would usually be split between the two lenses, i.e., 2^Δ BI each eye, to reduce weight and optical distortion. However, in the cases of esophoria and hyperphoria associated with signs and symptoms, clinical wisdom would recommend possibly neutralizing the entire angle of deviation with prisms or adds, if appropriate. For example, if 4^Δ esophoria and 2^Δ right hyperphoria were found by cover test in a symptomatic patient, the prism prescription may be: O.D. 2^Δ BO and 1^Δ BD; O.S. 2^Δ BO and 1^Δ BU.

Sheard

One of the oldest and most widely used clinical criteria for evaluating lateral phoria imbalance is *Sheard's criterion*. In 1929, Charles Sheard, a biophysicist at Ohio State University, suggested that the clinically significant relation in assessing vergence dysfunctions is the magnitude of heterophoria compared with the range of compensatory fusional vergence. He proposed that the compensating vergence "reserve" should be at least twice the demand (heterophoria) to be physiologically sufficient.[4] Therefore, the positive relative convergence (PRC) should be at least twice the magnitude of an exophoria and the negative relative convergence (NRC) should be at least twice the amount of an esophoria. Sheard's criterion proposes that if the reserve is less than this amount, a patient is likely to develop asthenopic symptoms with sustained visual activity (e.g., reading a book). If, indeed, a patient does report ocular symptoms and fails to meet Sheard's criterion, then compensating prisms (or a lens addition in some cases) may be considered. The goal is to prescribe sufficient relieving prism (or added lens) so the compensating relative vergence would be twice the demand. This can be done by either inspection of the graph or by calculation. The formula for calculating the Sheard's prism is: Sheard $\Delta = 2$ x Demand – Compensating Relative Vergence/3. That is, $\Delta = (2D-R)/3$.

Two examples are offered to demonstrate the use of Sheard's criterion. If a symptomatic patient has a nearpoint exophoria of 9^Δ and positive relative convergence ranges of 6/10/4 taken through the phoropter, then analysis would indicate that Sheard's criterion at nearpoint is not met. The demand is 9^Δ exophoria and the PRC (blurpoint) is 6^Δ. The reserve is much less than twice the demand. The PRC in this case should be 18^Δ BO to blur to satisfy Sheard's criterion. A prism can be prescribed to meet the theoretical criterion. Sheard's prism = $(2D^\Delta-R)/3$ or $[(2 \times 9)^\Delta-6]/3 = 12/3 = 4^\Delta$ base in. With 4^Δ BI in place, the measured phoria would be reduced from 9^Δ exo to 5^Δ exo and the reserve of 6^Δ would be increased to 10^Δ. This prism, therefore, satisfies Sheard's criterion, i.e., $2D = R$ or $2 \times 5 = 10$. In the spectacle prescription, the prism would be split, 2^Δ BI each eye. The patient may experience improved visual comfort and efficiency. There is evidence that Sheard's criterion is clinically effective, particularly in exophoric cases.[7] A better approach when feasible, in lieu of prism compensation, is to prescribe convergence vision training with the goal of building the PRC to at least 18^Δ base-out to blur; this would satisfy Sheard's criterion.

The second example is an esophoric patient, far and near, complaining of visually related headaches at the end of a workday. Phoropter findings indicate a far esophoria of 5^Δ with 3^Δ farpoint BI to break, and at near, esophoria of 7^Δ with an NRC of 5^Δ (to blur). Sheard's criteria are not met at either distance or near. The Sheard prism at far would be: $\Delta = (2D-R)/3 = [(10-3)/3] = 7/3 = 2.3^{\Delta}$ base-out. The Sheard prism for near would be: $\Delta = (14-5/3 = 3^{\Delta})$ base-out. One approach is to prescribe 3^{Δ} base out in single vision spectacles since this prism would satisfy Sheard's criterion at far and near. However, if the symptoms were related primarily to nearpoint work, another approach could be taken using plus added lenses. The Sheard's prism at near, 3^{Δ} BO, could be satisfied by prescribing a plus add for near, based on the gradient AC/A. If the gradient AC/A measured $4^{\Delta}/1D$ in this case, then a +0.75 D add would also balance the relationship between the demand and reserve to satisfy Sheard's criterion. [Sheard add = required Sheard prism/gradient AC/A ratio.] This add combined with the lens correction for any existing farpoint refractive error might be prescribed in single vision lenses for nearpoint, e.g., reading or computer work. A bifocal prescription could also achieve the desired results if appropriate for the work needs of the patient. Fusional divergence training should also be considered as either an alternate clinical approach in such cases, or combined with optical treatment.

Percival

Percival's criterion differs from the others in that it ignores the phoria position. Percival proposed that the clinically important relationship in the ZCSBV is the position of the *demand line* with respect to the limits of convergence and divergence blur lines.[8] He delineated a *zone of comfort* resting within the middle third of the ZCSBV, limited horizontally by the blur lines on either side and extending vertically from 0 to 3 diopters of accommodative stimulus. Percival believed that the demand line should ideally fall within or at a limit of this comfort zone. If it did not, then prism, added lens correction, or vision training was indicated. The clinician can assess whether Percival's criterion is satisfied by direct inspection of the plotted ZCSBV and by adding the NRC and PRC findings together and dividing by 3. This trisects the total range of fusional vergence and defines the zone of comfort, the

inner third. Does the demand line fall within the zone of comfort for all viewing distances? If not, the amount of prism necessary to shift the demand line to the nearest limit of the comfort zone can be easily determined from the graph. The amount may necessarily be different for near and far viewing.

Percival's criterion can also be applied by calculation. A useful formula is Percival's $\Delta = 1/3 L - 2/3 S$, where L = larger relative vergence range, and S = smaller relative vergence range. For example, if the PRC is 24^{Δ} (L) and the NRC is 9^{Δ} (S), the prism necessary would be:

$$\begin{aligned} \text{Percival's } \Delta &= 1/3 \, L - 2/3 \, S \\ &= 1/3 \, (24) - 2/3 \, (9) \\ &= 8 - 6 \\ &= 2^{\Delta} \text{ Base Out} \end{aligned}$$

A vision training approach in this case would call for fusional divergence training (also called base-in training) to increase the NRC to satisfy Percival's criterion.

FIXATION DISPARITY ANALYSIS

Besides evaluating the relation between heterophoria and vergence ranges, vergence disorders can be identified and managed using the clinical index of *fixation disparity*.

Definition and Features

Fixation disparity is a slight manifest misalignment of the visual axes (minutes of arc) even though there is single binocular vision with central sensory fusion. The misalignment can be horizontal, vertical, or torsional; however, the magnitude of the deviation is within Panum's fusional areas, resulting in a single binocular percept of a target. Ogle[9] suggested that the magnitude of the fixation disparity depends on the amount of the innervation to the extraocular muscles during fusion. This innervation is related to the magnitude of heterophoria, the strength of compensating fusional vergence, and the complexity and detail of the visual target.

Fixation disparity is not always considered abnormal. It possibly represents an individual's

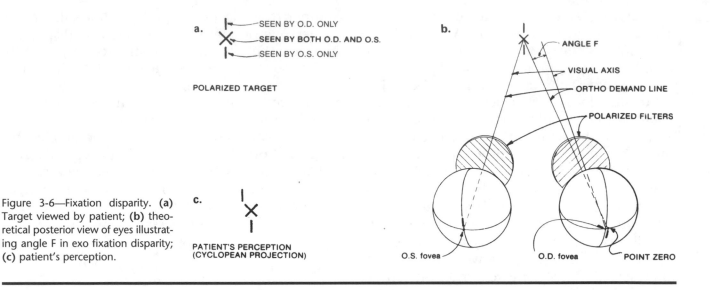

a.

— SEEN BY O.D. ONLY

— SEEN BY BOTH O.D. AND O.S.

— SEEN BY O.S. ONLY

POLARIZED TARGET

b.

ANGLE F

VISUAL AXIS

ORTHO DEMAND LINE

POLARIZED FILTERS

O.S. fovea   O.D. fovea   POINT ZERO

c.

PATIENT'S PERCEPTION
(CYCLOPEAN PROJECTION)

Figure 3-6—Fixation disparity. **(a)** Target viewed by patient; **(b)** theoretical posterior view of eyes illustrating angle F in exo fixation disparity; **(c)** patient's perception.

physiologic habitual set-point from which other binocular disparities are registered, e.g., for stereoscopic depth perception and as a stimulus for vergence eye movements. In fact, for fusional vergence error correction, it serves a useful purpose. Schor[10] indicated that fixation disparity may be a purposeful error signal that provides a stimulus to maintain a particular level of vergence innervation. Nevertheless, fixation disparity often indicates stress on the fusional vergence system and can be associated with excessive heterophoria, deficient fusional vergence compensation, and asthenopic symptoms.[11] Both abnormal and normal aspects of fixation disparity can, therefore, occur in the same individual. For example, a heterophoric patient with deficient vergence compensation can have a large fixation disparity, indicating vergence stress; but after vision therapy, there may be only a small residual fixation disparity that possibly indicates a normal set-point for that individual.

An example of an exo fixation disparity is illustrated in Figure 3-6. This is a posterior view of the eyes. If the error of vergence for the fixated X target is very small and fusion of X is possible because of Panum's areas, the X will appear to be single and not diplopic. The vertical lines (which are seen independently by each eye), however, will not be perceived by the patient as being in vernier alignment. This manifest deviation from exact alignment is too small to be detected by the cover test (i.e., unilateral cover test). For this practical reason, fixation disparity is not considered a small angle strabismus, despite a manifest misalignment of the visual axes. Morgan[12] summed up the quantification of fixation disparity by stating, "Normally, fixation disparity rarely exceeds 10 minutes of arc, although it may be somewhat greater when a substantial degree of heterophoria exists, and probably any deviation approaching 30 minutes should be considered abnormal." Since 30 minutes of arc is regarded as being a limiting value, and it is approximately the magnitude (0.9) of a prism diopter, it is practical to consider any manifest deviation of 1^Δ or greater as being a strabismus. If the deviation is less than 1^Δ and there is foveal fusion, the condition is a fixation disparity.

Clinical evidence suggests that excessive fixation disparity tends to reduce stereopsis. Cole and Boisvert[13] conducted a study and reported that the induction of fixation disparity on otherwise normal binocular subjects caused an increase in stereo threshold (decrease in stereoacuity). In another study, Levin and Sultan[14] neutralized existing fixation disparities in 12 subjects by means of prisms to determine the effect on stereoacuity. They found that ten of the subjects had an improvement in stereoacuity.

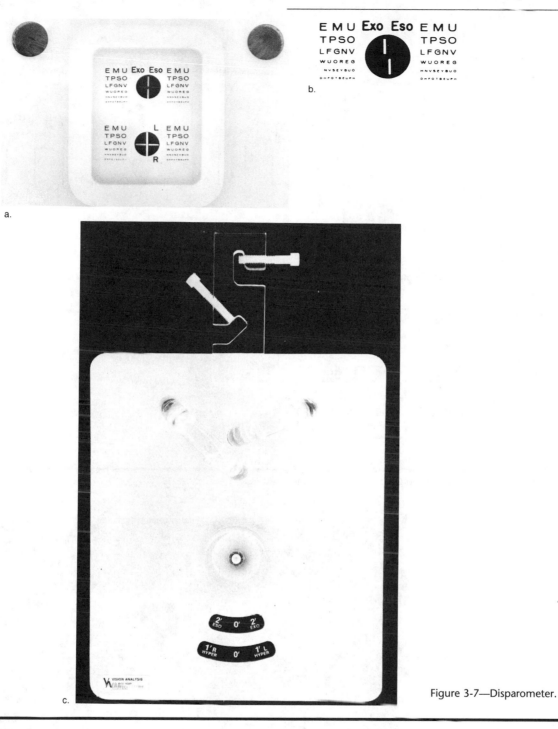

Figure 3-7—Disparometer.

Measurement

Fixation disparity testing can be done at both far and near. Instruments for such testing have the same general principles. The patient fuses a flat-fusion target under natural lighting conditions. Such tests incorporate vernier fiducials, clued to each eye by means of crossed polarizing filters. This is so the patient can report any noticeable misalignment. These vernier markings also serve as suppression clues. Central suppression is indicated if one line is not seen. Generally, two types of instruments are used; those that give a direct measure of fixation

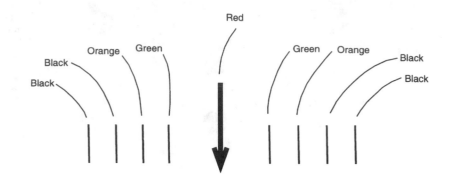

DISTANCE:	40 CM (16 INCHES)		25 CM (10 INCHES)
	↑	F.D. (MIN. ARC)	F.D. (MIN. ARC)
RED	0	0	0
	1/2	4.3'	6.9'
GREEN	1	8.6'	13.7'
	1-1/2	12.9'	20.6'
ORANGE	2	17.2'	27.5'
BLACK	3	25.8'	41.2'
BLACK	4	34.4'	55'

ESO F.D.:	ARROW TO LEFT
ESO F.D.:	ARROW TO RIGHT

Figure 3-8—Representation of the Wesson Card for fixation disparity testing.

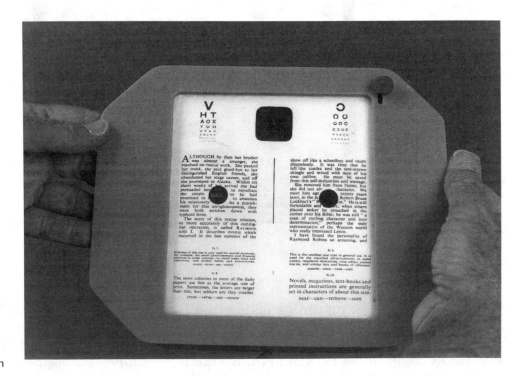

Figure 3-9—Mallett Unit for fixation disparity testing.

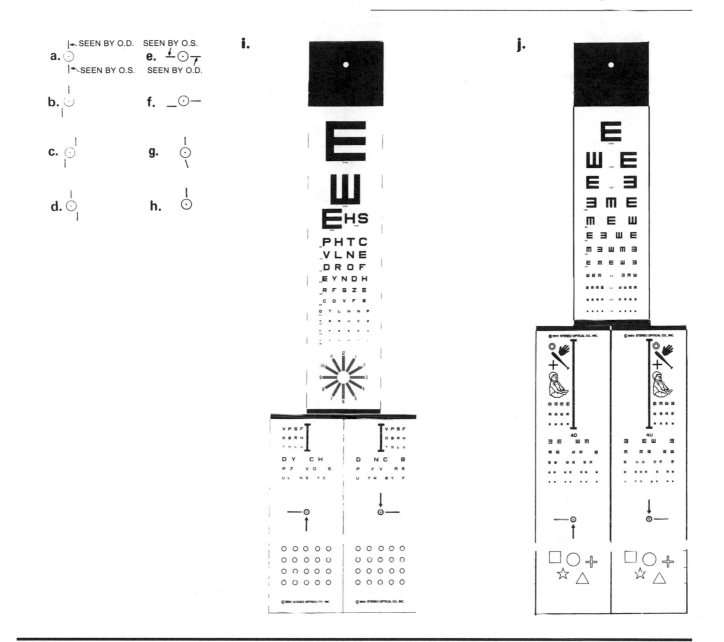

Figure 3-10—Results of fixation disparity testing with the Vectographic Slide. **(a)** No fixation disparity; **(b)** eso fixation disparity (O.D. dominant eye); **(c)** eso fixation disparity (mixed dominance); **(d)** exo fixation disparity (O.D. dominant); **(e)** no vertical fixation disparity; **(f)** hyperfixation disparity (O.D. dominant); **(g)** incyclo fixation disparity (O.D. dominant); **(h)** foveal suppression of O.S.; **(i)** adult version of the Vectographic Slide (courtesy Stereo Optical Co.); **(j)** children's version of the Vectographic Slide (courtesy Stereo Optical Co.).

disparity, e.g., Disparometer (Figure 3-7) and Wesson card (Figure 3-8) and those that measure only an *associated phoria,* e.g., Mallett Unit (Figure 3-9) and the Vectographic Slide (Figure 3-10).

The associated phoria is the minimum amount of prism that is necessary to neutralize a fixation disparity. Theoretically, this is the X intercept (XIN, pronounced "ZIN"). For exam-

ple, an exo fixation disparity would be neutralized with base-in prisms (Figure 3-11). Knowing the direction of fixation disparity and how much prism is required to reduce it to zero (measurement of the associated phoria) are of clinical importance. The XIN (associated phoria) should not be confused with the magnitude of the fixation disparity, theoretically the Y intercept (the YIN and pronounced as

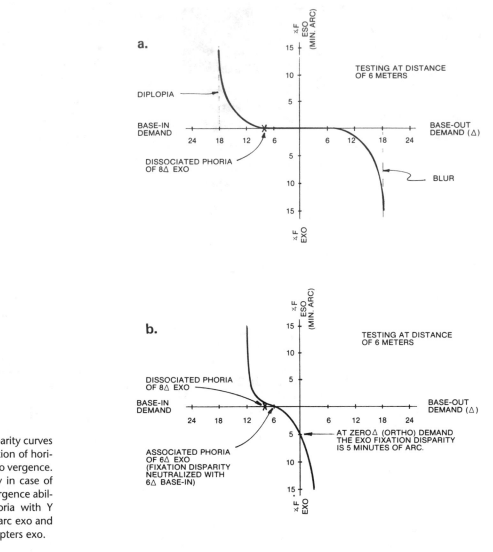

Figure 3-11—Fixation disparity curves plotting angle F as a function of horizontal prismatic demand to vergence. **(a)** Good vergence ability in case of 8$^\triangle$ exophoria; **(b)** Poor vergence ability in case of 8$^\triangle$ exophoria with Y intercept of 5 minutes of arc exo and X intercept of 6 prism diopters exo.

such). The XIN is measured by having the patient focus on the reading portion of the test and then look at the central target upon its being illuminated. The Vernier perception at that moment is used for clinical purposes. The prismatic power that produces alignment for the patient is the XIN measurement.

Fixation disparity targets similar to the Vectographic Slide (see Figure 3-10) are good for determining the farpoint associated phoria. The patient wears crossed-polarizing viewers and is instructed to keep fixation on the center of the "bull's-eye" target and to report any noticeable misalignment of the vertical or horizontal lines. If there is no misalignment, the clinician can

conclude that there is foveal fusion with no fixation disparity. If there is misalignment, compensating prisms are used to create vernier alignment. The power of the neutralizing prism is not the magnitude of the fixation disparity (YIN) but rather, the measurement of the associated phoria (XIN).

A good target for nearpoint fixation disparity testing is in the Mallett Fixation Unit[11] (see Figure 3-9). The unit is held by the patient at the preferred working distance and position as when reading. The centrally fused target is the X. The two vertical bars (one above and one below the binocularly seen X) are covered with mutually exclusive polarizing filters. One line is seen only by the right eye and the other only by the left eye. As in farpoint testing, any horizontal associated phoria (XIN) should be measured using the minimum amount of neutralizing prism. The fixation target may be constantly illuminated or intermittently illuminated for each measurement. The patient is instructed to look immediately from the reading material to the X. (Some clinicians prefer to have the patient continually fixate the X.) Any vertical associated phoria should also be measured using the target at the other location.

An associated phoria measuring 1^Δ or more may be clinically significant if accompanied by heterophoria and deficient fusional vergence ranges, particularly if the patient reports asthenopic symptoms. On the other hand, an associated phoria independent of symptoms or other signs may be clinically insignificant. Generally, the direction of the fixation disparity is consistent with the direction of the dissociated heterophoria, e.g., eso fixation disparity often occurs with esophoria. However, as Ogle[9] showed in his classic studies of fixation disparity, the two occasionally occur in opposite directions, e.g., an exophoric patient can show an eso fixation disparity. In such cases, the direction of the fixation disparity is considered to be the more important clinical indicator of the underlying oculomotor stress pattern. In such a case, prescription of base-out prism may be recommended to neutralize the eso fixation disparity, even though the patient has an exophoria (under dissociated testing conditions). Vision training to improve motor fusion ranges is, however, usually preferred in such cases, rather than prism prescription.

It is sometimes advisable to plot a *fixation disparity–forced vergence curve*, clinically called the *fixation disparity curve* (FDC). The Sheedy Disparometer (see Figure 3-7) was the first clinical instrument commercially available for this purpose.[15] This instrument has a series of pre-set vernier lines that allows direct measurement of the fixation disparity magnitude (YIN). The Disparometer can be attached to the nearpoint rod of a phoropter at the 40 cm viewing distance, although it can also be held by the patient with about the same accuracy.[16] Crossed-polarizing filters are used to clue the

fiducials to the right and left eyes. Fixation disparity is measured by the examiner dialing in the particular vernier lines for the patient's perception of exact alignment. The horizontal fixation disparity magnitude (YIN) can be determined to an accuracy of 2 minutes of arc, using the bracketing (method of adjustment) technique. The patient is asked to focus on the letters adjacent to the circular target containing the vernier lines. The vernier lines are transilluminated with a penlight by means of fiberoptic tubes. The examiner illuminates the lines intermittently and the patient is instructed to look from the letters to the illuminated vernier lines and report any misalignment of a line and its direction.

The FDC is plotted by measuring the magnitude of fixation disparity that corresponds with varying amounts of base-in and base-out prism. Risley prism increments of 3^Δ are advised to produce clinically useful curves. Fixation disparity is initially measured with an ortho demand. Subsequent measurements are taken in the following order: 3^Δ BI, 3^Δ BO, 6^Δ BI, 6^Δ BO, and so on. The limit of forced vergence in each direction is indicated when a prism results in either diplopia of the target or suppression of one fiducial. The instrument is designed for measurement of both horizontal and vertical fixation disparities.

The Wesson Fixation Disparity Card (see Figure 3-8) is a relatively inexpensive device but less precise than the Disparometer. It can be hand held or attached to a phoropter nearpoint rod; it also yields an approximate FDC. One study indicated that curves taken with the Wesson Card and Disparometer correlated highly if esophoric and exophoric subjects were analyzed separately.[17]

Figure 3-11**a** illustrates an FDC of a patient having normal binocular vision and Figure 3-11**b** shows an FDC of a patient with vergence dysfunction reporting asthenopic symptoms. Note the following clinically relevant features of the abnormal curve: (1) the significant fixation disparity at the ortho demand position, (2) the relatively large associated phoria (XIN), (3) the steep slope (exceeding 45°) of the curve at the ortho demand position, and (4) the limited range of fusional vergence. These features

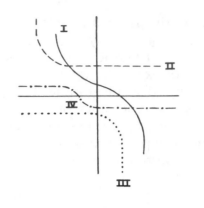

Figure 3-12—Four types of fixation disparity curves.

of the curve confirm the presence of a vergence dysfunction. Another feature of the FDC that has been suggested to be indicative of a vergence dysfunction is variability of the amount of fixation disparity and the curve over time, i.e., large day-to-day variation. In individuals having normal binocular vision, the FDC appears to be quite stable or reliable over time within a limited range of forced convergence and forced divergence.[18]

Four basic types of fixation disparity curves have been described by Ogle et al.[19] and are believed to have differential diagnostic value (Figure 3-12). The type I curve has a sigmoid shape and is considered to be the most prevalent, found in approximately 60% of the population. A type I curve having a steep slope (crossing at the ortho demand position) is often associated with visual complaints. In these cases, vision training is often successful in flattening the slope of the curve while increasing fusional vergence ranges, usually relieving symptoms due to vergence dysfunction. These cases have an excellent prognosis for improvement. Type II and type III curves have a flat segment that may or may not cross the x-axis (see Figure 3-12). Type II is often associated with esophoria (although occasionally exophoria) and is the second-most-prevalent type, found in approximately 25% of the population. Type III, often associated with exophoria (although occasionally esophoria), is found in about 10% of the population. It should be noted that all fixation disparity curves should be plotted from break to break (diplopia limits).

An FDC is sometimes incorrectly labeled as type II or III, when it is type I; this occurs when the examiner takes too few points and fails to find a segment that crosses the x-axis.

True types II and III often respond well to prism prescription. Many type III cases that are exo can be treated with fusional convergence training. Type IV cases, the least prevalent (approximately 5%), have the worst prognosis for a functional cure compared with the other FDC types. Figure 3-12 illustrates type IV exo fixation disparity, but eso is also possible. Individuals with this FDC type seem to adapt to prism so that the fixation disparity can never be permanently neutralized. In other words, there may be no stable XIN. Such binocular dysfunctions are not clearly understood. In heterophoria type IV, however, sensory and motor fusion disorders may be resistant to therapeutic attempts and the prism adaptation found during testing is characteristic of many strabismic patients. Vision therapy is frequently ineffective in such cases.

It is apparent that establishing the curve type and characteristics aids the clinician in making a diagnosis of a vergence dysfunction and points toward certain therapy options. The clinician needs to be aware that the type of curve can change from far to near fixation in many cases[19,20]; therefore it is important to evaluate the FDC at the distance the patient is experiencing binocular vision problems.

Ogle et al.[19] demonstrated that FDCs can also be generated using lens additions to stimulate forced vergence. By comparing the FDC found with prism stimulation and those found with lens stimulation, a "derived AC/A" can be computed. Following on this work, Wick and Joubert[21] found four FDC types induced by lens stimulation that are analogous to, but not totally consistent with, the types found by Ogle et al. who used prism stimulation. They suggested that these lens-induced curves have diagnostic value in some cases. Furthermore, the lens power that reduces the near fixation disparity to zero may help determine the proper near prescription, particularly with prepresbyopic patients. For example, if a +1.25 D addition lens reduces a nearpoint eso fixation disparity to zero, this could be the optimum prescription.

Although a Disparometer or Wesson card is recommended, the clinician can get a general sense of whether the FDC is normal or abnormal by merely measuring the associated phoria (e.g., using a Mallett unit) and evaluating the total range of fusional vergence. For example, if there is no fixation disparity induced over a relatively large range of base-in and base-out prism demand (e.g., 6^Δ BI and 9^Δ BO at near), then the clinician can assume there is a normal type I FDC. However, if eso fixation disparity and eso associated phoria are present with an ortho demand and the eso fixation disparity increases with relatively small amounts of base-in prism and an exo fixation disparity is induced with relatively small amounts of base-out prism, the clinician can visualize a steep FDC. A three dimensional model of fixation disparity, vergence, and accommodation can also be conceptualized (Figure 3-13).

Prescribing Prism

Two principal criteria have been recommended for the prescription of prism on the basis of fixation disparity: *Sheedy's criterion*[22] and the *associated phoria criterion.*[11] Sheedy's criterion for the prescription of prism is based on inspection of the fixation disparity curve. If the curve is steep where it crosses the y-intercept (ortho demand position) and the patient has fusional problems and symptoms, he recommends prescribing the least amount of prism that places the ortho demand position on the flattest portion of the curve. If, for example, the fixation disparity curve is steep at the ortho demand position but flattens out at the 4^Δ base-out location of the X axis, the prescription would be 4^Δ base-out prism. This would shift the ortho demand position to the flattest segment of the FDC, if there is no prism adaptation. We believe vision training is of great value in such cases, to flatten the curve near the ortho position.

The associated phoria criterion is the least amount of prism that neutralizes the fixation disparity (XIN). Typically, the targets used to make this clinical measurement are found with instruments similar to the Mallett Unit or Bernell Unit for near testing or the Vectographic Slide for far testing. These targets con-

tain both central and peripheral fusion contours; these are important in the assessment of the associated phoria. We believe a central fusion lock is necessary when the associated phoria criterion is used for the prescription of prism. It should be remembered that these instruments do not allow direct measurement of a fixation disparity (YIN), but only reveal the presence of fixation disparity. The associated phoria is determined by adding prisms until neutralization occurs. The patient should be instructed to determine whether vernier alignment is achieved with each prism power within a time limit of 20 seconds after the prism has been introduced. Beyond this time period, there may be significant prism adaptation to invalidate the measurement of the associated phoria.[10]

VALIDITY OF DIAGNOSTIC CRITERIA

Validity and reliability of diagnostic criteria need to be established before the clinician can securely apply them to patient management. However, most of the diagnostic criteria used in the prescription of prism and lens additions in cases of vergence dysfunction have not been subjected to rigorous tests of concurrent validity; their use has evolved slowly by experience in clinical practice. The rationale for the criteria of Sheard, Percival, Sheedy, and the associated phoria have a measure of face validity to them since they are all based on notions that have physiological credibility, but much of the evidence supporting their clinical use is anecdotal.

Graphical case analysis can be criticized on the basis of the subjective methods used in clinical testing of accommodation and vergence through a phoropter. Phorias, relative accommodation, and vergence endpoints can be influenced by a number of nonphysiologic factors: (1) patient's understanding of the instructions; (2) attention level; (3) cooperation level; (4) conscious effort expended; (5) rate and smoothness of prism or lens power induction by the examiner; (6) elapsed time between tests; and (7) the amount of central and peripheral contour in the fixation target. Also, how the

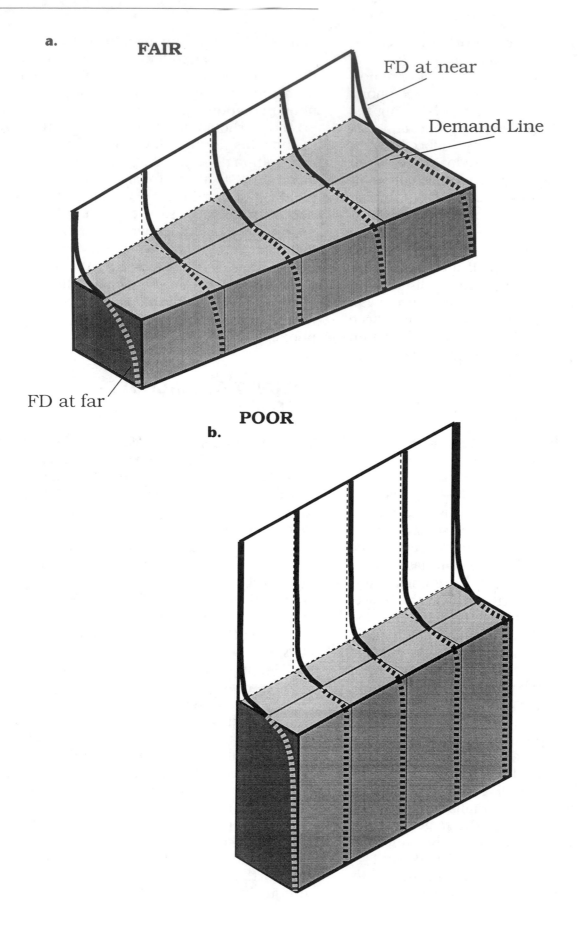

a. **FAIR**

FD at near

Demand Line

FD at far

b. **POOR**

c.   **GOOD**

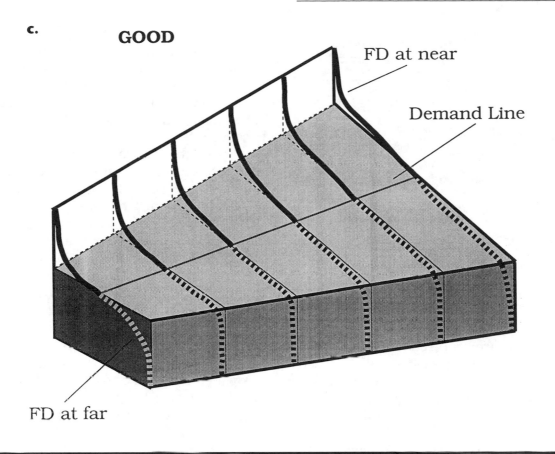

FD at near

Demand Line

FD at far

Figure 3-13—Three-dimensional models of binocular vision showing the relation among accommodation, vergence, and fixation disparity: **(a)** Indication of fairly good fusional vergences for clear, single, comfortable binocular vision; **(b)** poor fusional vergences indicating lack of good clear, single, comfortable, binocular vision; **(c)** good fusional vergences indicating excellent binocular status as to clarity and comfort.

instructions are phrased can make a significant difference in the measurement of vergences (e.g., "report when the image splits in two" versus, "try to keep the image single, but report when it doubles").[23] With several inherent sources of nonphysiologic variation and error, how can the examiner trust the validity and reliability of these clinical methods? More importantly, can any criterion for distinguishing a disorder from normal functioning, based on these endpoint measurements, be considered valid and reliable? Fortunately, these questions can be answered, at least for clinical purposes.

Morgan[23] found that tests for the farpoint phoria showed high reliability even when the time interval between tests was many years. Most standard clinical tests of far and near heterophoria have acceptable reliability and concurrent validity except for the Maddox rod test at nearpoint.[24] However, little has been reported on the test-retest reliability of Risley prism vergence ranges.

There is evidence to support the overall validity of graphical analysis and other clinical criteria of vergence assessment. Three different approaches to this problem are discussed: (1) a comparison of subjective and objective vergence measurements and analysis, (2) clinical criteria that discriminate subjects with and without binocular symptoms, and (3) prism prescription clinical trials.

Grisham[25] objectively recorded the dynamics of vergence eye movements in two groups of subjects; one group had clinically determined vergence dysfunctions and asthenopic symptoms and the other had normal binocular vision. An automated vergence stimulus was presented on a modified haploscope and an infrared eye monitor was used to record the

TABLE 3–4. *Ranking of Discriminating Factors between Symptomatic and Asymptomatic Subjects*[26]

Rank	Exophores	Esophores
1	Sheard's criterion	Phoria amount
2	Y intercept	FDC slope
3	X intercept	Recovery range
4	Vergence opposing phoria	Break range
5	Vergence recovery	Vergence opposing phoria

vergence responses. Vergence latency, velocity, and tracking rate were objectively determined variables that discriminated between the two clinical groups. He reported acceptable concurrent validity between the clinical and objective analysis of these subject groups and demonstrated that the objective analysis established the same categories of differential diagnosis as did a clinical analysis of vergence and heterophoria characteristics.

Sheedy and Saladin[26] also evaluated the validity of case analysis diagnostic criteria; however, they used the statistical technique of stepwise discriminant analysis to rank the effectiveness of many commonly used clinical criteria in differentiating symptomatic from asymptomatic nonstrabismic subjects. The symptomatic subjects all had clinically determined heterophoric and vergence disorders. Phorias, vergences, and fixation disparity curves were measured on all subjects. Sheard's criterion proved to be the best single discriminant variable for the entire population and particularly for the subgroup of exophoric subjects. For esophoric subjects, however, the magnitude of the deviation (phoria) was the most discriminating factor (Table 3-4). The power of these individual variables in successfully discriminating between the two subject groups (90% correct) supports the overall validity of binocular vision case analysis as an effective clinical approach.

One direct approach to assess the use of a particular clinical criterion for the prescription of prism is to allow the patient to choose between two comparable spectacle prescriptions, one including the particular prism amount and the other similar in all respects except for the prism. Worrell, Hirsch, and Morgan[27] were the first to use this technique when they assessed the prism prescribed by Sheard's criterion in 43 subjects with oculomotor imbalance and asthenopic complaints. They found that the Sheard prism was accepted at a statistically significant level in preference to no prism in esophoric subjects (particularly for farpoint viewing) and in presbyopic exophoric subjects. However, nonpresbyopic adults with exophoria did not prefer the prism beyond a chance level. Fortunately, vision therapy for increasing fusional convergence is very effective in such cases.

Payne et al.[28] provided two sets of lenses to ten patients with asthenopia and fixation disparity at near. The prism amount was determined by measuring the associated phoria using a nearpoint Mallett Unit and a double-blind research design was employed. By this criterion all patients (eight nonpresbyopic exophores and two esophores) chose to keep the prism prescription. Grisham[29] reported prism acceptance in a group of symptomatic presbyopic exophores using associated phoria as the prism criterion. Ten of the 12 patients chose to keep the prism that neutralized their fixation disparity at near. Based on theoretical considerations, some clinicians do not believe in the use of associated phoria alone for prism prescription. But the above evidence suggests that it has clinical utility, at least when determined by a test (e.g., Mallett Unit) that has a central fusion stimulus (i.e., "lock"). Unfortunately, not all fixation disparity tests have a central fusion stimulus.

The three approaches described above to evaluate the validity of graphical case analysis have all, in general, supported its clinical utility. However, any clinical analysis system based solely on subjective response indicators suffers from inherent limitations. In coming to a particular diagnosis of a binocular dysfunction, the clinician is advised to base judgment on a pattern of findings rather than on any specific attribute of the zone of clear, single, binocular vision. Several clinical criteria should be applied in case analysis when looking for a pattern of responses indicative of a functional binocular vision dysfunction. Fixation disparity analysis is an alternative system of evaluation that is often used in addition to the traditional, two dimensional, graphical analysis to establish the diagnosis and management of vergence disorders. A third dimension is added to the analysis.

An evaluation of fixation disparity and the attributes of the fixation disparity curve has become a popular mode of vergence case analysis. Ogle et al.[19] initially reported "good" reliability of fixation disparity measurements, and subsequent studies of the fixation disparity curve (FDC) with individuals having normal binocular vision indicated only a small amount of measurement drift over days and weeks.[30,18] Although increases in convergence or divergence fusional demand (prism demand) may result in some variability of the FDC, the overall shape and type of the FDC remain stable over time. This principle apparently applies to the vertical fixation disparity curve also. One study found that the shape of the vertical fixation disparity curve (approximating a straight line) remains stable over time whereas its slope varied significantly, more so over weeks and months than during the day.[31]

Variability in the FDC in patients with binocular problems has not been adequately studied. There are, however, indications that symptomatic patients with abnormal FDCs show increases in curve slope and magnitude of fixation disparity when reading for short periods of time.[32] Yekta et al.[33] found that a large fixation disparity (YIN) and associated phoria (XIN) are related to visual symptoms in patients of all ages, including presbyopes. They also reported that by the end of a working day, there is a significant increase in both of these indices that correlate with increased asthenopic symptoms.[34] Although more studies are indicated, it appears that several attributes of the FDC are clinically reliable and valid indicators of vergence dysfunction.

There are certain advantages and disadvantages associated with each particular clinical instrument used in the evaluation of fixation disparity. Both the Sheedy Disparometer and the Wesson card can be used to plot the fixation disparity curve (FDC). Several features of the FDC have clinical significance in identifying a vergence dysfunction, as reviewed previously. The FDC measured with a Disparometer appears to have acceptable concurrent validity with a laboratory horopter method for measuring the curve[35] and gives consistent information whether the device is mounted before a phoropter or is hand held.[16] Sheedy's criterion for the prescription of prism can be applied, therefore, with some assurance of a reliable and valid method of evaluation. We recommend using either the Disparometer or Wesson card as an adjunct diagnostic procedure in cases of suspected vergence dysfunction when applying Sheedy's criterion for the prescription of prism.

Dowley[36] concluded, however, that the associated phoria measured with a Disparometer (and by implication, the Wesson card), is not as reliable as the Mallett Unit. The Disparometer has a central fusion stimulus, an annulus, 1.5° in diameter, but no centered foveal binocular stimulus, which the Mallett Unit does have. Studies have demonstrated that the FDC is less variable and the associated phoria has a smaller magnitude if the target contains a foveal fusion stimulus.[37,38] Agreeing with Dowley, we recommend that a clinician should use either a Mallett Unit or a Bernell polarized nearpoint testing unit to measure the associated phoria if prisms or adds are to be prescribed by the associate phoria criterion. Our experience indicates that associated phoria prisms found by the Disparometer and prescribed are often excessive and rejected by patients. By contrast, the Mallett Unit prism amount that is prescribed is usually accepted by patients and proves beneficial if there are asthenopic symptoms and other signs of a vergence dysfunction. The foveal fusion lock prevents the measured XIN from being excessive, but it allows the clinically significant fixation disparity component due to fusional vergence stress to be revealed.

RECOMMENDATIONS FOR PRISM PRESCRIPTION

Other than the studies by Sheedy and Saladin,[26] there has been little research comparing the relative effectiveness of the various criteria for the prescription of prisms and adds to alleviate vergence dysfunctions. In the absence of abundant research data, clinicians adopt treatment preferences based on their own clinical experiences. From our experiences, we make the following recommendations regarding the relative effectiveness of prism prescription criteria (Table 3-5). Our initial bias in most cases of significant heterophoria, or intermittent strabismus, is to recommend vision training for improvement of fusional vergences. Prism compensation may also be necessary as a supplement to training. When vision training is an unacceptable alternative or training results are unsuccessful, prism therapy becomes the treatment of choice.

The *clinical wisdom criterion* for prism prescription works well for exophores, esophores, and hyperphores at both far and near. Generally speaking, exophores require less prism than esophores, angles of deviation being equal, due to the greater relative strength of fusional convergence. Prescribing a compensating prism that is 1/3 the angle of deviation is often appropriate for exophoria, up to 30^Δ. The prism can be split between the eyes and usually does not present a serious problem (i.e., optical distortion, weight, or cosmesis) if the eye size (spectacle dimension) is kept small. In symptomatic esophoria and hyperphoria cases, clinical wisdom calls for a prism equal to the angle of deviation as measured by the cover test. However, in cases of relatively great magnitudes, this criterion becomes impractical due to optical considerations. Lesser amounts of prism should be applied and evaluated empirically.

The studies of Sheedy and Saladin[26] and Worrell et al.[27] generally support the use of *Sheard's criterion* and conform to our clinical experience. We have found it useful in both eso and exophoria cases, but not for hyperphoric patients. It seems to be particularly valuable in cases of symptomatic presbyopic exophoria, a class of patients who are often neglected clini-

TABLE 3–5. Clinical Methods for Prescribing Prisms			
	Exop.	Esop.	Hyper
Clinical wisdom	3	3	3
Sheard's criterion	3	3	NA
Percival's criterion	1	2	NA
Associated phoria	3	3	3
Flat portion of FDC (Sheedy's Criterion)	2	2	NA
Prism confirmation procedure	3	3	3
Prism adaptation test	1	1	1

Key: 3 Best
2 Good
1 Fair
NA Not Applicable

cally. *Percival's criterion* is used less frequently than Sheard's criterion in clinical practice; although Sheedy and Saladin[26] found it may have validity in many esophoria cases. Prism, prescribed by the *associated phoria criterion,* however, has been shown to be accepted by symptomatic eso and exophoric patients in clinical studies,[27,28] but it is important that the test target has both central and peripheral fusion contours.

Sheedy's criterion (i.e., the flat portion of the FD curve) has clinical utility; however, we generally use it when the other criteria are inconsistent or they indicate unreasonable prismatic prescriptions. The measurement and plotting of the FDC are time consuming; although a valid procedure, this explains its lack of popularity among clinicians. Clinicians can work around this time-demanding obstacle by visualizing the FDC based on fairly routine findings, i.e., dissociated phoria, associated phoria, and fusional vergence ranges. (See the discussion of visualizing the FD curve in the section on Fixation Disparity Analysis.)

Diagnosis of a binocular vision dysfunction is rarely made on the basis of a single test; likewise, a prism prescription is seldom made unless a number of criteria indicate the necessity for it. The amount of prism power recommended by each criterion often varies and the clinician must use professional judgment. When there is coherence among criteria, that decision is relatively easy, but when there is wide variation, the validity of each should be questioned. Retesting or additional testing is often required. Particularly in these situations, a *prism confirmation procedure* should be carried out. We recommend the following procedure to test the suitability of any particular prism. Many patients with an oculomotor imbalance will immediately experience some relief of their symptoms when a compensating prism of appropriate magnitude is introduced. If an esophoric patient's symptoms are related to reading, for example, a reading test card is given to the patient to view. If, for example, the associate phoria criterion indicates 4^Δ base-out, a loose prism of this amount would be used in the confirmation test. With the prism in place, the patient is asked if the print appears clearer or if vision is more comfortable than without the prism. A valid prism prescription is indicated when there is a strong acceptance response by the patient. To check for a placebo effect, however, the prism direction is reversed surreptitiously and again tried. Validity is confirmed if there is strong rejection of the reversed prism. If, on the other hand, the patient accepts the reversed prism, further trials with different prisms are necessary. If no prism is accepted by this confirmation procedure, the prescription of prism is often unwarranted. Other approaches to resolving the patient's problem might be recommended (e.g., vision training, lens power additions, changing viewing conditions, or referral for general health examination).

If, after applying the above prism prescribing methods, a question still remains whether a prism is appropriate, a *prism adaptation test* may be helpful in resolving the issue. Heterophoric patients with normal binocular vision and no ocular symptoms typically show strong prism adaptation. After wearing a prism for approximately 10 minutes, they will often show the same, or nearly the same, phoria as originally measured. For example, if a 6^Δ exophoric patient with normal binocular vision wears 6^Δ BI (which initially neutralizes the angle of deviation) for a short time, the examiner typically finds the phoria to be increasing, resulting in another 4^Δ to 6^Δ of exo deviation. The prism would be ineffective because that patient reverts to the habitual phoria. Conversely, symptomatic patients with vergence problems usually benefit from prism compensation and do not typically show significant prism adaptation. If a prism, worn for 10 minutes, continues to neutralize the angle of deviation, then that prism establishes an acceptable physiological relation between the heterophoria and the compensating vergence, relieving the oculomotor stress. Complete prism adaptation, when it occurs, usually takes up to 24 hours to complete the full response, but most of the adaptation occurs within the first 10 minutes. This test is, therefore, a relatively quick clinical procedure. The results of this test are not always clear-cut and interpretation is often difficult. At times this is a good backup test of prism acceptance, but professional judgment is necessary.

VERGENCE ANOMALIES

The predominant classification system for vergence disorders is based on the tonic deviation of the eyes and the AC/A. It is used to describe both strabismic and heterophoric cases and has wide acceptance in optometry, ophthalmology, and by interested third-parties, e.g., insurance companies. Duane first proposed this model of classification, later amplified by White,[39] which was subsequently called the Duane-White classification. Schapero[40] also used the Duane-White model as a basis for his 10 case types. Duane proposed that at least a difference of 10^Δ between the far and near deviations was necessary before the patient should be described as one of his four original categories. Other writers have suggested 15^Δ difference between far and near and many clinicians use 5^Δ. We prefer to use a 5^Δ difference or greater between the deviations at far (6 m) and near (40 cm) to indicate the presence of an abnormally high or low AC/A. The larger values are typically used by ophthalmic surgeons when the desired level of accuracy in

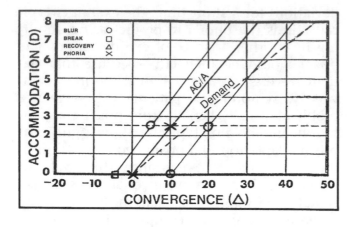

Figure 3-14—Convergence insufficiency represented graphically, classical graphic analysis that is a two-dimensional model of binocular vision in terms of the relation between accommodation and vergence.

surgical procedures is approximately 10^Δ. Compensation of the angles of deviation with prisms and added lenses, however, is more refined and often the therapy of choice. For example, if a symptomatic patient with an IPD of 60 mm manifests orthophoria at distance and 10^Δ esophoria at near, the calculated AC/A is $10^\Delta/1D$. This is convergence excess and is often treated with a bifocal add using the effect of the high AC/A to reduce the near deviation. However, if the same symptomatic patient measured ortho at far and 5^Δ esophoria at near, the calculated AC/A would be $8^\Delta/1D$, which is considered to be high by Morgan's normative data. Added lenses at near remain an ideal management approach. We believe a 5^Δ difference between near and far deviations is consistent with optical treatment approaches, and so we prefer this amount for the sake of clinical categories of vergence anomalies. This diagnostic classification assumes that symptoms and vision inefficiencies are caused by the vergence anomalies. Implicit in any of the Duane-White categories is poor compensatory fusional vergences. This classification system is usually based on angles of deviation measured by the alternate cover test, not phorometry. The angles of deviation should be measured in an open space environment. Instrument convergence and accommodation effects may invalidate the measurements of

tonic vergence and accommodative convergence. Although the categories apply to cases of strabismus as well as heterophoria, our following discussion of management recommendations is primarily for cases of heterophoria.

Convergence Insufficiency

Convergence Insufficiency (CI), or *convergence insufficiency exophoria* as it is sometimes called, is characterized by a low AC/A resulting in an increased exophoria at near viewing distances (Figure 3-14). A symptomatic patient showing orthophoria at far and 5^Δ exophoria at 40 cm would be an example. Other clinical findings associated with CI include a reduced PRC, a reduced NPC (poor gross convergence), and deficient accommodative responses.[41] Vision training is the treatment of choice for most CI cases. There is abundant evidence in the literature that this is effective.[41] Since the AC/A is low, added lenses (e.g., minus power) are of little value. Prism prescriptions have the disadvantage in these CI cases by inducing an esophoria at far. Sometimes it is advisable for patients presenting with accommodative insufficiency and CI to have a reading add together with base-in prism for nearpoint use only. However, these CI patients also respond well to vision training. Some CI cases present with a large exo (low tonic convergence) deviation at far combined with a low AC/A. These are the cases that most likely benefit from a base-in prism prescription (relieving the exo at far) in conjunction with vision training to improve the PRC at near.

Another similar CI case type, usually ignored in most classification systems, is *presbyopic exophoria*. Most aging presbyopes show increases in their exophoria at near. Often there is reduced PRC, and these patients develop classic symptoms of CI, e.g., tired eyes, sleepiness when reading, and avoidance of near work. Unfortunately, most clinicians and the patients interpret these symptoms as part of the normal aging process. If a young person presented with typical CI symptoms, vision training would likely be recommended. We believe that many symptomatic presbyopic patients with exophoria go undiagnosed or untreated. This neglect is inapproporiate considering the reports of successful treatment in the literature. Two extensive studies of symptomatic presbyopic exophores showed very positive outcomes with vision training.[42,43] Further evidence is supplied by Grisham et al.[29] who prescribed two pairs of bifocal spectacles to symptomatic presbyopic exophoric subjects; one pair had a prism amount equal to the associated phoria at near and the other was identical except there was no prism. The subjects wore the spectacles alternately for two weeks and then had to return one pair. Ten of the twelve chose to keep the prism spectacles for reasons of visual comfort, a result that illustrates our point. It was also found that the two individuals who returned the prism spectacles were uncomfortable because the prism, although helpful at near, had induced a significant esophoria at distance. Those two individuals would have been better managed with single vision reading lenses that included the base-in prism prescription.

Basic Exophoria

Basic exophoria (BX) refers to cases in which the tonic position is exophoric at far and the AC/A is normal. The far and near exo deviations are approximately equal in magnitude. An example would be a symptomatic patient who presents with 8^Δ exophoria at 6 m and 8^Δ exophoria at 40 cm (Figure 3-15). The BX patient may experience visual symptoms at both far and near. There is much clinical literature that indicates that significant exophoria is more prevalent in people with reading difficulties.[44] Since fusional convergence can easily be expanded, vision training for exophoria (and intermittent exotropia) is effective in these cases. Base-in prism is also effective in managing basic exophoria if there is little prism adaptation, since it reduces the convergence demand equally at all distances and the amount of needed prism is usually not excessive.

Divergence Excess

Divergence excess (DE) exophoria, is indicated when a significantly large exo deviation at far

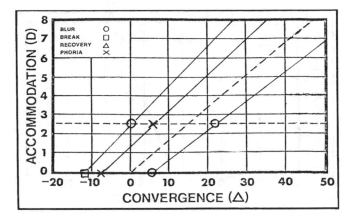

Figure 3-15—Basic exophoria represented graphically.

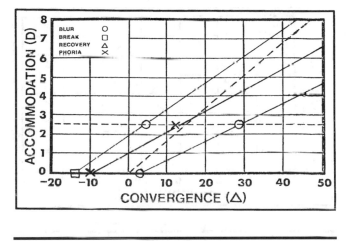

Figure 3-16—Divergence excess represented graphically.

is combined with a high AC/A. If a patient presents with 10^Δ exophoria at distance and 3^Δ exophoria at near, and after a prolonged occlusion test of 10 minutes the deviations do not significantly change, then divergence excess is indicated (Figure 3-16).

Some patients presenting with divergence excess actually have *simulated (pseudo) divergence excess*. For example, with prolonged occlusion, the nearpoint deviation of 3^Δ exophoria may increase to 10^Δ, exophoria. If the far exo deviation is 10^Δ, the correct diagnostic category would be basic exophoria. A spasm of fusional convergence at near is one possible explanation why the initial cover test gives a spurious result. Prolonged occlusion is necessary for convergence to decrease sufficiently to reveal the full

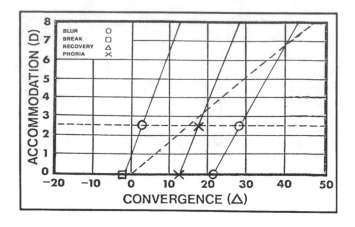

Figure 3-17—Divergence insufficiency represented graphically.

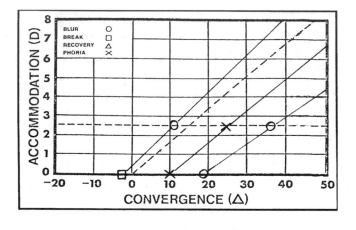

Figure 3-18—Basic esophoria represented graphically.

magnitude of the exo deviation at near. Therefore, these apparent cases of DE are called *simulated divergence excess,* also known as *pseudo DE.*

In the case of true divergence excess, which indeed has a high AC/A, the patient may experience esophoric problems at very near viewing distances (see Figure 3-16). If fusion is maintained most of the time at far and the AC/A is not extremely high, DE cases often respond well to vision training, but they are not generally as successful as the other types of exo deviations. In some cases, a minus add prescribed overall helps the patient control the far deviation, acting through the high AC/A ratio, but the amount of overminus must be carefully designed so not to induce an esophoric problem at near. Base-in prisms too may be useful,

but there remains the same reservation about inducing an eso at near. Many clinicians recommend plus-add bifocals along with vision training in the management of DE cases (see Chapter 14).

Divergence Insufficiency

Divergence insufficiency (DI) *esophoria* is the least prevalent of the eso cases. There is a significant esophoria (high tonic convergence) at far combined with a low AC/A. An example would be 12^Δ esophoria at far and 3^Δ esophoria at near (Figure 3-17). These patients can lapse into an occasional esotropia at far if fusional divergence is poor. Driving a vehicle, particularly at night, can be a problem.

Some cases of DI are difficult to manage successfully. One approach that seems moderately effective is possibly to prescribe base-out prism correction in single-vision lenses for general wear. For example, this may be 8^Δ BO if the far eso is 12^Δ. If there is no prism adaptation, the resulting distance esophoria would be 4^Δ, which considerably reduces the fusional divergence demand. However, with these spectacles in place, the near eso deviation would measure 5^Δ exophoria instead of 3^Δ eso. This amount is not excessive by Morgan's norms, but caution is needed in that an exo deviation at near is produced with the base-out prism. A vision training goal would be to increase divergence ranges. (Therapy for DI is discussed in Chapter 13.)

Basic Esophoria

Basic esophoria (BE) is characterized by a significant eso deviation at far and a moderate AC/A so that the far and near angles of deviation are approximately equal. An example would be esophoria of 10^Δ at all viewing distances (Figure 3-18). Other associated findings often include reduced NRC, a low PRA, and high NRA. Base-out prism is an obvious and safe treatment approach in BE and is usually effective since most symptomatic esophores do not prism adapt. Vision training is also useful in combination with prism prescription. However, without the prism, the divergence training often takes several months to complete and there can be frequent regression of fusional divergence skills. If the BE patient is symptomatic only at near due to work requirements (e.g., computer or desk work), a reading add (either single vision lenses or bifocals) may also be considered.

Convergence Excess

Convergence excess (CE) *esophoria* is the case that typically presents with little or no esophoria at far but with a high AC/A. An example would be orthophoria at far and 7^Δ esophoria at near (Figure 3-19). Patients with CE often complain of nearpoint problems because the esophoria increases dramatically as the viewing distance becomes closer. Eyestrain, blurring, and intermittent diplopia are often reported. These patients are vulnerable to developing an accommodative esotropia. Associated findings include low NRC, low PRA, high NRA, and possibly esotropia at very near fixation distances. Latent hyperopia is also frequently associated with CE; therefore, cycloplegic refraction is advisable in most cases of DE. Usually the full hyperopic refractive error needs to be corrected if it measures +1.00 D or more. Because of the high AC/A, plus-add bifocals are usually indicated for reading and other nearpoint activities. The amount of the add should be determined empirically by trying selected adds, measuring with the cover test, and listening for subjective reports of improvement of vision and comfort. Base-out prism may also be necessary if there is a significant eso deviation at far. Vision training is recommended to break any suppression and to expand the range and facility of fusional divergence. Frequent progress checks after training are usually indicated since there may be regression without an active home maintenance program of vision training.

Basic Orthophoria with Restricted Zone

Schapero[40] discussed *restricted zone* cases that he described as basic ortho with restricted fusional vergences, and the patient complains of visual symptoms. Heterophoria may be present, but its magnitude is insignificant at far and near. The

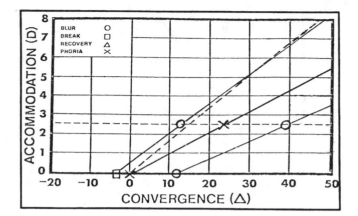

Figure 3-19—Convergence excess represented graphically.

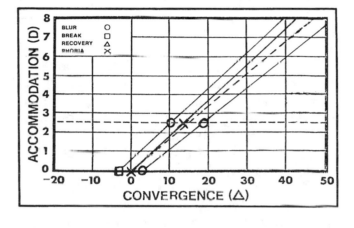

Figure 3-20—Restricted zone represented graphically.

NRC and PRC, one or both, are deficient, as can be the NRA and PRA. Sometimes the entire zone is found to be restricted (Figure 3-20). These patients often complain of visual fatigue after prolonged detailed visual activity and intermittent blurring, particularly when changing fixation distance. Reduced accommodative amplitude and facility are often found. The etiology is usually functional in that the patient's visual demands surpass their physiologic oculomotor and fusional capabilities. It must be kept in mind that the same clinical findings and visual symptoms can result from drug side effects and general health conditions (similar to those affecting accommodations that were discussed in Chapter 2). Careful case history is necessary for differential diagnosis. There may

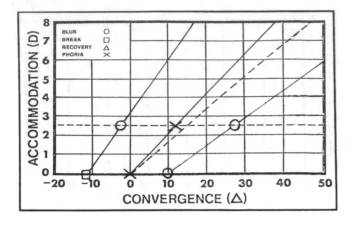

Figure 3-21—Symptomatic patient with normal zone of clear, single, binocular vision, represented graphically.

also be refractive causes of a restricted zone such as uncorrected astigmatism, uncorrected anisometropia, and aniseikonia. Optical management is indicated in these cases. If the condition is caused by accommodative and vergence dysfunctions, vision training is recommended. This mode of vision therapy is usually successful within a matter of a few weeks. The vision training goal would be to expand the range of the entire ZCSBV and improve the facility of all oculomotor functions.

Normal Zone with Symptoms

Schapero[40] also discussed the case of *symptoms, but no signs*. The patient presents with symptoms that sound uniquely binocular in nature; however clinical testing fails to find any component of the ZCSBV that is deficient by clinical standards (Figure 3-21). Accommodative and fusional amplitudes are normal. No significant heterophoria is measured and the NPC is within 8 cm of the bridge of the nose. The clinician needs to search for other possibilities before concluding that the patient has psychogenic problems, such as hysteria, malingering, or emotional instability, which are possible. Some questions and recommendations follow: Is there either latent hyperopia or pseudomyopia? Test for this with a cycloplegic refraction. Is there a latent phoria? Test for this with pro-

longed occlusion. Is there poor accommodation or vergence stamina? Test the patient at the end of the workday.

Are the symptoms really of binocular origin? Have the patient patch the nondominant eye for three days and keep a log of resulting symptoms. If symptoms decrease, some type of binocular dysfunction is indicated. If symptoms remain the same or increase, then other causes need to be identified (e.g., general health problems, drug reactions, or psychological distress). Sometimes diagnostic vision training can be given to determine if symptoms decrease. If the conclusion is that the symptoms are not of binocular origin, a referral for a medical or psychological evaluation is in the best interest of the patient.

BIOENGINEERING MODEL

Maddox[45] believed that the vergence system could be categorized by four additive components—tonic, accommodative, proximal (psychic), and fusional (disparity) vergence. Graphical analysis, based on this concept, was gradually developed by several notable individuals such as Percival, Sheard, Morgan, Fry, and Hofstetter. This became the scientific foundation for binocular case analysis. We have stressed the graphical analysis perspective in this chapter and adapted the Duane-White classification scheme to heterophoric disorders. We also applied Morgan's normative analysis, which is consistent with classical graphical analysis. In Chapter 2 the emphasis was on evaluating various oculomotor systems over time, with the dynamic components of each system tested. Accuracy, speed, and stamina were distinctive clinical features in that analysis. These two perspectives—graphical analysis and vision efficiency analysis—reinforce each other; however, each delineates visual functions, and disorders thereof, that the other may neglect. For example, disorders of accommodation, other than accommodative insufficiency, are ignored by classical graphical analysis. Vision efficiency analysis of accommodation, however, includes evaluation of lag of accommodation (accuracy), facility (speed), and stamina (sustainability).

Originating in the 1950s, fixation disparity analysis tended to reinforce and supplement the vergence evaluation of graphical analysis. Graphical analysis and fixation disparity analysis emphasized different aspects of vergence and accommodative dynamics, but the systems were intimately related since they both described the same underlying oculomotor physiology. What has become clear since the time of Maddox is that vergence and accommodative physiology, and disorders thereof, are substantially more complex than Maddox originally formulated. This realization has largely come to light through a bioengineering systems-control approach used in basic research.

One of the most useful research tools of bioengineers is to build mathematical control models of biological systems and then compare them with empirical physiological evidence. The model is modified until its features accurately simulate physiological responses and are consistent with what is known about the anatomy of the biologic system. Several important insights have evolved from the relation between control systems modeling and physiological evidence.

The accommodative system of the eyes and the vergence system are cross-linked and dynamically influence each another. Accommodation drives convergence (as evident by the AC/A). Conversely, convergence drives accommodation (as evident by the CA/C). (The CA/C abbreviation stands for convergence-accommodation per convergence.) When both systems are stimulated simultaneously, the cross-links interact and respond differently than when either system is stimulated in isolation.[46] Classical graphical analysis has not taken into account this dynamic relationship and has largely ignored the influence of the CA/C. Nevertheless, clinicians have long been aware that disorders of accommodation and vergence are often associated.

There are adaptive mechanisms for the AC/A, CA/C, and fusional vergence that, when stimulated, result in tonic changes in both accommodation and vergence. There are, therefore, both momentary and more lasting adaptations to prism and lens stimuli; a particular patient's physiologic responses to added lenses

or prisms cannot be accurately predicted in all conditions of clinical management. Schor[47] suggested that the lack of vergence adaptation is an important, if not the most important, characteristic of patients having vergence disorders. Clinical observations that are consistent with this viewpoint include finding that a steep fixation disparity curve is one indicator of poor prism adaptation. Also, prism adaptation does increase when vision training is successfully completed.[48]

The influence of proximal vergence on nearpoint vergence eye position has been largely ignored in classical case analysis, yet in some patients the amount of proximal vergence can significantly influence the associated phoria status, for better or worse.[49] Wick and London[50] proposed a version of the Hung-Semmelow model of interactions between accommodation and vergence that takes into account the influence of proximal convergence. They emphasized that one difficulty with the traditional system of binocular case analysis is that the vergence deviation that exists under binocular (associated) conditions is often not the same as that measured under dissociated viewing conditions (e.g., Maddox rod test). They joined Saladin[51] in a strong appeal for evaluating binocularity under closed loop (associated) conditions (e.g., fixation disparity testing). Wick and London[50] suggested that an improved graphical analysis approach would result from plotting and evaluating a graph of the *associated* gradient AC/A (derived from fixation disparity curves), the proximal vergence ratio, and far and near fixation disparity curves. Such an approach may indeed prove to be a significant improvement over traditional methods, but its incorporation into a practical clinical examination probably awaits technology that allows oculomotor measurements to be easily taken and transcribed directly into a computer program for analysis.

We have drawn our concept of a very simplified hypothetical model (Figure 3-22) adapted from various bioengineering models to illustrate the possible interaction between accommodation and vergence.

We believe it is expedient to evaluate binocular vision using the techniques of classical

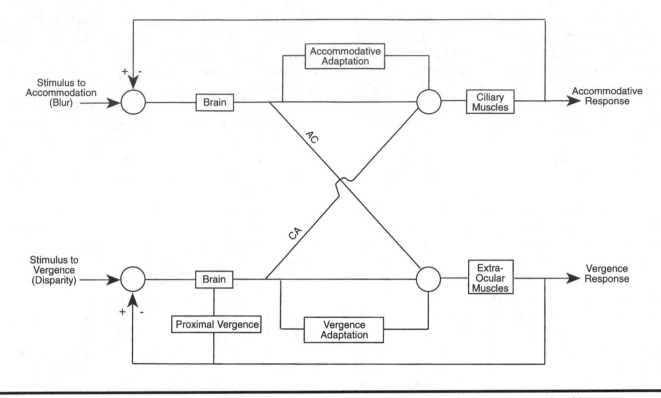

Figure 3-22—Theoretical bioengineering model illustrating interaction between accommodation and vergence in a closed-loop system.

case analysis and vision efficiency analysis. If clinical findings point to a dysfunction of accommodation, vergence, or their interactions, a complete fixation disparity evaluation is recommended. With this baseline clinical data and the analysis procedures recommended in this chapter, we believe the clinician has sufficient tools for successful and efficient treatment of the vast majority of nonstrabismic binocular anomalies. In cases that do not respond to vision therapy as expected, it is always prudent to retest, reevaluate, and reconsider other approaches to vision therapy, including referral to other professionals when indicated. Flexibility in the clinical approach is another lesson to learn from our new appreciation of the complexity of binocular vision interactions as suggested by bioengineering models.

References

1. Donders FC; Moore WD, trans. *On the Anomalies of Accommodation and Refraction of the Eye.* W.D. London: The New Sydenham Society; 1864.

2. Morgan MW. The Maddox classification of vergence eye movements. *Am J Optom Physiol Op.* 1980;57(9):537-539.

3. Flom MC: Treatment of Binocular Anomalies of Vision. In: Hirsch M, Wick R, eds. *Vision of Children.* Philadelphia: Chilton; 1963:216.

4. Sheard C. Ocular Discomfort and Its Relief. *E.E.N.T.* 1931;7.

5. Morgan MW. Analysis of clinical data. *Am J Optom Arch Amer Acad Optom.* 1944;21:477-491.

6. Morgan MW. Accommodation and convergence. *Am J Optom Arch Amer Acad Optom.* 1968;45:417-491.

7. Sheedy, JE, Saladin, JJ. Phoria, vergence, and fixation disparity in oculomotor problems. *Amer J Optom Physiol Optics.* 1977;54(7):474-478.

8. Percival AS. *The Prescribing of Spectacles.* Bristol, England: John Wright & Son; 1928.

9. Ogle KN, Martens TG, Dyer JA. *Oculomotor Imbalance in Binocular Vision and Fixation Disparity.* Philadelphia: Lea and Febiger; 1967:328-331.

10. Schor CM, Ciuffreda KJ, eds. *Vergence Eye Movements: Basic and Clinical Aspects.* London: Butterworths; 1983:467.

11. Mallett RFJ. The investigation of heterophoria at near and a new fixation disparity technique. *Optician.* 1964;148:547-551.

12. Morgan MW. Anomalies of Binocular Vision. In: Hirsch MJ, Wick RE, eds. *Vision of Children.* Philadelphia: Chilton; 1969:176.

13. Cole RG, Boisvert RP. Effect of fixation disparity on stereo-acuity. *Am J Optom.* 1974;51:206-213.

14. Levin M, Sultan B. Unpublished research. Ketchum Memorial Library: Southern California College of Optometry; 1972.
15. Sheedy JE. Fixation disparity analysis of oculomotor imbalance. *Am J Optom Physiol Optics*. 1980;57:623-639.
16. Frantz KA, Scharre JE. Comparison of Disparometer fixation disparity curves as measured with and without the phoropter. *Optom Vis Sci*. 1990;67:117-122.
17. Dittemore D, Crum J, Kirschen D. Comparison of fixation disparity measurements obtained with the Wesson Fixation Disparity Card and the Sheedy Disparometer. *Optom Vis Sci*. 1990;70:414-420.
18. Cooper J, Feldman J, Horn D, Dibble C. Reliability of fixation disparity curves. *Am J Opt Physiol Opt*. 1981;58:960-964.
19. Ogle KN, Martens TG, Dyer JA. *Oculomotor Imbalance in Binocular Vision and Fixation Disparity*. Philadelphia: Lea & Febiger; 1967:145-151.
20. Wick B. Forced vergence fixation disparity at distance and near in an asymptomatic young adult population. *Am J Optom Physiol Opt*. 1985;62:591-599.
21. Wick B, Joubert C. Lens-induced fixation disparity curves. *Am J Opt Physiol Opt*. 1988;65:606-612.
22. Sheedy JE. Actual measurements of fixation disparity and its use in diagnosis and treatment. *J Am Optom Assoc*. 1980;51:1079-1084.
23. Morgan MW. Anomalies of the visual neuromuscular system of the aging patient and their correction. In: Hirsch M, Wick R, eds. *Vision of the Aging Patient*. Philadelphia: Chilton; 1960:125.
24. Borish I.M. *Clinical Refraction*. 3rd ed. Chicago: Professional Press; 1970:808.
25. Grisham J.D. The dynamics of fusional vergence eye movements in binocular dysfunction. *Am J Optom Physiol Opt*. 1980;57:645-655.
26. Sheedy JE, Saladin J. Validity of dianostic criteria and case analysis in binocular vision disorders. In: Schor CM, Ciuffreda KJ, eds. *Vergence Eye Movements*. Newton, Mass.: Butterworth-Heinemann;1983:517-540.
27. Worrell BE, Hirsch MJ, Morgan MW. An evaluation of prism prescribed by Sheard's criterion. *Am J Optom Physiol Opt*.1971;48:373-376.
28. Payne CR, Grisham JD, Thomas KL. A clinical evaluation of fixation disparity. *Am J Optom Physiol Opt*. 1974;51:88-90.
29. Grisham JD. Treatment of binocular dysfunctions. In: Schor CM, Ciuffreda KJ, eds. *Vergence Eye Movements Newton, Mass.: Butterworth-Heinemann; 1983: 626 627*.
30. Daum KM. The stability of the fixation disparity curve. *Ophthal Physiol Opt*. 1983;3:13-19.
31. Rutstein RP, Eskridge JB. Studies in vertical fixation disparity. *Am J Optom Physiol Optics*. 1986;63:639-644.
32. Garzia RP, Dyer G. Effect of nearpoint stress on the horizontal forced vergence fixation disparity curve. *Am J Optom Physiol Opt*. 1986;63:901-907.
33. Yekta AA, Pickwell LD, Jenkins TCA. Binocular vision, age and symptoms. *Ophthal Physiol Optics*. 1989;9:115-120.
34. Yekta AA, Jenkins T, Pickwell D. The clinical assessment of binocular vision before and after a working day. *Ophthal Physiol Optics*. 1987;7:349-352.
35. Reading RW. Comparison of two fixation disparity determinations. *Optom Vis Sci*. 1989;66:612-615.
36. Dowley D. Fixation disparity. *Optom Vis Sci*. 1989;66:98-105.
37. Wildsoet CF, Cameron KD. The effect of illumination and foveal fusion lock on clinical fixation disparity measurements with the Sheedy Disparometer. *Ophthal Physiol Opt*. 1985;5:171-178.
38. Debysingh SJ, Orzech PL, Sheedy JE. Effect of a central fusion stimulus on fixation disparity. *Am J Optom Physiol Optics*. 1986;63:277-280.
39. Duane A. A new classification of the motor anomalies of the eyes based on physiologic principles. *Ann Ophthalmol Otolaryngol*. 1897;6:84.
40. Schapero M. The characteristics of ten basic visual training problems. *Am J Optom Arch Amer Acad Optom*. 1955;32:333-342.
41. Grisham JD. Visual therapy results for convergence insufficiency; A literature review. *Am J Optom Physiol Opt*. 1988;65:448-454.
42. Wick B. Vision training for presbyopic nonstrabismic patients. *Am J Optom Physiol Opt*. 1977;54:244-247.
43. Cohen AH, Soden R. Effectiveness of visual therapy for convergence insufficiency for an adult population. *J Am Optom Assoc*. 1984;55:491-494.
44. Simons HD, Grisham JD. Binocular anomalies and reading problems. *J Am Optom Assoc*. 1987;58:578-587.
45. Maddox EE. *The Clincal Use of Prisms and the Decentering of Lenses*. 2nd ed. Bristol, England: John Wright and Co; 1893.
46. Schor CM. Models of mutual interactions between accommodation and convergence. *Am J Optom Physiol Opt*. 1985;62:369-374.
47. Schor CM. Analysis of tonic and accommodative vergence disorders of binocular vision. *Am J Optom Physiol Opt*. 1983;60:1-14.
48. North R, Henson DB. Adaptation to prism-induced heterophoria in subjects with abnormal binocular vison or asthenopia. *Am J Optom Physiol Opt*. 1981;58:746-752.
49. Wick B. Clinical factors in proximal vergence. *Am J Optom Physiol Opt*. 1985;62:1-18.
50. Wick B, London R. Analysis of binocular visual function using tests made under binocular conditions. *Am J Optom Physiol Opt*. 1987;64:227-240.
51. Saladin JJ. Convergence insufficiency, fixation disparity, and control system analysis. *Am J Optom Physiol Opt*. 1986;63:645-653.

Chapter 4 / Strabismus Testing

History   97
   Time of Onset   98
   Mode of Onset   98
   Duration of Strabismus   100
   Previous Treatment   100
   Developmental History   100
   Summary of Clinical Questions   101
Measurement of Strabismus   101
   Direct Observation   101
   Angle Kappa   102
   Hirschberg Test   102
   Krimsky Test   103
   Unilateral Cover Test   104
   Alternate Cover Test   104
   Four Base-out Prism Test   106
   Brückner Test   107
Comitancy   107
   Causes   107
   Criteria and Terminology   108
   Primary and Secondary Deviations   109
   Ductions   111
   Versions   112
   Three-step Method   112
   Recording Noncomitant
     Deviations   115

Spatial Localization Testing   115
Signs and Symptoms   116
   Diplopia   116
   Abnormal Head Posture   116
Subjective Testing   117
   Single-object Method   117
   Two-object Method   118
Frequency of the Deviation   121
   Classification   122
   Evaluation   123
     Case History   123
     Testing   123
Direction of the Deviation   123
   Classification   123
   Objective Testing   124
   Subjective Testing   124
Magnitude of the Deviation   125
   Classification   126
   Testing Procedures   127
AC/A   128
Eye Laterality   128
Eye Dominancy   129
Variability of the Deviation   129
Cosmesis   130

When the status of a patient's strabismus is evaluated, the first step is to make a diagnosis of the deviation. Much information about the strabismic deviation can be obtained by a careful case history. After that, objective testing can verify nine important diagnostic variables: comitancy, frequency, direction, magnitude, AC/A, variability, cosmesis, eye laterality, and eye dominancy.

HISTORY

Besides giving tentative determination for each of the above variables, case history is necessary to assess the time of onset of a manifest deviation, its mode of onset, its duration, previous treatment, and results, along with pertinent developmental history that may have a bearing on the binocular status of the patient.

Time of Onset

A vital part of any strabismus diagnosis is to ascertain whether the strabismus is congenital. More correctly, this term should be referred to as *essential infantile* strabismus because, in many such cases, the manifest eye turn is not present at the time of birth. In cases of essential infantile strabismus, clinical experience with vision therapy, including surgery, has shown that the prognosis for normal binocular vision is very poor unless there is very early treatment.

We believe that the age of 4 months is the critical cutoff between *essential infantile* and *early acquired* strabismus because by that time the accommodation has developed to a large degree. The classification of *late acquired* pertains to the occurrence of strabismus beyond the age of 2 years. For example, an infant with intermittent esotropia at 6 months of age may have an accommodative convergence component resulting in the strabismus. For infants, aged 2 years and younger, parents should be questioned to determine the specific month of onset. For example, an essential infantile esotropia at birth probably has a lower prognosis for cure with early treatment (e.g., surgery before age 2) than if the onset were at 4 months of age. In the latter case, the infant has presumably had 4 months of normal cortical development for binocular vision.

To be completely sure of the time of onset, a complete report of previous professional examinations should be obtained. Unfortunately, this is not always possible, and information from parents, relatives, and friends is often erroneous. Pseudostrabismus can be confused with true strabismus; the appearance of esotropia can be simulated by epicanthal folds, negative angle kappa, narrow interpupillary distance, and other cosmetic factors. Such factors can cause parents to believe their baby had esotropia, when in fact there was only pseudostrabismus. Further confusion as to time of onset is introduced when a pseudostrabismus later becomes an acquired strabismus. Case history from parents cannot always be relied on for an accurate timing of the onset. Parents can also be misled by the poorly coordinated eye movements usually present in the early postnatal period. This can cause a report of congenital strabismus when, in fact, the infant's binocular status was normal in respect to age.

We believe the prevalence of infantile esotropia is approximately 25% of all who have constant esotropia. The majority of all esotropes have an onset after the age of 4 months, usually before 6 years, but occasionally later. Since time of onset is important in the prognosis for functional cure, the clinician must differentiate infantile from later acquired esotropia. When history fails to pinpoint the onset of esotropia, certain testing may indicate whether the esotropia was essential infantile or acquired. Some possible characteristics of essential infantile esotropia can be compared with those of acquired esotropia (Table 4-1). These findings are useful when case history is insufficient.

The prevalence of essential infantile esotropia is less than that of infantile esotropia. Onset of acquired exotropia, however, may be early, often before 2 years of age.

Mode of Onset

It is important to know whether the strabismus was intermittent or constant when the strabismus became apparent. An intermittent strabismus is relatively more noticeable than one of equal magnitude that is constant and unchanging. An intermittent strabismus may cause cosmetic concern but it has less deleterious effect on binocular function than one that is constant. Even if treatment had been delayed, it can be assumed that the child with an intermittent manifest deviation did not completely give up central binocular fusion as would happen in constant strabismus. This is a particularly important point to consider in cases of small angle esotropia with monofixation pattern. Even though the eyes are apparently "straight" a small constant esotropia is present. It is only when peripheral fusion breaks down and the larger eso component is manifest that the esotropia may be cosmetically noticeable. This seemingly intermittent esotropia is, nevertheless, constant.

Exotropia, on the other hand, tends to be either purely intermittent or constant; the deviating eye is likely to be either all the way out or all the way aligned for bifoveal fixation. Mode of onset history is usually more reliable in cases of exotropia than esotropia. Early acquired exo deviations tend to be intermittent compared with eso deviations, which tend to have a sudden constant mode of onset. It is typical for an intermittent exo deviation with an onset at age around 2 years to continue being intermittent for many months. Frequently, however, intermittent exotropia in young children gradually becomes more frequent and may become constantly exotropic with time. This is so unless vision therapy is instituted. An eso deviation of comparable magnitude, however, often begins as a constant strabismus.

Whether the deviation was alternating or unilateral at the time of onset is an important question to answer, especially in evaluation of amblyopia. An alternating strabismus is less likely to cause amblyopia than strabismus that is unilateral. The onset of amblyopia, therefore, cannot be equated with the onset of alternating strabismus; a case history of unilateral strabismus is more definitive in regard to time of onset of amblyopia.

Reports of noticeable variations of the strabismus angle may be useful. Changes of magnitude in different positions of gaze suggest an acquired paresis as the probable cause of strabismus. If, however, the angle in the primary position was reported to vary from time to time, the deviation may have been comitant and due to physical illness, emotional disturbances, or other causes affecting the tonic angle of convergence. For example, psychogenic strabismus, either eso or exo, is a possibility, although psychogenic esotropias are much more frequent than those of exotropia. The conceivable way an exophoric individual could have a psychogenic exotropia is by letting go of fusion to allow the latent deviation to lapse into an exotropia. This usually occurs in individuals who use this means to get their way, receive sympathy, or for other reasons designed to gain something from others.

In the event the patient has not been examined previously by another ophthalmologist or optometrist and reports of the patient's refrac-

TABLE 4-1. *General Guidelines for Possible Differentiating Characteristics Between Essential Infantile and Later-Acquired Esotropia*

Essential Infantile Esotropia (Birth to 4 Months)	Acquired Esotropia
1. Alternating deviation (often a midline switch)	1. Unilateral deviation (in majority of cases)
2. Possible lack of any correspondence (often unable to prove any correspondence with testing)	2. Presence of correspondence (either normal or anomalous)
3. Often no awareness of diplopia (only alternate perception of images)	3. Diplopic awareness possible (true simultaneous perception)
4. Double hyperdeviation and often excyclo rotation of covered eye (dissociated vertical deviation, DVD, in majority of cases)	4. No double hyperdeviation (dissociated vertical deviation, DVD, possible, but rare)
5. Insignificant refractive errors (occurring occasionally but as a separate component of the strabismus)	5. Significant refractive errors (e.g., hyperopia causing accommodative esotropia)
6. Normal or low AC/A (may be high but usually normal)	6. High AC/A (e.g., high ratio causing nearpoint accommodative esotropia)
7. Little or no functional amblyopia (alternating fixation preventing unilateral amblyopia)	7. Unilateral functional amblyopia (constant unilateral strabismus causing amblyopia)

tive, visual acuity, and binocular status are unavailable, the practitioner must depend largely on the patient or parents' statements for any case history. A good line of questioning directed to parents of young patients is the following: "When the turning of the eye was first noticed, did the eye turn out toward the ear or in toward the nose? Was it always the same eye that turned, or did the other eye turn some of the time? Was the turning more noticeable at different times of the day? Was it more noticeable when the child looked up, down, to the left or right?" Answers to these questions may indicate the mode of onset of strabismus.

Duration of Strabismus

The duration of time elapsing between the onset of a manifest deviation and therapy is a crucial factor in the re-education and recovery and/or further development of normal binocular vision. This is particularly so in the child below the age of 6 years. Clinical experience indicates that several months without bifoveal fusion can cause irreparable loss of central fusion to the infant or very young child, if treatment is delayed. When the duration is inordinately long and vision therapy is delayed, peripheral fusion may also be irrecoverable.

The duration time factor is not as critical in the ages above the developmental years as it is in the plastic years below age 6. Nevertheless, loss of the faculty of bifoveal fixation is not uncommon in adults who have had to give up bifoveal fixation over a long period for one reason or another (e.g., unilateral cataract of long-standing or acquired strabismus of many years due to paresis). It is not always possible to regain bifoveal fusion even though the obstacles may cease to exist (e.g., good visual acuity after a cataract operation).

Duration must be differentiated between the total duration (from time of onset to patient's current age) and the time elapsing from onset to treatment. While both time periods are important determinants in prognosis for functional cure, the period between the time of onset and the beginning of treatment is usually more important. If effective therapy is wisely and immediately instituted, the chance for recovery of binocularity is greater than if treatment is delayed. This is not meant to imply that treatment (e.g., surgery) should be performed instantly with reckless abandon; but rather, caution and discretion should be observed in all cases. It is very unwise just to let things be, losing valuable time. For instance, a case where the onset is early and there is constant unilateral esotropia, alternate occlusion might be prescribed as a measure to prevent amblyopia. Also, base-out prisms (e.g., Fresnels) should be considered as a holding action, particularly if the patient is below the effective orthoptic training age (under 4 years). In certain cases this may be done in conjunction with plus-lens therapy. If good binocularity cannot be recovered after a reasonable period, extraocular muscle surgery may be the recommended treatment.

Previous Treatment

After questioning is completed regarding time, mode, and duration of onset, another important answer to determine from case history is the extent and type of previous treatment the patient has actually received. Unfortunately, it happens all too often that treatment was recommended but not done sufficiently. Treatment is usually in the form of patching an eye, but not adequately undertaken in many cases. Not only does the lack of proper occlusion therapy impede recovery, but a history of the patient having been patched can lead to erroneous conclusions by a subsequent doctor seeing the patient. The second doctor may mistakenly conclude that everything possible had been done for the patient and that any existing amblyopia cannot be eliminated by means of patching, since it had been tried without success. Therefore, to avoid such wrong assumptions, questions regarding previous treatment must be pursued in depth. This rule applies not only to occlusion therapy, but to any of the other treatments for binocular anomalies. Table 4-2 lists desired information when there has been extraocular muscle surgery.

Developmental History

The purpose of taking a developmental history is to determine the important milestones at different ages in the child's life. This is related to the physical, mental, and emotional development of the individual, mainly in the plastic years below age 6. A developmental history may explain why a patient has a particular binocular anomaly.

TABLE 4-2. *History of Extraocular Muscle Surgery*

1. Age when surgery performed
2. Eye having operation
    Right
    Left
    Both
3. Muscle(s) having operation
4. Technique (e.g., recession, resection)
5. Cosmetic appearance
    Before surgery
    Immediately after surgery
    Later after surgery
6. Functional results (much depending on professional reports)
7. Repeat above information for additional surgeries

TABLE 4-3. *Typical Questions in Case History Regarding Time and Mode of Strabismus Onset*

1. When was the eye turn first noticed?
2. Was it an inward or outward turning?
3. Was it just one eye, or did either eye turn?
4. If either eye turned, what percentage of time did the right eye turn, and what percentage did the left eye turn?
5. Did the turning take place all the time or just some of the time?
6. If the turning was just some of the time, how often was it?
7. Was there any particular time or activity that caused the eye turn?
8. Has the eye turn gotten worse, more frequent, or larger?
9. What treatment was given and what were the results?
10. What are the cosmetic concerns, symptoms, or other problems?

TABLE 4-4. *Objective Testing Procedures for Detection of Strabismus*

Less Sensitive	Direct Observation
—	Hirschberg Test
—	Krimsky Test
—	Four Base-out Prism Test
—	Unilateral Cover Test
Most Sensitive	Brückner Test

Fisher[1] stated that gross neurologic dysfunction has been found in almost 25% of patients with infantile esotropia. On the other hand, the prevalence of such coexisting anomalies is low in cases of acquired esotropia. History of neurological signs may indicate infantile strabismus. A mild lag in neurological development may produce detrimental factors in the development of good binocularity. A developmental history may be important in many cases of strabismus.

Summary of Clinical Questions

Table 4-3 outlines sample questions on a typical clinical form for the purpose of strabismus diagnosis. Each of these questions can be explored in depth, but the basic format is similar in most cases when strabismus testing is begun.

MEASUREMENT OF STRABISMUS

Several methods may be used for detection of strabismus. Some are more sensitive than others, meaning that detection is more likely. For example, the unilateral cover test is more likely to detect strabismus than direct observation. Objective methods are listed in Table 4-4 with relative sensitivity shown.

Direct Observation

Horizontal manifest deviations greater than 20^Δ can often be detected by observation alone, because they are cosmetically noticeable in most cases. Deviations less than 10^Δ are usually not detectable by direct observation alone. Moderately sized angles may or may not be noticeable, depending on other factors such as angle kappa and epicanthal folds. A great problem with reliance on direct observation is that pseudostrabismus is often confused with true strabismus. More sensitive testing is required, such as the Hirschberg test, which involves evaluation of angle kappa.

Angle Kappa

Angle kappa is the angle between the visual axis and the pupillary axis. It is practically the same as angle alpha, which is the angle formed at the first nodal point by the intersection of the optic axis and the visual axis. Since angle alpha cannot be measured by clinical means, angle kappa is the traditionally designated clinical term; although technically, the clinician is measuring angle lambda (the angle subtended at the *center of the entrance pupil* of the eye by the intersection of the pupillary axis and the visual axis).

The magnitude of angle kappa (actually lambda) is customarily referred to in terms of millimeters rather than prism diopters or degrees. Although the normally expected magnitude is from 1/4 mm positive (nasalward) to 1/2 mm positive, there is nothing abnormal about a larger or smaller angle kappa (even a negative, or temporalward, angle), provided the magnitude is the same for each eye.

The distance in millimeters between the corneal relection of the fixated penlight and the center of the pupil determines the magnitude (Figure 4-1).

Testing is done monocularly under dim room illumination. The patient fixates a penlight at a distance of approximately 50 cm. The examiner's sighting eye must be directly behind the light source. The position of the corneal light reflection in relation to the center of the pupil is observed and estimated. For example, 1 mm nasal is written as 1 mm positive angle kappa for the eye (+1 mm). The same procedure is repeated for the other eye. The usual causes for an observable difference in angle kappa of each eye are: (1) large eccentric fixation of an eye; (2) displaced pupil (corectopia); (3) displaced fovea (macular ectopia).

Hirschberg Test

Julius Hirschberg introduced a quick and practical test in the latter part of the nineteenth century. The procedure has been the same but interpretation of the test has varied. The Hirschberg test is performed by directing a small light source, such as a penlight (Hirschberg used a candle flame), onto the patient's eyes. From behind the light the examiner sights the eyes while the patient is fixating the light. The examiner's dominant eye for sighting is directly behind the light, preferably less than 10 cm from the light source. Hirschberg recommended about 30 cm distance between the light and the patient, although this may be increased to 1 m with accuracy maintained. We recommend a range of 0.5 to 1 m for clinically measuring an angle of strabismus.

Hirschberg attempted to quantify the strabismic angle by comparing the first Purkinje image (clinically referred to as the corneal reflex) located in the entrance pupil of the fixating eye with the apparent location of the corneal reflex on the deviating eye. Since the cornea acts as a small convex mirror, a virtual image of the bulb of the penlight is formed. The reference points for judging the position of the reflection on the strabismic eye include the center-of-the-pupil, the pupillary margin, and the limbus. Guidelines for quantification were

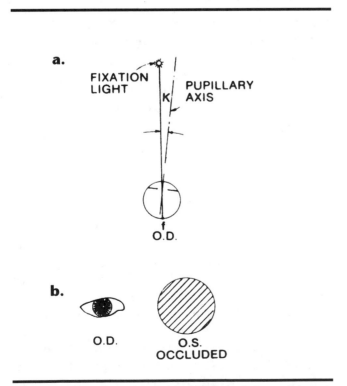

Figure 4-1—Illustrations of angle kappa ("K" stands for angle kappa). **(a)** Top view of right eye, illustrating a positive angle kappa. **(b)** Front view of right eye, illustrating a positive angle kappa. The light reflection is displaced nasally by approximately 1 mm.

used in the past. For example, a reflex appearing to be on the temporal limbus of the deviating eye was estimated to represent 100^Δ of esotropia. This method is not reliable because factors of corneal size, corneal steepness, and angle kappa must be taken into account for accurate measurement.

Various clinicians proposed simple ratios for measuring the magnitude of strabismic deviations. In the past the commonly accepted ratio was 12^Δ per 1 mm displacement of the reflex of the deviating eye, relative to its location on the fixating eye. A much higher ratio of 22^Δ/1 mm was proposed by Jones and Eskridge.[2] Griffin and Boyer[3] used photographic means to study subjects with known magnitudes of strabismus. The position of each corneal reflex in the photographs was determined by microscopic analysis. Their results concurred closely with those of Jones and Eskridge.

Interpretation of the Hirschberg test is illustrated in Figure 4-2 in which a 22/1 ratio is assumed and the pupil size is 4 mm. In Figures 4-2a and 4-2b, angle kappa (more correctly angle lambda) is zero. In Figures 4-2c and 4-2d angle kappa is +1 mm, and in Figure 4-2e angle kappa is −1 mm. The importance of accounting for angle kappa for Hirschberg testing is evident in these illustrations. Angle kappa is normally between +0.5 and +1.0 mm and a zero angle kappa is the exception. Therefore, the center of the pupil and the corneal light reflection are usually not in conjunction; rather, the reflex is usually displaced nasalward from the center-of-the-pupil.

The sensitivity of the Hirschberg test is limited to approximately 5^Δ for horizontal deviations.[4] A convenient clinical ratio is 20^Δ/1 mm, which means that a relative displacement of 1/4 mm of the corneal reflex on the deviating eye represents 5^Δ. This is the best a clinician can expect since a displacement less than 1/4 mm is almost impossible to discern.

Krimsky Test

The Krimsky test has slightly more sensitivity than the Hirschberg test, and it is similar, with one exception. Prisms are used to reposition the

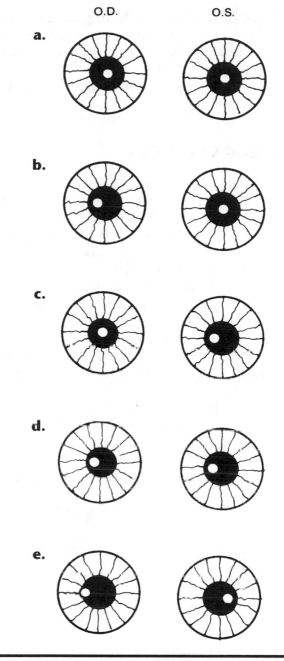

Figure 4-2—Interpretation of the Hirschberg test in five examples. **(a)** Bifoveal fixation, zero angle kappa, **(b)** O.S. fixating, zero angle kappa and 22^Δ esotropia of O.D.; **(c)** O.S. fixating, +1 mm angle kappa, and 22^Δ esotropia of O.D.; **(d)** O.S. fixating, +1 mm angle kappa, and 44^Δ esotropia of O.D.; **(e)** O.S. fixating, −1 mm angle kappa, and 22^Δ esotropia of O.D.

corneal light reflex of the deviating eye to the same relative location as the reflex on the fixating eye. The magnitude of the prism necessary to accomplish this is the measurement of the angle of strabismus. A confounding factor in the Krimsky test is the possibility of prism adaptation. Therefore, the testing time must be brief, 2 to 3 seconds at most. For this reason and because the Krimsky test is more complicated and less natural for the patient, we routinely use the Hirschberg test more often than the Krimsky test.

Unilateral Cover Test

The unilateral cover test is also known as the cover-uncover test. Its main purpose is to detect strabismus by distinguishing it from heterophoria. For example, assume a patient has an esophoria and the cover is placed before the patient's right eye. The left eye would continue to fixate, but the right eye would move in a nasal direction behind the occluder (Figure 4-3). When the occluder is removed from the right eye, the eye would move in a temporal direction for resumption of bifixation. Similarly, when the occluder is placed before the left eye, that eye will move inwardly behind the cover; when the cover is removed, the left eye will move outwardly in case of esophoria.

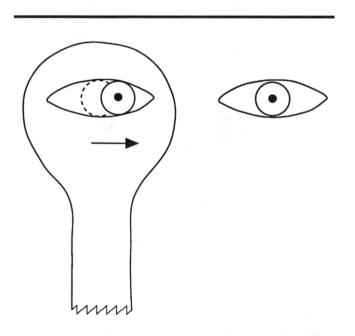

Figure 4-3—Unilateral cover test in an example of esophoria. A translucent cover paddle (as depicted here) may be used for observation of the eye behind the occluder; or, if an opaque occluder is used, the examiner can look around the paddle to observe the occluded eye.

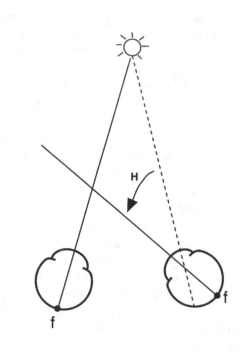

Figure 4-4—Schematic illustration of esotropia of the right eye. The letter H represents the magnitude of the horizontal angle of strabismus.

An example of an esotropia of the right eye is illustrated in Figure 4-4. If the cover is placed before the right eye, there will be no movement of either eye because only the left eye is fixating. When the cover is placed before the left eye, however, the right eye will have to move outwardly to fixate the target. Also, the left eye will make an inward movement and be in an eso posture behind the occluder (Figure 4-5). The movement of the uncovered eye is the distinguishing feature of strabismus on the unilateral cover test.

Alternate Cover Test

The alternate cover test is also referred to as the Duane cover test. It may be used with prisms to measure the angle of deviation of either a strabismus or phoria. Although a very sensitive method for detecting a deviation of the visual axis, a limitation of the alternate cover test is that it cannot differentiate between heterotropia and heterophoria (i.e., strabismus versus phoria) as can the unilateral cover test. This is

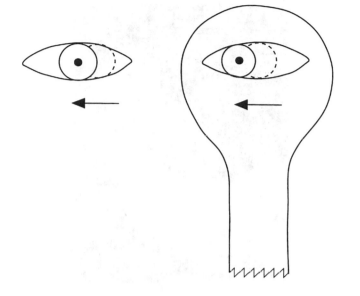

Figure 4-5—Examiner's view of eye movements on the unilateral cover test when the occluder is placed before the fixating left eye. If an opaque occluder is used the examiner must look behind the occluder to see the movement of the covered eye.

because, during the procedure, only one eye is fixating at any given moment; the eyes are in a state of dissociation, making fusion impossible. The alternate cover test cannot determine whether a deviation is concealed by fusion.

The test is performed by alternately occluding one eye and then the other while watching for any conjugate movement of the eyes; this indicates a deviation. The greater the conjugate movement, the greater is the deviation (either strabismic or phoric). An exo deviation will result in conjugate movement in the same direction as the movement of the occluder ("with" motion). An eso deviation causes an "against" motion during the alternate cover test.

Testing procedure is explained by using an example. Assume the patient in this example has an esotropia of the right eye of 25^{Δ}. The first step is to occlude the eyes alternately at a rate of 1 to 2 seconds per occlusion to determine if there is an eso, exo, and/or hyper deviation. The direction and magnitude of the conjugate movement of the eyes indicate the direction and magnitude of the deviation.

Assuming the unilateral cover test had been done previously, certain information

about the deviation of the visual axes is already known, i.e., whether the deviation is strabismic or phoric, the dominant eye preferred for fixation, the direction, and estimated magnitude of the deviation. With that knowledge from the unilateral cover test together with observation of the patient's eyes during alternate occlusion, the next step is to occlude the nondominant deviating eye. In this example the right eye is occluded and no movement of either eye is expected, since the left eye remains the fixating eye and is motionless. When, however, the occluder is switched to the left eye the right eye takes up fixation that causes a conjugate eye movement to the patient's right-hand side.

The next step is to switch the occluder to the right eye and place a prism between the eye and the occluder. The occluder is next switched to the left eye and any conjugate movement is noted; if there is none, the prismatic power represents the magnitude of the deviation (Figure 4-6). If there is an "against" motion, the base-out neutralizing prismatic power is insufficient, with a residual eso deviation. If there is a "with" motion the prismatic power is over-

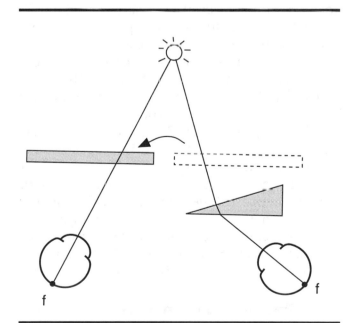

Figure 4-6—Occluder is switched to the left eye. In this example, no eye movement is seen because the base-out prismatic power is equal to the magnitude of the strabismic deviation, i.e., neutralization of the conjugate movement on the alternate cover test.

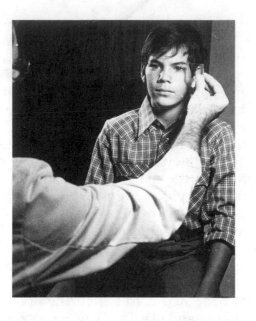

Figure 4-7—Preparing for the four base-out prism test in the case of a small esotropia of the right eye.

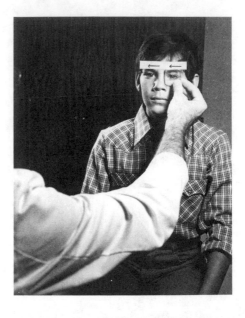

Figure 4-8—When the 4^Δ base-out prism is placed before the fixating left eye it adducts (toward the apex of the prism), and the esotropic right eye abducts. This is dextroversion but no convergence in this case of strabismus. If the patient were heterophoric rather than strabismic, a convergence would follow the initial dextroversion.

correcting the eso deviation (as though the patient has an exo deviation).

A pitfall of the cover test is that its validity is vitiated if there is eccentric fixation. (Refer to discussion of eccentric fixation in Chapter 5.) For example, suppose the patient has nasal eccentric fixation of 5^Δ of the right eye and the patient has an esotropia of the right eye of 5^Δ. The *measured* magnitude on the cover test would be zero. If, in another case, the *true* angle of esotropia is 8^Δ, the cover test would yield a magnitude of 3^Δ eso deviation. Eskridge[4] gave rules to differentiate between the measured and true deviation. Nasal eccentric fixation causes the measured angle H to be smaller than the true angle H in esotropia but larger than the true angle H in exotropia. In contrast, temporal eccentric fixation causes the measured angle H to be larger in esotropia but smaller in exotropia (Table 4-5).

Four Base-out Prism Test

When an esotropic angle is small (10^Δ or less), the four base-out prism test may be helpful in detecting a microstrabismus. Assume a patient

TABLE 4-5. *Effects of Eccentric Fixation on Measurement Results of the Cover Test*

Direction of Deviation	Nasal Eccentric Fixation	Temporal Eccentric Fixation
Eso	Smaller measurement	Larger measurement
Exo	Larger measurement	Smaller measurement

has a small unnoticeable esotropia of the right eye and the 4^Δ prism is placed in a base-out orientation before the fixating left eye. The right eye will abduct. The right eye will move approximately 4 prism diopters (Figures 4-7 and 4-8). Conversely, if the base-out prism is placed before the strabismic right eye, no movement of either eye is expected, presumably because of suppression of the deviating eye. Exceptions to the above result may occur in very small esotropic angles, less than 4$^\Delta$, since the prism power is larger than the angle of deviation. This is because peripheral (extramacular) fusion may allow a convergence response to the prism, although usually not the full 4$^\Delta$ of convergence.

If the deviation were esophoric rather than esotropic, the left eye, and later the right eye, would be expected to adduct. Clinical results from this test and the unilateral cover test provide information on tropia versus phoria, assessment of suppression in an objective manner, and indicate which eye tends to be strabismic. As with both tests, analysis of the patient's eye movements requires keen observation. These tests appear to be very simple but they probably require more clinical acumen than other tests for assessing binocular vision.

Brückner Test

An extremely sensitive, although not always reliable, method for detecting strabismus is the Brückner test[5,6] It is performed by using an ordinary direct ophthalmoscope held at approximately 75 cm from the patient's eyes with the beam of the ophthalmoscope directed to the bridge of the nose and equidistant from each eye. The examiner observes the fundus (red) reflex and compares the brightness between the two eyes. The strabismic eye, as a rule, will appear brighter (Figure 4-9). There are frequent exceptions to this rule. Pigmentary difference, unequal pupil size, and anisometropia invalidate the Brückner test (i.e., the fixating eye may appear brighter than the deviating eye in such cases). Nevertheless, the Brückner test is a good adjunct method for detection of microstrabismus.

COMITANCY

All deviations are classified as being either "comitant" or "noncomitant." (The correct etymological terms are *concomitant* and *nonconcomitant,* but the shortened words are generally preferred for ease in clinical usage.) Comitancy means that the angle of deviation of the visual axes remains the same throughout all positions

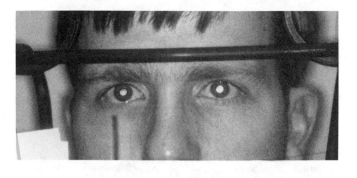

Figure 4-9—Example of a patient with esotropia of 3$^\Delta$ of the left eye in which the fundus reflex is brighter on the Brückner test.

of gaze. This implies there are neither abnormal underactions nor overactions of any of the 12 extraocular muscles controlling eye movements. On the other hand, noncomitancy means that the magnitude of the deviation changes when the eyes move from one position of gaze to another. Thus, there is either abnormal restriction to movement or overaction of one or more of the extraocular muscles.

Causes

Underactions are the result of one of three basic reasons. First, the extraocular muscles themselves may be paretic as in cases of direct traumatic injury. Second, and more frequently, mechanical reasons such as faulty muscle insertion and ligament abnormalities may restrict ocular motility. Third, and most frequently, the extraocular muscle paresis responsible for underactions is caused by innervational deficiencies due to impairment of the cranial nerves (3rd, 4th, and 6th), which innervate the muscles. Nerve impairment is commonly attributable to vascular problems, such as hemorrhages, aneurysms, and embolisms in older patients. Infectious diseases that affect the central nervous system also are frequent causes and should be suspected, particularly in young patients.

Overactions may be due to mechanical reasons, such as a faulty muscle insertion giving mechanical advantage to the particular muscle. More often, however, the overaction can be explained by Hering's law of equal innervation to two yoked muscles. This law states that the

TABLE 4-6. Yoked Muscles

Right lateral rectus (RLR) and left medial rectus (LMR)

Right medial rectus (RMR) and left lateral rectus (LLR)

Right superior rectus (RSR) and left inferior oblique (LIO)

Right inferior rectus (RIR) and left superior oblique (LSO)

Right superior oblique (RSO) and left inferior rectus (LIR)

Right inferior oblique (RIO) and left superior rectus (LSR)

contralateral synergists are equally innervated when a movement is executed by both eyes. If, for example, the right lateral rectus muscle is paretic and requires an abnormally high level of innervation to abduct the right eye, the equally high level of innervation is sent to the medial rectus of the left eye (the yoke muscle of the lateral rectus of the right eye) (Table 4-6). This results in an overaction of the left medial rectus, which further increases an eso deviation due to the paretic right lateral rectus. If this overaction continues for several months, a permanent state of contracture may result whereby the tissues of the left medial rectus eventually become fibrotic and nonelastic. This worsens the prognosis for cure of an eso deviation. In this example of a paretic right lateral rectus the right medial rectus (homolateral antagonist) can also become spastic, and eventually fibrotic. Precautions and appropriate therapy in such cases are discussed in Chapter 15.

Criteria and Terminology

Few individuals have perfect comitancy in the strictest sense when the term is used to mean that the angle of deviation remains exactly the same throughout all positions of gaze. The frequent lack of perfect comitancy occurs because the basic deviation of most individuals varies slightly from one direction of gaze to another. Therefore, some allowance must be made so that the term "noncomitancy" is not misleadingly overused. For clinical purposes, the amount of change of deviation allowable is five prism diopters, thus providing for the deviation to be classified as comitant. If the change in deviation in any of the various gazes is greater than five prism diopters, the deviation is considered to be noncomitant. The severity of noncomitancy can be evaluated by applying the following qualifications:

Mild: 6^Δ to 10^Δ change in deviation

Moderate: 11^Δ to 15^Δ change in deviation

Marked: 16^Δ or more change in deviation

A noncomitant deviation of the visual axes may or may not be paretic. Paresis is an etiological term whereas noncomitancy is a descriptive term. Unless there is absolute certainty of the etiology, it is wise to avoid using the word "paresis" or similar terms such as "palsy" or "paralysis." This is because noncomitancy can also be due to a mechanical problem, such as restriction due to faulty muscle insertion. When there is uncertainty as to the etiology, it is best to state the condition as noncomitant or to use a synonymous term, such as "incomitant" until the exact cause is established.

The term "paresis" is used in this text rather than paralysis. Although these are used synonymously in the literature, paralysis seemingly denotes total loss of function; however, the

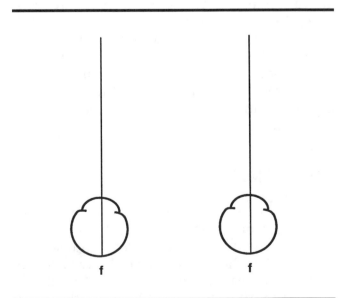

Figure 4-10—The orthophoric posture of the eyes in the primary position of gaze.

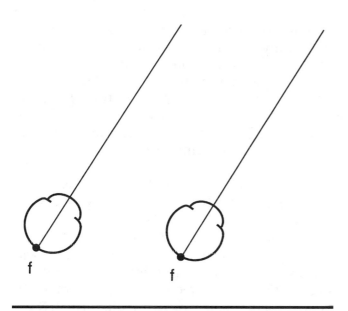

Figure 4-11—The orthophoric posture on dextroversion.

of dextroversion. Each eye made an equal movement to the right so that the ortho posture was maintained. Another helpful way of illustrating eye posture is by showing a confrontation view. Nine diagnostic positions of gaze are shown in Figure 4-12. These illustrations depict the patient's eyes in the orthophoric posture as seen by the examiner.

To illustrate a noncomitant deviation, Figure 4-13 shows the eyes not in the ortho posture with dextroversion. The left eye made a nasal movement (adduction) larger than the temporal movement (abduction) of the right eye. Assuming the left eye is the fixating eye, this results in an esotropic deviation of the right eye in right gaze. This same deviation is clinically depicted in Figure 4-14. This indication of noncomitancy is even more evident when Hirschberg testing is used (Figure 4-15).

complete loss of function may not always be the case. If there is total loss of muscle function due to nerve lesions, paralysis would be an appropriate term. This may also be called "complete paresis." As a rule, when in doubt as to the totality of loss of function, paresis is probably the preferred term to use.

In testing for noncomitancy, it is important to know the relationship of the visual axis of one eye to that of the other. If the axes are parallel, the eyes are postured in the ortho position. Figure 4-10 illustrates parallelism with the eyes being in the primary position of gaze. Similarly, Figure 4-11 shows the eyes in the ortho posture in the secondary position of gaze

Primary and Secondary Deviations

Measurements of the primary and secondary deviations are customarily made in the straight-ahead gaze (primary position), using the alternate cover test with prisms, usually at far (6 m) but may also be done at near (e.g., 40 cm). The magnitude of one angle is compared with the magnitude of the other. If a patient has a paretic muscle in one eye but not the other, the primary angle of deviation is the angle measured when the nonparetic eye fixates. The secondary angle is the angle measured when the paretic eye fixates.

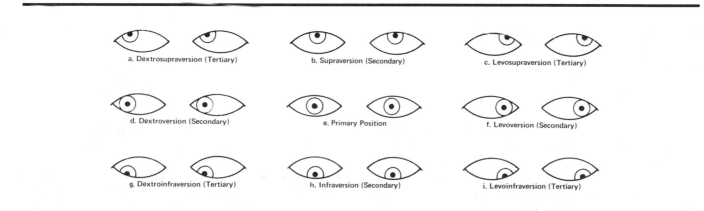

Figure 4-12—The nine diagnostic positions of gaze for conjugate eye movements, with secondary and tertiary positions indicated.

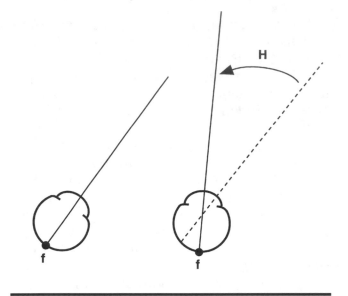

Figure 4-13—Esotropia of the right eye on dextroversion (right gaze).

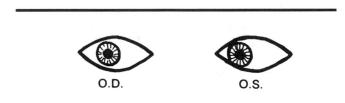

O.D.   O.S.

Figure 4-14—Direct observation of esotropia of the right eye on dextroversion due to insufficient abduction; the left eye is fixating.

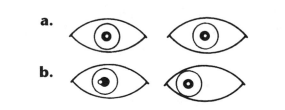

a.

b.

Figure 4-15—Hirschberg test in primary and dextroversion. (a) Ortho posture in the primary position of gaze; (b) esotropia of the right eye in right gaze.

The literature too often obfuscates the true meaning of the secondary angle by implying that it is the angle measured when the non-dominant eye (or the deviating eye in strabismus) is fixating. This can be misleading, since the nondominant eye may possibly be the non-

paretic eye and the dominant eye the paretic one. Under such circumstances, the primary angle of deviation would be the one measured when the nondominant eye is used for fixation. For this reason, we prefer to restrict the use of "primary" and "secondary" deviations to the question of comitancy rather than commingling the issue of dominancy (discussed later in this chapter).

The secondary angle of deviation is almost always significantly larger than the primary angle. This is because of Hering's law of equal innervation. Figures 4-16 and 4-17 are examples of paresis of the right lateral rectus muscle. The excessive innervation involved in contracting the right lateral rectus is carried over to the yoke muscle, the left medial rectus. The left eye is turned inwardly to an excessive degree, thus causing the eso deviation to be larger when the paretic eye is fixating.

Differences between the primary and secondary deviations may be due to noncomitancies caused by other reasons than paresis. A faulty muscle insertion may test positive in this regard. However, the difference between primary and secondary angles is usually less remarkable than when a paretic muscle is involved. The

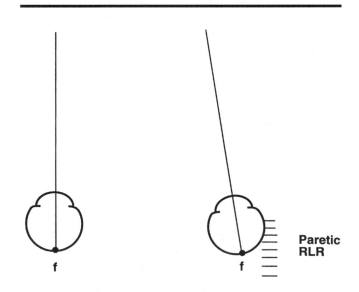

Paretic RLR

Figure 4-16—Esotropia of the right eye in a case of paresis of the right lateral rectus muscle. The nonparetic eye is fixating a distant target, revealing the primary angle of deviation.

disparity is usually greater in the case of a newly acquired paresis than in one of long duration. (There is a tendency for a noncomitant deviation of very long duration to evolve toward comitancy, but not completely comitant in almost all cases.)

If there is a difference greater than 5 prism diopters between the primary and secondary angles, a noncomitancy should be suspected. Although a lack of difference would indicate comitancy, there may be exceptions. Mild noncomitancies not caused by nerve impairment are often overlooked since they may not produce a significant difference in the deviations. Even some paretic muscles with nerve impairment etiology may show a false negative (appear normal) when they are of long duration. Conversely, a false positive (appearing to be abnormal when in fact not) finding of noncomitancy sometimes occurs in cases of uncorrected refractive errors. For example, a patient fixating with the right eye that is plano may be orthophoric, but the patient may have an eso deviation when fixating with the left eye that is 2.00 D hyperopic. In general, however, positive findings tend to be true indications of noncomitancy.

Ductions

There has been confusion in clinical terminology between "ductions" and "vergences." Technically, ductions are monocular eye movements (Table 4-7). The common interchanging of the two terms probably arose from clinicians who used the term "ductions" when they meant vergence.

Duction testing is useful when evaluating noncomitancy. It is not as sensitive, however, as version testing, but ductions can be very informative if the extraocular muscles are tested in their diagnostic action fields (Table 4-8). Each diagnostic action field (DAF) is evaluated by having the patient look in the appropriate direction. This may be either a voluntary saccadic eye movement or a following pursuit to the gaze testing point. To test the integrity of the right lateral rectus, for example, the left eye is occluded while the patient fixates a target with the right eye in

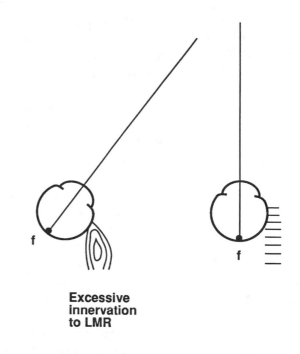

**Excessive
innervation
to LMR**

Figure 4-17—Esotropia of the left eye is illustrated in a case of paresis of the right lateral rectus muscle when the right eye is fixating. This secondary angle of deviation is much larger than the primary angle.

TABLE 4-7. Classification of Ductions and Vergences

Ductions	Vergences
Horizontal	*Horizontal*
Adduction (Nasal)	Convergence
Abduction (Temporal)	Divergence
Vertical	*Vertical**
Supraduction (Elevation)	Positive
Infraduction (Depression)	Negative
Torsional	*Torsional*
Incycloduction (Intorsion)	Incyclovergence
Excycloduction (Extorsion)	Excyclovergence
Tertiary Positions	
Dextrosupraduction	
Levosupraduction	
Dextroinfraduction	
Levoinfraduction	

*This is also referred to as vertical divergence. It is positive if the right eye elevates and negative if the left eye elevates.

right gaze. To test the right superior oblique in its DAF, the patient's right eye fixates a target that is to the left and down. Any underaction indicates a restriction, possibly due to paresis.

Distinction between a true paresis and a mechanical, or anatomical, problem is often difficult to make. In many cases, this can be ascertained by a good case history, combining results obtained from the various methods of testing and by careful observation during duction evaluation. A more involved fast eye movement that is limited probably indicates a mechanical problem. A limited and slow eye movement probably indicates paresis. A differential diagnostic procedure requiring local anesthesia to the conjunctiva is the forced duction test. If, for example, the right lateral rectus is paretic, the doctor can use forceps to hold a small portion of the conjunctiva and abduct the patient's eye. The patient's passive eye movement indicates no restriction from mechanical causes but, rather, the likelihood of paresis. To help verify a paresis, the doctor holds the patient's eye in the primary position as the patient is asked to make a voluntary saccadic movement in the DAF, right gaze in this example of RLR paresis. If no pulling (tugging) is felt by the doctor, paresis is assumed. On the other hand, if a tugging is felt and the forced duction is restricted on passive rotation, a mechanical restriction is indicated.

Versions

Versions are conjugate movements of both eyes. Testing for noncomitancy is more sensitive with versions than with ductions. This is because a change in the deviation of the visual axes from one position of gaze to another can be measured fairly precisely. This is in contrast to duction testing when only one eye is being examined; a restriction or overaction must be relatively larger to be observed. Observation of a change in the deviation under binocular seeing conditions during versions, however, is relatively easy to detect. For example, assume the patient has a mild paresis of the RLR. On duction testing the patient may be able to abduct the right eye with a large excursion, making the diagnosis of noncomitancy difficult. Dextroversion testing, however, would probably detect the restriction in the DAF of the right lateral rectus in this case, because an eso deviation would increase dramatically on right gaze.

The three objective methods of version testing ranging from least to most sensitive are: (1) direct observation; (2) Hirschberg test; and (3) the alternate cover test with prism. Each method may be used in the nine diagnostic action fields illustrated in Figure 4-12. For example, with dextroversion the DAFs are for the right lateral rectus and the left medial rectus. If the RLR is paretic, esotropia is likely on right gaze; if the LMR is paretic, exotropia is likely.

Three-step Method

The eight cyclovertical muscles are ordinarily more difficult to analyze than the four horizontally acting recti. A useful paradigm taking into account a vertical deviation was introduced by Parks[7] for identifying an isolated paretic cyclovertical muscle. The three basic steps of this method are shown in Table 4-9 for each cyclovertical muscle.

The three-step method is best explained by using as an example a known paretic muscle and then proceeding to the three differentially diagnostic steps. Suppose the patient has a paretic right superior oblique. This muscle's main action is infraduction, and secondarily intor-

---

TABLE 4-8. *Diagnostic Action Field of Each Extraocular Muscle*

Right Eye Muscle	Gaze	Left Eye Muscle	Gaze
RLR	R	LLR	L
RMR	L	LMR	R
RSR	R & Up	LSR	L & Up
RIR	R & Down	LIR	L & Down
RSO	L & Down	LSO	R & Down
RIO	L & Up	LIO	R & Up

TABLE 4-9. *The Three-Step Method*

Right or Left hyper eye in primary position	Hyper deviation greater on either Right or Left gaze	Hyper deviation greatest on either Right or Left tilt	Paretic Muscle
R	R	R	LIO
R	R	L	RIR
R	L	R	RSO
R	L	L	LSR
L	R	R	RSR
L	R	L	LSO
L	L	R	LIR
L	L	L	RIO

Key: R = right or rectus; L = left; I = inferior; S = superior; O = oblique

sion. In the primary position the superior oblique has a slight action of abduction, but this can be considered negligible for purposes of the discussion here. When the patient fixates in the primary position of gaze, the right eye is likely to have a small degree of hyper deviation. This could be either hypertropia or hyperphoria depending on the results of the unilateral cover test. The likelihood of a right hyper deviation occurring is because of weakened depressing (infraduction) action of the paretic superior oblique. The magnitude of the right hyper deviation may be estimated objectively, either by direct observation or with the unilateral cover test. For the exact measure of magnitude the alternate cover test with base-down prism before the right eye is used.

The first column of Table 4-9 lists hyper deviations of either the right or left eye. The fourth column gives the answers by listing the eight cyclovertical muscles. When there is a right hyper deviation in the case of an isolated paretic muscle, any of three other muscles besides the right superior oblique may be the cause. They are the left inferior oblique, the right inferior rectus, and the left superior rectus. A paretic left inferior oblique could cause a hyper deviation because its yoke muscle, the right superior rectus, receives excessive innervation (Hering's law). Besides that, the left inferior oblique is an elevator, and the weakened mus-

cle would cause the left eye to have a hypo deviation (relative right hyper). The same reasoning applies to a paretic left superior rectus with its yoke muscle, the right inferior oblique, receiving excessive innervation to cause a right hyper deviation. Similar explanations can be used for the other cyclovertical muscles.

The number of four possibilities can be narrowed to two by having the patient fixate in two lateral positions of gaze approximately 30 degrees each way. In right gaze, the amount of the hyper deviation is measured with the alternate cover test and base-down prism. The same procedure is performed in left gaze. If the hyper deviation of the right eye increases in left gaze, the paretic muscles are narrowed to two possibilities, right superior oblique and left superior rectus. This is because both have an isolated vertical action in left gaze.

Theoretically, the right superior oblique becomes a pure depressor only when the right eye is adducted 51 degrees, and the left superior rectus, a pure elevator, only when the left eye is abducted 23 degrees. (Refer to Chapter 1.) For clinical purposes, however, 30 degrees in each lateral gaze is a satisfactory and workable compromise. When the possibilities are narrowed to two muscles, the Bielschowsky head tilt test is necessary (Figure 4-18). The patient is instructed to tilt the head about 40 degrees toward the right shoulder. Next, the same instructions are given for head tilt to the left shoulder. An *increase* in an existing hyper deviation is the important observation. Usually the upshooting of the hyper eye is obvious on right head tilt in this example of RSO paresis. If fusion is strong and the vertical deviation remains latent, the alternate cover test must be used to dissociate the eyes and assess the hyper deviation. A subjective measurement of the hyper deviation can be misleading because the tilting itself produces a "hyper" eye that should not be confused with a true hyper deviation that can be seen objectively. Because of this artifact, subjective testing is unreliable. The examiner must make this assessment by objective means. This is best accomplished by both the examiner and the patient tilting their heads in the same direction (e.g., toward patient's right shoulder and toward doctor's left shoulder). In this orientation, the alternate cover test with prisms can be performed as though both the doctor and patient were facing each other with their heads in the upright position. A small fixation light (if testing is done at near) may be held by either the patient or an assistant since the doctor may

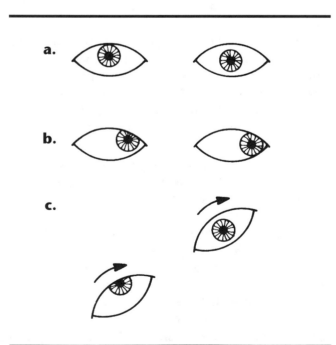

Figure 4-18—The three-step method for diagnosing an isolated paretic cyclovertical muscle. The right superior oblique is affected in this example. **(a)** Right hypertropia in the primary position; **(b)** hypertropia increases in left gaze; **(c)** further increase of the hypertropia when head is tilted toward patient's right shoulder. Arrows indicate direction of compensatory torsional movements.

require both hands to hold the occluder and loose prisms. The tip of the doctor's nose is also a convenient and satisfactory target for this purpose.

In case of a right superior oblique paresis, the hyper deviation increases with a right head tilt due to postural reflexes causing compensatory torsional eye movements. At the same time, the left eye must make an excycloduction movement. The impulse to keep the visual fields upright is compelling; that is why the head tilt test is definitive in so many cases. In the case of a right superior oblique paresis, the other intorter is called upon to help incycloduct the eye, and that is the right superior rectus. The action of this elevating muscle is the principal reason the right hyperdeviation increases with a right head tilt. Another reason involves the fellow eye. The left inferior rectus is the yoke muscle of the right superior oblique. Because of Hering's law, a hypodeviation of the left eye is produced (making the right eye relatively more hyper).

The responses of the other cyclovertical muscles on the Bielschowsky head tilt test can be analyzed similarly by accounting for the torsional action of each muscle. The rule to remember is that the superior muscles intort, and the inferior ones extort. The mnemonic expression "inferior people extort" may help in remembering the torsional actions of the eight cycloverticals. For clinical purposes, the four lateral recti have no significant torsional action.

The chief advantage of the three-step method is that it is an objective means of testing requiring little participation by the patient, other than fixating a target and tilting the head. If the patient has a large enough hypertropia to be noticeable, direct observation (with or without Hirschberg testing) may be all that is required. If the deviation is either latent (phoric) or the hypertropia is too small to discern, the alternate cover test is used.

Bajandas[8] suggested a fourth procedure for the three-step method. This involves having the patient look in upward and downward positions of gaze. If results are questionable and a clear differential diagnosis cannot be made between, for example, a right superior oblique and a left superior rectus, the downward gaze will tend to increase the right hyper and, thus, implicate the right superior oblique. Conversely, an increasing vertical deviation on upward gaze would implicate the left superior rectus. Similar reasoning applies for the other cycloverticals when analyzing this fourth step.

Because there tends to be an evolution toward comitancy (clinically often referred to as "spread of comitancy") in many cases of noncomitancy, the three-step method may give nebulous results. Therefore, it is most useful when there is a newly acquired paresis of a cyclovertical muscle, and it may not be differentiating in cases of long duration. Also, mechanical problems do not always provide a clear-cut diagnosis as in cases of newly acquired paresis. Furthermore, if more than one cyclovertical muscle is involved, the three-step method is not valid.

Recording Noncomitant Deviations

Jampolsky[9] recommended a direct and efficient system of evaluating and recording the motoric aspects of a strabismus. The objective testing and recording procedure can be divided into four parts. The evaluation is done with the patient wearing the habitual refractive correction to ascertain the current oculomotor status. If the examination indicates a significant change in refractive error, spectacles are prescribed and the patient is scheduled for an additional examination after adapting to the lenses. *Step 1:* Without correcting for head posture, the presenting deviations at far and near are measured with a prism bar or loose prisms and recorded. *Step 2:* With the patient holding fixation with the dominant eye on a distant target (6 m), the patient's head is rotated by the examiner so the eyes move to the extreme position in up, down, left, and right fields of gaze. The deviation at each horizontal or vertical position is neutralized with prisms and recorded on a diagram illustrated in Figure 4-19. If necessary, the primary deviation is again measured and recorded on the diagram without allowing the patient to assume the habitual head posture. *Step 3:* The patient's head is rotated to extreme tilted positions, right and left, and any resulting hyper deviation is measured. The results of the head tilt test are simply recorded close to the diagram. *Step 4:* The patient is instructed to follow a penlight or toy as it is moved into eight extreme DAFs. The examiner qualitatively grades any observed overaction or restriction in each field of gaze on a ranking scale as illustrated in Figure 4-20. Restrictions are graded and recorded on the diagram in the affected field of gaze. An advantage of this method of recording (compared with the Lancaster test, for example) is the direct and easy visualization of the affected fields of gaze and comitancy pattern.

Spatial Localization Testing

Patients who have a newly acquired paresis usually have spatial localization errors as evidenced by past pointing. For example, assume the right superior oblique is paretic. This muscle should be tested in its DAF (levoinfraduction). The left eye is occluded. With the right eye fixating, the patient is instructed to look at a penlight (or any suitable target) located in

OD Fixating				OS Fixating		
2 eso	5 eso	20 eso		5 eso	15 eso	35 eso
2 eso	5 eso	20 eso		5 eso	15 eso	35 eso
2 eso	5 eso	20 eso		5 eso	15 eso	35 eso

Figure 4-19—Recordings in a case of left lateral rectus paresis (examiner's view).

Grading of Restriction
of LLR

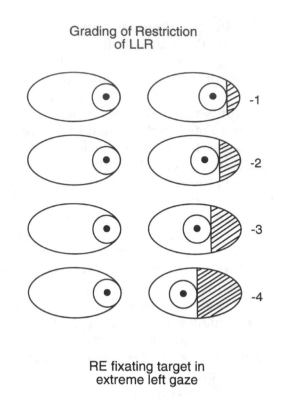

RE fixating target in
extreme left gaze

Figure 4-20—Grading of Ocular Motility on a ranking scale similar to that of Jampolsky, with –1 being the most mild and –4 being the most marked in severity.

the DAF position (to the patient's left and down) and then to touch it with an index finger. Although testing distance is not critical, approximately 40 cm is recommended. The patient is told to move a hand quickly from behind the shoulder (out of view) and to touch the light. This must be done rapidly; otherwise, judgment corrections may be made and the patient will touch the target accurately (although slowly). Unless the procedure is done correctly, localization may falsely appear to be normal. Correctional judgments of localization are learned in time; this is why sensitivity of this test diminishes in cases of paresis of long duration.

If testing is done correctly in a newly acquired case of a paretic right superior oblique, the patient will likely miss the target by pointing to the left (patient's left) of the target and below it. All 12 extraocular muscles can be tested in this manner, in the DAF of each. Clear-cut evidence of spatial localization error implicates a newly acquired paresis as the cause of noncomitancy.

Signs and Symptoms

Noncomitancy may or may not cause noticeable problems or complaints. In young children, the deviations have to be obvious before many parents will have their child examined by an eye care professional. Subjective complaints arising from noncomitancy are relatively infrequent in children under the age of 7. The situation is most often that of the parent noticing signs of intermittent deviation rather than the child complaining of diplopia. Likewise, other subjective complaints, such as nausea and vertigo, are thought to be more frequent in adults.

Diplopia

Young children complain infrequently of diplopia. We have seen many children who, when examined and asked, said, "I thought everybody sees double." The lack of life experience and their difficulty in articulating what is and what should be is one reason complaints of diplopia may not be heard from many young children who are strabismic. Another reason is that they can usually suppress the aggravating image caused by the deviation eye. This is more difficult to achieve with maturity. Most adults have trouble coping with diplopia resulting from a manifest deviation of sudden onset, such as from a newly-acquired paretic muscle. Diplopia is the main reason for the office visit. If, however, a patient has always had poor binocular vision with deep suppression, diplopia may not be noticed and would not be a warning of a newly-acquired paresis.

Abnormal Head Posture

An affected extraocular muscle can often be determined by merely observing the head posture of the patient. Interpretation of abnormal posture is made easy by realizing that the patient's face points to the same direction as the diagnostic action field (DAF) of the affected muscle (Tables 4-8 and 4-10). For example, a paretic right superior oblique causes a patient to turn the head abnormally to the left and to lower the chin. (The RSO is in its DAF when the right eye is turned to the left and down.)

Another similar rule explains why there is also an abnormal head tilt. A paretic right superior oblique, for example, causes the head to tilt toward the left shoulder in habitual natural seeing conditions. Since the RSO is an intorter, it moves the top of the eye in a leftward direction. Because the muscle is weak, the patient's head tilts in the leftward direction as compensation. The rule to remember is that the compensatory abnormal head tilt is in the same direction as the torsional movement of the eyeball that would result from the contracting muscle.

Diagnosis is complicated when more than one muscle is affected. Nevertheless, the patient is likely to have an abnormal head posture, and one that tends to be biased toward the DAF of the most severely affected muscle. Multiple pareses require careful analysis, as with the Hess-Lancaster method (discussed later in this chapter). Unlike past pointing, the mere passing of time does not tend to compensate for head posture abnormalities when the muscle (or muscles) remains paretic. Consequently, it is likely that a noncomitancy of long duration can be detected by means of head posture observation.

Subjective Testing

Subjective comitancy testing, when feasible, is usually more precise than by objective testing methods. The patient may be able to notice a very small displacement of two images resulting from misalignment of the visual axes. Small deviations are sometimes difficult for the examiner to observe, making objective testing less sensitive. This is particularly true for cyclo deviations where subjective testing must often be used for accurate diagnosis.

There are, however, disadvantages to subjective testing. This type of examination is greatly dependent on the cooperation of a capable and aware patient. An uncooperative, dull, or unperceptive patient gives either invalid or no results. Objective testing has to be relied on in such cases. The presence of anomalous retinal correspondence (ARC) also may invalidate subjective findings because the objective and subjective angles are different.

TABLE 4-10.   *Abnormal Head Posture Related to Affected Extraocular Muscles*

Muscle	Position of Face		
	Turn	Elevation	Tilt
RLR	R	—	—
RMR	L	—	—
RSR	R	Up	L
RIR	R	Down	R
RSO	L	Down	L
RIO	L	Up	R
LLR	L	—	—
LMR	R	—	—
LSR	L	Up	R
LIR	L	Down	L
LSO	R	Down	R
LIO	R	Up	L

Moreover, the subjective angle itself is often variable when ARC is present. (ARC is discussed in Chapter 5.)

Single-object Method

The traditional way to make the patient aware of pathological diplopia is by using a single target. (Refer to Chapter 1.) If the patient has an exotropic deviation, a bright penlight in a darkened room should be perceived as a double image. A deviating right eye sees the image of a light to the left of the fixated light seen by the left eye. This is heteronymous (crossed) diplopia and the type normally expected with exo deviations. On the other hand, homonymous (uncrossed) diplopia is normally expected with eso deviations. There are two rules when testing for noncomitancy using the single-object method. The patient should perceive the target seen by the deviating eye in an opposite direction from that in which the eye is deviating. An exotropic right eye sees the image to the left; an esotropic right eye sees the image to the right. The other rule is that the distance between the diplopic images becomes greater when there is an increase in either an underaction or an overaction during versions. Neutralization with loose prisms, however, can determine the direction and magnitude of the subjective angle of directionalization. This is the same as the objective angle of deviation of the visual axis *if* there is normal "retinal" correspondence (NRC).

The subjective angle of directionalization (angle *S*) can also be measured by using a black tangent screen and can be done in all nine diagnostic positions of gaze. The examiner marks on the screen the separation of the diplopic images reported by the patient. If a 1-meter test distance is used, each centimeter displacement of the images represents one prism diopter. Nevertheless, many practitioners find the single-object method confusing, because they have to think in reverse as to direction of the deviating eye and the diplopic image. This confusion is eliminated by employing the two-object method.

Two-object Method

Two fixation targets are required for this method. Special filters, usually red and green, are utilized. The right eye sees only one target (customarily through a red filter) and the left eye sees the other target (customarily through a green filter). The Hess-Lancaster test may be custom made by drawing red lines on a white board to form a grid. This is a rectangular coordinate tangent screen with a white background and red lines and red fixation spots (Figure 4-21). The red lines and spots are invisible to the eye wearing the red filter. This is because the white background is more intense than the red lines and spots; they are, consequently, washed out. They are visible, however, to the eye having the green filter. The lines and spots appear as dark gray, because the red hue is not transmitted by the green filter, but the white background is. A convenience when interpreting the results is that the directions in which the flashlights are pointed correspond to those of the visual axes. Figure 4-22 illustrates a recording chart for the Hess-Lancaster test. The separation between the lines represents approximately seven prism diopters. The fixation spots are five squares from the center; therefore, they are 35^Δ (almost 20°) laterally displaced. The spots are placed 28^Δ vertically above and below the level of the central fixation spot. Because of changing tangent values, the magnitude represented by each separation of lines is variable. The prism diopter value becomes less as fixation changes from the primary position to the periphery. In spite of this mathematical variable, it is generally unnecessary to compensate for these changes for clinical purposes. The mathematical error amounts to only one or two prism diopters within the range of the test. Fixations would have to be much greater than 35^Δ away from the primary position before tangent values would create a signifi-

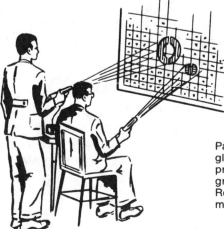

Figure 4-21—Testing procedure with the Hess-Lancaster test. The patient is instructed to place the projected green spot (seen by the left eye) on the projected red spot (seen by the right eye).

Patient wearing green and red glasses (provided) is given hand projector and directed to place green dot inside red circle. Relationship of dot to circle makes diagnosis possible.

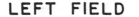

LEFT FIELD   **RIGHT FIELD**

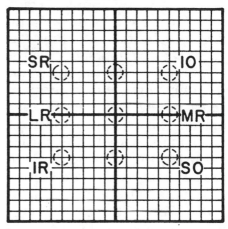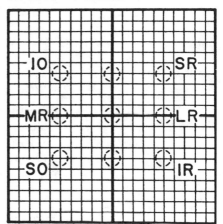

Figure 4-22—Form used for charting results of the Hess-Lancaster test. Chart on the left is used when right eye is fixating; chart on the right is used when the left eye is fixating.

cantly invalidating factor. The chart also includes the names of the 12 extraocular muscles. The location of each represents the DAF for those particular muscles.

The following procedure is recommended for performing the Hess-Lancaster test. To evaluate the right field (meaning the muscles of the right eye are to be tested) the patient puts on red-green spectacles with the red filter over the right eye. This stays in place throughout testing for both the right field and the left field. The room is dimly illuminated. While the examiner holds the green projecting flashlight, the patient holds the red one. Test distance from the patient to the center of the screen is one meter. The deviation in the primary position is measured first. The examiner projects the green light onto the central spot. The patient attempts to superimpose the projected red spot of light (being seen only by the right eye) with the green spot, which is seen and fixated only by the left eye. An exotropic, or exophoric, patient with a deviating right eye will point the red flashlight to the right of the central target to achieve the perception of superimposition of the red and green images (Figure 4-23).

If the patient is esotropic (or esophoric) the red spot should be projected to the left of the fixated green spot. The rule is that the patient projects the light in the same direction as that of the deviating eye. This is direct foveal projection; interpretation is facilitated by not having to think in reverse, as in the single-object method.

If the patient does not understand this testing procedure, often in cases of young children, it is instructive to remove the colored spectacles and ask the patient to superimpose the projected spots. Since there is no binocular demand, this should be accomplished easily. It is wise to allow the parent of a young child to watch this procedure. When the child feels confident about superimposing the spots, the red-green spectacles are put on. Since fusion is broken and the eyes are now dissociated, the visual axes must be in ortho alignment for superimposition to occur. When a deviation is present, the child will have the perception that the spots are actually superimposed on the screen, but the parent can see that they are actually separated. This observation is helpful in explaining the nature of a deviation to the parent of a child patient.

After measuring the subjective angle in the primary position of gaze, the other eight positions should be similarly tested. For right field testing, the left eye remains the fixating eye. For left field testing, however, the examiner exchanges the flashlights with the patient. The examiner directs the red spot to the central fixation circle. The patient fixates with the right eye and tries to superimpose the green spot with the red. All nine positions of gaze are measured for the left field following the procedure used in testing the right field. It is impor-

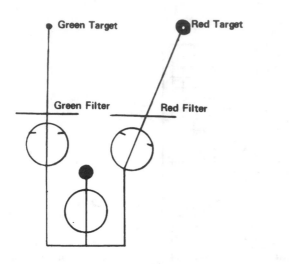

Figure 4-23—Diagram showing patient's perception of superimposition on the Hess-Lancaster test in an example of an exo deviation of the right eye. This could be either an exotropia of the right eye or an exophoria, that is decompensated by the dissociating red and green filters, and one in which the left eye is the dominant eye.

tant that the red filter remain over the right eye and the green over the left so this method can be followed consistently; otherwise, interpretation of results may be confusing. This is particularly true when two or more affected muscles are involved.

Examples are given to explain interpretation of the measured deviations. Figure 4-24 shows the charting of a paretic right lateral rectus. In right gaze the paretic right lateral

rectus is in its DAF and is underacting. The left medial rectus is in its DAF and is overacting (Hering's law). The X's represent the positions of the spots seen by the deviating eye; the circles represent the fixation spots for the fixating eye. An outline of the eight outside X's is made by connecting them to form an enclosure. The area of the enclosure of each field is compared. In this example, the right enclosure is smaller than the left. This means that the paresis causing the underaction is in the right eye. The left enclosure is larger, indicating overaction by the left eye, thus graphically illustrating the effect of Hering's law. For clarification with a contrasting example, an exotropic deviation due to paresis of the right medial rectus is shown in Figure 4-25. The area of the enclosure for the right field is much smaller than for the left. The overaction of the left lateral rectus is large when the paretic right medial rectus is in its DAF.

This method of charting is very useful when two or more muscles are affected. Figure 4-26 illustrates an example of paresis of both the right lateral rectus and the right superior oblique. Besides the similar effect of the paretic lateral rectus, there is also an underaction in the DAF of the right superior oblique, which results in an overaction of its yoke muscle, the left inferior rectus. The two underacting muscles of the right eye cause the enclosure of the right field to be much smaller

LEFT FIELD   **RIGHT FIELD**

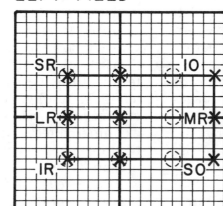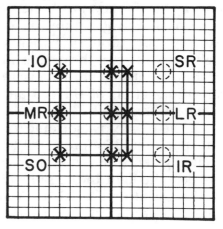

Figure 4-24—Chart of the results of the Hess-Lancaster test in the case of a paretic right lateral rectus.

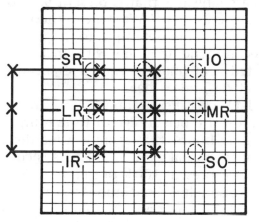

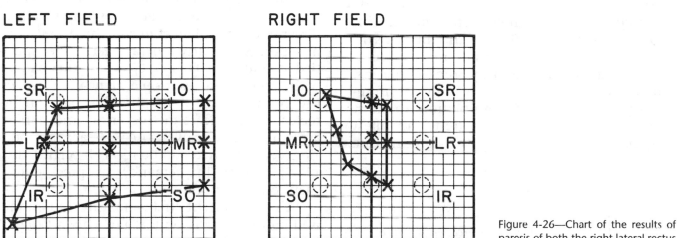

Figure 4-25—Chart of the results in the case of a paretic right medial rectus.

Figure 4-26—Chart of the results of paresis of both the right lateral rectus and the right superior oblique.

than that of the left field. Visual inspection of muscle field charting facilitates diagnosis of the affected muscles.

The Hess-Lancaster test is the most sensitive of all clinical tests for noncomitancy. There are, however, some pitfalls including ARC, deep suppression, and poor cooperation by the patient. If any of these exist, testing may have to be performed entirely by objective means. Furthermore, results of one test should confirm the results of another; therefore, it is wise to perform different types of tests on a patient when noncomitancy is suspected. Management

of cases of noncomitancy is discussed in Chapters 7, 8, and 15.

FREQUENCY OF THE DEVIATION

Next in importance to comitancy evaluation is determination of the frequency of a manifest deviation. This knowledge helps the practitioner assess the status of a patient's binocularity. For example, a patient who is strabismic 95% of the time has poorer control on bifoveal fusion than does a patient who is strabismic only 5% of the time.

Classification

Frequency refers to the amount of time a deviation is manifest. This may range from 1% to 100%. If a strabismus is not present any of the time under natural habitual seeing conditions, the patient is necessarily classified as either orthophoric or heterophoric (if there is a latent deviation of the visual axes). More patients are heterophoric than orthophoric because there is usually at least some deviation present, even though it may be small. Any latent deviation, one prism diopter or greater, is classified as heterophoria. As in strabismus, the heterophoric deviation may be horizontal, vertical, or torsional.

Strabismus is classified as intermittent if it is present from 1% to 99% of the time. A synonymous term for intermittent is "occasional." This term is used by some clinicians, but we believe it implies a state of infrequency. The semantic connotation to most practitioners is that the deviation is manifest only occasionally. This may not state the true

situation. It would be misleading, for example, to refer to a strabismus that is present 95% of the time as "occasional." We believe the term "intermittent" is more neutral as to frequency, and we recommend it along with including the estimated percentage of time a strabismus is present at far and at near.

Table 4-11 classifies frequency of strabismus, based on the percentage of time (during normal waking hours) that there is a manifest deviation of the visual axes. Strabismus is constant when it is present 100% of the time. Synonymous terms include continuous strabismus, permanent strabismus, and absolute strabismus. We prefer the term "constant."

An intermittent strabismus may be either periodic or nonperiodic. In most cases, it is the latter. If a strabismus is to be called periodic, its occurrence must be predictable and regular. A periodic intermittent strabismus may be either direct or indirect. Direct means that the strabismus occurs regularly only at near, under specified conditions. This is typically the patient with intermittent esotropia at near caused by the combination of esophoria at far, uncorrected hyperopic refractive error, and a high accommodative-convergence to accommodation (AC/A). Accommodation brought into play for nearpoint demands can precipitate a manifest deviation.

An intermittent strabismus that is periodic and indirect occurs only at far. This is typified by the patient who has intermittent exotropia at far but is exophoric at near. Such a patient usually has a high ACA ratio that allows the deviation to be less at near. At far, however, the individual may regularly lapse into an exotropia unless there is strong compensatory fusional ability.

Another cause for periodicity may be noncomitancy. For example, a patient with complete paresis of the right lateral rectus has a marked noncomitancy. This would likely result in the patient always having esotropia in right gaze.

In the majority of cases, however, the intermittent regularity of strabismus is uncertain and cannot be absolutely predicted. This is why most cases of intermittent strabismus are nonperiodic.

TABLE 4-11. Classification of Frequency of the Deviation

Constant Strabismus	100%*
Intermittent Strabismus	1% to 99%*
Periodic	
Direct (strabismus atnear)	
Indirect (strabismus at far)	
Certain cases of noncomitancy	
Nonperiodic (unpredictable intermittency)	
Nonstrabismus	0%*
Heterophoria (deviation always latent under normal seeing conditions)	
Orthophoria	

*Percentage of time the deviation is manifest

Evaluation

There are two principal ways to evaluate the percentage of time there is a manifest deviation of the visual axes: case history, and results of testing procedures.

Case History

Case history information can come from knowing how others see the patient. Parents of young children may give such reports as "cross-eyed about half the time, especially when he is tired" or "wall-eyed when she looks out the window or is daydreaming." This information is important since young patients seldom complain of diplopia.

Older children and adults may give an index to the frequency of strabismus by reporting the amount of time diplopia is noticed. This, however, is not always highly correlated with the frequency of strabismus, because the individual may use the antidiplopia mechanisms of suppression and ARC. Questioning the patient's self-perceived appearance of the eyes and the observations of family and friends must therefore be pursued.

Testing

Estimation of frequency of strabismus is not made by a rigid system of testing. Rather, it is done by using professional judgment based on impressions from case history and results of various testing procedures. Some guidelines for testing are given below.

It is better to observe the patient before dissociative testing is begun than afterwards. The eyes are not dissociated when making direct observation, either with or without the Hirschberg test.

The cover test, however, fully dissociates the eyes. When the cover is removed, any refusion movements should be noted and evaluated. A slow recovery rather than a quick recovery indicates the frequency of strabismus is relatively high.

Diplopia testing reveals the patient's ability to notice pathological diplopia. If it is easily noticed when the patient becomes strabismic, the frequency of strabismus is relatively low. If

diplopia is seldom perceived when the deviation is manifest, the frequency is relatively high. This is because compensatory fusional vergence tends to be better when suppression is less. In other words, diplopia is not likely to be noticed in most cases of constant strabismus (because of suppression and ARC).

Many other sensory and motor fusion tests (Chapters 2, 5, and 6) can contribute to the overall estimation of frequency of a manifest deviation. This estimation should be determined for far and near fixation distances.

DIRECTION OF THE DEVIATION

The direction of a deviating eye may be horizontal, vertical, or torsional, or a combination of these. Table 4-12 lists the directions in which an eye may deviate.

Classification

Horizontal deviations in the majority of cases are isolated, without a vertical or torsional component, when all strabismus and phoria cases are considered. On the other hand, vertical deviations are different in that they often have a horizontal component, e.g., esotropia with hypertropia. Torsional (cyclo) deviations al-

TABLE 4-12. *Classification of Direction of Deviation*

Deviation	Direction of Deviating Eye When Fixating Eye Is in the Primary Position
Horizontal	
Eso	Inward rotation of eye
Exo	Outward rotation of eye
Vertical	
Hyper	Upward rotation of eye
Hypo	Downward rotation of eye
Torsional	
Incyclo	Inward rotation of top of eye
Excyclo	Outward rotation of top of eye

most always have vertical and horizontal components.

Some clinicians speak only of hyper deviations, thus avoiding the term "hypo." We believe this is misleading. For example, it is preferable to call a constant unilateral downward deviation of a nonfixating right eye a "right hypotropia" rather than a "left hypertropia." In this case the left eye is the fixating eye and is not deviating upward, which invalidates the diagnosis of left hypertropia.

Testing procedures to determine the direction of deviation may be either objective or subjective (Table 4-13).

Objective Testing

When there is a manifest deviation, direct observation, the Hirschberg test, or the Krimsky test are useful if the strabismus is large enough to be noticeable. If it is either small or latent, the cover test is necessary for diagnostic purposes. Unilateral occlusion is good for detecting the direction of deviations for lateral and vertical components. It has limitations, however, for determining cyclo deviations. (Subjective methods are more sensitive.) In the case, for example, of a right exotropia combined with right hypertropia and right excyclotropia, covering the left eye would result in the following movements: The right eye would be seen to move inward and downward with the top of the eye (the 12 o'clock position on the limbus) moving inward. This is the required movement the right eye must make to go from the deviated position to the position of fixation. Unilaterally covering the strabismic right eye would result in no movement. If, however, there is an exophoria combined with a right hyperphoria and an excyclophoria, occlusion of the right eye would result in the following: the anterior segment of the right eye would drift outwardly and upwardly, and the top of the eye would rotate outwardly.

The alternate cover test is also a good method for determining the direction of the deviation. Neutralizing prisms will give the answer. When the lateral (horizontal) component is neutralized, either with base-out or base-in prism, the vertical component is then much easier to observe. If the vertical component is also neutralized with either base-up or base-down prisms, it may be possible to isolate and observe cyclo deviations as small as three degrees. Smaller cyclo deviations usually need to be detected and measured by subjective means.

Subjective Testing

The subjective angle of directionalization may be determined with two targets (e.g., Hess-Lancaster test) or, more commonly, a single target. This may be done with several methods for either phorias or tropias. The horizontal subjective angle is easily determined with the von Graefe method using vertical prism dissociation. This is done routinely in measurement of phorias in primary eye care examinations. As the patient sees the diplopic images of the single target (e.g., penlight), the examiner introduces a sufficient horizontally oriented prism, either base-in or base-out, to create vertical alignment of the two images. This is the subjective angle of directionalization.

Colored filters can be used in conjunction with the von Graefe method; or, they can be used without the vertical dissociation. If, for example, a red lens is placed before a right esotropic eye that is being suppressed, the filter creating a color difference between the eyes may serve to break the suppression. In some cases when suppression is very deep in the de-

---

TABLE 4-13. *Examples of Testing Procedures to Determine the Direction of a Deviation of the Visual Axes*

Objective Procedures
  Direct Observation
  Hirschberg Test
  Krimsky Test
  Unilateral Cover Test
  Alternate Cover Test
Subjective Procedures
  von Graefe (vertical prism dissociation)
  Colored filters
  Maddox rod
  Phi phenomenon

viating eye, the red filter should be switched to the fixating eye. This reduces the intensity of the light entering the eye and acts as a mild occluder giving an advantage to the deviating eye. In any event, assuming NRC, the patient should perceive homonymous (uncrossed) diplopia when there is an eso deviation. If the patient has an exo deviation, the perception should be heteronymous (crossed) diplopia.

The Maddox rod can also be used to determine the direction of the subjective angle. Although the original design by Maddox was a single elongated cylindrical lens, most clinicians prefer multiple rods for dissociative testing. This, however, is referred to as the Maddox "rod," rather than rods. If the Maddox rod is placed with its axis at 180 degrees (rod horizontal) before the right eye, the eye should see a vertical streak. If, for example, the patient is exotropic (or exophoric), the vertical streak should be seen to the left of the fixation light. If the patient has an esotropia (or esophoria), the vertical streak should be seen to the right of the fixation light.

Cyclo deviations require the use of two Maddox rods. If one Maddox rod is placed before the right eye with its axis at 180 degrees and another rod, with its axis at 180 degrees, is placed before the left eye, two vertical streaks may be seen (assuming a horizontal deviation is also present to prevent the superimposition of the two vertical streaks). If a cyclo deviation is not present, the streaks appear parallel. If, however, the right eye is exotropic and excyclotropic, the top of the leftward streak (seen by the right eye in this example) will appear inclined away from the vertical streak seen by the fixating left eye. In regard to the direction of the perceived slant, the rule is that the patient perceives the streak as slanting in the direction opposite to the cyclo deviation of that eye. This is illustrated and clarified in Figure 4-27.

Another subjective method to determine the direction of the deviation is the use of the phi phenomenon. This is seen when the patient perceives movement of a stationary single target during rapid alternate occlusion. The apparent movement is perceived when a deviation of the visual axes is present. The phi phenomenon is based on disparate retinal points being stimulated and not on eye movements. Refer to Figure 4-4 where the right eye is shown to be esotropic. Upon rapid alternate occlusion, the right eye can be briefly exposed by shifting an occluder from the right eye to the left eye. The fixated target will appear to move to the right (opposite movement from that of the occluder). When the occluder is shifted back to the right eye, the target will appear to move to the left (opposite direction).

In cases of exo deviations, the shift of the phi phenomenon is the same as the motion of the occluder. In vertical deviations, when the hyper eye is exposed, the apparent movement is downward. If the patient has a torsional deviation, a vertical line is used for fixation and a shift in the inclination during alternate occlusion reveals a cyclo deviation. If, for example, a patient has an excyclotropic eye, the top of the line will appear to move in the same direction as the occluder. If the eye has an incyclo deviation, the top of the line will appear to move in the opposite direction.

If there is no deviation of the visual axes, a phi phenomenon movement should not be perceived. There may also be no perception of the phi phenomenon if the alternate occlusion is too rapid so that the patient is allowed to see as though looking through the blades of a rotating fan. We recommend switching the occluder approximately every 0.5 seconds to achieve the most reliable results for the phi phenomenon.

MAGNITUDE OF THE DEVIATION

Unless otherwise specified, the magnitude of the deviation customarily refers to the angle of deviation of the visual axes when fixation is in the primary position. This should be measured for both the farpoint (optical infinity) and the nearpoint. The most frequently used fixation distances are 6 m (20 feet) for far and 40 cm (16 inches) for near. There must be careful control of accommodation, particularly at near, if measurements of horizontal deviations are to be valid (because of effects of accommodative convergence). The best objective test for measuring the magnitude of deviations for distance or near is the alternate cover test combined with loose prisms. There is an advantage of using loose

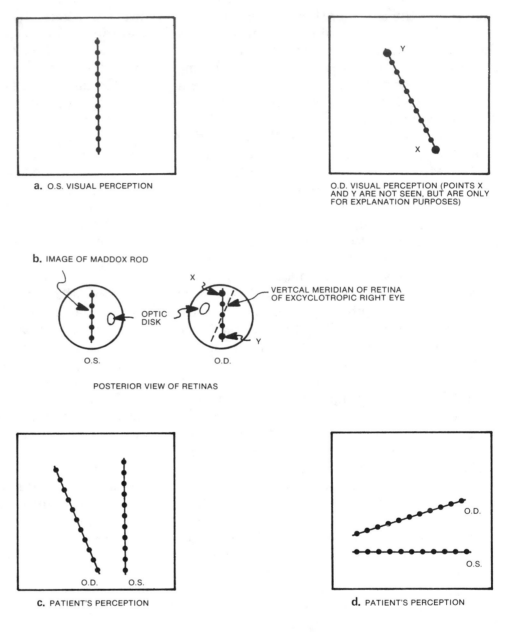

Figure 4-27—Explanation of cyclodeviation testing using Maddox rods. **(a)** The patient perceives the imaged line as being vertically oriented for the fixating left eye. However, the line seen by the right eye appears to be slanting, with the top oriented in a leftward position. **(b)** Posterior view of the eyeballs, illustrating the excyclo deviation of the right eye. The analogy of visual fields and retinal projection is used here for clarification. Point X stimulates the superior nasal retina and is therefore projected into the inferior temporal field. Likewise, point Y on the inferior temporal retina is projected into the superior nasal field. **(c)** The slanted line seen by the right eye is seen to the left of the vertical line because of a horizontal exo deviation of the right eye. **(d)** Many practitioners prefer to place the axis of the rods at 90 degrees so the patient sees horizontal streaks (in this example, by the left eye). If a vertical prism is placed base-down before the right eye, the excyclo deviation causes the perceived streak for the right eye to slant upward in the temporal field and downward in the nasal visual field. The vertical prism is necessary to create the doubling so that one line is above the other. This may be unnecessary if the patient has an existing vertical deviation.

a. O.S. VISUAL PERCEPTION

O.D. VISUAL PERCEPTION (POINTS X AND Y ARE NOT SEEN, BUT ARE ONLY FOR EXPLANATION PURPOSES)

b. IMAGE OF MADDOX ROD

VERTCAL MERIDIAN OF RETINA OF EXCYCLOTROPIC RIGHT EYE

OPTIC DISK

O.S.   O.D.

POSTERIOR VIEW OF RETINAS

c. PATIENT'S PERCEPTION

d. PATIENT'S PERCEPTION

prisms rather than prism racks because both the horizontal and vertical components of a deviation can be conveniently measured simultaneously. In addition, the prism rack is bulky making measurement of more than one component awkward. For example, to use the prisms in measuring an esotropia of the right eye that also has a hypertropia, two loose prisms, one base-out, the other base-down, are placed together between the occluder and the right eye.

Classification

Classification of the magnitude of heterophoric deviations is somewhat nebulous in that the deviation is latent and, thus, not cosmetically noticeable. Although cosmesis is not of concern, binocular function may sometimes be related to magnitude. In general, a very large deviation tends to cause symptoms and may affect performance in school, work, and play. There are many exceptions, however. For example, a small esophoria may play havoc with an individual's comfort and performance when reading if fusional divergence is inadequate and there is an eso fixation disparity. On the other hand, we have seen patients with relatively large esophoria who are comfortable and perform well at school, work, or play, possibly because of excellent fusional divergence and no fixation disparity being present. The factors discussed in Chapter 2 on vision efficiency skills must be taken into account when correlating magnitude of heterophoria with comfort and performance. Nevertheless, the magnitude classifications that follow for strabismus may also be useful as guidelines in heterophoria.

The question of what is small and large strabismus needs answering. The classification of von Noorden was cited by Press,[10] stating that acceptable surgical results in infantile strabismus are less than 20 prism diopters, which is classified as small. Unacceptable results are greater than 20^Δ, which is classified as large angle strabismus. This was based mainly on cosmetic evaluation, and we concur with the classification of large being greater than 20^Δ since the deviation is usually noticeable and may be a cosmetic problem. This is somewhat in accord with our recommendations. Classification of strabismus magnitude based on cosmetic acceptability is given in Table 4-14. Horizontal strabismic deviations greater than 20^Δ are often not acceptable cosmetically, vertical strabismus greater than 15^Δ is often cosmetically unacceptable.

Another aspect of magnitude classification is the functional cure approach (Table 4-15). The question involves the predicted outcome if nonsurgical means are used to cure the strabismus, i.e., prism or lens compensation and/or vision training procedures. An esotropia greater than 20^Δ may require surgical reduction. This is because excessive prismatic power is needed to compensate for the deviation. Comfort and cosmetic acceptance may be problems as well as fusional divergence training often not effecting the desired result in large strabismic deviations. A greater magnitude is allowed in exotropia because fusional convergence is more robust

than fusional divergence in most cases and it can usually be increased sufficiently with functional training procedures. However, patients with an exo deviation greater than 25^Δ should be considered as possible candidates for surgery. Vertical deviations cannot be improved greatly with training in most cases and they may require prismatic compensation. Hypertropia greater than 10^Δ is, therefore, considered large. These are only general guidelines for a functional description and there are many exceptions in clinical practice.

Testing Procedures

Testing for magnitude can be done with those procedures listed in Table 4-13 that determine the direction of a deviation of the visual axes. Although the magnitude may be measured by

TABLE 4-14. *Magnitude of Strabismic Deviation Considering Cosmesis (Prism Diopters)*

	Esotropia and Exotropia	Hypertropia
Small (usually acceptable)	1–15	1–10
Moderate (sometimes unacceptable)	16–30	11–20
Large (usually unacceptable)	>30	20

TABLE 4-15. *Magnitude of Strabismic Deviation Considering Prognosis for Functional Cure (with prism compensation and/or training procedures)*

	Esotropia	Exotropia	Hypertropia
Small	1–10	1–15	1–5
Moderate	11–20	16–25	6–10
Large	>20	>25	>10

subjective and objective methods, there are times when measurement by subjective means is preferable. This is because objective testing may lack necessary precision, as in cyclo deviation. Subjective testing, however, is not always reliable, especially when there is deep suppression, ARC, or the patient is a poor observer.

Subjective methods designed for the determination of the magnitude of deviation are variations of either the single-object method or the two-object method. The measuring tools are either prisms or calibrated scales. The scales may be in true space. For example, in the Hess-Lancaster test, the patient directly views the test targets and their separation can be converted into prism diopters by using the measurement lines on the screen. On the other hand, when haploscopes such as the major amblyoscope (discussed in subsequent chapters) are used, the deviation is measured from scales on the instrument.

AC/A

The accommodative-convergence to accommodation ratio (AC/A) means that for every diopter of accommodative response, a certain amount of accommodative convergence is brought into play, depending on the value of the ratio. For example, if the AC/A is 6^Δ per 1.00 D of accommodative response, a patient who accommodates 2.50 diopters will have an increased convergence of 15 prism diopters. In strabismus cases, the *calculated* AC/A is determined in the same manner as described in Chapter 3. However, a *gradient* AC/A in strabismic patients is usually not determined using phoropter measurements, but it may be arrived at by finding the effect of spherical lenses on convergence (with alternate cover testing). At the farpoint, minus lenses are used for this purpose. At the nearpoint, either plus or minus lenses will give the value. Regardless of the testing distance, the AC/A should be determined with the patient wearing full-plus farpoint refractive correction, i.e., CAMP lenses (Chapter 2).

The following is an example of the gradient method. Assume the patient has an exotropia of 15^Δ at far. A spherical lens of −2.50 D is placed before each eye in free space and the patient is instructed to focus and clear the fixation target while looking through the lenses. When the target is reported to be clear, another measurement of the angle of deviation is made (e.g., alternate cover test). If the lenses cause the angle to change from 15^Δ exo to ortho, the AC/A is 6/1. This is determined by dividing the change in magnitude of the deviation by the change of accommodative stimulus.

EYE LATERALITY

In cases of strabismus, eye laterality refers to whether only one eye is able to maintain fixation, or if either eye is able to do so. This determination should be made at far and near fixation distances. If only one eye is able to fixate, the strabismus is classified as unilateral. If either eye can fixate, it is an alternating strabismus (Table 4-16). Alternation should be classified as either habitual or forced. Habitual alternation means the patient switches fixation naturally, without being aware of doing so. Forced alternation is when the patient must be aware or instructed to alternate. The degree of forcing indicates the patient's tendency to alternate or not alternate. This important information should be included in the evaluation of eye laterality.

Evaluation is made by means such as the Hirschberg, unilateral cover test, case history, and direct observation of the patient. Judgment is made whether the patient fixates with either

TABLE 4-16. *Classification of Alternation of Strabismus at Far and Near*

Unilateral:	Strabismic right eye
	Strabismic left eye
Alternating:	Habitual alternation
	Right eye preferred for fixation
	Left eye preferred for fixation
	Forced alternation

eye (and how frequently with each) or if fixation is confined to one eye. An interesting characteristic of many strabismics is alternation of fixation upon lateral versions. The clinician can observe whether or not the patient switches fixation at the midline with lateral pursuits to the right and left. For example, in left gaze an esotropic patient may prefer the right eye for fixation, while in right gaze, the left eye may be preferred. The presence of such a midline switch should be recorded. This is often associated with infantile esotropia and/or ARC. The midline switch is also referred to as a cross-fixation pattern. Although each eye is used at various times, this is not truly an alternating strabismus in regard to switching fixation in the primary position of gaze.

EYE DOMINANCY

Eye dominancy refers to the superiority of one eye over the other. This may be in either the motor or sensory realm. Sighting tests that determine the eye preferred for fixation are examples in the motor realm. In strabismus, the terms *eye preference* and *eye dominancy* are used synonymously. The unilateral cover test can be used to determine the fixating eye in strabismus. If the deviation is large enough to be observed, the Hirschberg test is a practical means for this evaluation.

In heterophoria, where the deviation is latent and not observable except upon dissociation, sighting tests such as the hole-in-the-card test should be used. With both hands, the patient holds, at arm's length, a card having a small hole in the center and sights a distant fixation target. The clinician alternately occludes each eye to determine which eye the patient is using to sight the target.

The nearpoint of convergence is another means of determining which eye is superior in motoric functioning. The eye that stops first in following the advancing target is considered to be nondominant at least for very near fixation distances. Testing of accommodative facility (monocularly) and fixation disparity are other indices of motor dominancy (Chapters 2 and 3).

Dominancy testing in the sensory realm includes retinal rivalry, color fusion, and suppression; this applies to cases of heterophoria. In strabismus evaluation, eye dominancy is generally based on determining which eye is preferred for fixation. This should be determined at far and near, as there may be a difference when fixation distance is changed. This is an example of mixed dominancy, meaning that one eye is preferred for some functions but not for others.

In evaluation of heterophoria, eye dominancy is determined by testing for both sensorial and motoric superiority between the two eyes. In the past, great interest was shown in crossed dominancy (i.e., the dominant eye and the dominant hand being on opposite sides of the body). The relation between crossed dominancy and learning disabilities was once considered by some to be significant, although modern thinking tends to disregard this association.

VARIABILITY OF THE DEVIATION

There are many influences on tonic convergence that, in turn, affect the magnitude of a deviation. According to Maddox (Chapter 1), tonic convergence is one of the four components of convergence; the other three are accommodative, fusional (reflex), and proximal (psychic).

In cases of heterophoria, changes in tonic convergence are not obvious, unless dissociative testing is performed and the findings are compared with each other from day to day. However, significant changes in cases of strabismus may be observable and can have a striking effect on the patient's appearance when the deviation changes from being slightly noticeable to very noticeable. Cosmetic appearance of a strabismus is often the patient's greatest concern. It is important to understand this and have empathy for the patient's feelings in this regard.

Changes in the magnitude of deviation may occur for various reasons. Fatigue, emotional stress, medication, illness, and other factors may be involved. Variation in the magnitude of

TABLE 4-17. *Anatomical Factors in Cosmesis of Strabismus*

Favorable for Esotropia Unfavorable for Exotropia	Favorable for Exotropia Unfavorable for Esotropia
Positive angle kappa	Negative angle kappa
Narrow bridge of nose	Wide bridge of nose
Absence of epicanthus	Presence of epicanthus
Large interpupillary distance	Small interpupillary distance
Narrow face	Wide face

the angle of deviation may cause a latent deviation to become manifest. A case of intermittent strabismus is usually more noticeable than if it were constant. It should be noted, however, that intermittency is not usually the result of a change in tonic convergence. Intermittency, in most cases, probably involves the power of compensatory fusion, whereby a deviation may or may not be held latent.

COSMESIS

In addition to magnitude, variability, and strabismic intermittency, there are certain anatomical factors affecting cosmesis. These are listed in Table 4-17 indicating those that are favorable and those unfavorable to the appearance of patients with esotropia or exotropia.

Clinicians should not judge cosmesis exclusively on the magnitude of the deviation. All factors must be considered. For example, the recommendation to undergo surgery for cosmetic reasons may be given a patient having an esotropia of 20 prism diopters. This may not be necessary for cosmetic reasons if the patient has

a large positive angle kappa, a narrow bridge, no epicanthal folds, a large interpupillary distance, and a narrow face. Under these conditions, the eyes are likely to appear cosmetically straight. It is possible that the eyes would appear exotropic if the eso deviation were significantly reduced by means of surgery. Consequently, it is always wise to observe the patient carefully and weigh the various factors influencing appearance before reaching any conclusion regarding extraocular muscle surgery.

The effect of eyewear on cosmesis should also be taken into account. A certain spectacle frame may either help or hinder the strabismic individual's appearance. Trial of different sizes and patterns and keen observation of the patient's appearance are the rules to follow.

REFERENCES

1. Fisher NF. General principles of esotropia. *Audio Digest Ophthalmology.* 1972; 10(18); side B;Sept. 14, 1972.
2. Jones R, Eskridge JB. The Hirschberg test : a re-evaluation. *Am J Optom Arch Am Acad Optom.* 1970;47:105-114.
3. Griffin JR, Boyer F. Strabismus: measurement with the Hirschberg test. *Optom Weekly.* 1974;75:863-866.
4. Eskridge JB. The complete cover test. *J Am Optom Assoc.* 1973; 44:601-609.
5. Griffin JR, Cotter S. The Brückner test: evaluation of clinical usefulness. *Am J Optom Physiol Opt.* 1986;63:957-961.
6. Griffin JR, McLin L, Schor CM. Photographic method for Brückner and Hirschberg testing. *Optom Vision Sci.* 1989;66:474-479.
7. Parks MM. Isolated cyclovertical muscle palsy. *Arch Ophthalmol.* 1958;60:1027-1035.
8. Bajandas FJ, Kline LB. *Neuro-Ophthalmology Review Manual.* Thorofare, NJ: SLACK Inc; 1987:103.
9. Jampolsky A. A simplified approach to strabismus diagnosis. In: *Symptoms on Strabismus,Transaction of the New Orleans Academy of Ophthalmology.* St Louis: CV Mosby Co, 1971:34-92.
10. Press LJ. Topical review: strabismus. *J Optom Vision Development.* 1991;22:5-20.

Chapter 5 / Sensory Adaptations to Strabismus

Suppression   131
  Characteristics of Suppression   132
  Testing for Suppression   135
    History   135
    Red Lens Test   136
    Worth Dot Test   136
    Amblyoscope Workup   137
Amblyopia   138
  Classification   139
    Strabismic Amblyopia   140
    Anisometropic Amblyopia   140
    Isoametropic Amblyopia   141
    Image Degradation Amblyopia   141
  Amblyopia as a Developmental
    Disorder   142
  Case History   144
  Visual Acuity Testing   145
    Snellen Charts   146
    Bailey-Lovie Chart   147
    Psychometric Charts   148
    Tumbling E and Picture Cards   149
    Infant Visual Acuity Assessment   152
    Visually Evoked Potential   154

Interferometry   155
Fixation Evaluation   156
  Description of Eccentric Fixation   157
  Visuoscopy   158
  Haidinger Brush Testing   159
  Refraction Techniques   160
  Eye Disease Evaluation   161
Anomalous Correspondence   163
  Classification   163
  Characteristics   166
    Horopter in ARC   166
    Horror Fusionis   171
    Etiology of ARC   171
    Depth of ARC   172
    Prevalence   173
Testing   173
  Dissociated Red Lens Test   173
  Afterimages   173
  Bifoveal Test of Cüppers   177
  Major Amblyoscope   178
  Bagolini Striated Lenses   181
  Color Fusion   182

Several anomalous conditions can develop secondary to the onset of a developmental strabismus, particularly of early origin. These include suppression, amblyopia, and anomalous correspondence. These conditions and their appropriate testing methods are discussed in this chapter. Although it is customary to think in terms of the deviation causing these adaptive conditions, it is also possible that the process may work in reverse. In other words, the strabismus may be the result rather than the cause of the anomalous sensory conditions.

SUPPRESSION

When a strabismus occurs the individual may experience pathological diplopia and/or confusion. Suppression is usually the defense mechanism first attempted by an individual to eliminate these perceptual annoyances. *Suppression* is the lack of perception of normally visible objects in all or part of the field of vision of one eye, occurring only under binocular viewing conditions and attributed to cortical inhibition.[1] In normal binocular vision, *physiological*

Figure 5-1—Confusion and diplopia in an example of esotropia of the right eye and the resulting pathological suppression. (a) Cyclopean perception of confusion and pathological homonymous diplopia. The fixation starlike object is seen diplopically. The nonfixated circle falling on the fovea of the deviating right eye causes confusion. Although the circle could possibly be seen diplopically, it is not usually noticed since attention to it is not being paid by the patient. (b) Theoretical posterior view of the eyes showing the suppression zone that could result from the esotropic right eye. (c) Theoretical ophthalmoscopic view of the right fundus illustrating the shape and location of the suppression zone.

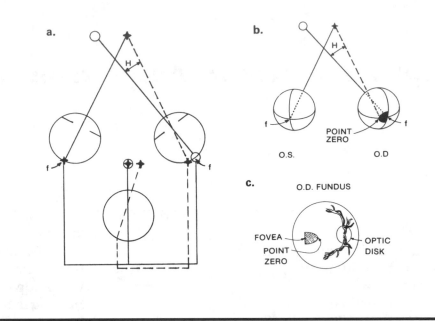

suppression naturally occurs, particularly, for all objects falling outside the singleness horopter. The suppressed image can usually be brought to consciousness by directing attention to it. On the other hand, *pathological suppression* is a binocular anomaly. In the presence of strabismus, for example, a suppressed image is not easily perceived by merely directing one's attention to it. There is, apparently, active cortical inhibition of the suppressed eye's image that may not be under volitional control. Von Noorden[2] noted that even retinal rivalry disappears in strabismic patients. Retinal rivalry (see Chapter 1) and suppression both occur in the visual cortex, although they may be mediated by other neural processes.[3]

Characteristics of Suppression

The precise neurological mechanism for suppression is not thoroughly known, but the phenomenon can be easily demonstrated by diagram. Figure 5-1 illustrates the concept of diplopia and confusion and the resulting zone of suppression. The fixation target is imaged on the fixating left eye. An esotropia of the right eye causes the target's image to fall on the nasal retina. Cyclopean projection shows the patient perceiving two images. When the diplopic image is seen on the same side as the eye that deviates (e.g., right eye seeing the diplopic image in the right field), the diplopia is called homonymous, also referred to as uncrossed diplopia. If, however, the diplopic image were to fall on the temporal retina of the deviating eye, heteronymous (crossed) diplopia would occur. For the redundant ocular image to be eliminated, the target point on the nasal retina of the right eye must be suppressed. Jampolsky[4] referred to this location as the "zero measure" point (*point zero*). This point and its adjacent area must be suppressed to avoid diplopia. Peripheral diplopia may occur if the deviation is larger than Panum's fusional areas in the peripheral binocular field, but the combined influence of low resolution, suppression, and selective attention to the fixated target usually prevents the perception of double images in these distant locations.

While point zero (the target point, sometimes designated as "T") is usually suppressed, the fovea in the deviating eye is suppressed even more intensely. If this were not the case, then two dissimilar images would be superimposed since each fovea is pointing to a different location within the binocular visual field. This intolerable situation is called *confusion*. Suppression of the fovea of the deviated eye occurs more quickly and deeply than at the target point (point zero) since foveal vision is usually the location of attention. Clinically, strabismic individuals usually do not complain of confusion, but many do have symptoms of diplopia.

It is probable that suppression begins first at the fovea when a horizontal deviation of the visual axes becomes manifest as in Figure 5-1; then, later, point zero (the target point) is also suppressed. Afterwards, a pathological zone of suppression encompasses the area between the fovea and the target point of the deviating eye. The vertical dimension of this zone is usually smaller than the horizontal. The shape of the zone resembles the letter D, according to Jampolsky[4]; and the vertical demarcation at the fovea resembles a hemianoptic visual field defect. While this is a theoretical model of the suppression zone, clinical findings suggest that these demarcations are not always that clear cut. Pratt-Johnson and MacDonald[5] showed that suppression does not exclusively involve the nasal retina in esotropes and the temporal retina in exotropes, but it may extend in both directions regardless of the direction of the deviation. The shape and size of the suppression zone depend on the targets used and how the test is performed. The suppression "scotoma" is, therefore, considered *relative* rather than absolute, appearing more extensive and deep in the hemiretina toward the target point. In some cases, however (e.g., a large-angle strabismus with amblyopia of long-standing), it appears that most or all of the binocular visual field of the deviating eye is pathologically suppressed.

How does the suppressing strabismic patient perceive visual objects in space? Such a patient does experience continuity of visual space across the visual field similar to the individual having normal binocular vision (Figure 5-2a). However, there may be a slight decrease or increase in the horizontal size of the visual field depending on whether the deviation is esotropic (Figure 5-2b) or exotropic (Figure 5-2c), respectively. Fortunately, a strabismic patient who is free of ocular pathology perceives no gaps (missing portions) in the visual field. Suppression of the turned eye only occurs within the binocular overlap area. Suppression is not obvious to the individual except indirectly, possibly because of deficient stereopsis. A vivid spatial sense of

three dimensionality is often missing, depending on the extent and depth of the suppression zone. The extreme peripheral lateral fields of each eye are, however, normal. These temporal crescents, approximately 30 degrees on each side, cannot be suppressed. The crescents are neurally subserved only by monocular fibers from the nasal retina of each eye. The suppressed eye is unresponsive to binocular stimulation but is responsive to the "monocular" stimulation of the peripheral nasal retina.

Foveal suppression may also be found in nonstrabismic patients. Anisometropia may cause image size difference on the retina of each eye (aniseikonia) and also a difference in clarity. Suppression is, therefore, necessary to eliminate the confusion arising from the resulting superimposition of dissimilar ocular images (i.e., one image being larger than the other). The suppression zone in such cases is relatively small and encircles only the fovea since there is no extrafoveal point *zero*. Therefore, confusion, and not diplopia, is the problem. Foveal suppression is also found in patients with large heterophoria if fusional vergence compensation is poor. The mechanism is not fully known, but it is likely that vergence stress and/or a large fixation disparity can possibly initiate a suppression response.

Suppression may be classified by size and intensity. In regard to size, suppression is referred to as being either central or peripheral. If a patient has central suppression, the edge of the suppression zone can extend to 5° from the center of the fovea. Beyond this limit, suppression is considered to be peripheral (Table 5-1). It must be remembered that the limits of the suppression zone depend on the testing conditions and the size of the targets used.

Intensity of suppression varies on a continuous scale from shallow to deep (Table 5-2). This is necessarily a qualitative determination. It is made by finding the ease with which suppression can be broken by utilizing various testing procedures. The more unnatural the environment (laboratory type of testing conditions), the less likely is suppression. For example, the Worth dot test using red-green filters in a dark room is relatively unnatural and serves as a strong stimulus to break through suppres-

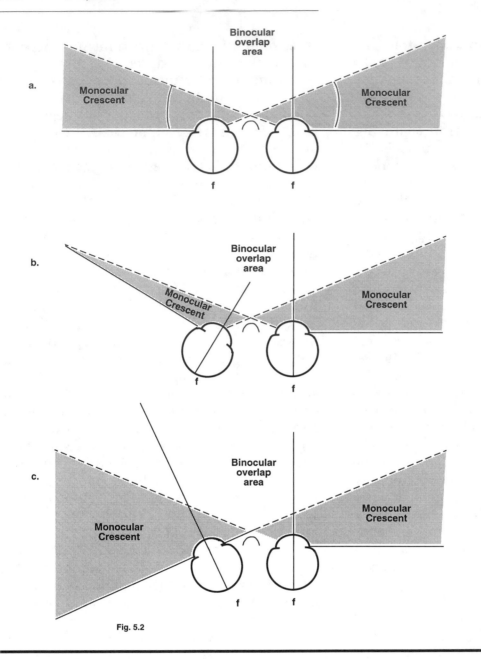

a.

Binocular overlap area

Monocular Crescent

Monocular Crescent

f   f

b.

Binocular overlap area

Monocular Crescent

Monocular Crescent

f   f

c.

Binocular overlap area

Monocular Crescent

Monocular Crescent

f   f

Fig. 5.2

Figure 5-2—Horizontal visual field limits. **(a)** Orthophoria. **(b)** Esotropia of the left eye. **(c)** Exotropia of the left eye.

TABLE 5-1. Size of Suppression Zone in Either Superimposition or Fused Targets

Classification	Separation from Target Center to Suppression Clue
CENTRAL	5° or less
Foveal	1° or less
Parafoveal	3° or less (but >1°)
Paramacular	5° or less (but >1°)
PERIPHERAL	>5°

sion. Conversely, in more natural seeing conditions (e.g., Pola-Mirror), the patient will more likely suppress an eye. Illuminated targets, such as penlight or worth lights, become less natural by lowering room illumination.

In effect, intensity is described in terms of the testing procedure that is required to break (eliminate) the suppression response. Some of the methods commonly used to test the intensity of suppression are listed in Table 5-2. The more natural tests appear at the top of the list, with the less natural following in descending

TABLE 5-2. *Tests for Intensity of Suppression*

Naturalness of Testing	Method of Testing	Instrumentation	Intensity of Suppression
Natural	Diplopia in free space	Ordinary objects	Shallow
		Penlight	
	Vectographic methods	Pola-mirror	—
—		Vis-a-Vis	
		Vectograms°	
—	Septums	Turville test	—
		Bar reading	
—	Septums with optical systems	Brewster stereoscope	—
		Wheatstone stereoscope	
—	Colored filters	Red lens test	—
Unnatural		Worth 4-dot test	Deep

order. Using this as a guide, it is reasonable to assume, for example, that a strabismic patient who notices pathological diplopia when viewing a penlight in an illuminated room has shallow suppression. On the other hand, if the room must be darkened and the patient must wear red-green filters to perceive diplopia, then the suppression would be deep.

Several attributes of the strabismic deviation affect the suppression response. Magnitude of the deviation is one. Generally, the larger the deviation, the larger and deeper is the suppression zone. The intensity of suppression, however, is not always correlated with the magnitude. It may be that a patient with a constant, small-angle esotropia will have a small suppression zone, but one that is suppressed very deeply. Another factor is eye laterality. If the strabismus is alternating, the suppression is also likely to alternate from eye to eye. If the strabismus is unilateral, suppression is confined to the deviating eye. Frequency of the strabismus is also an important variable. The more frequent the strabismus, the more likely deep suppression will be found. If anomalous correspondence (ARC) is present, these relations do not necessarily apply since ARC is also an antidiplopia mechanism that partially obviates the need for suppression.

Suppression is usually shallow in noncomitant strabismic patients. Intensity is less because the magnitude of the deviation is continuously changing as fixation shifts from one field of gaze to another. This means that point zero (the target point) is not at a fixed site on the retina; thus, diplopia is more likely to be perceived. Fortunately, the accompanying diplopia with noncomitant deviations can warn individuals of possible neurological problems that require immediate health care attention.

Testing for Suppression

The number of tests for suppression is legion. Only some of the basic methods are presented here for assessing suppression associated with strabismus. All of these, except the major amblyoscope, are readily available to the primary eye care practitioner. The patient should be wearing the correct optical correction (CAMP lenses) if needed.

History

Strabismic patients should be questioned if they notice diplopia under natural viewing conditions. Are the double images only at a particular distance or in a certain field of gaze? Are the double images present at all times or

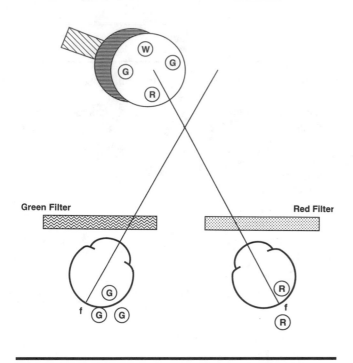

Figure 5-3—Worth 4-dot test in a case of esotropia of the left eye.

just occasionally? Is diplopia only noticed when the patient is thinking about it and ignored at other times?

Red Lens Test

The patient views a fixation light in a normally illuminated testing room at a distance where the strabismus is manifest. Ask if the patient sees one or two lights. Seeing two lights under these conditions indicates that the suppression is either relatively shallow or not present at all. If one light is reported, insert a red lens or filter before the fixating eye. Ask if the patient sees one red light (a suppression response), one pink light (a fusion response), or both the red and white (indicating diplopia). Strabismic individuals having anomalous correspondence may report seeing some variation of a pink light, simulating a normal fusion response. Patients who suppress and have alternating strabismus will report seeing the light change from red to white. If only one red light is seen, the depth of suppression can be assessed by sequentially adding other red lenses to the dominant eye to increase filter density until diplopia can be noticed. When multiple filters are necessary to elicit diplopia, deep suppression is indicated. Another method for assessing the intensity of suppression, is to dim the room light until diplopia of the penlight image is noticed. If no diplopia is seen in a dark room, the suppression can be considered to be deep.

Worth Dot Test

The Worth dot test is similar to the red lens test, but it is more popular. Red-green filters are worn by the patient over any needed spectacles. By convention, the red filter is placed before the right eye and the green before the left. The test is administered under two lighting conditions, full room illumination and in the dark. A Worth flashlight is held with the white dot (of the four dots) oriented on the top (Figure 5-3). The examiner stands across the room from the patient and asks how many lights are perceived. A report of two red dots indicates suppression of the green filtered eye. A report of three green dots means suppression of the red filtered eye. A 4-dot response suggests second-degree sensory fusion at that testing distance and under those particular test conditions. Alternate suppression is indicated if the patient reports switching between two and three lights. A report of five dots (two red and three green) indicates diplopia. The examiner notes the response at far and then slowly moves toward the patient. The patient reports any changes in the perception of the dots as the examiner advances the Worth flashlight to 10 cm from the patient. It is customary to record the patient's responses at least at far (6 m) and at 40 cm. If the initial test was done with the room lights on, it is again repeated with the lights off.

The interpretation of test results can be complex. The Worth dot test at far assesses central sensory fusion because the angular subtense of the dots is less than 10°. As the flashlight is advanced toward the patient, peripheral fusion can be assessed. Also as the flashlight is moved forward, the intensity of the lights on the retina increases, which tends to overcome suppression. For these reasons, the Worth dot test at near, particularly in a dark room, is a strong stimulus to break suppression. The clinician must also consider any change in the patient's strabismic deviation from distance to near that has previously been measured on the cover test. Another problem in interpretation is that a light is not a good stimulus for accommodation, and therefore an accommodative response may be inadequate thereby affecting the magnitude of strabismic deviation. It must also be recognized that red-green filters tend to dissociate the eyes and may cause a latent deviation to become manifest. Dark room conditions exaggerate this tendency because the only effective fusion stimulus is the small, single, white dot. Despite these complications, an experienced clinician can obtain much information about a patient's suppression and sensory fusion. For example, suppose that a patient has a comitant, intermittent exotropia of 15^Δ at far and 18^Δ at near. In a lighted room, the Worth dot responses are 3 dots at far and 4 dots at near. These responses indicate that the patient is suppressing the red filtered eye at far but sensorily fusing at near. In the dark room, the report is 5 dots at far and at near. The patient is showing a relatively shallow central suppression. This is indicated by suppression at far in the lighted room with a small retinal image and diplopia in the darkened room. Inadequate fusional convergence is also indicated if there was the fusion response at near in a lighted room, yet fusion was broken in a darkened room.

Amblyoscope Workup

The major amblyoscope (e.g., Synoptophore) has the advantage that various targets can be placed precisely at the strabismic angle of deviation. Superimposition, flat fusion, and stereofusion targets (i.e., first-degree, second-degree, and third-degree, respectively) are used to assess the patient's sensory fusion ability. If the patient has second-degree fusion, vergence ranges can be measured relative to the strabismic angle. In addition, the extent and intensity of suppression can be easily evaluated.

The Synoptophore (Clement Clarke) is one of the most popular major amblyoscopes (Figure 5-4). Each tube of the Synoptophore has a mirror placed at 45° and a +7 diopter eyepiece lens. Test targets are placed at optical infinity. Figure 5-5 shows the direction of movement of a carriage arm to create base-in and base-out prism demands. Typical first-degree (superimposition) targets for sensory fusion assessment are shown in Figure 5-6 and

second-degree in Figure 5-7. The carriage arms are aligned to the patient's measured subjective angle of directionalization (discussed later in this chapter).

Initially, superimposition targets are placed in the amblyoscope with the illumination equal for the two eyes. If one of the targets is not seen, suppression is indicated. Regarding suppression zone size, slide G48 (the fish tank) subtends angular dimensions of 1.5° vertical and 2° horizontal and are useful for foveal and parafoveal suppression testing (see Figure 5-6). The G2 slide (sentry box) subtend angles of 15° vertical and 9.5° horizontal. The soldier and the house slides, therefore, are useful for testing peripheral suppression. The other superimposition targets in these examples, X and square, test for foveal suppression.

An excellent example of second-degree targets containing both peripheral and central suppression clues are those illustrated in Figure 5-7. Again, the targets are placed in the amblyoscope at the subjective angle with the illumination equal for the two eyes. A normal fusion response would be the report of seeing a single bug having 4 wings and 3 dots on its body. Any missing dots would indicate central suppression, and missing wings would indicate peripheral suppression. If suppression is noted, intensity can be assessed by simply changing the relative illumination of the targets. The target of the dominant eye can be dimmed until the patient sees the missing clues with the suppressing eye. The larger the difference in illumination between the two eyes, the deeper is the suppression. Flashing and moving the suppressed target can also provide an index to the intensity of suppression. (These methods for breaking suppression are discussed under therapy procedures in Chapter 12.) Subsequent to this evaluation, the extent and depth of the suppression zone are recorded.

When third-degree fusion slides are employed, the targets should be positioned again at the patient's subjective angle. If stereopsis is not perceived, suppression should be suspected. Some patients, however, have been found to be stereoanomalous, where a certain class of stereodisparity detectors (e.g., crossed disparity detectors) is congenitally missing; this is independent of suppression.

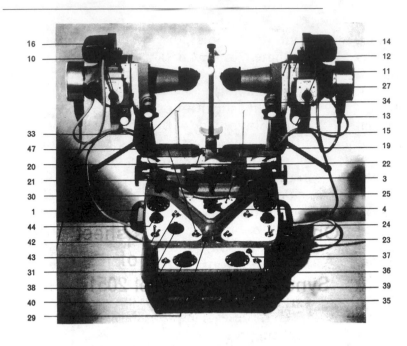

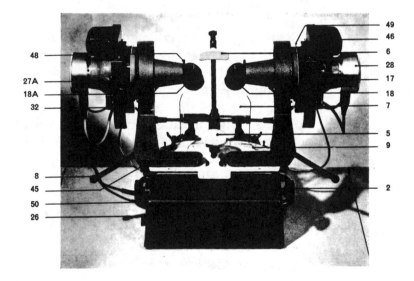

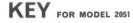

MECHANICAL

1. Carrying handles (2).
2. Interpupillary distance selection controls (2).
3. Interpupillary distance scale.
4. Chinrest height control.
5. Chinrest.
6. Forehead rest.
7. Breathshield.
8. Handles for adjustment of horizontal angle between tubes (2).
9. Horizontal deviation scales (2).
10. Vertical deviation scales (2).
11. Vertical deviation controls (2).
12. Torsional deviation scales (2).
13. Torsional deviation controls (2).
14. Elevation and depression scales (2).
15. Elevation and depression controls (2).
16. Slide carriers (2).
17. Slide ejectors (2).
18. Auxiliary lens holders (2).
18A. Eyepiece lens (removable) (2).
19. Horizontal vergence scale.
20. Horizontal vergence controls (2).
21. Tube locking controls (horizontal) (2).
22. Central lock.
32. Lever for swivelling opal screen from optical pathway (2). (Model 2052 only.)

ELECTRICAL

23. On/Off switch.
24. Mains current input plug and socket.
25. Indicator lamp.
26. Voltage selector.
27. 6V. Lampholders (slide illumination) (2).
27A Lamphouse locking lever (2).
28. 12V. Lampholders (after-images and Haidinger's brushes).

29. Hand flashing switches (2).
30. Dimming rheostats (2).
31. Selector switch.

33. Plug and socket connections to 6V. lamps (2).
34. Plug and socket connections to 12V. lamps (2).

Automatic Flashing (Models 2051 and 2052 only).

35. Automatic flashing unit.
36. On/Off switch.
37. Indicator lamp.
38. Rapid/Variable switch.
39. Simultaneous/Alternating switch.
40. Light and dark phases controls (2).
50. Fuse.

Haidinger's brushes (Model 2051 only).

42. On/Off switches.
43. Reversing switches (2).
44. Speed controls (2).
45. Plug and socket connections to motors (2).
46. Motors and rotating polaroid discs (removable from instruments) (2).

47. Haidinger's brush illumination switches (2).
48. Blue filters (removable) (2).
49. Iris diaphragms (2).

Figure 5-4—Clement Clarke Synoptophore Model 2051 with key for labeled parts. (Courtesy of Clement Clarke.)

AMBLYOPIA

Amblyopia is defined as the condition of reduced visual acuity, usually unilateral, not correctable by refractive means and not attributable to obvious structural or pathological ocular anomalies.[6] The word *amblyopia* literally means "dullness of vision." In general, best correctable visual acuity worse than 20/30 (6/9) is considered to meet a descriptive criterion for amblyopia. Generally speaking, amblyopia of 20/30 - 20/70 is mild (shallow); 20/80 - 20/120 is moderate; worse than 20/120 is marked (deep).

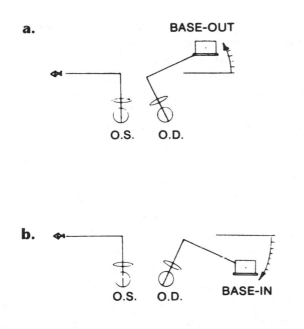

a.

BASE-OUT

O.S.   O.D.

b.

O.S.   O.D.   **BASE-IN**

Figure 5-5—Schematic of a major amblyoscope. (**a**) Carriage arm moved toward examiner results in a base-out demand. (**b**) Carriage arm moved away from the examiner results in a base-in demand.

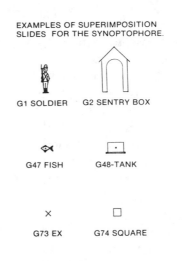

EXAMPLES OF SUPERIMPOSITION
SLIDES FOR THE SYNOPTOPHORE.

G1 SOLDIER   G2 SENTRY BOX

G47 FISH   G48-TANK

G73 EX   G74 SQUARE

Figure 5-6—Superimposition (first-degree fusion) slides used in the Synoptophore. G1 and G2 test for peripheral suppression. G47 and G48 test for parafoveal suppression. G73 and G74 test for foveal suppression.

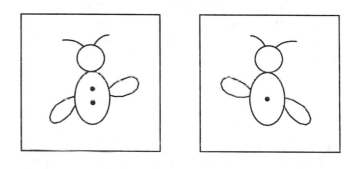

Figure 5-7—Target designed to test second-degree fusion while monitoring peripheral suppression (wings) and central suppression (dots).

Amblyopia is also defined by a difference in visual acuity between the two eyes. For clinical purposes, if the acuity difference is two lines of letters on the Snellen chart, amblyopia of the poorer eye may be present. For example, if the better eye is 20/15 (6/4.5) and the poorer eye is 20/25 (6/7.5), this aspect of the definition is met. Ciuffreda, Levi, and Selenow[7] make the important point that amblyopia is not merely any reduction of visual acuity, but the etiology of the acuity loss must be some recognized amblyogenic factor, e.g., constant unilateral strabismus, anisometropia, or high refractive error bilaterally (isoametropia). Amblyopia refers to a developmental loss of acuity during early childhood due to one or more of the above etiological factors. For consistency with health science classifications, amblyopia needs to be described by the etiological factors.

The prevalence of any condition depends on how the condition is defined and the sampling characteristics of the surveyed population. For these reasons, there is considerable variation in the reported prevalence of amblyopia in the professional literature. In a major review of the topic by Ciuffreda, Levi, and Selenow,[7] their most accurate estimates were 1.6% for military personnel, 1.8% for preschool and school-aged children, and 2.3% for clinical patients seeking vision care.

Classification

Amblyopia is usually considered to arise from a deprivation of form vision, abnormal binocular interaction (i.e., suppression), or both during early development, probably before 7 years of age. The form deprivation can be either unilateral or bilateral, but most often occurs unilaterally. Those patients in whom visual acuity is reduced significantly due to obvious ocular disease, or if there is proven pathology in the visual pathways, are classified as having *low vision,* in contradistinction to amblyopia. *Organic amblyopia,* rather than low vision, is the term customarily used in certain cases of reduced vision in which ocular pathology is not obvious (even though there may be a small central scotoma in some cases). Examples include a reduction of acuity from nutritional, tobacco, alcohol, salicylates, and other etiologies. Another type of reduced visual acuity that is often referred to as *psychogenic amblyopia* is due to causes such as hysteria or malingering. It is fairly common in children and adolescents, and sometimes in adults, who are in stressful situations. Perimetric studies usually reveal tubular fields. This text, however, will discuss developmental amblyopia due to form deprivation and suppression rather than organic and other causes of reduced visual acuity.

A current classification system for amblyopia is based on the specific etiology of the condition: strabismic amblyopia, anisometropic amblyopia, isoametropic amblyopia, and image degradation amblyopia.

Strabismic Amblyopia

Amblyopia may occur as a result of long-standing suppression when there is constant unilateral strabismus at all viewing distances during early childhood. The foveal area is suppressed to prevent confusion. Subsequently, there is active cortical inhibition of point zero (target point) in the deviating eye and often the entire binocular overlap area in the amblyopic eye. Stereopsis is usually severely reduced or absent in strabismic amblyopia. The suppression mechanism may be similar in strabismic and anisometropic amblyopia, but it may be more intense in strabismic amblyopia. The acuity loss in strabismic amblyopia tends to be worse than in anisometropic amblyopia, but the severity of amblyopia is not consistently correlated with the size of the strabismic deviation.[8] When both conditions coexist, strabismus and anisometropia, the amblyopia tends to be deeper than if only one of the conditions is present.

Since constant unilateral esotropia is much more prevalent than constant unilateral exo-

tropia, amblyopia is more frequently associated with esotropia. Most esotropic patients have constant strabismus and most exotropes are intermittent. Helveston[9] found amblyopia in 80% of his sample of esotropes, but only 17% of the exotropes were amblyopic. If reduced unilateral acuity is associated with intermittent strabismus, in the absence of anisometropia, the clinician should suspect an organic cause.

Strabismic amblyopia is highly associated with eccentric fixation. When the amblyopic eye is forced to pick up fixation, the time-averaged position of fixation is not the fovea, but an extrafoveal point. The patient's sense of "straight ahead" or oculocentric direction has also shifted to the extrafoveal point or area used for fixation; this may be why eccentric fixation initially develops.

Anisometropic Amblyopia

Some clinical studies indicate that anisometropia is the most common cause of amblyopia.[9,10,11] However, a more recent retrospective study of 544 amblyopes by Flynn and Cassady[12] that assessed microtropia found pure anisometropic amblyopia to be the least prevalent type. They reported 20% due solely to anisometropia, 48% were purely strabismic, and 32% were both anisometropic and strabismic. Anisometropia deforms foveal images in a different way than strabismus. In strabismus the two foveas are presented with two different images (confusion), a disparity of form perception, thus causing suppression. In anisometropia, the suppression is less intense; the dissimilarities of the foveal images are in relative clarity, size (aniseikonia), and contrast.

The amount of anisometropia directly influences the depth of amblyopia and its incidence. One diopter difference in refractive error is considered to define anisometropia, but this amount does not usually cause amblyopia to develop. However, Tanlamai and Goss[13] found an incidence of 50% for hyperopic anisometropes of 2 diopters and 100% incidence for 3.5 diopters or greater. Most investigators have found a strong correlation between the amount of hyperopic anisometropic and severity of amblyopia.[4,14,15] It is, however, possible for a patient with only a small amount of anisometropia and no strabismus to have deep amblyopia.[16]

Myopic anisometropia does not generally result in deep (or as prevalent) amblyopia as does the hyperopic variety. The uncorrected hyperopic anisometrope typically focuses to the level of the least hyperopic eye, leaving the more hyperopic eye permanently deprived of a clear image. The uncorrected myopic anisometrope, on the other hand, often alternates fixation, since each eye is independently in focus at a different near distance. Tanlamai and Goss[13] reported the incidence of 50% amblyopia among myopic anisometropes of 5 diopters and 100% incidence for those 6.5 diopters and greater. If reduced unilateral visual acuity is found associated with a small degree of myopic anisometropia (e.g., OD: −2.00 20/60 and OS: plano 20/20) and strabismus is absent, then the clinician should suspect an organic or other cause of reduced acuity until proven otherwise.

Generally, anisometropic amblyopia is not highly associated with eccentric fixation, although there are many exceptions. In most cases, the fixation is central, but unsteady. There appears to be increased spatial uncertainty regarding visual direction, but the time averaged position of fixation usually is not shifted away from the fovea.

Uncorrected astigmatic anisometropia of 1.50 D cylinder or greater early in life can also result in amblyopia for sharp contours in the deprived meridional orientation. *Meridional amblyopia* is usually not severe. Patients frequently show significant improvement after a few weeks or months after wearing the appropriate spectacle or contact lens correction. Part-time occlusion of the dominant eye often promotes rapid progress in these cases.

Isoametropic Amblyopia

This form of amblyopia is relatively rare, about 0.03% of army draftees.[17] It is secondary to high symmetric refractive error (hyperopia, myopia, and/or astigmatism) that remained uncorrected

TABLE 5-3. Common Causes of Image Degradation Amblyopia
Congenital cataracts
Ptosis
Corneal opacities
Other media opacities
Occlusion (iatrogenic cause)

during early childhood before age 7 years or so. These patients typically have a mild impairment of acuity, 20/30 to 20/70, in each eye when the ametropia is first optically corrected.[18] Due to the bilateral nature of this type of amblyopia, it is usually detected earlier than anisometropic amblyopia, since the child cannot see clearly with either eye. Because the images are equally blurred, there is little or no suppression.[19] This is probably why, in part, the effect of a bilateral loss of acuity is less severe than with anisometropia and, consequently, the condition usually responds well to vision therapy. Fortunately, visual acuity often improves spontaneously after wearing spectacles or contact lenses for a few weeks or months. Vision training often proves useful too and, frequently, normal or almost normal visual acuities are achieved.

Image Degradation Amblyopia

Reduced vision caused by a physical obstruction to clear vision during early childhood resulting in severe light and form stimulus deprivation may be referred to as *image degradation amblyopia*. The most common cause is congenital cataracts that are removed much later in life (Table 5-3). Because of abnormal binocular interactions, unilateral light or form deprivation results in deeper amblyopia than binocular deprivation for the same time period.[20] Stimulus deprivation of one or both eyes before age 1 can lead to profound and permanent visual acuity loss as well as nystagmus. Early and effective treatment is absolutely critical for remediation of acuity.

Amblyopia as a Developmental Disorder

Amblyopia may be considered to be a developmental disorder of spatial vision caused by some type of visual form deprivation during early childhood.[21] If anisometropia, strabismus, or other causes of form deprivation occur relatively late in life, amblyopia does not develop. If there is no impedance to clear retinal imagery or binocular coordination of the eyes, visual acuity develops quite rapidly from the time of birth. There is a rapid increase of (Visually Evoked Potential) acuity to near-adult levels within 8 months of age, which actually reaches an adult level by 13 months.[22] The receptive field organization of foveal vision (retinal, LGN, and cortical) undergoes a little understood process of neural tuning to higher spatial frequencies of contours at all orientations in the environment. However, the consolidation of these neural processes takes considerable time, probably 5 to 7 years. Anisometropia, constant strabismus, high refractive error, and visual form deprivation can all interrupt the normal process of acuity development and consolidation within this time period.

Nearly a century ago, Worth[23] referred to the acuity loss due to lack of development as *amblyopia of arrest* and the acuity loss due to interference with consolidation as *amblyopia of extinction.* He believed the former to be irrecoverable by patching or other therapy and the latter to be reversible through proper treatment. This view of amblyopia still strongly influences many clinicians and scientists alike, although aspects of it do not seem to be supported by recent evidence. Although there is significantly more information on the specific nature of the visual deficits in amblyopia, Worth provides a conceptual framework that still guides clinical decisions, for better or worse, and serves as a reference for addressing research questions.

Reduced visual acuity is the best known clinical feature of amblyopia. There does not appear to be a leveling or dip of acuity at the fovea as once was thought. In most cases, acuity still peaks at the fovea as with the normal eye; however, the resolution capacity of the peak is lower. The resolution capacity of peripheral retinal re-

TABLE 5-4. Visual Deficiencies Associated with Amblyopia

Sensory Testing:
   Decreased visual acuity
   Decreased contrast sensitivity for fine detail
   Spatial uncertainty
   Monocular spatial distortion
   Increased perception and reaction times
   Suppression
   Reduced stereopsis

Motor Testing:
   Unsteady fixation: increased drift amplitude
   Eccentric fixation
   Defective saccades: increased latency, reduced
      peak velocity, inaccuracy
   Defective pursuits: jerkiness
   Reduced and asymmetric OKN responses
   Subtle afferent and efferent pupillary defects
   Defective accommodation: increased latency,
      inaccurate dynamic responses, inconsistent
      responses, poor sustaining ability
   Deficient accommodative convergence with the
      amblyopic eye fixating
   Deficient or absent disparity vergence

gions in an amblyopic eye, on the other hand, is approximately the same as in the nonamblyopic eye. The implication is that the foveal receptive field organization in amblyopia is coarser than normal due in part to lack of development.

Reduced visual acuity is not the only visual deficit found in amblyopia (Table 5-4). A large body of research data has accumulated in recent years describing visual characteristics in various types of amblyopia. Ciuffreda, Levi, and Selenow[24] wrote an extensive, in-depth analysis of the literature. They regard amblyopia as a developmental anomaly involving primarily those cortical mechanisms involved in form and shape perception. There is insufficient evidence supporting the concept of "receptor amblyopia," i.e., a fundamental defect in retinal rods and cones. A defining defect in both strabismic and anisometropic amblyopia is reduced photopic contrast sensitivity for high spatial frequencies (i.e., fine detail), with little or no loss at low spatial frequencies (i.e., coarse forms). This loss of contrast detection for fine detail in central vision increases with the severity of the amblyopia and appears to have a neural basis, rather than, for example, optical or oculomotor. In anisometropic amblyopia, this deficit persists throughout the binocular visual field of the amblyopic eye, which is consistent with retinal image defocus. In strabismic amblyopia, however, the deficits in contrast sensitivity are often asymmetrically distributed across the visual field in a way consistent with the pattern of suppression found in strabismics.

Amblyopia is also characterized by marked spatial uncertainty according to a review by Ciuffreda, Levi, and Selenow.[24] The amblyopic eye has a relative inability to judge position, width, and orientation of detailed forms. In anisometropic amblyopia, the loss in spatial judgment is consistent with the reduced resolution and contrast sensitivity of the amblyopic eye. In contrast, strabismic amblyopes show an extra loss in positional acuity, often accompanied by monocular distortions (i.e., contractions and expansions) of space perception. The reviewers suggested that this intrinsic cortical spatial distortion in strabismic amblyopia may be due either to loss of neurons or to scrambling of signals secondary to the abnormal binocular interactions found in constant developmental strabismus. One interesting implication of this concept is that there may be a causal relation between ARC, monocular distortions, and eccentric fixation in strabismic amblyopia.

A survey of anatomic and physiologic studies of the visual pathways of animals and humans with amblyopia indicates markedly disturbed cortical function.[24] In anisometropic amblyopia, the specific cortical dysfunction appears related to those neurons subserving contrast sensitivity. In strabismic amblyopia, there is a dramatic loss of cortical connections for the amblyopic eye. The LGN often shows shrinkage of cells in layers connecting the amblyopic eye, a defect believed to be secondary to the cortical changes through retrograde degeneration. Electroretinogram (ERG) studies suggest that retinal abnormality is not a fundamental characteristic of amblyopic eyes. Amblyopia apparently results from the effects of at least two mechanisms during early visual development: (1) cortical competition for connections from the two eyes, and/or (2) cortical inhibition (suppression) when there is asymmetric binocular input to cells.

Besides the sensory deficits in visual acuity, contrast sensitivity, and spatial temporal processing, an amblyopic eye has several deficiencies in monocular eye movements, some of which are characteristic of the condition. One characteristic feature found in most amblyopic eyes is an unsteady fixation pattern. Normal fixation appears steady only by gross inspection. With magnification, normal fixation is seen actually to be composed of microdrifts from perfect fixation, corrective microsaccades, and physiologic tremor. The abnormal component of micro eye movements in an amblyopic eye appears to be the microdrifts that have an increased amplitude and velocity.[25] Flom and Schor[26] proposed that there is an increased "dead zone" for corrective saccades in amblyopia. There is reduced detection of a fixation error so the amblyopic eye drifts from foveal fixation farther and faster (due to increasing velocity with distance) than a normal eye. Therefore, one component to reduced visual acuity in amblyopia can be the reduced and variable resolution of nonfoveal retinal points.

Eccentric fixation is considered to be an extrafoveal time-averaged position of fixation. Rarely does one find a perfectly steady eccentric fixation pattern in strabismic amblyopia when fixation is attempted with the amblyopic eye. In most cases of strabismic amblyopia, unsteady eccentric fixation is the usual observation. It is also seen, unexpectedly, in some patients solely having anisometropic amblyopia. In cases of eccentric fixation, patients believe they are looking directly at the target, although they are, in fact, fixating with an extrafoveal point or area. The principal visual direction (PVD) of the amblyopic eye (also called the straight ahead direction) has shifted away from the fovea. The monocular spatial distortions found in strabismic amblyopic eyes described by Bedell and

Flom[27] may be the pathophysiologic basis for an eccentric fixation pattern. The monocular spatial distortions occur only when both amblyopia and strabismus are present; they have not been found in amblyopes without strabismus or strabismics without amblyopia.[28,29]

Saccadic and pursuit eye movements of an amblyopic eye are usually defective as one might suppose. In amblyopic eyes, three abnormalities of the saccadic system have been reported: (1) increased latency, (2) reduced peak velocity, and (3) dysmetria (inaccuracy). The increased latency (slower reaction time) often exceeds 100% and is considered by Ciuffreda et al.[24] to reflect a slowing in the sensory pathways that process visual information subsequently used by the oculomotor system in generating saccadic eye movements. Large horizontal and vertical saccades of an amblyopic eye are usually hypometric (undershoots), multiple, and variable. Pursuit eye movements of an amblyopic eye often break down into a series of saccades suggesting reduced and variable gain in the neurologic control process. Consistent with these anomalies, the OKN responses of an amblyopic eye often appear defective since they are composed of both saccadic and pursuit components. An asymmetry in the OKN responses may be seen in strabismic amblyopia. For example, temporalward stimulation of the amblyopic eye may show a reduced response compared with nasalward stimulation.

The triad responses of accommodation, pupil, and accommodative convergence are also affected in amblyopia. Both static and dynamic accommodation show response abnormalities. One would expect, therefore, that accommodative vergence responses with the amblyopic eye fixating would be correspondingly reduced. There is research evidence supporting this prediction.[30] With regard to dynamic accommodation, response abnormalities include increased latency, reduced gain, increased response variability, and poor sustaining ability.[24] The site of the accommodative dysfunction seems to be in the sensory controller rather than the motor controller. Besides the sensory deficit, accommodation responsivity is further reduced by such factors

as abnormal fixational eye movements, defective contrast sensitivity, and eccentric fixation. Fortunately, the deficient accommodative responses found in amblyopia can usually be improved significantly with vision training.

There are often subtle afferent pupillary defects in many amblyopic eyes; response latencies may be increased and amplitude decreased.[24] Clinical testing with a penlight can, in many cases, indicate an afferent defect as seen with the swinging flashlight test. There is evidence that these defects normalize with successful amblyopia therapy.[31,32]

Fusional or disparity vergence is often found deficient or absent in cases of amblyopia.[30,33,34] The deficient disparity vergence responses appear to be related to the depth and extent of suppression associated with amblyopia and strabismus. Strabismic individuals having defective disparity vergence frequently substitute accommodative vergence to shift their eyes to a new target position.

Case History

An in-depth case history should be conducted on every amblyopic patient. Diagnostic conclusions often depend on this evidence. Questioning should relate to strabismic history, refractive history, and social history.

The time of onset of amblyopia often coincides with that of strabismus; therefore, it is vitally important to know the age of onset of the strabismus. In general, the earlier the onset and the later the therapeutic intervention, the deeper the amblyopia and the more difficult it is to treat successfully. Eccentric fixation is also less likely to develop if the onset is after the child is 3 years old.

The mode of onset of strabismus can influence the prognosis. A constant strabismus from the onset is more likely to produce deeper amblyopia than one that is intermittent. The depth of amblyopia is probably related to both the duration and intensity of suppression, which would be greater in a constant deviation at all distances. Another important question regarding mode of onset is concerned with eye laterality, i.e., was the strabismus unilateral or alternating? As a

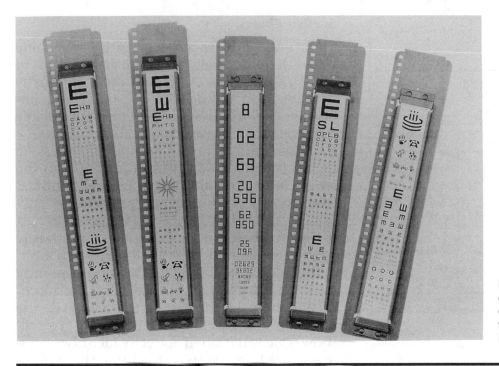

Figure 5-8—Examples of a Snellen chart designs in which there is neither an adequate number of larger letters compared with smaller letters nor is there control for interletter spacing.

rule, if the child alternates, the likelihood of amblyopia diminishes. Even in some esotropic cases that appear to be unilateral in onset, a child may use a form of alternation. Some esotropic infants and children learn to cross fixate without any alternation in the primary position of gaze. For example, a constant unilateral left esotropic eye may be used to view objects in the right field of gaze. Each eye, consequently, gets adequate visual stimulation monocularly to prevent the development of amblyopia.

Previous treatment should be questioned very carefully. If occlusion was prescribed, try to establish if the wearing schedule was adhered to faithfully. Frequently, careful questioning reveals that patching was done only as a token gesture. If extraocular muscle surgery was performed, complete information about the strabismic deviation before and after the operation should be obtained, if possible. The duration of amblyopia can be assumed to be about the same as the length of time the patient has had a constant unilateral strabismus. It is unlikely that amblyopia developed during the period of time the strabismus was either intermittent or alternating.

The two most important factors from the case history in determining the prognosis for successful treatment of amblyopia are the best estimate of the time of onset and the time appropriate treatment for amblyopia began. Table 5-5 summarizes theoretical prognostic expectations based on these factors that reflect our clinical experience in working with patients. The later the onset of amblyopia, the less profound is the loss of acuity during the critical period of acuity development. The earlier the appropriate treatment begins after the onset of amblyopia, the better and faster is the outcome. The importance of early detection and treatment of amblyopia can not be over emphasized. We recommend that all children have a complete eye examination within the first year of life to check for the host of visual conditions that can affect visual development.

Visual Acuity Testing

Departure from customary visual acuity measuring is often required when an amblyopic eye is being tested. This is because of the wide variation of responses when an ordinary chart of Snellen optotype is employed.

TABLE 5-5. Prognostic Factors in Amblyopia from Case History (Age In Years)

Onset of Amblyopia	Begin Tx	Prognosis
Birth to 1	1	Good
Birth to 1	2	Fair to good
Birth to 1	3-4	Fair
Birth to 1	5-6	Fair to poor
Birth to 1	≥7	Poor
1 to 2	2-3	Good
1 to 2	4-5	Fair to good
1 to 2	6	Fair
1 to 2	≥7	Fair to poor
2 to 4	4-6	Good
2 to 4	≥7	Fair to good

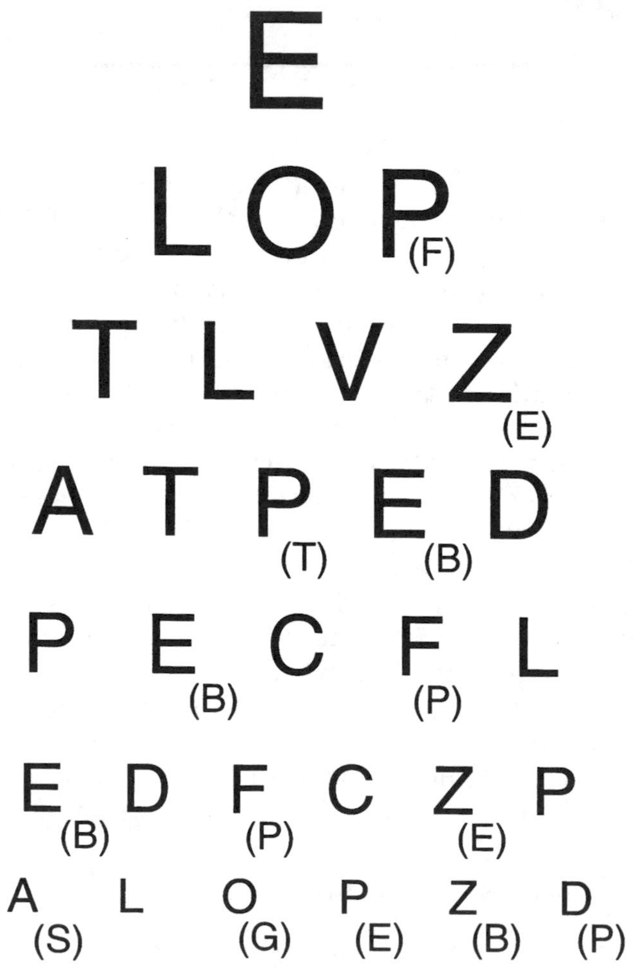

Figure 5-9—Typical responses with testing of an amblyopic eye. Patient's incorrect calls are shown parenthetically.

Snellen Charts

These tests have remained essentially the same since Herman Snellen first devised them in 1862. (Figure 5-8.) A Snellen chart is usually adequate for testing the acuity of nonamblyopic eyes but it is not designed for reliable interpretation of visual acuity in amblyopia.

A standard clinical criterion for assessing the acuity threshold is that at least 50% of the letters in a particular line must be identified correctly. There is usually no problem in determining this level in a nonamblyopic eye. A myopic patient, for example, will consistently identify smaller and smaller letters up to a certain point. Beyond that, letters are consistently missed if an attempt is made to guess the appropriate letters. In contrast to this response, the patient reading with an amblyopic eye will show wide variation in correctly identifying different-sized letters (Figure 5-9). The typical response is to read one or two letters correctly in each of several lines with no clear-cut threshold. The patient often properly recognizes the first and last letters of any particular line, whereas the ones in between are not correctly recognized.

One reason often given for such differences between amblyopic and nonamblyopic test responses is the effect of contour interaction, sometimes referred to as the "crowding phenomenon," in which neighboring contours impair the resolution of the fixated letter. Contour interaction reportedly affects amblyopic eyes more than normal eyes. Using Landolt Cs and movable interacting bars, Flom et al.[35] found that contour interaction started to affect resolution of the gap in the C when the bar spacing equaled the size of the letter. Maximum effect occurred when the bar spacings were 4/10 of the letter size. Flom et al.,[35] however, challenged the conventional wisdom that amblyopic eyes are more affected by contour interaction. They maintained that the effect is approximately equal at threshold visual acuity levels for both normal and amblyopic eyes. The letter spacing varies on each line on the Snellen Chart and so does the crowding phenomenon. On the 20/20 (6/6) line of a typical Snellen Chart slide, the spacing is large, well beyond

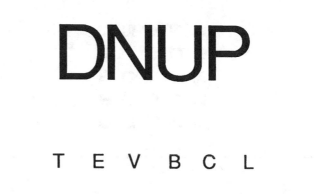

Figure 5-10—Larger Snellen letters having smaller spacing to cause greater crowding effect than the smaller Snellen letters.

the distance causing contour interaction. However, the spaces between the letters in some Snellen charts are relatively reduced for larger letter sizes in the threshold acuity range of many amblyopes. They would show significant contour interaction effect, whereas a person having 20/20 acuity would not (Figure 5-10).

It is common observation that amblyopic visual acuity is better for isolated letters, or possibly for a single line of letters, compared with full Snellen chart acuity. This phenomenon is may also be explained on the basis of the impaired "aiming" ability of an amblyopic eye rather than due to contour interaction. In a complex detailed visual field, amblyopic spatial uncertainty and unsteady fixation result in an increased number of fixation errors. A restricted field with fewer letters is less confusing to an amblyopic observer; therefore, each letter can be fixated more easily.

When testing with the Snellen chart, the clinician should suspect amblyopia if: (1) letters are missed on several lines using the full chart, (2) letters in the middle of a line are more frequently misread than those at the ends of the line, (3) letters are transposed in position, and (4) isolated letter acuity is better by one or two lines than single-line or full-chart acuity.

Bailey-Lovie Chart

The Bailey-Lovie visual acuity chart (a cardboard, freestanding chart) was designed specifically with low vision patients in mind but it can be used effectively with many amblyopic patients (Figure 5-11). On this chart, the number of letters on each line (five) and letter spacing are consistent. This is a distinct improvement over the traditional Snellen chart. Many times it is desirable to test a patient at closer distances than 20 feet (6 m); the acuity may be worse than 20/200 (6/60) or the patient may be an uncooperative child or an older patient who is a malingerer. The steps in letter size are based on a logarithmic scale of the minimum angle of resolution or *logMAR*. This scale allows for easy determination of Snellen equivalent visual acuity at testing distances other than 20 feet. This consistency of optotype spacing and flexibility of use at nonstandard distances makes the

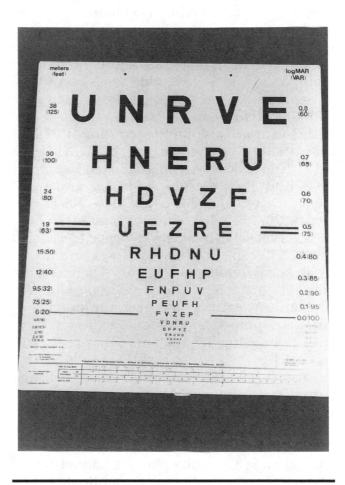

Figure 5-11—Bailey-Lovie chart. (Courtesy of the School of Optometry, University of California, Berkeley)

Bailey-Lovie chart particularly suited for amblyopia assessment. Several different optotype versions of the chart are available to minimize memorization of letters on repeated testing.

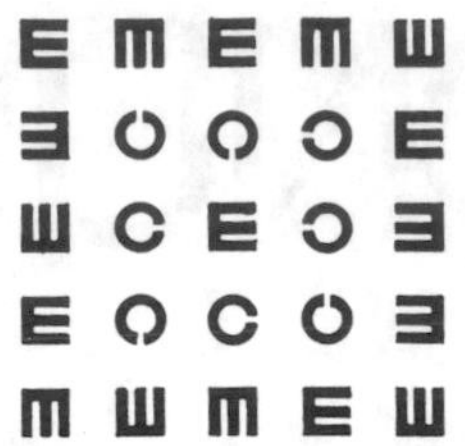

Figure 5-12—Psychometric chart of Flom.

Psychometric Charts

The psychometric chart, also referred to as the "S-chart," was designed by Flom[36] and takes the crowding phenomenon into account as well as the problem of an indefinite acuity threshold in amblyopes. The S-chart slide series consists of 21 separate 35 mm projected slides. Each slide contains eight Landolt Cs of a particular size with the "gap" randomly appearing in one of four positions: up, down, left, or right (Figure 5-12). The slides come in graduated sizes from 20/277 to 20/9, descending in 5% visual efficiency increments (e.g., 20/20 = 100% efficiency; 20/200 = 20% efficiency). At each of the 21 acuity levels, the interletter spacing is equal to the letter size, and each letter is surrounded by an equal number of contours. Therefore, the contour interaction effects on each slide are constant. At each acuity level, the number of correct responses is recorded on the test form with eight being the maximum number of correct calls.

The visual acuity threshold for a particular patient is determined by psychometric analysis. After the series is completed, a "best fit" sigmoid curve is drawn on a chart (Figure 5-13a) representing the data. (See Figure 5-13b illustrating the S-chart visual acuity plot of a normal and an amblyopic eye.) Note that the ordinate of the recording graph represents the acuity threshold and the abscissa, the number of correct responses. The intersection of the sigmoid curve with the abscissa value of 5 determines the visual acuity threshold value. The criterion for acuity is the 50% level of correct responses. Intuitively, four of eight correct responses would represent the 50% level, but this does not take guessing into account. Merely by guessing,

the patient has a one in four chance of a correct call for each Landolt C, which is why five of eight represents the adjusted 50% level.

Testing and recording of visual acuity by means of the S-chart proceed as follows:

1. The patient wears CAMP lenses during testing in a darkened room.
2. The nonamblyopic eye is tested first.
3. The examiner begins with sufficiently large-lettered slides so that the patient properly identifies all Landolt Cs in the correct orientations.
4. The patient is asked to begin making calls starting with the upper left-hand C proceeding in a clockwise direction for the remaining seven Cs. The patient must call the orientation of each C, even if this requires strictly guessing; this is a forced choice procedure. On the recording form, the correct orientations are listed. The examiner indicates each correct call with a slash mark. For each incorrect call, the examiner indicates the patient's response with a subscript (see Figure 5-13).
5. The examiner tests the patient using slides of decreasing size until only two, or less, correct calls are consistently made, indicating that the patient is merely guessing.
6. The number of correct calls is plotted on the adjacent graph. The "best fit" sigmoid curve is then drawn on the graph by visual inspection of the data points (see Figure 5-13).
7. The above procedure is repeated for the amblyopic eye.
8. The acuity thresholds for the normal and amblyopic eyes are indicated by the intersection of the sigmoid curve and the abscissa value of five correct responses (50% threshold corrected for guessing).

Davidson and Eskridge[37] modified the S-chart test to make it easier to use with young children by removing the Landolt Cs but leaving eight Es. Less detail is intended to be less confusing. They reduced the interletter spacing to 1/2 the letter size to increase the effect of contour inter-

Name _____ OD OS OU   Date _____

Eccentricity _____   w/ Rx

Duration _____   w/o Rx

	A									**B** 0	1	2	3	4	5	6	7	8	
1.	9	L	D	R	D	U	D	R	U	110									
2.	15	D	U	L	D	R	U	L	U	105									
3.	20	R	L	U	L	D	R	U	L	100									
4.	26	U	L	D	R	L	R	D	R	95									
5.	32	L	D	R	U	L	D	U	D	90									
6.	38	D	U	L	D	R	U	L	U	85									
7.	45	U	R	L	R	U	L	D	R	80									
8.	52	U	L	D	R	L	R	D	R	75									
9.	60	L	D	R	U	L	D	U	D	70									
10.	68	R	U	D	U	R	U	L	D	65									
11.	77	U	R	L	R	U	L	D	R	60									
12.	87	D	R	U	L	D	L	R	L	55									
13.	97	L	D	R	D	U	D	R	U	50									
14.	109	U	R	L	R	U	L	D	R	45									
15.	122	D	U	L	D	R	U	L	U	40									
16.	137	D	R	U	L	D	L	R	L	35									
17.	155	R	U	D	U	R	U	L	D	30									
18.	175	L	D	R	U	L	D	U	D	25									
19.	200	R	L	U	L	D	R	U	L	20									
20.	232	U	L	D	R	L	R	D	R	15									
21.	277	D	R	U	L	D	L	R	L	10									

Figure 5-13— **(a)** Custom made recording chart for psychometric visual acuity testing. The first column (1, 2, 3 . . .) is the slide number. The second column (9, 15, 20 . . .) represents 20/9, 20/15, 20/20, etc. The columns following indicate the correct response (L = left, D = down, R = right, U = up). The last column (110, 105, 100 . . .) represents percent of visual efficiency. In summary, the A column is for visual acuity and the B column is for visual efficiency. *(Continued on following page.)*

action compared with the S-chart, which has an interletter spacing equal to the letter size. They reported this test to be reliable in the assessment of visual acuity (Figure 5-14). It is used essentially in the same way as the S-chart. (A convenient handheld series of S-charts of this design is available from Dr. Michael Wesson, University of Alabama, School of Optometry, Birmingham, AL 35294.)

Tumbling E and Picture Cards

Handheld tumbling E cards are a popular acuity test for young children or older patients who are illiterate or who do not know the Roman alphabet. Two sets of cards are available, one with contour interaction bars and one set without (Figure 5-15). The acuity levels range from 20/20 to 20/200 in eight steps. Visual acuity threshold is established by finding the threshold distance for a letter of particular size. For example, the examiner can start testing a child at 3 feet with a 10-foot letter. The patient is to indicate the correct orientation of the E at an 80% (4 of 5) correct criterion. "In which direction are the legs of the E pointing—up, down, left, or right?" The patient's responses can be verbal or nonverbal. A child may be more comfortable using fingers to indicate the direction of the tumbling E. If 4 of 5 responses are correct,

Name _____ (OD) (OS) OU   Date _____

Eccentricity   1 degree nasal O.D.   (w/ Rx)

Duration   Most of life, right eye amblyopia   w/o Rx

1.	9	L	D	R	D	U	D	R	U	110	
2.	15	D	U	L	D	R	U	L	U	105	
3.	20	R	L	U	L	D	R	U	L	100	
4.	26	U	L	D	R	L	R	D	R	95	
5.	32	L	D	R	U	L	D	U	D	90	
6.	38	D	U	L	D	R	U	L	U	85	
7.	45	U	R	L	R	U	L	D	R	80	
8.	52	U	L	D	R	L	R	D	R	75	
9.	60	L	D	R	U	L	D	U	D	70	
10.	68	R	U	D	U	R	U	L	D	65	
11.	77	Ø	R$_U$	L$_R$	R$_L$	U$_D$	Ø	D$_R$	R$_L$	60	
12.	87	D$_L$	Ø	U$_R$	L$_R$	D$_R$	L$_U$	R$_L$	Ø	55	
13.	97	Ø	D$_U$	Ø	Ø	U$_L$	Ø	Ø	U$_L$	50	
14.	109	U$_D$	Ø	Ø	Ø	U$_R$	Ø	D$_R$	Ø	45	
15.	122	Ø	U$_L$	Ø	Ø	Ø	Ø	Ø	Ø	40	
16.	137	Ø	Ø	Ø	Ø	Ø	L$_R$	Ø	Ø	35	
17.	155	Ø	Ø	Ø	Ø	Ø	Ø	Ø	Ø	30	
18.	175	Ø	Ø	R$_D$	Ø	Ø	Ø	Ø	Ø	25	
19.	200	Ø	Ø	Ø	Ø	Ø	Ø	Ø	Ø	20	
20.	232	Ø	Ø	Ø	Ø	Ø	Ø	Ø	Ø	15	
21.	277	D	R	U	L	D	L	R	L	10	

Left eye

Right eye amblyopic

Figure 5-13 (continued)—**(b)** Graphical results for an amblyopic patient who had reduced vision in the right eye (lower curve) and normal vision in the left eye (upper curve). Large charts are used initially to ensure that 2 consecutive ones are all correct, i.e., 8 of 8 calls. Target size is reduced in 5% visual efficiency steps until 2 or less correct calls are made for 2 consecutive charts. The best fit curve is drawn for the plotted data. Visual acuity is determined by the place the curve crosses the line representing 5 of 8 correct calls. In this example the left eye has 20/9 acuity and the right eye has 20/107 acuity.

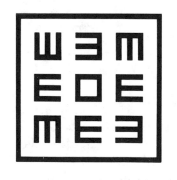

Figure 5-14—Psychometric acuity test design of Davidson and Eskridge.

then the examiner backs away a few steps and retests at that distance. This process continues until a distance is found where the patient cannot achieve the 80% correct criterion. The farthest distance from the patient in which 80% correct calls were made represents the visual acuity threshold. If that distance is 7 feet away from the patient using a 10 foot letter, the acuity is 7/10 or approximately 20/30.

Amblyopia is suspected if the patient is fully corrected optically and, yet, shows poorer acuity in one eye than the other. In a young child, there is often a question of whether reduced acuity is due to psychological variables (e.g., inattention, poor cooperation, hysteria). The contour interaction tumbling E cards can add further evidence in cases of suspected amblyopia. If a child has shown relatively poor acuity in one eye, the threshold should be remeasured using the interaction bar E cards. If that acuity is further significantly reduced using the bar cards, it suggests that developmental amblyopia is present and does not have a psychological basis. Contour interaction occurs maximally when threshold letters are used.[35]

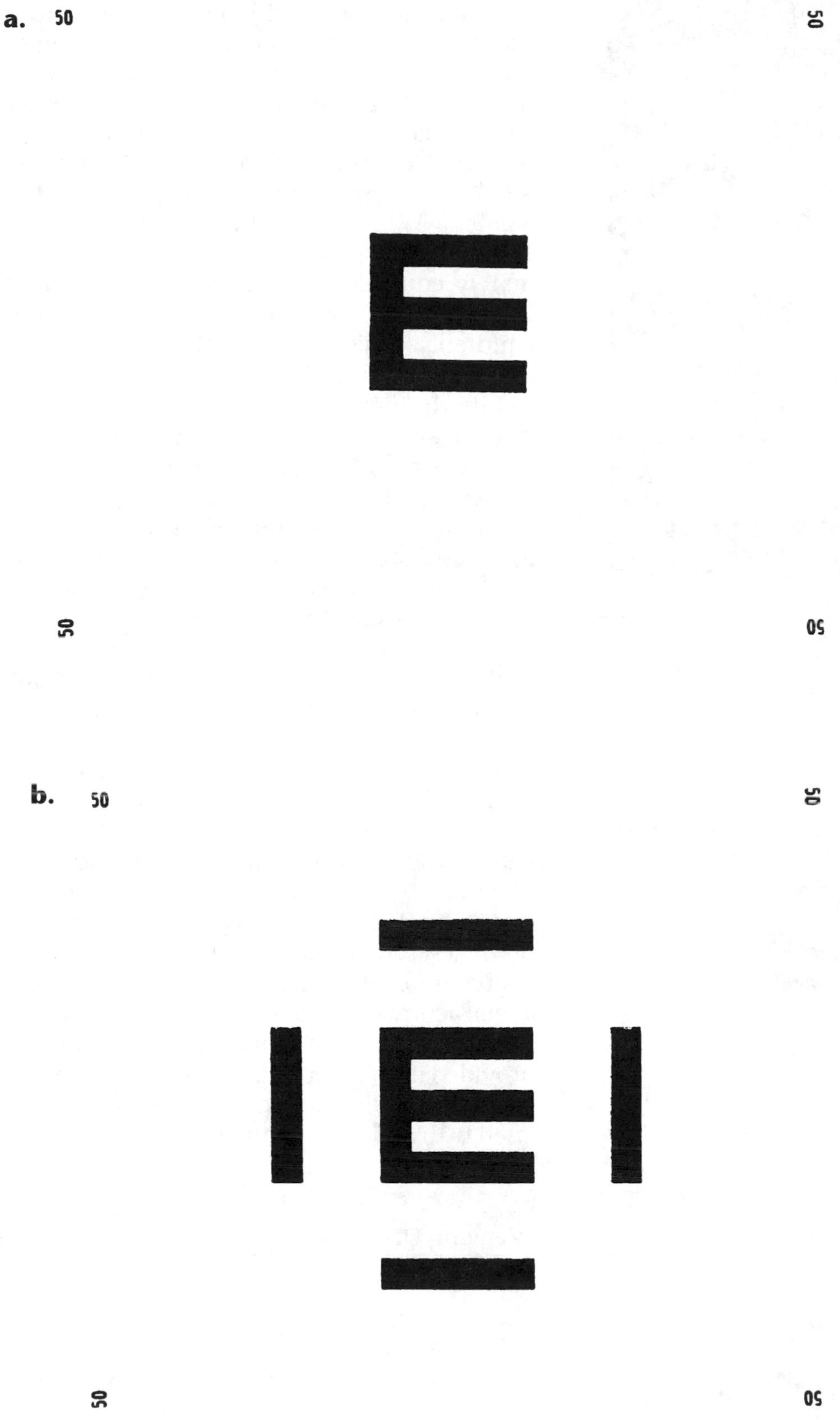

a. 50   50

b. 50   50

Figure 5-15—Tumbling E cards: **(a)** no interaction bars, **(b)** interaction bars surrounding the letter.

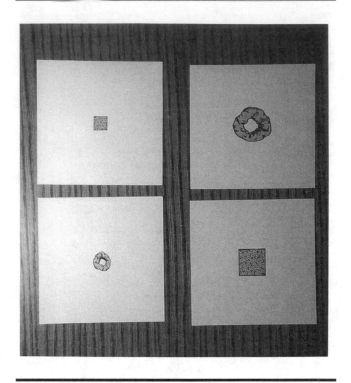

Figure 5-16—Cereal test for visual acuity.

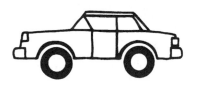

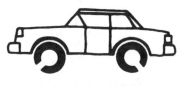

Figure 5-17—Broken Wheel test for visual acuity.

Several other sets of visual acuity test cards are suitable for preschoolers, aged 2 through 5 years. But unlike the tumbling Es, they do not have contour interaction bars to aid in amblyopia identification. Each has, however, its own particular advantages and limitations. See Figure 5-16 showing the Cereal test and Figure 5-17 showing the Broken Wheel test. These visual acuity test targets are approximately equivalent to Snellen optotype in angular size and are very appealing to preschool children. They all are considered to be *recognition* acuity tasks in which the child is asked to discriminate a test form from among a small set of similar shapes known to the child. (Figure 5-18 shows examples of symbols of The Lighthouse Flash Card Test.)

A sophisticated group of visual acuity charts for preschool children is the LH (lighthouse) symbol tests. This series of charts has some advantages over other children's charts. The four symbols (ball, box, house, apple) communicate well to children and, when indistinct or out of focus, appear to have the same overall shape, that of a circle. The symbols on the charts are equally spaced and arranged in a logMAR progression. Various test layouts are available: single symbol book, symbol charts from 8 to 14 lines, near vision card, simulated reading card (crowded, textlike format), and domino cards for matching. There are also two low contrast forms of the test for contrast sensitivity testing. The far charts are calibrated for testing at 10 feet, but actual acuity values at other test distances can be quickly determined using the conversion table provided in the manual. The actual visual acuity at other test distances can also be simply calculated by using the formula:

$$VA = \frac{\text{Viewing Distance (feet)} \times VA \text{ value for 10 feet}}{10 \text{ feet}}$$

For example, $\dfrac{5 \times 20/20}{10} = \dfrac{5}{10} = \dfrac{20}{40}$ or $\dfrac{6}{12}$

Infant Visual Acuity Assessment

Amblyopia screening in infants relies primarily on objective techniques to identify the specific

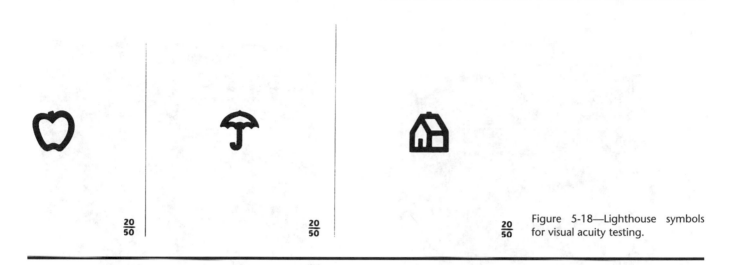

$\frac{20}{50}$ $\frac{20}{50}$ $\frac{20}{50}$ Figure 5-18—Lighthouse symbols for visual acuity testing.

amblyogenic cause, i.e., usually constant strabismus or anisometropia. However, an informal inferential assessment of visual acuity can also be used for amblyopia screening for infants and children under 2 years of age, when visual acuity charts and card sets are inappropriate. The examiner simply observes the infant's behavior with one eye covered or patched compared with the behavior when the other eye is occluded. For example, if the child consistently objects to having one eye occluded versus the other, unilateral visual impairment is suspected. If the child's reaching behavior is less accurate with one eye patched than the other, impairment is again suggested.

Preferential looking methods for visual acuity threshold determination offer a means to study or test *behavioral* visual acuity development of the infant. The examiner exposes two targets, side by side, to the infant. One target is a spatial frequency grating of a particular acuity level and the other is a blank gray field that has the same average luminance as the grating. Infants from the time of birth prefer to look at patterns rather than at a blank field, if they can resolve the pattern. With repeated presentation of the targets, in random left-right order, the examiner watches the patient's eyes and judges whether the infant sees the grating. This is done by observing which target the infant views more frequently. The 80% correct "looking" criterion is often used to indicate that the infant does indeed resolve a particular spatial frequency grating. Only monocular testing is usu-

ally done using this technique. This technique usually works well with infants under 1 year of age, since they innately prefer to look at detail. Older children, however, need more interesting targets or operant conditioning rewards to get reliable responses. Two popular preferential looking tests, designed for clinical use, are the PL 20/20 Infant Vision Tester (Figure 5-19) and the Teller Preferential Looking Cards, a hand-held series of cards.

Optokinetic nystagmus (OKN) has been used to establish visual acuity thresholds in infants, but its validity is questionable, and this technique in not used very often in clinical practice. However, directional asymmetries to OKN stimulation have been reported in patients having infantile strabismus or amblyopia. If visual development proceeds normally, each eye monocularly shows equal amplitude responses to nasalward and temporalward OKN drum rotation by about six months of age. If the infant develops amblyopia or strabismus, responses are typically less vigorous (i.e., lower amplitude and frequency) when the striped stimuli are moving in a temporal direction than in a nasal direction. Schor and Levi[38] investigated this phenomenon and suggested that the asymmetric OKN was due to incomplete development of binocular vision. This may explain why some patients show OKN asymmetry of the nonamblyopic as well as the amblyopic eye. However, there does not seem to be a direct relation between the degree of OKN asymmetry and the depth of the

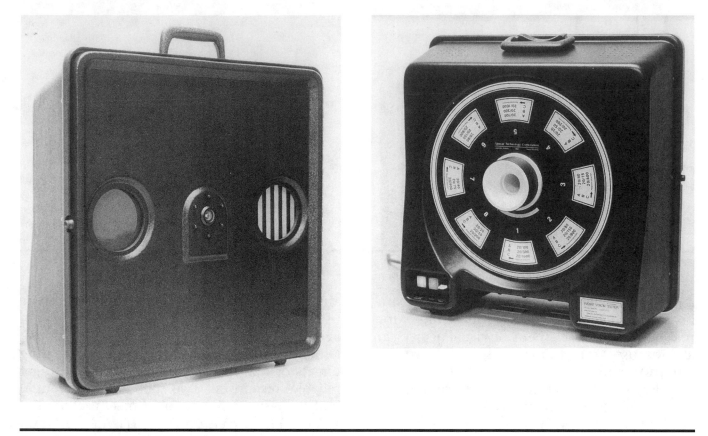

Figure 5-19—PL 20/20 Infant Vision Tester. **(a)** Front view; **(b)** back view showing examiner's peephole and dial for stimulus presentations. Photo courtesy of Optical Technology Corporation, Lawrence, Kansas.

amblyopia, although deeply amblyopic eyes tend to have increased asymmetry.[24]

This observation of OKN asymmetry can be used clinically to screen for amblyopia or strabismus in infants and young children. One eye is occluded while the other is tested using a striped drum rotating at a slow frequency of 8 to 10 RPM (revolutions per minute). The examiner evaluates the responses to nasalward and temporalward motion of the stimulus, and also compares responses of the right eye with the left eye. Although there are pediatric OKN drums with colored pictures, we have found the standard striped drum more effective in assessing of OKN asymmetries (Figure 5-20).

Visually Evoked Potential

In infants where amblyopia is indicated by these direct observations, preferential looking methods, or other clinical assessments, it may be valuable to evaluate acuity further by visually evoked potential (VEP) methods.

The early works by White and Eason[39] on evoked cortical potentials in the occipital lobe have led to great interest in evaluation of vision by electroencephalographic means. By analyzing the VEP displayed graphically as a plot of amplitude against time, visual acuity can be determined. The visually evoked potential is also known as the visually evoked response (VER) or the visually evoked cortical potential (VECP).

One of the most important uses of VEP is determining whether a patient has an organic lesion resulting in decreased visual acuity. Harding[40] believed that organic causes can be ruled in or out by use of formless flash stimuli. Transient VEP, which is a stroboscopically presented stimulus, will elicit a graphical representation of the electrical activity of the visual cortex. This pattern is evaluated in terms of (1) amplitude,

(2) latency of occurrence of the major positive peak response, and (3) general waveform morphology. A computerized recording showing a reduced amplitude indicates there is a lesion somewhere in the visual pathways. Amplitude reduction may indicate optic atrophy (Figure 5-21). Latency differences between each eye may indicate optic nerve demyelination as found in multiple sclerosis (Figure 5-22).

Another type of VEP is that of pattern stimuli of black and white checks that exchange places at a rapid rate. The black checks become white and vice versa, as in Sherman's procedure.[41] The sustained response with this type of VEP allows assessment of visual acuity and aids in the diagnosis and prognosis of amblyopia. The VEP recording of each eye can be compared for differences in visual acuity. This comparison helps establish the diagnosis of amblyopia in the absence of an organic lesion, particularly with those patients who do not respond reliably to optotype acuity tests. Figure 5-23 illustrates how visual acuity is estimated by looking at the peak VEP amplitude for different spatial frequency checkerboard patterns. It is a common clinical observation that VEP acuity is often superior to that found when using optotype in cases of amblyopia. We consider this observation to be a favorable prognostic sign. This suggests that there is sensory potential for the improvement of visual acuity, often to the level indicated by the VEP. Besides the sensory reduction of acuity, amblyopes often have a motor disorder, e.g., eccentric fixation. The VEP reveals the visual acuity independent of the "aiming error" in the amblyopic eye.

Interferometery

The interferometer is a useful instrument to predict the possible visual acuity achievement of an amblyopic patient. It uses the principle of interference fringes, as with a laser, to produce a spatial frequency line grating that is projected onto the patient's retina. A dial is turned on the instrument to change the spatial frequency of the grating over a large range, each setting corresponding to Snellen visual acuity. The advantage of using a coherent light source is that the projected image is not affected by minor opaci-

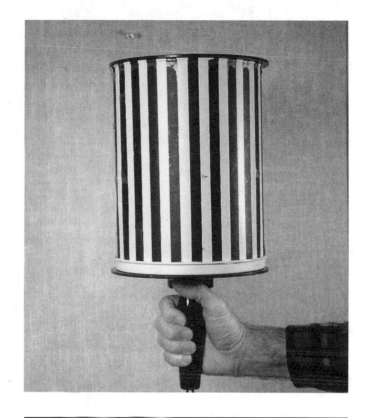

Figure 5-20—Optokinetic Nystagmus (OKN) drum used to detect amblyopia.

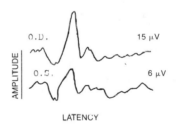

Figure 5-21—Transient VEP graph showing normal latency for each eye and normal amplitude for the right eye but reduced amplitude for the left eye, as in optic atrophy.

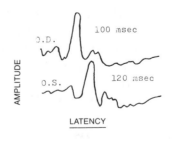

Figure 5-22—Transient VEP graph showing normal amplitude for each eye and normal latency for the right eye but increased latency for the left eye, a difference indicative of optic nerve demyelination as in multiple sclerosis.

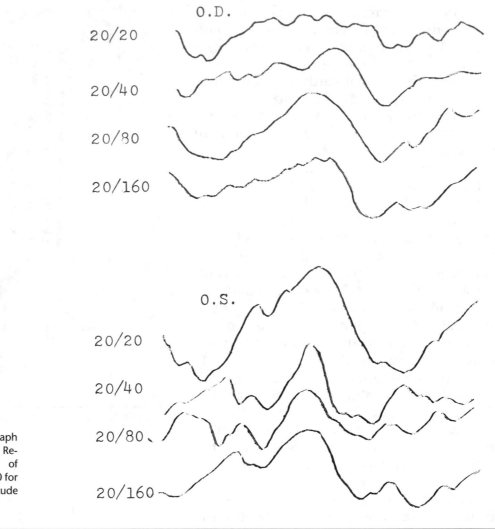

O.D.

20/20

20/40

20/80

20/160

O.S.

20/20

20/40

20/80

20/160

Figure 5-23—Sustained VEP graph for visual acuity assessment. Responses indicate visual acuity of 20/80 for the right eye and 20/20 for the left eye, judging from amplitude comparisons.

ties of the media or refractive errors. The acuity determination is quick and is done by asking the patient to identify the orientation of the grating (vertical, horizontal, or diagonal) at the various acuity settings. The acuity determination is independent of eccentric or unsteady fixation, similar to the VEP. Therefore, in cases of amblyopia, the acuity estimate can be useful in making the diagnosis and possibly in estimating the prognosis for success of therapy. Selenow et al.[42] compared pretherapy interferometry visual acuity with pre- and post-therapy optotype measures of visual acuity in a group of 37 patients with amblyopia. They found that in most cases the pretherapy interferometry acuity and the post-training Snellen acuity closely agreed: 90% were within two acuity

lines of each other and 75% were within one line. If further investigations support these impressive results, interferometry may become an important prognostic tool in the assessment of amblyopia. A popular available clinical instrument is the SITE IRAS Interferometer (Figure 5-24). Interferometers typically use four-choice targets (Figure 5-25).

Fixation Evaluation

Fixation is normal when the center of the fovea is used for fixation and when fixation is steady. If any other area of the retina is used (eccentric fixation), or if there is significant unsteadiness, fixation is considered to be abnormal. *Eccentric fixation* (EF) then is considered to be an abnormality of monocular fixation in which the time-averaged position of the fovea is off the fixation target. Unsteadiness refers to the presence of nystagmoidlike oscillations (usually irregular flicks and drifts) of the affected eye. They are often noticeable upon careful direct observation, but more easily observed during visuoscopy. An eye with 20/20 (6/6) or better visual acuity necessarily has central fixation that is relatively steady, while an eye with poor visual acuity may have eccentric and/or unsteady fixation.

Ciuffreda, Levi, and Selenow[24] considered eccentric fixation to be caused in many cases by a shift in sensory spatial direction away from the fovea and was probably related to the impaired directional sense found in the central retina of amblyopic eyes. Bedell and Flom[27] found monocular spatial distortion, spatial uncertainty, and direction error to be associated with strabismic amblyopia. Monocular spatial distortion can be described as a monocular asymmetry in spatial values between nasal versus temporal retinal loci. This sensory spatial asymmetry and uncertainty results in a motor fixation pattern in which the time-averaged position of the fovea is off the fixation target and appears unsteady.

Description of Eccentric Fixation

The fixation pattern of an amblyopic eye is described with reference to the centricity, direction, and the degree of steadiness. The following scale can be used to describe centricity where the fixation point is based on the time-averaged position of an eye (Table 5-6).

A description of eccentric fixation includes reference to the direction and distance from the fovea to where the eccentric point (or time-averaged position) is located on the retina. The

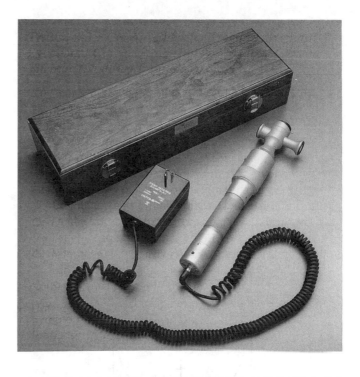

Figure 5-24—SITE IRAS Interferometer. (Courtesy of Bernell Corporation.)

direction of EF is referred to one of eight locations: nasal, temporal, superior, inferior, superior nasal, inferior nasal, superior temporal, and inferior temporal. We have found that nasal eccentric fixation is generally the rule in strabismic amblyopia, particularly esotropia, and often has a vertical component, but smaller than the horizontal component. Temporal eccentric fixation is the exception in strabismic amblyopia, even in exotropia.

Unsteadiness of fixation can be associated with central or eccentric fixation. It is clinically relevant to describe the amplitude of unsteadiness if it exists. The degree of unsteadiness is indicated as a ± amplitude from the fixation

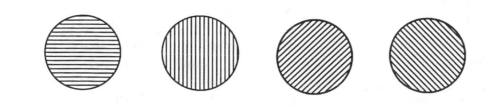

Figure 5-25—Typical orientations of grating targets of interferometers.

TABLE 5-6. *Classification of Centricity of Fixation*

Central fixation	—foveal
Eccentric fixation	—parafoveal (between fovea and 2° EF)
	—macular (2° to 5° EF)
	—peripheral (beyond 5° EF)

a.   WELCH-ALLYN

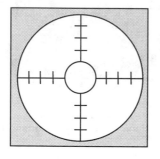

b.   PROPPER

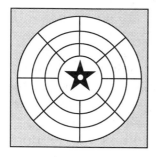

c.   KEELER

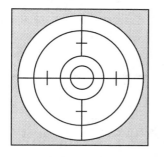

Figure 5-26—Examples of reticules of direct ophthalmoscopes for visuoscopy: **(a)** Welsh Allen, **(b)** Propper, **(c)** Keeler.

locus (time-averaged position). For example: 3° nasal, unsteady (±1°) eccentric fixation. A more common clinical way of recording this would be unsteady, nasal, 3° eccentric fixation ±1°.

Visuoscopy

Visuoscopy for evaluating fixation is done by using an ophthalmoscope with a graduated reticule in place. The doctor observes a projected image of the reticule on the patient's fundus while the patient is asked to look directly at the center of the projected pattern and to hold fixation as steady as possible (Figure 5-26). The separations in reticules are generally of a magnitude representing one prism diopter. This can be verified by projecting the target onto a wall at a distance of 1 meter, at which each separation (e.g., circle) would be 1 cm apart. Because fixation must be tested under monocular conditions, the patient must have one eye occluded when testing. A practical way of doing this is by asking the patient to cover the nontested eye with a hand or an occluder. For very small pupils, dilation (with mydriatic drops) is often necessary to locate the fovea and make visuoscopic observations. A dilated fundus examination should be done initially in any case of suspected amblyopia to rule out organic lesions; this is a convenient time to perform visuoscopy.

During visuoscopy, four clinical observations are routinely made:

1. Does the fovea and macular area look normal? The clinician must carefully inspect the fovea and macula for lesions and developmental anomalies. Is there a well defined foveal light reflex or not? Are there reflexes? If other macula look abnormal in any way, then a 60 or 90 diopter lens examination on a slit lamp is recommended to rule out or identify an organic lesion.
2. Is there central or eccentric fixation? If there is eccentric fixation, then what is the direction and magnitude?
3. Is there steady or unsteady fixation? If there is unsteady fixation, what is the amplitude and type of occillations?

4. Is there faulty localization associated with eccentric fixation?

Figure 5-27 shows examples of the visuoscopic patterns of fixation in different cases of eccentric fixation and their associated clinical description. These examples for the right eye depict nasal and inferior eccentric fixation with the fovea (represented by the starlike spot) being temporal to the fixated center of the visuoscopic reticule.

Haidinger Brush Testing

Haidinger brush is a retinal entoptic phenomenon that can be used clinically to indicate if the fovea is functionally intact and to determine the position and steadiness of the fovea as the patient attempts to fixate a target. There are several instruments available for producing a Haidinger brush, but the most practical, we believe, is the Bernell Macular Integrity Tester-Trainer (MITT) (Figure 5-28). This instrument has a motor-driven rotating polarized filter behind a transparent slide imprinted with fixation targets. Perception of the Haidinger brush requires the patient to look at the rotating polarized filter through a deep cobalt blue filter in front of the eye being tested. This is a monocular technique; the nontested eye is occluded. The patient should see a pair of brushlike "propellers" that appear to radiate from, and to rotate about, the point of foveal fixation. The entoptic image of the fovea is believed to be caused by double refraction by the radially oriented fibers of Henle around the fovea.[43] Since these radial fibers converge on the fovea, the center of the perceived pattern represents the center of the fovea.

In cases of amblyopia, the perception of the Haidinger brush is sometimes difficult to elicit. If perception of the entoptic phenomenon can be evoked in the amblyopia eye, it represents a good prognostic sign. The fovea is then considered to be functionally intact and, practically speaking, a foveal tag is available for training proper foveal fixation reflexes. The lack of perception of the Haidinger brush does not necessarily mean the macula is either dysfunctional or diseased. Some individuals with normal retinas have difficulty seeing this entoptic image.

RIGHT EYE

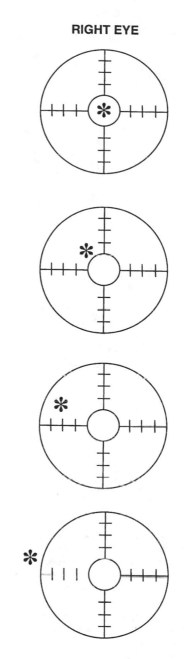

Figure 5-27—Visuoscopic patterns of fixation in an example of right eye being tested. **(a)** Central fixation; **(b)** parafoveal eccentric fixation; **(c)** eccentric fixation within the macular area; **(d)** peripheral. The direction of eccentric fixation in these examples is nasal and inferior.

An amblyope may have a particular problem seeing the brush if there is eccentric fixation, because it does not appear where the patient is fixating. The "straight ahead" direction is usually associated with the eccentric point, not the fovea. The brush will appear, when it is per-

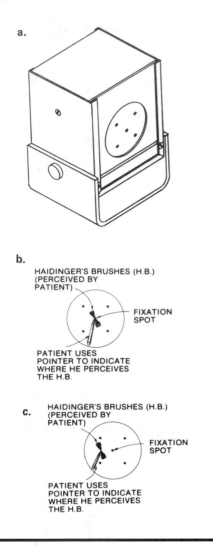

b.

HAIDINGER'S BRUSHES (H.B.)
(PERCEIVED BY
PATIENT)

FIXATION
SPOT

PATIENT USES
POINTER TO INDICATE
WHERE HE PERCEIVES
THE H.B.

c.

HAIDINGER'S BRUSHES (H.B.)
(PERCEIVED BY
PATIENT)

FIXATION
SPOT

PATIENT USES
POINTER TO INDICATE
WHERE HE PERCEIVES
THE H.B.

Figure 5-28—The Bernell Macular Integrity Tester-Trainer. **(a)** Drawing of the instrument, clear slide with fixation spots placed before the illuminated circular window. **(b)** Example of central fixation in which case the patient sees the Haidinger brush and the fixation spot superimposed. **(c)** Example of eccentric fixation whereby Haidinger brush and the fixation spot are not superimposed. This response would indicate nasal eccentric fixation of the right eye. If this response were found when testing the left eye, temporal eccentric fixation would be indicated.

ceived, off to one side of the fixation target on the MITT.

When an amblyopic patient is having difficulty observing the brush, several techniques may help to elicit its perception: (1) Demonstrate what the Haidinger brush looks like using the patient's normal eye; the entoptic image should be relatively easy to appreciate. (2) Lower the background room illumination to increase the contrast of the MITT screen and use double (two) cobalt blue filters over the amblyopic eye, occluding the dominant eye, to intensify the perception of Haidinger's brush. (3) Add a high-plus trial case lens (e.g., +10 D) in front of the cobalt filter. This blurs out all extraneous contours and shadows, but leaves the entoptic image unaffected. (4) To confirm that the perceived image is indeed the Haidinger brush, insert a piece of cellophane or plastic wrap before the amblyopic eye to see if the direction of brush rotation is reversed. The cellophane acts as a quarter wave plate and should reverse the perceived direction of rotation of the entoptic image.

Besides establishing macular integrity, the Haidinger brush can be used to evaluate the fixation pattern of an amblyopic eye. Most characteristics of the fixation pattern that are observed by visuoscopy can also be assessed using the brush if the patient is a reliable observer. The patient is instructed to fixate a suprathreshold target on the MITT at exactly a 40 cm distance from the instrument. After the correct perception of the entoptic image is established, the following assessment of fixation can be made: Is there central or eccentric fixation? If there is eccentric fixation, what is the direction and magnitude? (Note: at 40 cm fixation distance, 4 mm lateral displacement on the screen represents 1^Δ.) Is there steady or unsteady fixation? If there is unsteady fixation, what is the amplitude between fixated locations? Is the fovea included within the range of unsteadiness? Is there faulty localization associated with eccentric fixation or is the patient eccentrically viewing? Visuoscopy, of course, has a major advantage over the MITT as an assessment technique since it is objective; however, the MITT can be immediately employed in the remediation of faulty fixation associated with amblyopia. Both instruments, the visuoscope and the MITT, are important and useful in the management of eccentric fixation.

Refraction Techniques

Subjective refractive techniques are usually unreliable when testing an amblyopic eye due to the abnormal fixation pattern and the deficient spatial resolution. Consequently, cycloplegic retinoscopy is often necessary for determining the refractive error. We generally use one drop of 1% cyclopentolate preceded by a drop of 0.5% proparacaine. In most patients, the cycloplegic effect is sufficiently strong to reveal the full amount of hyperopia, if it exists. We prefer not to use a phoropter in cases of amblyopia or strabismus. It is easier to monitor the fixation by directly viewing the patient. The refractive error is determined with trial case lenses or a lens bar. To ensure accuracy, care must be taken that the retinoscopic beam on the amblyopic eye is directly on axis. The correct visual axis can be estimated with a penlight by moving to a lateral position where angle kappa of the amblyopic eye equals that of the normal eye. In cases of amblyopia associated with esotropia, on-axis retinoscopy is easily accomplished by scoping the amblyopic eye from the opposite side, e.g., in a case of a right esotropic amblyopic eye, scoping from the patient's left side. In cases of anisometropic or strabismic amblyopia, the full refractive error is usually prescribed even when a patch is to be worn. Undercorrecting hyperopia can be a mistake since the accommodative responses of an amblyopic eye are usually deficient.

Eye Disease Evaluation

Before the diagnosis of amblyopia is made, the clinician needs to investigate the possibility that ocular pathology may be the direct cause of the reduction in visual acuity. It is prudent to be suspicious of eye disease or pathology affecting the visual pathways in all cases of unexplained reduction of visual acuity, even in cases associated with anisometropia and strabismus; it is not uncommon for organic eye disease to coexist with amblyopia. The following procedures provide the basis for making a clinical distinction between a pathologic loss of acuity and developmental amblyopia.

Ophthalmoscopy

A dilated fundus examination may be necessary for careful inspection of the macular and foveal region of the amblyopic eye. However, retinal lesions can sometimes be difficult to detect. Besides using direct and indirect ophthal-

moscopy to examine an amblyopic eye, we recommend a careful slit-lamp inspection of the macula and fovea using high magnification; for example, using a 60 D or a 90 D lens.

Visual Fields

Automated visual field testing is usually unsuccessful or unreliable due to the poor fixation responses of an amblyopic eye. Ordinary tangent screen field testing has some advantages over the automated techniques. Unsteady fixation of the amblyopic eye can be reduced if no central fixation target is used. As an alternative, four strips of masking tape or paper can be applied to the tangent screen at the 3, 6, 9, and 12 o'clock positions, approximately 10° away from the center of the screen; this pattern indicates a virtual fixation point (Figure 5-29). The patient holds the amblyopic eye steady on the virtual point where the four lines would theoretically intersect; then the field testing of the blind spot, periphery, and central areas proceeds in the usual manner. Testing with a 1 or 2 mm white target at 1 meter is generally sufficient to determine whether a scotoma exists. During this procedure, the patient should wear spectacles, contact lenses, or trial case lenses to correct fully any significant refractive error. The visual field of the amblyopic eye is compared with that of the normal eye.

Amsler grid testing for central field defects is also recommended. As in tangent screen testing, the visual fields of the two eyes are compared for consistency. When testing an amblyopic eye, we recommend a +2.50 D

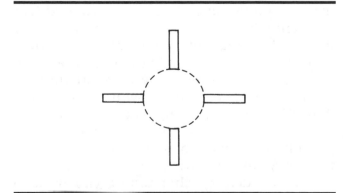

Figure 5-29—Paracentral fixation lock for testing the integrity of the central visual field on a tangent screen.

nearpoint add (a trial case lens) be used along with any needed spectacle correction because monocular accommodation of an amblyopic eye is usually deficient. Even if there is significant unsteady eccentric fixation, the fovea will usually fall somewhere on the grid pattern and a central visual field defect, if it exists, may be noticed by the patient.

Schapero[44] believed that detection of a central absolute scotoma (no light perception within the scotomatous area) indicates an organic lesion or amblyopia with an organic component, and that the prognosis for attaining better acuity is limited by the potential acuity of the retinal area surrounding the absolute scotoma. A relative central scotoma (depressed sensitivity), however, indicates a functional reduction of acuity that is potentially recoverable. Irvine[45] reported a more optimistic view in this regard, based on his findings that some functional cases of deep amblyopia apparently exhibited an absolute central scotoma.

Neutral Density Filters

Ammann[46] proposed that differential diagnosis of organic (pathologic acuity loss) and developmental amblyopia is possible by comparing the visual acuity measured in normal and reduced illumination. There is an expected decrease of visual acuity when target illumination is reduced for both the normal and the amblyopic eye. Visual acuity normally decreases under mesopic and scotopic conditions. However, if the cause of acuity loss is pathological (e.g., macular degeneration, optic atrophy, central pathway lesion), the decrease in visual acuity with decreased illumination is sudden and dramatic. Caloroso and Flom[47] demonstrated that at essentially all luminance levels, visual acuity in the functional amblyopic eye was less than that of the normal eye. At the lowest levels of luminance, however, it was approximately equal. In contradistinction, von Noorden and Burian[48] have convincingly shown that in cases of macular organic lesions, visual acuity dropped precipitously as illumination decreases, thus confirming Ammann's observations.

Neutral density filter testing can be used clinically when a patient presents with unexplained monocular reduced acuity and differential diagnosis is needed. Either a 2.0 or 3.0 log unit neutral density filter, such as a Kodak Wratten filter #96, should be utilized. We recommend measuring the visual acuity of each eye under normal photopic room lighting conditions by means of an S-chart. If a Snellen chart must be used, the acuity thresholds should be converted to Snell-Sterling visual efficiency scale (e.g., 20/20 = 100%; 20/50= 76%). The patient's eyes are then partially dark adapted, approximately 5 minutes, to a mesopic level. The appropriate neutral density filter is placed over the projector's objective lens. The poorer eye is occluded while the visual acuity of the better eye is quickly remeasured. Switching the occluder, the clinician then determines the acuity threshold of the poorer eye. Under mesopic conditions, the visual acuity of the better eye may have decreased from 20/20 to 20/40, about 15% reduction in Snell-Sterling visual efficiency, for example. An organic lesion would be suspected if the visual acuity of the poorer eye decreases from 20/50, for example, to 20/200, about a 55% decrease in visual efficiency. The rate of decrease is much faster in cases of macular pathway lesions compared with functional amblyopia. If the poorer eye, however, showed only a 20% or less decrease in visual efficiency with the ND filter, functional amblyopia would be indicated. (See visual acuity/visual efficiency conversion scales in the Appendices.)

Tests of Retinal Function

Two other tests may be helpful in making the distinction between a pathological reduction of acuity and functional amblyopia. These are monocular color vision and ERG. Several diseases of the retina and optic nerve result in subtle monocular color vision defects. Retinal disease tends to produce subtle blue-yellow defects whereas acquired optic atrophy often results in subtle red-green defects. Monocular color vision can be tested in most children ages 10 years and older using the Farnsworth panel D-15 test. Unfortunately, a good differential diagnostic test for younger children is not commercially available at this time. The color vision responses of each eye are inspected for differences that ordinarily are not found. If a defect is found with this test, it represents a strong defect. The desaturated panel D-15 may be necessary to pick up the initial signs of color vision defects due to pathology.

Another test of retinal function that may help in differential diagnosis when needed is the electroretinogram (ERG). Although the research literature is very mixed, consistent differences are not apparent in the ERG responses between normal and amblyopic eyes.[49] If abnormal ERG responses or significant differences between the eyes are found, the condition is unlikely to be developmental amblyopia. For example, the *pattern ERG* is abnormal in cases of Stargardt's macular dystrophy (a juvenile rod-cone dystrophy) that may be confused with amblyopia during its early stages. The ERG procedure usually requires referral to a visual functions testing clinic at a medical or optometric center since most primary care doctors do not have the relatively expensive instruments used for this evaluation. The expense of this test is often justified when a reasonable suspicion of retinal disease exists, since patching the sound eye can be frustrating for a patient even when the chance of functional improvement is good. Useless patching is to be avoided.

ANOMALOUS CORRESPONDENCE

Anomalous correspondence is a sensory defense mechanism against diplopia that preserves rudimentary binocular vision in response to a strabismus of early onset. It is defined as the binocular condition in which the two foveas and all other homologous retinal loci do not correspond to each other in regard to directional values. The primary visual direction in the deviating eye has shifted to a nonfoveal location to be in accord with that of the fixating eye. This shift of directional value allows at least some sensory integration of the two eyes so the strabismic individual is not "monocular." Although the correspondence actually takes place in the cortex of the occipital lobe, clinicians refer to "retinal" correspondence because the retinas are the reference locations for angular measurements. Consequently, ARC (anoma-

lous retinal correspondence) is used throughout this book; this is the traditionally recognized abbreviation.

Classification

ARC is an antidiplopic sensorial adaptation that is prevalent in developmental strabismus. Its presence indicates a significant difference between the horizontal *objective angle of deviation* (*H*) and the subjective *angle of directionalization* (*S*). The difference between these two angles is the angle of anomaly (*A*). Some measurement error must be allowed; otherwise, a false-positive diagnosis may result, i.e., the clinician making a diagnosis of ARC when there is normal "retinal" correspondence (NRC). In small angle strabismus, allowance of 1^Δ to 2^Δ error may be necessary and up to 5^Δ should be allowed for large angles of strabismus when comparing *H* and *S*. The larger the strabismus, therefore, the more allowance for measurement error is made. In theory, angles *H* and *S* should be exactly the same in NRC (angle *A* being zero in magnitude). Clinical measurements, however, are not always precise; this necessitates the allowance for measurement error. This is particularly so when the patient is an uncooperative child or a poor observer.

An example of normal correspondence is illustrated in Figure 5-30. Angles *H* and *S* are the same in this case of esotropia with NRC.

Example: $H = 25^\Delta$ eso, $S = 25^\Delta$ eso
$A = 25^\Delta - 25^\Delta$
$A = 0^\Delta$

In free-space natural viewing, diplopia is likely to occur when there is a strabismus of recent onset and NRC. Point *zero*, the "target" point, is stimulated peripherally and produces homonymous diplopia, unless there is strong peripheral suppression. Suppression is likely to take place at the fovea of the deviating eye to prevent overlapping of the two different foveal images (i.e., confusion). ARC would be the more parsimonious antidiplopic adaptation since there is the added advantage of preserving rudimentary peripheral binocularity and possibly gross stereopsis in small angles of strabismus. However, ARC can probably only develop

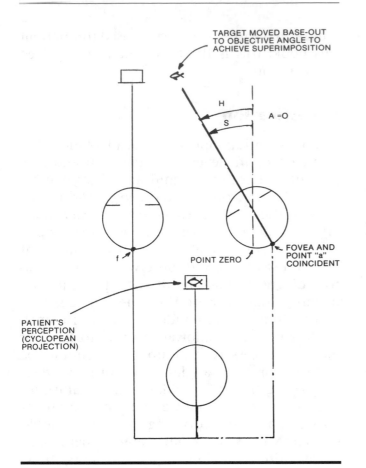

Figure 5-30—Illustration of normal correspondence.

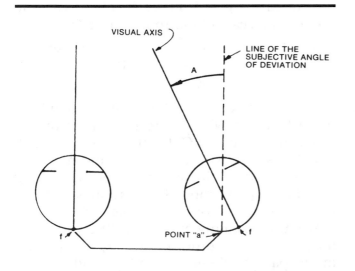

Figure 5-31—Angle of anomaly in which the fovea of the left eye corresponds to point "a" of the right eye. Angle A is subtended at the center of rotation of the eye by the visual axis and the line of the subjective angle of deviation.

in response to strabismus during early childhood when there is cortical plasticity with respect to binocular visual direction.

Three angles are involved in ARC. The following relation between these angles applies: $H = A + S$ or solving for A; $A = H - S$. Angle A is the angle subtended at the center of rotation of the eye by the fovea (f) and the anomalous associated point (a) (Figure 5-31). The fovea of the fixating eye corresponds with point a in the deviating eye when there is ARC. Point *a* is strictly functional; there is no retinal landmark as there is for point *f*.

The type of ARC occurring most frequently in natural seeing conditions is harmonious ARC (HARC). An example of this is illustrated in Figure 5-32 in which S is 0^Δ and A has the same magnitude as H. Such strabismic patients often give "orthophoric" responses during routine phorometry. This is because point *a* is in the *same* location as point *zero*. The fovea of the fixating left eye in this example corresponds to point *a* of the right eye, which happens to be coincident with point *zero,* the "target" point. Clinicians, therefore, should be on guard if phorometry indicates $S = 0$ or a value close to zero when a strabismic deviation is present. HARC is suspected in such cases.

Example of HARC (Figure 5-32)
$$H = 25^\Delta, S = 0^\Delta$$
$$A = 25^\Delta - 0^\Delta$$
$$A = 25^\Delta$$

Not all cases of ARC are harmonious. Assume a patient has an esotropia of the right eye of 25^Δ and that S is 12^Δ (as measured by subjective tests such as the dissociated red lens test). The fact that H and S are different suggests ARC. Figure 5-33 illustrates this example by depicting points *f, a,* and *zero* (also called point *o* or the "target" point in the deviating eye). This example represents a case of *unharmonious ARC (UNHARC) in which H* is larger than *S,* and point *a* lies between point *f* and point *zero.*

Example of UNHARC (Figure 5-33)
$$H = 25^\Delta, S = 12^\Delta$$
$$A = 25^\Delta - 12^\Delta$$
$$A = 13^\Delta$$

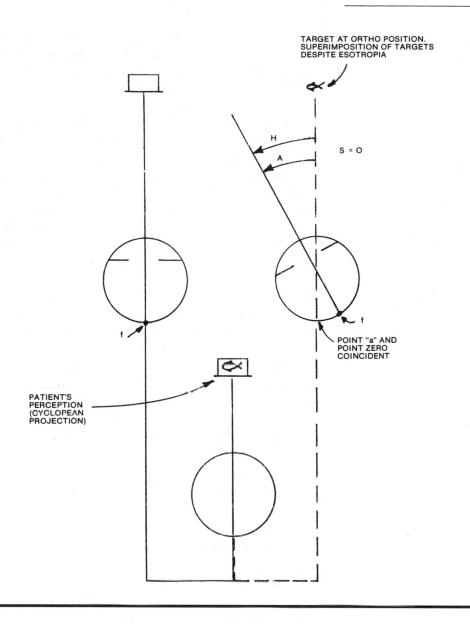

TARGET AT ORTHO POSITION.
SUPERIMPOSITION OF TARGETS
DESPITE ESOTROPIA

H

A

S = O

POINT "a" AND
POINT ZERO
COINCIDENT

PATIENT'S
PERCEPTION
(CYCLOPEAN
PROJECTION)

f

f

Figure 5-32—Illustration of harmonious anomalous correspondence.

There are relatively rare types of ARC that occur secondary to changes in the angle of deviation (*H*) which can result in some unusual measurements of the subjective angle (S). An example of paradoxical ARC type one (PARC I) is illustrated in Figure 5-34. In such a case the patient subjectively directionalizes, under binocular viewing conditions, as if there were exotropia, even when *H* indicates esotropia. This condition often occurs when the original angle of esotropia was greater before extraocular muscle surgery than afterwards. In this example, the deviation was reduced by surgery, but not enough to make the visual axes parallel. Assume that before surgery there had been HARC, so that point *a* was originally at point *zero*. The outward rotational movement of the deviating eye with surgery caused point *a* to be moved from the ortho demand point to another point farther in the nasal retina. Stimulation of the post-surgical point *zero*, which is temporal in respect to point *a*, causes S to be in the exo direction.

Example: $H = 25^\Delta$ (eso), $S = -28^\Delta$ (exo)
$A = 25^\Delta - (28^\Delta)$
$A = 53^\Delta$

Paradoxical type two ARC often occurs following a surgical overcorrection of exotropia.

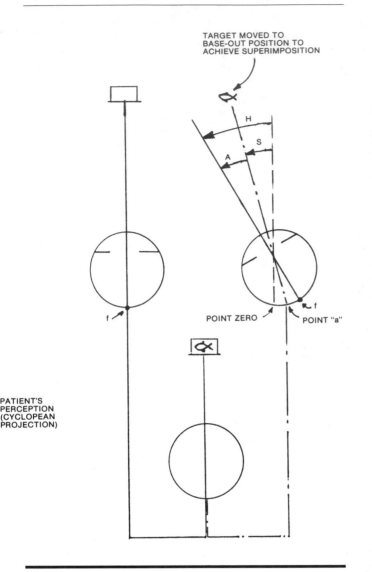

TARGET MOVED TO
BASE-OUT POSITION TO
ACHIEVE SUPERIMPOSITION

H

S

A

f

POINT ZERO   POINT "a"

f

PATIENT'S
PERCEPTION
(CYCLOPEAN
PROJECTION)

Figure 5-33—Illustration of typical unharmonious anomalous correspondence.

For example, a patient with an exotropic right eye and HARC before surgery may have an esotropic right eye after surgery (Figure 5-35). Point *a* would be moved from point *zero* to a location temporalward in relation to point *zero*. Stimulation of point *zero* would then cause the patient to have *S* more eso in direction than before surgery. (*S* is more eso in magnitude than *H*.)

Example: $H = 17^\Delta$ (eso), $S = 30^\Delta$ (eso)
$A = 17^\Delta - 30^\Delta$
$A = -13^\Delta$

Other causes than extraocular muscle surgery may alter the magnitude of *H* to result in unharmonious or a paradoxical type of ARC.

Plus lenses, for example, may reduce an eso deviation, and minus an exo deviation. Prisms may optically affect these angular relationships as well as the possibility of vision training procedures producing changes. There appears to be wide variation in how patients having HARC as the initial adaptation to their strabismus sensorially readapt to a new angle of deviation post-surgically or after optical and training manipulations of the angle H. In some cases HARC and its consequential advantages to fusion reestablishes itself; at other times, paradoxical ARC results along with the undesirable, but fortunately rare, consequence of intractable diplopia.

In summary then, the conceptual basis for the classification of normal and anomalous correspondence is the location of the anomalous associated point (*a*) in the deviating eye (Figure 5-36). If point a of the deviating eye is anywhere other than at the fovea, then there is ARC. If point *a* is at the target point (zero), there is HARC; if between the fovea and the target point (zero), there is UNHARC; if nasal to the target point, PARC type I; and if temporal to the fovea, then PARC type II. See Table 5-7 to review the relations between angles *H*, *S*, and *A* that serves to classify types of correspondence.

Characteristics

Horopter in ARC

Flom[50] demonstrated that the identical visual direction horopter in strabismic patients having ARC has an irregular shape that may help to explain many of the characteristics of the

TABLE 5-7. *Classification of Normal and Anomalous Correspondence by Mathematical Formulas*

NRC	H = S; A = O
ARC	H ≠ S
HARC	H = A; S = O
UNHARC	H>S; H>A
PARC Type I	A>H; S opposite direction to H (S <zero)
PARC Type II	S>H; A opposite direction to H (A <zero)

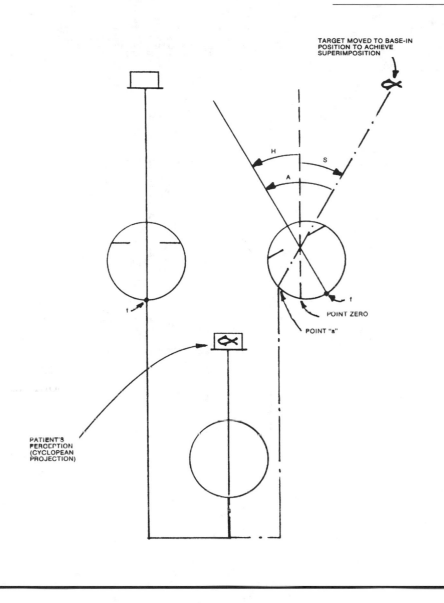

Figure 5-34—Paradoxical type one unharmonious anomalous correspondence.

condition. The peripheral horopter in ARC cases was similar in shape and location to nonstrabismic patients with NRC, and in that sense these patients can be said to have peripheral "fusion" (Figure 5-37). The nonstrabismic's horopter goes through the point of fixation. When an intermittent esotrope with NRC lapses into a strabismic deviation, the horopter shifts from the plane of the target to a point where the visual axes cross (the centration point). Images then in the plane of the target, including the target, appear to be diplopic if there is no suppression (Figure 5-37b). However, if there is esotropia with ARC, the horopter beyond the area between the visual axes,

remains in the plane of the target of regard and the world appears fused even though there may be some central suppression (Figure 5-37c). This is a very convenient adaptation for the strabismic patient because diplopia is eliminated, peripheral stereopsis may be present if the deviation is not very large and fusional vergence eye movements can still occur (Figure 5-37d).

Another remarkable feature of the ARC horopter is its abrupt and radical change in direction within the space subtended between the visual axes (Figure 5-37c). Flom[50] referred to this area as the "notch" in the horopter. One might ask how does the patient process binocular information within the visual axes when the

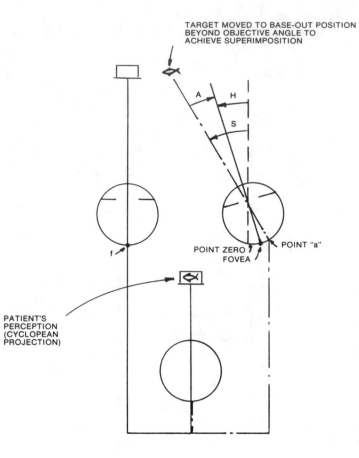

Figure 5-35—Paradoxical type two unharmonious anomalous correspondence.

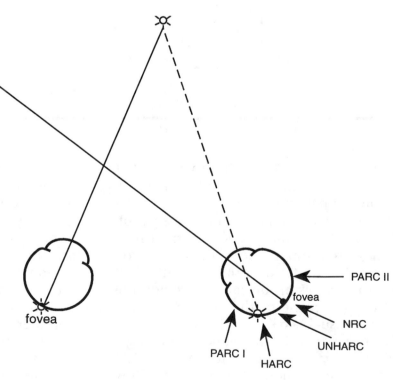

Figure 5-36—ARC classification based on the location of point "a" indicated by arrows pointing to the retinal site on the right eye.

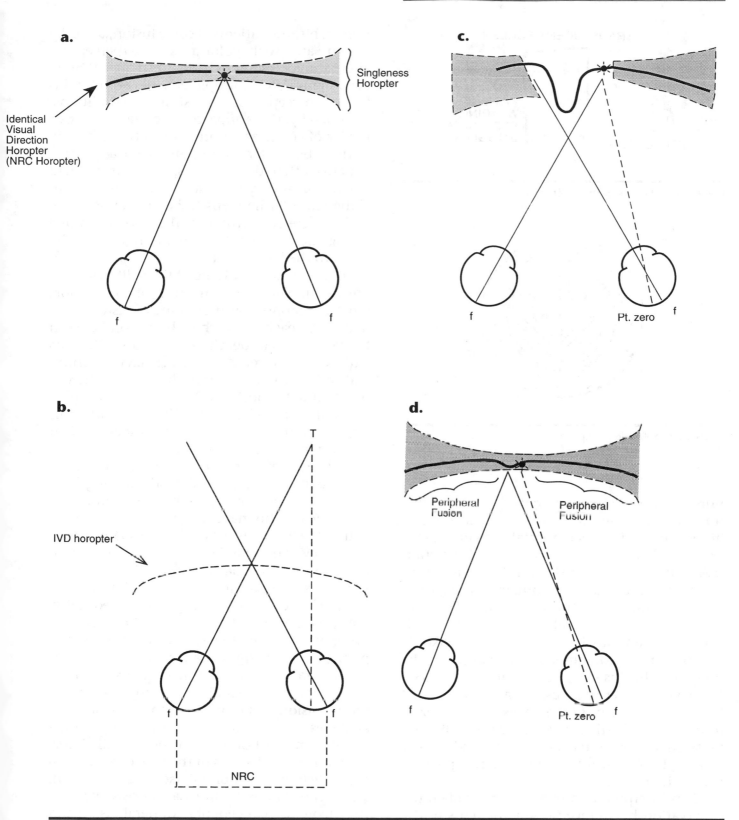

Figure 5-37—Identical visual direction horopter. **(a)** Bifixating person with horopter passing through the centration point and the location of the target. **(b)** Esotropic person with normal correspondence having the identical visual direction horopter passing through the centration point but not through the location of the target. **(c)** Esotropic person with HARC having the central notch approaching the centration point but the peripheral portion of the horopter passing through the location of the target. **(d)** Same as **c** but the magnitude of the esotropia is small, allowing for an almost normal binocular field of fusion.

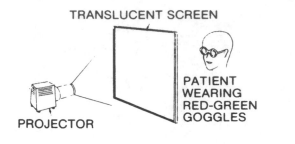

Figure 5-38—Stimulus apparatus for color fusion.

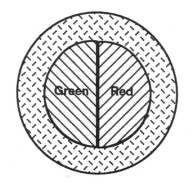

Figure 5-39—Split field perception.

horopter is so extremely skewed? One possible notion is that this area between the axes is not binocular at all under normal viewing conditions. A skew in the identical visual direction (IVD) horopter in nonstrabismic subjects usually means there is aniseikonia and the greater the skew, the greater the aniseikonia. The radical skew of the central portion of the ARC horopter could possibly mean that aniseikonia is too extreme for binocular disparities to be processed. In this case, the patient may be said to have no central fusion and the visual information within the axes is processed monocularly. Furthermore, there is usually suppression in the notch area subtended by the angle between the fovea and the target point of the deviating eye.

This interpretation may help to explain the observation by strabismic ARC patients of the *Swann split field effect*. Red-green glasses are worn by a nonstrabismic subject and the patient views a detailed target against a white background (Figure 5-38). The usual report in nonstrabismus patients is color fusion, a murky brown, and with color rivalry (a percept of alternating, moving red and green areas). However, many ARC esotropic patients report a different percept under similar conditions. Peripherally, there appears to be the melding or rivalry of colors as reported by patients having normal binocular vision, but centrally, ARC patients often describe a split bipartite field where half is purely red and half purely green. If the red filter happens to be on the right eye and the green on the left, the patient reports seeing the red hemifield to the right and the green to the left. Sometimes they report a seam running down the middle of the split field (Figure 5-39). These central areas of pure colors represent monocular processing of visual information by each eye within the region between the visual axes under these conditions. Patients with ARC are often described as having peripheral fusion, the implication being that there is no "central fusion." The Swann split field effect is an important example that supports this interpretation of the status of binocularity in strabismic patients having ARC.

ARC appears to be more prevalent in patients having small and moderate angles of constant strabismus (e.g., 30^Δ or less) compared with those who have larger angles.[51,52] Some patients with small deviations, usually under 10^Δ, show considerable sensory fusion capability. It is not unusual to find 200 seconds of stereopsis when testing with the animals of the Stereo Fly stereograms, but poorer stereoacuity, if any, can be found with the Wirt circles. Also fusional vergence ranges may be fairly normal particularly if prism demands are introduced at a slower rate than in routine vergence testing.[53] Presumably, peripherally sized targets allow for motor fusion to be possible. In cases of small angle esotropia with ARC, there is a small "notch" in the horopter so the overall shape, location, and thickness of the singleness horopter appear nearly normal (see Figure 5-37d). These clinical observations are consistent with the theoretical concept of peripheral fusion and central suppression as a general mechanism in ARC where the size of the angle of deviation determines, in part, the binocular capabilities of the strabismic patient.

Horror Fusionis

Cline et al.[54] define horror fusionis as "the inability to obtain binocular fusion or superimposition of haploscopically presented targets, or the condition or phenomenon itself, occurring frequently as a characteristic in strabismus, in which case the targets approaching superimposition may seem to slide or jump past each other without apparent fusion or suppression." In the past, horror fusionis has been associated with "macular evasion,"[55] patients needing psychotherapy,[56] intractable diplopia,[57] and aniseikonia.[58] Not much has been published on this condition, and the mechanism has been uncertain. We believe this condition is almost always associated with ARC. An inspection of the horopter in ARC gives a clue to the nature of this binocular anomaly. Aniseikonia, indeed, appears to be a factor. The fovea of the fixating eye seems to be associated with many points in the strabismic eye and vice versa. For example, as shown in Figure 5-37c, it is as though the fovea of the left eye is associated with a series of points between point zero (same location as point *a* in HARC) and *f* of the right eye, creating an intolerable magnification effect.

Flom[50] explained horror fusionis in subjects with esotropia and ARC as nonuniform relative distributions of corresponding retinal points (irregularly shaped horopter). He explained the horror fusionis movement of the images when superimposition is attempted, as in the Synoptophore. A sudden movement occurs when the target of the deviating eye is moved across a limb of the notch of the horopter; it is not due to any eye movements. Flom explained, "This jumping phenomenon is commonly observed by strabismics with ARC when viewing constantly illuminated first-degree targets, one of which is moved toward the other to obtain superimposition."[50]

Etiology of ARC

The neurophysiologic basis for ARC is unknown, but most authorities assume the visual cortex mediates binocular visual direction. The binocular striate neurons seem capable of comparing the images from the two eyes, detecting disparities between them, and linking corresponding retinal points.[59] The traditional view is that normal correspondence is innate. Anomalous correspondence is an acquired sensorial adaptation to a strabismus during early development when the cortex is still malleable and capable of establishing a new coupling of noncorresponding cortical elements. Visually mature individuals, past age 6 years or so, who acquire a strabismus later in life are almost always incapable of developing ARC. Burian[60] stated that "ARC is acquired by usage . . . the acquisition of an anomalous correspondence represents an adaptation of the sensory apparatus of the eyes to the abnormal position of the eyes." The earlier the onset of the strabismus and the longer an individual "practices" ARC (a learned response), the deeper the ARC adaptation is established. This view has become known as the "adaptation" theory of ARC. This theory would predict that one would tend to find ARC in early onset, constant, comitant strabismus and less often in late onset, intermittent, and/or noncomitant strabismus. There is substantial clinical evidence confirming this prediction.

Morgan[61] proposed that ARC is a motor phenomenon (rather than merely a sensorial adaptation) and stated, "Thus anomalous correspondence might depend not on a sensory adaptation to a squint but rather on whether the basic underlying innervational pattern to the extraocular muscles was one which registered itself in consciousness as altering egocentric direction, or whether the pattern was one that was 'nonregistered' in consciousness as altering egocentric direction." A nonregistered innervation would imply NRC, while a registered pattern would imply ARC. This notion is called the "motor" theory of ARC. This theory implies that at the time of strabismus onset, the moment the eye turns, an abnormal neural circuit allows the change in vergence eye position to be "registered" in the perceptual mechanism subserving visual direction.

Ordinarily version eye movements are "registered" and vergences are not, but an abnormal reflex, possibly genetically determined, links vergence to the perceptual apparatus. ARC localization is, therefore, immediate and complete, all or none. This view dispenses with the concepts of depth, learning, and adaptation and suggests that ARC is a neural reflex possibly mediated by the neurology responsible for the well-documented phenomenon of ARC *covariation*. Hallden[62] demonstrated that strabismic patients with ARC have some daily variation in their angle of deviation (H) and that the angle of anomaly increases and decreases in tandem with it. Such covariation in ARC also has been reported in some patients with A-V patterns in which the strabismic angle changes in up and down gaze.[63] Correspondence can also be demonstrated to change synchronously with fusional vergence eye position in many cases of strabismus. It is not unusual to find an intermittent exotrope who shows normal correspondence and excellent stereopsis when fusing and ARC when strabismic. As the deviation becomes manifest, angle A increases simultaneously with angle H. Therefore, the subjective angle stays the same (zero) during the motor movement. Far from being a rigid, hard-wired adaptation, ARC is found to vary considerably with changes in vergence eye position.

These two theories of ARC etiology lead to different ideas about its remediation. The adaptation theory suggests that early intervention is critical. NRC must be relearned by realigning the eyes with early surgical and optical means or by stimulating bifoveal localization using vision training procedures, often applied in an amblyoscope. The motor theory, however, suggests that it is necessary to train realignment of the eyes using fusional vergence, thus stimulating covariation. If the eyes can be straightened by fusional vergence, then covariation will change the correspondence from anomalous to normal; NRC will persist as long as the eyes remain straight. This approach is easier to apply to exotropes than to esotropes since fusional convergence is fairly easy to train.

Many investigators and clinicians tend to advocate either one etiology or the other. We believe there is reasonable and substantial evidence that supports each theory. It may well be that there are two or more etiologies for ARC and a complete description of the condition will require appreciating at least both developmental sensory and reflex motor aspects. The clinical challenge may be to determine which mechanism is primarily responsible for ARC in a particular patient. Vision therapy related to the cause or causes can then be more appropriately prescribed for efficacious treatment.

Depth of ARC

Those who espouse the adaptation theory of ARC believe it is clinically useful to evaluate the depth of the condition. Testing the depth of ARC is analogous to testing the intensity of suppression; if testing conditions are very unnatural, suppression is not likely to be found. Burian[60] promoted the concept that ARC is an acquired sensorial adaptation to a motor deviation and that this adaptation may be either deep or shallow. This may explain the more frequent clinical finding of ARC on Bagolini striated lens testing than on other less-natural clinical tests, such as afterimages. The principle is that the more natural the testing environment, the more likely it is that ARC will be found. Conversely, the more unnatural the environment, the more likely it is that NRC will be found.

Flom and Kerr,[64] espousing the motor theory, rejected the concept of depth of anomalous correspondence. They contended that disagreement among various tests can be attributed to measurement error, unsteady fixation, or changes in the relative position of the eyes from one test to another. They employed several different tests in their study which included: (1) the Maddox rod-cover test, (2) major amblyoscope, (3) Hallden test using red-green filters and afterimage to measure *H, A,* and *S,* and (4) the Hering-Bielschowsky afterimage test. These testing methods, however, were unnatural in many respects. The Bagolini striated lens test (a relatively natural test) was not included in their study. In contrast, Bagolini and Tittarelli[65] found harmonious ARC in 83% of their strabismic patients using the striated lenses, but only 13% on the amblyoscope. Von Noorden[66] reported similar results suggesting that ARC has a depth characteristic.

We believe it is prudent to perform several tests for ARC as part of a strabismus examination and if the clinical findings support a depth effect, then use this information in forming the diagnosis and prognosis. Prognosis for elimination of ARC and ultimate cure of strabismus is generally more favorable for those patients giving an ARC response on only one test than when it is found on all tests. Further research, however, is needed to resolve the issue of depth of ARC.

Prevalence

Statistics on prevalence of ARC are variable; this is often due to the unanswered questions of which type of ARC was being considered, what testing was done, and who did the testing. A study of 295 strabismics reported ARC in 45% of the cases. Of the esotropes, 53% were found to have ARC and only 16% of the exotropes.[67] These results were based solely on major amblyoscope findings, and possibly the rates would be lower if more unnatural tests, such as afterimages, had been used and higher with more natural tests. Similarly, Hugonnier[68] reported that in 98 cases of strabismus, the Bagolini striated lens test revealed 84 cases of ARC, the Synoptophore yielded 64 cases of ARC, and with afterimages there were only 35 cases of ARC. In general, ARC is more prevalent in infantile strabismus versus late onset, constant angles versus intermittent, small versus large angles, and esotropia versus exotropia. ARC due to vertical deviations may be possible, but are rare from our clinical experience.

Testing

Correspondence can be assessed indirectly by comparing the measured angles H and S. The angle of anomaly (A) is simply calculated by subtracting the subjective angle (S) from the objective angle (H). It is often convenient clinically to use the alternate cover test results for angle H and the dissociated red lens test results for angle S. The angle of anomaly (A) can also be measured directly without reliance on calculation from H and S. Entoptic phenomena, such as Haidinger's brush and Maxwell's spot may be used, but instruments for these tests are not commonly found in the primary care practice. The most frequently used direct measure of A is done with afterimages. Next in frequency is

visuoscopy performed with the patient under binocular viewing conditions (discussed later in the section on bifoveal test of Cüppers). Most other clinical tests for ARC determine A indirectly by calculating the difference between H and S.

Dissociated Red Lens Test

The dissociated red lens test was recommended by Flom[69] for assessing correspondence as part of the minimal strabismus examination for primary eye care practitioners. This test determines the subjective angle (S) for distance viewing and is compared with the objective angle (H) measured by cover test at the same distance and under similar lighting conditions. A red filter is held together with a 10^Δ base-down loose prism before the dominant eye in a normally illuminated room. The fixation target is a bright "muscle" light (e.g., penlight). Most strabismic patients, even with considerable suppression, will then perceive vertically displaced diplopic images of the light, red on top and white on the bottom. The horizontal angle S is measured using sufficient horizontal prism placed before the nondominant eye until the two images appear to the patient to be vertically aligned. The method of limits (bracketing) should always be used to increase measurement accuracy. In the presence of a strabismus, if angle S is found to be zero or close to zero, HARC is indicated. If angle S is significantly different from zero but less than angle H, UNHARC is suggested. If, however, angles H and S are essentially the same (within the limits of measurement error), then NRC is present.

Afterimages

The Hering-Bielschowsky test is the most frequently used afterimage method of ARC testing and directly measures the angle of anomaly (A). An ordinary electronic flash attachment to a camera can be modified to serve as an afterimage generator (Figure 5-40a). The face of the flash is masked off with opaque tape to produce a long narrow slit. A small piece of tape also is placed across the middle of the slit, which serves as a fixation target. The unit is held at a distance of approximately

Camera Flash Attachment

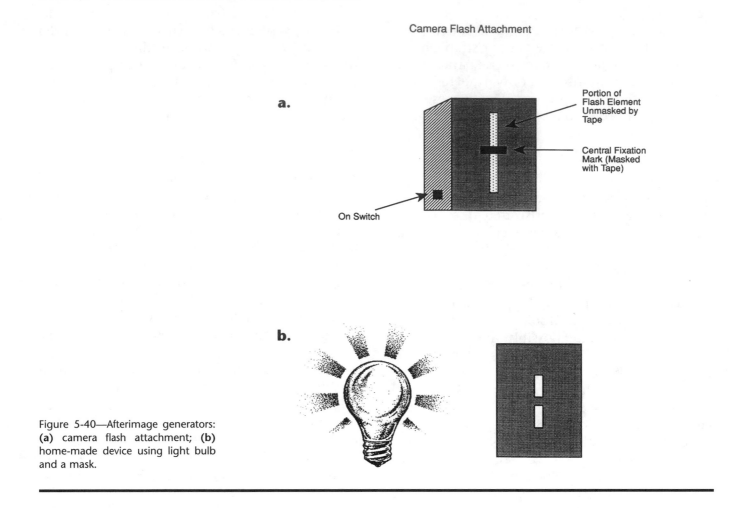

a.

Portion of Flash Element Unmasked by Tape

Central Fixation Mark (Masked with Tape)

On Switch

b.

Figure 5-40—Afterimage generators: **(a)** camera flash attachment; **(b)** home-made device using light bulb and a mask.

40 cm (16 inches) from the patient when the flash is triggered. A 100 watt lightbulb can also be modified if a sustained stimulus is desired (Figure 5-40b). The patient should fixate the masked lightbulb for 30 seconds to produce a vivid, sustained afterimage for each eye. The procedure is as follows:

1. Occlude the nondominant eye while the patient fixates a central mask on a *horizontal* line strobe flasher or a masked lightbulb. The exact center should be opaque to produce a small gap in the afterimage (AI) for the purpose of identifying the position of the fovea.

2. After the horizontal AI is applied occlusion is switched to the dominant eye, and then an AI is applied in the same manner to the nondominant eye, except it is now oriented *vertically*.

3. Uncover the eye and instruct the patient to fixate a small discrete target (e.g., black spot) on a blank (e.g., gray) wall with the dominant eye so that the gap in the horizontal AI is centered on the target. A recommended testing distance is one meter to facilitate measurement of angle A.

4. Alternately lowering and raising the room illumination (approximately every 3 seconds) helps the patient perceive and sustain both the horizontal and vertical afterimages.

5. The negative AI is more reliable in routine testing than is the positive AI. The negative AI is seen in a lighted room and the positive AI is seen in a darkened room. The patient is asked to pay attention to the negative AI as the room illumination is increased.

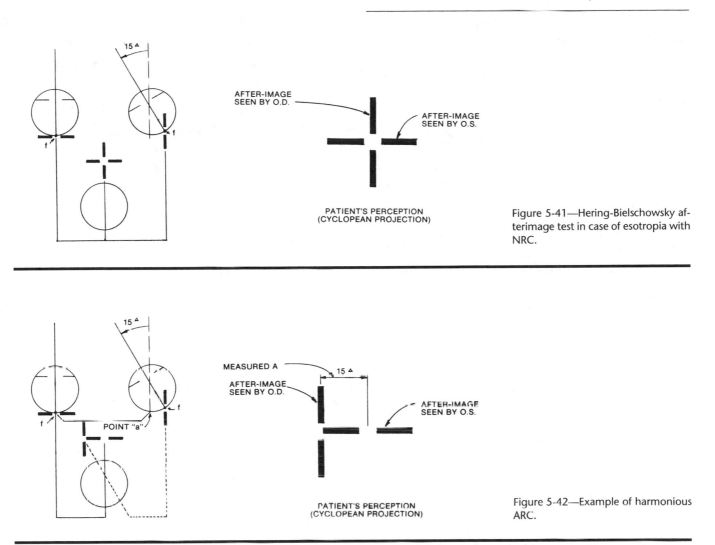

Figure 5-41—Hering-Bielschowsky afterimage test in case of esotropia with NRC.

Figure 5-42—Example of harmonious ARC.

6. The patient is asked to describe the location of the vertical AI in relation to the gap in the horizontal AI. If the vertical AI is perceived as crossing the horizontal AI any place other than the exact center of the target, the examiner measures the perceived displacement with a centimeter ruler and converts it to prism diopters.

Interpretation of results is made by measuring the displacement of the vertical AI from the central gap of the horizontal AI. If the patient reports seeing a perfect cross, there is presumption of NRC, since this represents an A of zero (Figure 5-41). Whether the eyes are straight (ortho posture) is irrelevant if a perfect cross is perceived and reported. Each fovea has been stimulated; if there is normal correspondence between the two foveas, a cross will be perceived regardless of the direction in which each eye is positioned.

An example of a noncross perception is shown in Figure 5-42. The right eye is esotropic with ARC. Point a is the representational point that corresponds to the fovea of the left eye. Cyclopean projection shows the vertical afterimage being seen to the left, since point a has the directional value of zero, and the fovea projects as a temporal retinal point.

The Hering-Bielschowsky AI test is not valid unless the effect of a coexisting eccentric fixation is taken into account. Figure 5-43 illustrates this by taking the same case as in the above examples and adding to it the condition of nasal eccentric fixation of the right eye. A perfect cross is perceived if the angle of eccentric fixation (E) and A are the same in direction and magnitude. Points a and e are in the same

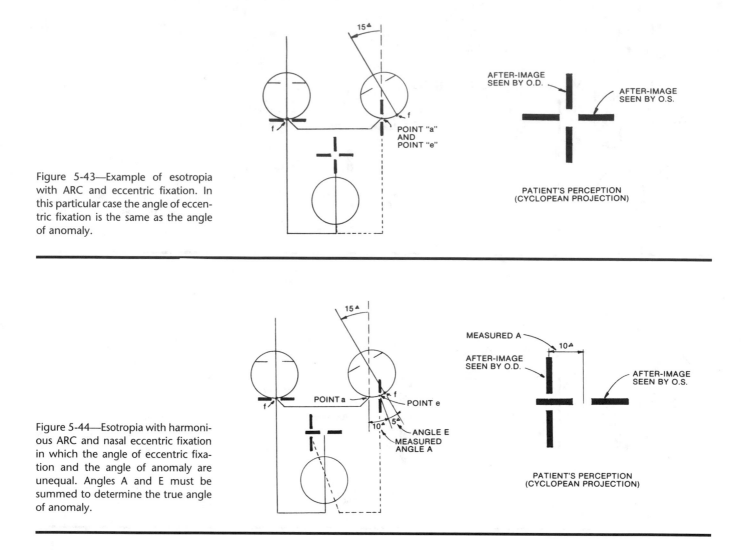

Figure 5-43—Example of esotropia with ARC and eccentric fixation. In this particular case the angle of eccentric fixation is the same as the angle of anomaly.

Figure 5-44—Esotropia with harmonious ARC and nasal eccentric fixation in which the angle of eccentric fixation and the angle of anomaly are unequal. Angles A and E must be summed to determine the true angle of anomaly.

location on the retina. In such a case, the patient has point e stimulated with the vertical AI during monocular fixation with the right eye. Because this is the same point on the retina that corresponds to the fovea of the left eye, the patient will project the vertical afterimage in the same direction as the gap in the horizontal line. This is an exceptional case and not the rule; E and A are usually not of the same magnitude, although most often in the same direction (e.g., points a and e at different locations on the nasal retina). Therefore, unless they are in the identical location, a noncross will be perceived.

In an evaluation of correspondence when eccentric fixation is present, the first step is to measure E using a graduated reticule in an ophthalmoscope. Angle A may then be deter-

mined by measuring the separation between the vertical AI and the center of the gap of the horizontal AI and adding the magnitude of E to this. Assume, for example, an E of 5^Δ is found (Figure 5-44). If the patient looks at the afterimages at 1 m, each centimeter displacement represents 1^Δ. The patient then reports seeing the vertical AI off to the left by 10^Δ. This is the *measured A*, but not the *true A*. The magnitude of E (5^Δ in this example) must be added to this measured A to arrive at the true angle of anomaly. It is easily seen that the angle between the fovea and point a is equal to 15^Δ (not the 10^Δ as measured).

It is not always necessary to use an AI for each eye as in the Hering-Bielschowsky test. The Brock-Givner afterimage transfer test is another means of measuring A. Only one AI is

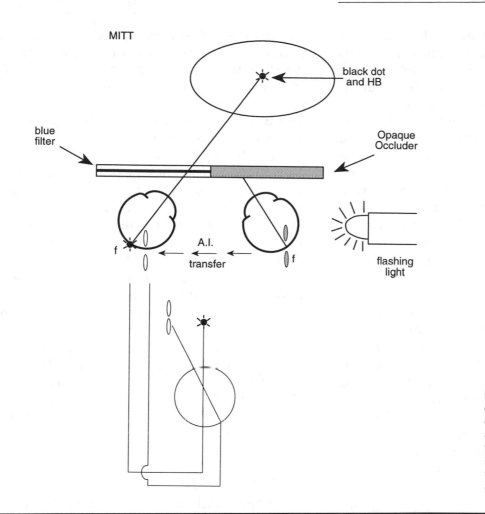

MITT

black dot
and HB

blue
filter

Opaque
Occluder

A.I.

transfer

f

f

flashing
light

Figure 5-45—Combination of Haidinger brush superimposed on the black dot (seen by left eye) and a vertical afterimage (also seen by left eye but transferred from the right eye). Flashing light near right eye enhances the transferred afterimage seen by the left eye.

applied to the fovea of the dominant eye, which is then occluded. The projection of the AI is transferred intracortically to point *a* of the strabismic eye. Assume for example that the left eye is occluded and the right eye is stimulated with the vertical AI. The occluder is switched to the right eye and the left eye fixates a black spot on a gray wall at 1 m. The displacement of the AI from the fixated spot from the AI represents the angular subtense of *A*. It is only when there is no eccentric fixation (*E* = O) that the displacement between the fixated spot and the perceived AI represents the true *A*. Angle *E* must be added to the measured *A* to calculate the true *A*. Thus, True *A* = measured *A* + the magnitude of eccentric fixation (*At* = *Am* + *E*).

Conveniently, *A* and *E* measurements can be combined into one procedure by using a Haidinger brush (HB) and an AI (Figure 5-45).

The separation between the AI and HB represents *A*. In this example there is no eccentric fixation. If there were eccentric fixation, the HB would be displaced from the fixated black dot, the magnitude representing that of *E*. In summary, *E* is measured by the displacement between the dot and the HB, whereas *A* is measured by the distance between the AI and the HB.

Bifoveal Test of Cüppers

Most tests for ARC have one or more shortcomings, the most common being the contamination of eccentric fixation. The bifoveal test of Cüppers can eliminate this possibly invalidating factor. It is particularily useful in assessing correspondence in cases of strabismic amblyopia. Testing is done by performing visuoscopy under *binocular* seeing conditions for the measurement of the angle of anomaly (*A*). This should not be confused with the procedure for measurement of the angle of eccentric fixation (*E*) under *monocular* seeing conditions.

The bifoveal procedure is illustrated in Figure 5-46. Suppose the patient has an esotropia of the right eye. An angled mirror (or a large base-out prism of approximately 40$^\Delta$) is placed before the patient's dominant left eye to fixate a penlight off to the side from a distance of 2 to 3 meters (see Figure 5-46a). This is necessary so the patient can maintain seeing under binocular conditions without one eye being occluded by the examiner's head during visuoscopy. The next step is for the examiner to look into the patient's right (amblyopic) eye and observe the image of the star that is projected on the patient's retina. If mydriatics are not used for pupil dilation, a darkened room is recommended. At the same time, the patient is asked to look into the instrument for the star on the grid of the ophthalmoscope (visuoscope). The patient should be aware of both the penlight and the star, unless suppression is very deep and extensive. If so, a red filter can be used to produce a red light stimulus to the left eye. This almost always breaks through any existing suppression. The examiner's next step is to project the star directly onto the fovea and ask the patient to report the direction in which the targets are seen. If there is NRC, the patient should report that the penlight and the star are superimposed (see Figure 5-46b) because both foveas correspond to each other. If, however, the foveas do not correspond (ARC), as in Figure 5-46c, the patient will report that the star and penlight appear separated in space, even though both foveas are being stimulated. In this case, the examiner should move the star nasalward to find point *a* so that the penlight and the star are superimposed (see Figure 5-46d). This is necessary because point *a* corresponds to the fovea of the left eye. The distance from point *a* to the center of the fovea (*f*) represents the magnitude of *A*. This distance can be measured by using projected concentric circles of a reticule. If a direct ophthalmoscope without a reticule is used, retinal landmarks, such as the optic disk (disc), can be observed to estimate the magnitude of *A*. Knowing that the

center of the disc is normally 15.5° from the center of the fovea helps in the estimation of the distance from the star to the fovea. Likewise, if the width of the disc is 5.5° the first margin of the disc would be 12.75° (23$^\Delta$) and the outer margin 18.25° (33$^\Delta$) from the center of the fovea (Figure 5-47).

The bifoveal visuoscope test, therefore, takes much of the guesswork out of measuring *A* compared with other more subjective methods of testing. In addition to this advantage, the presence of eccentric fixation does not need to be taken into account (assuming the dominant eye is centrally fixating, which is almost always the case). This is because testing is done under binocular conditions, thereby vitiating any effect of eccentric fixation that would otherwise come into play if testing were done under monocular conditions. The disadvantage of the bifoveal visuoscopic test is that a high level of patient cooperation must be maintained; otherwise, testing is either impossible or results are unreliable. Testing is sometimes not feasible in young children.

Major Amblyoscope

The major amblyoscope can be used to detect and calculate the angle of anomaly (*A*). The Synoptophore (see Figure 5-4) has a long history in the field of strabismus diagnosis and therapy and is still in use today. Each tube of the Synoptophore has a mirror placed at 45° and a +7 diopter eyepiece lens. Test targets are placed at optical infinity. (Sketches showing the direction of movement of the carriage arm to create horizontal prismatic demands are presented in Figure 5-5.)

The procedure for measuring the objective angle of deviation (called *alternate exclusion method*) using this instrument is as follows:

1. Turn on the main power switch and have the patient look into the instrument. Properly adjust the chin and forehead rests and the interpupillary distance setting for the patient. Adjust the illumination for each tube by setting the rheostat to approximately #8.
2. Use first-degree targets that are central in size (see Figure 5-6). For example, place

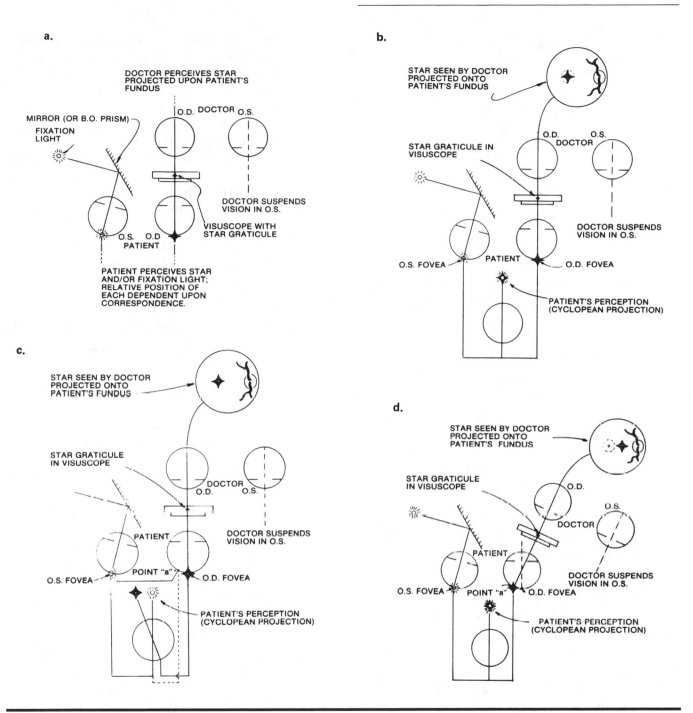

Figure 5-46—The bifoveal test of Cüppers. **(a)** Doctor's right eye views the patient's right eye by means of visuoscopy. The star is seen by the doctor and the patient. An angled mirror (or a large base-out prism) before the patient's left eye avoids obstruction to seeing by left eye. **(b)** Example of normal correspondence. **(c)** Example of anomalous correspondence. **(d)** Star must be projected onto point "a" for a patient with ARC to achieve superimposition of the penlight and the star.

the X target in one tube and the square target in the other. Instruct the patient always to look at the center of each target.

3. Alternately douse (occlude) each tube light by means of the two small button switches near the front of the control panel. The alternate dousing of each target makes this an "alternate cover test" in an instrument, rather than in true space.

4. The examiner neutralizes the lateral movement of the eyes by adjusting the

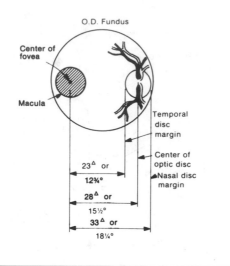

O.D. Fundus

Center of
fovea

Macula

Temporal
disc
margin

Center of
optic disc

Nasal disc
margin

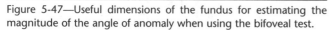

23△ or

12¾°

28△ or

15½°

33△ or

18¼°

Figure 5-47—Useful dimensions of the fundus for estimating the magnitude of the angle of anomaly when using the bifoveal test.

position of the tube of the nondominant eye. Keep the tube for the dominant eye placed on zero (primary position of gaze). When the conjugate movement is neutralized using a bracketing technique, the objective angle (H) is determined. The magnitude is read directly from the prism diopter scale. The direction of the deviation, eso or exo, is noted by observing the final positions of the tubes as illustrated in Figure 5-5.

Hirschberg testing can also be performed with a Synoptophore by observing the positions of the corneal reflections of the light from the two tubes. This method is particularly appropriate for determining the objective angle (H) when amblyopia is present in one eye and monocular fixation is inaccurate. For this procedure, the instruments lights should be turned up to the maximum intensity and the room lights dimmed. The patient must be properly positioned so the examiner has a good view of the patient's eyes to judge the positions of the corneal light reflexes. The accuracy of the technique is limited to about five prism diopters. A recommended procedure follows:

1. Use only one target placed before the dominant eye and direct the patient's fixation to the center of that target (e.g.,

the fish target). Be sure that the tube is in the primary position (zero on the scale).

2. Estimate angle kappa (K) of the fixating eye. Adjust the tube of the nondominant eye so the corneal reflection is positioned in the same relative position in each eye. (The position of the reflex should look like angle K.) The examiner should sight from behind the tube to assure the greatest accuracy.

3. Use the method of limits (bracketing technique) to determine the symmetric position of the corneal reflections. Read the magnitude of the objective angle (H) directly from the prism diopter scale of the nondominant eye.

The procedure for finding the horizontal subjective angle (S) with the Synoptophore is as follows:

1. After the instrument has been adjusted properly for the patient, insert two first-degree targets, one before each eye, of sufficient size to avoid or minimize suppression (e.g., the fish and tank targets). This is a binocular test; neither eye is occluded.

2. Instruct the patient to maintain fixation constantly on the center of the dominate eye's target (e.g., fish), which is set to the zero position on the scale.

3. The patient (or the examiner if necessary) adjusts the position of the nondominant eye's tube (e.g., with the tank) until the two targets appear superimposed (i.e., the fish inside the tank). If suppression occurs, the illumination can be increased for the suppressing eye or dimmed for the dominant eye.

4. The magnitude of the subjective angle (S) is read directly from the scale and the measurement taken several times approaching angle S from both sides (bracketing technique) to increase accuracy.

Determining the subjective angle is sometimes difficult due either to deep suppression or horror fusionis. Vertical dissociation can sometimes overcome these obstacles allowing the measurement of angle S. Using the vertical adjustment, the Synoptophore target to the nondominant eye is elevated 10^Δ or more above the other target. The nondominant eye's target is then moved horizontally until one appears above the other. This value represents the subjective angle. Another effective procedure uses a large first-degree target before the nondominant eye while the patient is fixating a small target with the other eye (e.g., the X and the sentry box) (see Figure 5-6).

After angles H and S are measured on the Synoptophore, it is a simple matter to calculate angle A ($A = H - S$). Measurement accuracy must be taken into account when determining the presence of ARC. Allowance of 1^Δ to 2^Δ error may be necessary for small angles and up to 5^Δ should be allowed for large angles of strabismus in comparing H and S.

Another quick check for ARC on the Synoptophore is the unilateral *douse target test.* This is done after angle S has been measured and the targets appear to be superimposed. The examiner simply shuts off (douses) the illumination to the target of the dominant eye and watches for movement of the nondominant eye. If the nondominant eye makes a horizontal movement in order to fixate the center of the target, ARC is presumed to be present, and there is a difference between angles S and H. This test, in effect, is a "unilateral cover test." The size of the movement represents the magnitude of angle A.

For example, a patient has a 15^Δ right esotropia (angle H), i.e., 15^Δ base-out by alternate exclusion as measured on the Synoptophore. The fish and the tank, however, appear to be superimposed at 9^Δ base-out (angle S) which represents a significant difference from the measured objective angle. ARC is, therefore, suspected. On the douse target test when the left eye is doused, the examiner observes an outward movement of the right eye of approximately 6^Δ to pick up fixation on the target. This is a positive douse target test, confirming the presence of ARC. (As discussed previously, however, any eccentric fixation must be taken into account.)

Bagolini Striated Lenses

The Bagolini striated lens test is a quick, simple, and informative clinical test for ARC in strabismic patients. Striations in Bagolini lenses are so fine that the patient is unaware of them, therefore making the test a fairly natural one for the subjective angle (S). The striations cause a streak of light to be visible when the fixation target is a bright spot of light, similar to the effect of a Maddox rod (Figure 5-48). A patient bifoveally fixating a penlight will see the penlight at the intersection of the streaks, as in Figure 5-48c. If the patient has a manifest strabismic deviation whereby bifoveal fixation is not taking place, diplopic images of the light occur, unless suppression is too intense and extensive. Often, however, only a portion of one line will be missing, as in Figures 5-48d and e. An esotropic patient is normally expected to have homonymous diplopia and reports seeing the lights above the intersection of the streaks (see Figure 5-48f). An exotropic patient with heteronymous diplopia, would be expected to report seeing the lights below the intersection (see Figure 5-48g). The above examples presume NRC. However, if an esotrope has ARC of the harmonious type, the patient is expected to report seeing one light centered at the intersection of the streaks (see Figure 5-48c), as would be the report of a patient who is nonstrabismic and bifixating. The reason for the strabismic's "normal" response is that angle S is zero in HARC. The clinician will not be misled if the manifest deviation is observed while listening to the patient's report of seeing the light centered at the intersection of the two streaks. This is obviously a case of ARC since S is zero and H is of a conspicuous magnitude. If, however, the strabismus is small and difficult to detect by direct observation, the unilateral cover test is necessary. (This is analogous to the douse target test using the major amblyoscope.) The clinician watches for any movement of the uncovered nondominant eye when the dominant eye is occluded. A significant movement means that H is greater than zero; this confirms the presence of ARC.

Von Noorden and Maumenee[70] suggested that the Bagolini test is not useful in diagnosing cases of unharmonious ARC in which S is a magnitude other than zero. We believe, however, the following procedure is useful in UN-HARC cases. First, find out from the patient

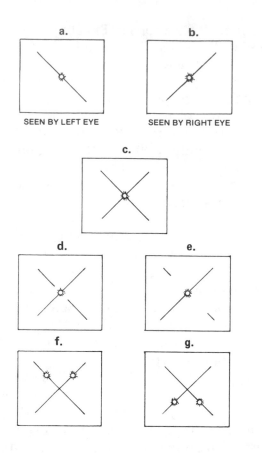

a.   b.

SEEN BY LEFT EYE   SEEN BY RIGHT EYE

c.

d.   e.

f.   g.

Figure 5-48—Patient's view when looking through Bagolini striated lenses and fixating a penlight. **(a)** Orientation of streak seen by left eye. **(b)** Orientation of streak seen by the right eye. **(c)** Perception when the patient is bifoveally fixating, indicating fusion. This same perception indicates harmonious anomalous correspondence if there is a manifest deviation. **(d)** Central suppression of the left eye. **(e)** Peripheral suppression of the left eye. **(f)** This indicates esotropia with normal correspondence, but it may also mean there is a manifest subjective eso deviation in a case of unharmonious anomalous correspondence. **(g)** This means there is an exotropia with normal correspondence. This type of response could also occur in an exotropia with unharmonious correspondence.

where the streaks intersect. If they cross below the lights, as in an eso deviation, base-out prism is increasingly introduced until the patient reports that the light is centered at the intersection of the streaks. At this time the unilateral cover test is done to see if there is any movement of the uncovered eye. The patient has UNHARC if there is any significant movement. In this case *S* is equal to the base-out prism power necessary for attainment of the centered pattern. (When the patient is strabismic and *S* is not zero, the ARC is

unharmonious.) The estimated magnitude of *A* is represented by the magnitude of the movement of the uncovered eye on the unilateral cover test during this procedure. This test should be done quickly to avoid possible contamination of prism adaptation.

The great majority of strabismic patients with ARC show HARC on the Bagolini test. Harmonious ARC is an ideal antidiplopic adaptation for a strabismic individual in natural seeing conditions at school, work, or play; some peripheral binocularity with its many benefits is often preserved. The Bagolini test is relatively natural; clinicians find the highest prevalence of ARC using this test compared with other less-natural clinical methods.

Color Fusion

Color fusion is also referred to as luster. The most efficacious way to evaluate whether color fusion is present is by having the patient wear colored filters (usually red OD and green OS) while viewing a brightly illuminated translucent gray screen containing no contours. Normally the patient reports a mixture of the red and green, perceived as a muddy yellow or brown with some color rivalry taking place. Testing at the centration point helps to elicit this response in many esotropic patients. The centration point addition lens (add) in diopters is calculated by dividing the objective angle at far (Hf) by the interpupillary distance in cm.

$$D_{cpa} = \frac{Hf}{IPDcm}$$

Key: D_{cpa} is the centration point
       add in diopters.
       Hf is the horizontal objective angle
       in prism diopters at 6 meters.
       IPDcm is interpupillary distance
       in centimeters.

For example, a 24^Δ constant right esotropic patient having a 6 cm IPD would require at least a +4.00D add to bring targets into focus at the position in space where the eyes cross. Wearing this high plus add in a trial frame and moving to a distance of 25 cm from the screen, this esotropic patient has the optimum conditions to demonstrate true color fusion. (High base-in prisms may help achieve perception of color fusion in an exotropic patient.) Color fusion is determined by alternately occluding each eye to demonstrate what a monocular response looks like, i.e., purely red or purely green. Under binocular conditions, the patient is then asked if the percept looks "different" compared with monocular viewing. Color fusion is indicated if the patient reports a yellowish or brownish blending of colors.

A split field is not true color fusion but is indicative of ARC (see Figure 5-39). This is the Swann split field effect described previously. We have found that patients who give an evenly split response often have HARC, whereas a field not split evenly down the middle suggests UNHARC. Although color fusion testing is not completely reliable, it does seem to have some diagnostic and prognostic value. For example, a patient who shows a Swann split field effect when no contours are in the visual field, has a poorer prognosis for successful treatment of ARC than a patient reporting color fusion over the entire field.

REFERENCES

1. Cline D, Hofstetter HW, Griffin JR. *Dictionary of Visual Science.* 4th ed. Radnor, Penn: Chilton Book Co; 1989:664.
2. Von Noorden GK. *Binocular Vision and Ocular Motility.* 4th ed. St Louis: CV Mosby Co; 1990:202.
3. Smith EL, Levi DM, Manny R, Harwerth RS, White JM. The relationship between binocular rivalry and strabismic suppression. *Invest Ophthalmol Vis Sci.* 1985;26:80-87.
4. Jampolsky A. Characteristics of suppression in strabismus. *Arch Ophthalmol.* 1955;54:683-696.
5. Pratt-Johnson JA, MacDonald AL. Binocular visual field in strabismus. *Can J Ophthalmol.* 1976;11:37-41.
6. Cline D, Hofstetter HW, Griffin JR. *Dictionary of Visual Science.* 4th ed. Radnor, Penn: Chilton Book Co; 1989:21.
7. Ciuffreda KJ, Levi DM, Selenow A. *Amblyopia: Basic and Clinical Aspects.* Boston: Butterworth-Heinemann; 1991:13-17.
8. Von Noorden GK, Frank JW. Relationship between amblyopia and the angle of strabismus. *Am Orthopt J.* 1976;26:31-33.
9. Helveston EM. The incidence of amblyopia ex anopsia in young adult males in Minnesota in 1962-63. *Am J Ophthalmol.* 1965;60:75-77.
10. Glover LP, Brewer WR. An ophthalmologic review of more than twenty thousand men at the Altoona Induction Center. *Am J Ophthalmol.* 1944; 27:346-8.
11. Schapero M. *Amblyopia.* Philadelphia: Chilton; 1971:60-62.
12. Flynn JT, Cassady JC. Current trends in amblyopia therapy. *Ophthalmology.* 1978;85:428-450.
13. Tanlamai T, Goss DA. Prevalence of monocular amblyopia among anisometropes. *Am J Optom Physio Opt.* 1979;56:704-715.
14. Kivlin JD, Flynn JT. Therapy of anisometropic amblyopia. *J Pediatr Ophthalmol.* 1981;18:47-56.
15. Ingram RM, Walker C, Wilson JM, Arnold PE, Lucas J, Dally S. A first attempt to prevent amlyopia and squint by spectacle correction of abnormal refractions from age 1 year. *Br J Ophthalmol.* 1985;69:851-853.
16. Ciuffreda KJ, Levi DM, Selenow A. *Amblyopia: Basic and Clinical Aspects.* Newton, Mass: Butterworth-Heinemann; 1991:24.
17. Agatston H. Ocular malingering. *Arch Ophthalmol.* 1944;31:223-231.
18. Ciuffreda KJ, Levi DM, Selenow A. *Amblyopia: Basic and Clinical Aspects.* Newton, Mass: Butterworth-Heinemann, 1991:26.
19. Pratt-Johnson JA, Wee HS, Ellis S. Suppression associated with esotropia. *Can J Ophthalmol.* 1967;2:284-291.
20. Brent HP, Lewis TL, Maurer D. Effect of binocular deprivation from cataracts on development of Snellen acuity. *Invest Ophthalmol Vis Sci.* 1986;27 (suppl):51.
21. Ciuffreda KJ, Levi DM, Selenow A. *Amblyopia: Basic and Clinical Aspects.* Newton, Mass: Butterworth-Heinemann, 1991:43.
22. Norcia AM, Tyler CW. Spatial frequency sweep VEP: Visual acuity during the first year of life. *Vision Res.* 1985;25;1399-1408.
23. Worth CA. *Squint: Its Causes, Pathology and Treatment.* Philadelphia: Blakiston, 1903.
24. Ciuffreda KJ, Levi DM, Selenow A. *Amblyopia: Basic and Clinical Aspects.* Boston: Butterworth-Heinemann, 1991:43-136.
25. Ciuffreda KJ, Kenyon RV, Stark L. Increased drift in amblyopic eyes. *Br J Ophthalmol.* 1980;64:7-14.
26. Schor CM, Flom MC. Eye position control and visual acuity in strabismus amblyopia. In: Lennerstrand G, Bach-y-rita P, eds. *Basic Mechanisms of Ocular Motility and Their Clinical Implications.* New York: Pergamon Press; 1975:555-559.
27. Bedell HE, Flom MC. Monocular spatial distortion in strabismic amblyopia. *Invest Ophthalmol Vis Sci.* 1981;20:263-268.
28. Levi DM, Klein SA. Difference in discrimination for gratings between strabismic and anisometropic amblyopes. *Invest Opthalmol Vis Sci.* 1982;23:398-407.
29. Bedell HE, Flom MC. Normal and abnormal space perception. *Am J Optom Physiol Opt.* 1983;60:426-435.
30. Kenyon RV, Ciuffreda KJ, Stark L. Dynamic vergence eye movements in strabismus and amblyopia: asymmetric vergence. *Br J Ophthalmol.* 1981;65:167-176.
31. Greenwald MJ, Folk ER. Afferent pupillary defects in amblyopia. *J Pediatr Ophthalmol Strabismus* 1983;20:63-67.
32. Kase M, Nagata R, Yoshida A, Hanada I. Pupillary light reflex in amblyopia. *Invest Ophthalmol Vis Sci* 1984;25:467-471.

33. Boman DR, Kertesz AE. Fusional responses of strabismics to foveal and extrafoveal stimulation. *Invest Ophthalmol Vis Sci.* 1985;26:1731-1739.

34. Boonstra FM, Koopmans SA, Houtman WA. Fusional vergence in microstrabismus. *Doc Ophthalmol.* 1988;70:221-226.

35. Flom MC, Heath GG, Takahashi E. Contour interaction and visual resolution: Contralateral effects. *Science* 1963;142:979-980.

36. Flom MC. New concepts on visual acuity. *Optom Weekly* 1966;53:1026-1032.

37. Davidson DW, Eskridge JB. Reliability of visual acuity measures of amblyopic eyes. *Am J Optom Physiol Opt.* 1977;54:756-766.

38. Schor CM, Levi DM. Disturbances of small-field horizontal and vertical optokinetic nystagmus in amblyopia. *Invest Ophthalmol Vis Sci.* 1980;19:668-683.

39. White CT, Eason RG. Evoked cortical potentials in relation to certain aspects of visual perception. *Psychology Monogram* 1966;80, Number 24.

40. Harding GFA. The visual evoked response. *Adv Ophthal.* (Karger, Basal) 1974;28:2-28.

41. Sherman J. Visual evoked potential (VEP): basic concepts and clinical applications. *J Am Optom Assoc.* 1979;50:19-30.

42. Selenow A, Cuiffreda KJ, Mozlin R, Rumpf D. Prognostic value of laser interferometric visual acuity in amblyopia therapy. *Invest Ophthalmol Vis Sci.* 1986;27:273-277.

43. Hallden U. An explanation of Haidinger's brushes. *Arch Ophthalmol.* 1957;57:393-399.

44. Schapero M. *Amblyopia.* Philadelphia: Chilton, 1971:162.

45. Irvine SR. Amblyopia exanopsia. Observations on retinal inhibition, scotoma, projection, sight difference, discrimination, and visual acuity. *Trans Am Ophth Soc.* 1948; 46:531.

46. Ammann E. Einige Beobachtunger bei den Funtion sprufungen in der Spechsturde: Zentrales Sehensehen der glaukomatosen-schen der Amblyopen. *Klin Monatsbl Augenheilkd.* 1921;66:564-573.

47. Caloroso E, Flom MC. Influence of luminance on visual acuity in amblyopia. *Am J Optom Physiol Opt.* 1969;46:189-195.

48. Von Noorden GK, Burian HM. Visual acuity in normal and amblyopic patients under reduced illumination: II. The visual acuity at various levels of illumination. *Arch Ophthalmol.* 1959; 62:396-399.

49. Von Noorden GK. *Binocular Vision and Ocular Motility,* 4th ed. St. Louis: CV Mosby Co; 1990:339.

50. Flom MC. Corresponding and disparate retinal points in normal and anomalous correspondence. *Amer J Optom Physiol Opt.* 1980;57:656-665.

51. Flom MC. Treatment of binocular anomalies in children. In: Hirsch MJ, Wick RE, eds. *Vision of Children.* Philadelphia: Chilton, 1963:197-228.

52. Burian HM, Luke N. Sensory retinal relationships in 100 consecutive cases of heterotropia. A comparative clinical study. *Arch Ophthalmol.* 1970;84:16.

53. Burian HM. Fusional movements in permanent strabismus. A study of the role of the central and peripheral retinal regions in the act of binocular vision in squint. *Arch Ophthalmol.* 1941;26:626.

54. Cline D, Hofstetter HW, Griffin JR. *Dictionary of Visual Science.* 4th ed. Radnor, Penn: Chilton Book Co; 1989:318-319.

55. Lyle TK, Wybar K. *Practical Orthoptics in the Treatment of Squint.* 5th ed. Springfield, Ill: Charles C Thomas; 1967:617.

56. Kramer M. *Clinical Orthoptics.* 2nd ed. St Louis: CV Mosby Co; 1953:337.

57. Krimsky E. *The Management of Binocular Imbalance.* Philadelphia: Lea and Febiger; 1948:204.

58. Bielschowsky A. Congenital and acquired deficiencies of fusion. *Am J Ophth.* 1935;18:925-937.

59. Nelson JI. Binocular vision: disparity detection and anomalous correspondence. In: Edwards K, Llewellyn R. eds. *Optometry, London.* Newton, Mass: Butterworth-Heinemann; 1988:217.

60. Burian HM. Anomalous retinal correspondence, its essence and its significance in prognosis and treatment. *Am J Ophth.* 1951;34:237-253.

61. Morgan MW. Anomalous correspondence interpreted as a motor phenomenon. *Am J Optom.* 1961;38:131-148.

62. Hallden U. Fusional phenomena in anomalous correspondence. Copenhagen, Ejnar Munksgaard, *Acta Ophthalmol.* 1952;37(suppl).

63. Helveston EM, von Noorden GK, Williams F. Retinal correspondence in the A and V pattern. *Am Orthopt J.* 1970;20:22.

64. Flom MC, Kerr KE. Determination of retinal correspondence, multiple-testing results and the depth of anomaly concept. *Arch Ophthal.* 1967;77:200-213.

65. Bagolini B, and Tittarelli. II. Sensorio-motorial anomalies in strabismus (anomalous movements). *Doc Ophthalmol.* 1976;41:23.

66. Von Noorden GK. *Binocular Vision and Ocular Motility.* 4th ed. St Louis: CV Mosby Co; 1990:252-253.

67. Enos MV. Anomalous correspondence. *Am J Ophthalmol.* 1950;33:1907-1913.

68. Hugonnier R, Hugonnier S, Troutman S. *Strabismus, Heterophoria, Ocular Motor Paralysis.* St Louis: CV Mosby Co; 1969:199.

69. Flom MC. A minimum strabismus examination. *J Am Optom Assn.* 1956;27:642-649.

70. Von Noorden GK, Maumenee A. *Atlas of Strabismus.* St Louis: CV Mosby Co; 1967:84.

Chapter 6 / Diagnosis and Prognosis

Establishing a Diagnosis   185
Prognosis   186
   Functional Cure of Strabismus   186
    Prognostic Variables of the
      Deviation   189
    Associated Conditions   191
    Other Factors   192
   Cosmetic Cure of Strabismus   193
   Heterophoria   195
Modes of Vision Therapy   196
   Lenses   197
   Prisms   197
   Occlusion   197
   Vision Training   197
   Extraocular Muscle Surgery   198
    General Approach   198
    Adjustable Suture Procedure   200
    Surgical Considerations   200
   Pharmacological Treatment   201
   Botulinum Toxin   202

Other Approaches   202
Case Examples   202
   Poor Prognosis   203
    Case no. 1   203
    Case no. 2   203
    Case no. 3   204
   Poor-to-Fair Prognosis   204
    Case no. 4   204
    Case no. 5   205
   Fair Prognosis   206
    Case no. 6   206
   Fair-to-Good Prognosis   206
    Case no. 7   206
    Case no. 8   207
    Case no. 9   207
   Good Prognosis   208
    Case no.10   208
    Case no.11   208
    Case no.12   209

A valid prognosis cannot be made unless there is a complete diagnosis. Most of this chapter is devoted to the diagnosis and prognosis of strabismus rather than to heterophoria. This is because there is a full range of prognosis, from poor to good, in cases of strabismus (Table 6-1). The prognostic range is more limited in cases of heterophoria, which has relatively few complications (e.g., ARC, lack of fusional vergence, and deep and extensive suppression) that adversely affect successful treatment. Since the prognosis to achieve a functional cure is generally good, only a brief discussion is given to the prognosis of heterophoria.

ESTABLISHING A DIAGNOSIS

The first part of a complete diagnosis of strabismus is the test results of each of the nine variables of the deviation of the visual axes, i.e., comitancy, frequency, direction, magnitude, AC/A, variability, cosmesis, eye laterality, and eye dominance. The next portion includes associated conditions, i.e., suppression, amblyopia, abnormal fixation, ARC, horror fusionis, and any deficient visual skills.

Case history also helps establish the exact diagnosis and is necessary for a valid prognosis. Furthermore, time of onset, mode of onset, duration of strabismus, refractive history, what

TABLE 6-1. *Range of Prognosis in Strabismus and Chance of Functional Cure*

1. Poor	0%–20%
2. Poor to fair	21%–40%
3. Fair	41%–60%
4. Fair to good	61%–80%
5. Good	81%–100%

treatment was given, and developmental history of the patient are all vitally important in determining the prognosis. The doctor must also assess the results of additional evaluative procedures such as prism adaptation, special cover testing, vertical and cyclo deviation testing, prolonged occlusion, and testing for sensory fusion at the centration point.

A good diagnostic statement is not a listing of clinical data, but rather, one that is succinct and understandable that includes the distinguishing features and nature of the condition. The diagnostic statement must be well written in clinical records and reports, not only for conceptual clarity, but also for medical-legal purposes. One acid test of a good diagnostic statement is whether it can be communicated completely and concisely. Examples are given in this chapter to illustrate succinct diagnostic clarity.

PROGNOSIS

Prognosis is the prediction for success by a specified means of treatment. As to binocular anomalies, prognosis pertains to the chance for a favorable outcome by the use of lenses, prisms, occlusion, vision training, surgery, medication, mental effort, or any combination of these methods of treatment. After all necessary testing has been completed and a thorough diagnosis has been made, the doctor makes a prognosis of the case. From this, appropriate recommendations for the patient can be made. There are two types of prognoses depending on the goal of treatment of strabismus. The doctor can describe either the chances for a *functional* cure or a *cosmetic* cure.

Functional Cure of Strabismus

The Flom criteria for functional cure of strabismus has been the standard for assessing success in vision therapy for many years.[1] His criteria made it feasible to compare results of one study to another. Flom,[2] however, later modified the criteria for clinical purposes. In the past, the criteria for functional cure of strabismus, according to Flom,[1] were that there must be clear, comfortable, single, binocular vision present at all distances, from the farpoint to a normal nearpoint of convergence. There should be stereopsis, but a stereoacuity threshold was not specified by Flom. The patient should achieve normal ranges of motor fusion. The deviation may be manifest up to 1% of the time, providing the patient is aware of diplopia whenever this happens (i.e., feedback so patient knows the deviation is not latent but manifest at that time). This should mean that the strabismus may occur only about 5 to 10 minutes per day and that the patient has clear, single, comfortable binocular vision the rest of his or her normal waking hours. Corrective lenses and small amounts of prism may be worn; however, prismatic power is limited to 5^Δ. In a later publication, Flom dropped the requirement of stereopsis, diplopia awareness, normal ranges of motor fusion, and the limit of 5^Δ compensation. He stated that "a reasonable amount of prism" meets the criteria.[2]

Flom listed another category of cure, called "almost cured." The criteria are that there may be stereopsis lacking, the deviation may be manifest up to 5% of the time. Fairly large amounts of prism may be used as long as there is comfortable binocular vision. Otherwise, the other criteria for functional cure must be met. The third category was called "moderate improvement." The stipulation here was that there must be improvement in more than one defect. The fourth category of cure, according to Flom, was "slight improvement." This means improvement in only one defect, such as amblyopia reduced. The final category was "no improvement" as a result of therapy.

Flom's current criteria for a functional cure are listed as follows: (1) maintenance of bifoveal fixation in the ordinary situations of life 99%

of the time; (2) clear vision that is generally comfortable; (3) bifixation in all fields of gaze and distance as close as a few centimeters from the eyes; (4) corrective lenses and a reasonable amount of prism can be worn.[2]

We concur with the new cure criteria set forth by Flom, which can incorporate his former category of "almost cured." We recommend keeping Flom's categories of "moderate improvement" and "slight improvement."

Although not included within the stated cure criteria, we believe the level of stereopsis is clinically useful in evaluating functional success. Manley[3] indicated that a stereothreshold of 67 sec. of arc (for *contoured* tests) is the differentiating value between monofixation pattern and bifoveal fusion and, for example, that on the Stereo Fly tests "central fusion (bifixation) must be present for circles 7 to 9 to be answered correctly." This compares closely with the findings on the Pola-Mirror in which there was central suppression found in all patients who had worse than 60 sec. of arc stereoacuity on *contoured* tests, whereas all those with better than 60 sec. passed the Pola-Mirror test.[4] Therefore, we believe the cutoff value of 60 sec. of arc is reasonable, and it should be included in the criteria. This can be one of the means of determining if the strabismus is completely eliminated (i.e., when there is bifoveal fixation without suppression). A realistic cutoff for *noncontoured* stereoacuity tests would be 100 sec. of arc. Although there are exceptions, the general rule is that stereoacuity is the "barometer" of binocular status.

It should be pointed out that a patient who has made either "moderate improvement" or "slight improvement" may or may not be much better off from a practical standpoint. These labels are sometimes nothing more than academic, since they are useful only in statistical analyses of reported studies. For example, suppose ARC is temporarily eliminated, but the patient still has esotropia, suppression, etc. The important question that should be answered by the doctor is whether the patient is actually any better off as a result of having had an "improvement." There are, however, possible psychological benefits for these patients when they feel they have been helped. These results

should be evaluated and put in their proper perspective.

It is unfortunate that most reported studies giving rates of cure have not incorporated such complete and definitive criteria as those of Flom.[1,2] Consequently, it is difficult to evaluate their significance. One of the exceptions, however, is the survey by Ludlam.[5] In this study of 149 strabismic patients the previous criteria of Flom were strictly adhered to. Treatment did not include surgery or drugs as methods of therapy. This kept the study "clean" in comparison with most others in which the effects of surgery cannot be delineated from nonsurgical methods. According to Ludlam, the reported functional cure rate was 33%. The almost-cured rate was 40% with the remaining percentage being distributed among the other categories.

Ludlam's study took place at a large teaching clinic with many inherent disadvantages for efficient and effective functional vision training (e.g., frequent change of doctors, poor patient control, group therapy). A higher rate of success was reported by Etting[6] who surveyed a random sampling of 42 case results of an optometrist in private practice. There were 20 exotropes, 6 of whom had constant strabismus, and 22 esotropes, 18 of whom had constant strabismus. Using Flom's criteria, the overall functional cure rate was 64%. It was 85% for exotropia and 45.4% for esotropia. Seven patients were known to have had surgery prior to training, but there was no subsequent surgery for any of the patients in this study.

A well-documented strabismus report in which surgery was the dominant method of therapy is the study by Taylor.[7] He found that in cases of congenital esotropia there was not one instance of functional improvement when surgery was accomplished after the second birthday. However, he did believe it possible to achieve functional cure in such cases with early surgery (meaning before 2 years of age), particularly if diligent (minimum of 5 years) follow-up care is given. Surgery must result in a deviation that is 10^Δ or less horizontally, and 5^Δ or less vertically in order for there to be any hope for functional results. In a selected sample of 50 such patients having early surgery, 30 were later found to have stereopsis ranging from 40 to 400 seconds. Of those 30 patients, 4 had stereo-acuity of 40 sec. of arc on the Stereo Fly test. Taylor, therefore, advocated early surgery in cases of congenital esotropia believing that late surgery is hopeless in respect to achieving a functional cure. Early surgery is currently considered the most efficacious means of treatment in cases of infantile esotropia, particularly if it is congenital. This also applies to infantile constant exotropia although it is less prevalent than infantile constant esotropia.

Cases of acquired strabismus are usually helped by some or all of the other methods of therapy. The possible use of surgery for achieving functional cure in cases of acquired strabismus should be considered in those cases that fail to respond to nonsurgical means of therapy. Table 6-2 classifies these types of strabismus according to *time of onset*. An expected prognosis is listed for each category, but it is in no way meant to apply to all cases within each category. (Further classification of types of strabismus is discussed in Chapter 7).

Most cases of comitant *nonaccommodative acquired* strabismus are idiopathic (unknown cause). Although there are genetic trends in many cases, the etiology of this type of strabismus remains uncertain. Some causes are clinically well established. For example, a sensory obstacle to fusion, such as either a unilateral cataract or anisometropia usually results in an esotropia in young children. On the other hand, exotropia is likely in older individuals as a result of sensory obstacles to fusion. Psychogenic causes of strabismus can also occur; these cases are almost always esotropic but psychogenic exotropia is possible. For example, an emotionally disturbed child with a large exophoria may learn how to let his or her deviation become manifest, purposefully, for the sake of gaining attention, recognition, or sympathy.

Accommodative strabismus is usually esotropic and often due to uncorrected hyperopia and high AC/A. However, there can be accommodative exotropia in cases of divergence excess. This is the condition in which the exo at far is much greater than the exo deviation at near, indicating a high AC/A. For example, a patient with uncorrected moderate hyperopia may be orthophoric at near but exotropic at far. This type, therefore, can be thought of as an indirect type of accommodative strabismus.

The prognosis in most cases of accommodative strabismus is usually good, providing effective treatment is administered without delay. A long duration of constant strabismus makes the prognosis considerably worse. If the sensorial adaptive anomalies (e.g., suppression, amblyopia, or ARC) become deeply embedded, the prognosis may be only fair, or even poor. An example of a deteriorated accommodative esotropia is the case in which the onset was at age one. Many years of constant esotropia that go by without treatment make it almost impossible to effect a functional cure by means of therapy. When optical therapy is applied later in life, a micro-esotropia may be the best result that can be attained. Bifoveal fixation achieved in such cases of long duration is the exception. In some cases of untreated accommodative esotropia, the magnitude of the esotropia increases with time; extraocular muscle surgery may be recommended for cosmetic improvement.

The reports on prognosis in strabismus by Flom[1,2] included certain factors that he found favorable and those that he found unfavorable for functional cure. A modification of this list giving general rules is given in Table 6-3. Flom presented a quantitative scheme for determining the prognosis for a given case (Table 6-4). Note that his term for strabismus is "squint"

TABLE 6-2. Classification of Strabismus According to Time of Onset and Prognosis for Functional Cure	
Type	Prognosis
Infantile (onset 6 months of age or earlier)	Poor (unless early surgery)
Acquired (onset after 6 months of age)	
1. Nonaccommodative	Fair (depending on circumstances and therapy used)
2. Accommodative	Good (unless strabismus of long duration)

and for intermittent it is "occasional." In Flom's scheme the three most important prognostic factors are *first,* direction of the deviation (eso or exo); *second,* constancy of the deviation (intermittent or constant); and *third,* correspondence (ARC or NRC). We explain Table 6-4 with the following example. In a case of intermittent esotropia with NRC, the basic probability for functional curve is 60%. If there is good second-degree sensory fusion, family history of strabismus, and no amblyopia, the prognosis would improve by 10+10+10 (total of 30%) yielding a prognosis of 90% chance for achieving a functional cure by any and all means of vision therapy, which may include surgery. If in the above case there is deep suppression, the prognosis would be lowered to 80%. If there are also marked noncomitance and deep amblyopia, the prognosis would be 60%.

The second significant factor is frequency. For example, intermittent esotropia with NRC would have a 60% chance for functional cure compared with 30% for constant esotropia with normal correspondence. While this scheme has instructional value for students and can serve as hypothetical guidelines for practitioners, we believe it is unwise to depend entirely on statistical models to make a prognosis for a particular patient with strabismus. Instead, the doctor must take into account all the variables, associated conditions, and other factors and then use professional judgment to arrive at the most correct prognosis for the patient. This requires an item analysis of each factor in the prognosis and evaluation of the total combined effect (possible only after extensive clinical experience).

Prognostic Variables of the Deviation

An important prognostic factor is the *direction* of the deviation. Exo deviations are ordinarily easier to treat than eso deviations. Vertical deviations present more of a challenge, and torsional deviations even more so.

In regard to *frequency* of the deviation, there is general agreement that an intermittent strabismus has a more favorable prognosis than one that is constant. However, there are differences in favorability from one intermittent

TABLE 6-3. *General Rules for Prognosis for Functional Cure of Strabismus by Means of Vision Therapy (Modified from Flom)* [1,2]

Favorable Factors

1. Good cooperation
2. Intermittent strabismus
3. Exotropia better than esotropia
4. Small angles of deviation rather than large angles
5. Comitancy better than noncomitancy
6. Family history of strabismus
7. Patient's age between 7 and 11 years
8. Late onset
9. Early treatment
10. Strabismus of short duration

Unfavorable factors

1. Eccentric fixation
2. Amblyopia in esotropia, but not as bad in exotropia
3. Cyclotropia
4. ARC in esotropia but not an unfavorable factor in exotropia
5. No motor fusion range (unfavorable in esotropia but not unfavorable in exotropia)
6. Suppression in esotropia, but not as bad in exotropia
7. Constant strabismus
8. Early onset
9. Delay of treatment
10. Strabismus of long duration

case to another. A deviation that is manifest 95% of the time is obviously more difficult to treat than one present 5% of the time. The less time the deviation is present, the better is the prognosis.

The factor of *comitancy* must be considered. Comitant strabismus is generally regarded to have a better prognosis than noncomitant strabismus, but many exceptions may occur. Noncomitancy caused by a recently acquired paresis in which remission is quite likely would not follow the general rule; the outcome in such a case is often favorable if the patient is managed properly.

Although there is some correlation between the *magnitude* of the deviation and prognosis,

TABLE 6-4. *Model for Estimating the Probability of Functional Correction of Different Types of Squint and Associated Factors. (Courtesy of M.C. Flom.)*

Esotropia					Extotropia			
Occasional NRC	Occasional ARC	Constant NRC	Constant ARC	Eight Basic Squint Types	Constant ARC	Constant NRC	Occasional ARC	Occasional NRC
0.60	0.50	0.30	0.10	Basic Probabilities + FACTORS (ADD 0.1)	0.40	0.50	0.70	0.80
( )	( )	( )	( )	Good second-degree fusion	(——)	(——)	(——)	(——)
( )	( )	( )	( )	Family history of squint	(——)	(——)	(——)	(——)
( )	( )	( )	( )	No amblyopia	( )	( )	( )	( )
(——)	(——)	( )	( )	Deviation <16Δ – FACTORS (SUBTRACT 0.1)	(——)	(——)	(——)	(——)
( )	( )	( )	(——)	Marked suppression	(——)	(——)	(——)	(——)
( )	( )	( )	(——)	Marked incomitance	( )	( )	( )	( )
( )	( )	( )	( )	Deep amblyopia	( )	( )	( )	( )
( )	( )	( )	( )	Estimated Probability	( )	( )	( )	( )

the relationship is not always close. It is generally assumed that the larger the angle, the worse is the prognosis. This rule, however, is often refuted in cases of small-angle strabismus. Wybar[8] stated that "microtropia is unlikely to prove responsive to therapeutic measures." Likewise, Parks[9] concluded that the prognosis for bifoveal fixation in the patient with monofixation pattern is poor.

The effect of the *AC/A* has to be considered in regard to the particular case in question. Generally speaking, a normal AC/A is more favorable than either a high or low AC/A. However, a high ratio can be either a blessing or a curse, depending on the circumstances. It may be the principal cause of esotropia at near, or exotropia at far. However, the mechanical advantage of a high ratio when using lenses may greatly reduce deviations, e.g., plus lenses for nearpoint esotropia and minus for farpoint exotropia. It is difficult, therefore, to make prognostic generalizations about the AC/A.

In regard to *variability* of the deviation, it may be favorable if the magnitude of the deviation changes occasionally. Sensorily, this may keep suppression and ARC from becoming too deeply embedded, but it cannot be assumed to be so in many cases. Motorically, however, a greatly variable magnitude can be a surgeon's nightmare. Similarly, the factor of *cosmesis* can be a blessing or a curse. If cosmesis is good, this is a blessing for the patient. This, unfortunately, causes complacency and is often the reason such patients do not enthusiastically try for a functional cure; this is a curse for the doctor treating the strabismus.

As to *eye laterality,* traditional thinking is that treatment of an alternating strabismus is more difficult than treating one that is unilateral. This conclusion has been prevalent because alternate fixation is common in cases of infantile esotropia. This group of patients has led to equating alternation with poor prognosis. Most recent studies show that alternation is not a deterrent and may be slightly favorable when all types of strabismus are considered.[1,2] One reason may be that individuals with alternating strabismus do not become amblyopes.

Eye dominancy is probably not a factor in strabismus prognosis. However, it can be a consideration regarding the strabismic's perceptual adjustment to everyday seeing and may be related to certain eye-hand or eye-foot coordination tasks.

Associated Conditions

As with diagnostic variables of the deviation, it is difficult to pin down what influence each of the associated conditions has on the overall prognosis.

Peripheral and deep *suppression* may cause the prognosis to be worse than if it is only central and shallow. Although this is generally true, there are many exceptions. For instance, there could be an esotropia with ARC in which suppression is very shallow. The prognosis may be poor because of the ARC in spite of the apparent favorable factor of the almost negligible suppression. Since there is always an interplay among the many factors that go into making a prognosis, it is difficult to speak in terms of absolutes for any one factor. Generally speaking, though, suppression alone is only slightly unfavorable.

The presence of *amblyopia* is, however, a stumbling block to the successful treatment of strabismus. Fortunately, amblyopia can be detected and treated at early ages. Once amblyopia is eliminated, strabismus therapy is facilitated.

We agree with Winter[10] who suggested that practically all cases of strabismic amblyopia or anisometropic amblyopia can be cured by direct occlusion alone, providing the child is less than 4 years old, and that from ages 4 to 6 the prognosis is often good. However, extensive treatment may be required. Aust[11] similarly stated that occlusion therapy can lead to a cure of amblyopia in more than 90% of the cases, whether or not fixation is central; this can occur up to the fifth year of life. Goodier[12] used direct occlusion for 46 amblyopic patients up to age 9. An improvement in fixation and visual acuity was reported in 44 cases. It was concluded that the use of inverse occlusion did not appear to be as efficacious as direct occlusion.

Many disagree with the contention that direct occlusion is always the best method of occlusion therapy. If a patient older than age 5 has eccentric fixation, direct occlusion is thought to cause the abnormal fixation to become even more deeply embedded. If this happens, very specialized pleoptic therapy utilizing afterimages and entopic foveal "tags" may be necessary to treat the abnormal fixation. The contention is that inverse occlusion would have prevented the degree of embeddedness that resulted from direct occlusion. Kavner and Suchoff[13] reported that prognosis is poorer when there is a stable eccentric fixation as opposed to one that is unstable. They recommended inverse occlusion and specialized pleoptic training when dealing with this condition.

We believe that direct occlusion is the procedure of choice in amblyopic patients up to 6 years of age. In patients older than six, direct occlusion should be tried if fixation is central, or if there is unstable eccentric fixation. The prognosis may be fair or good depending upon the circumstances. However, in cases of steady eccentric fixation above the age of five, the prognosis for eliminating the eccentric fixation and amblyopia by means of direct occlusion alone may be poor. What so often happens when direct occlusion is used in this type of condition is an immediate small improvement in visual acuity, but no further gain afterward. This may be because the eccentric fixation becomes very entrenched, making it difficult to reduce it any further. Therefore, the contention is that the prognosis may be somewhat better if indirect occlusion is initially tried.

Chavasse[14] introduced the concepts of amblyopia of arrest and amblyopia of extinction. Amblyopia of arrest is a failure in the development of visual acuity due to strabismus, anisometropia, or other conditions (e.g., cataract). In any event, the development of visual acuity is arrested at the time of onset of the causative condition. The prognosis for improving visual acuity in a documented case of amblyopia of arrest is considered very poor. This is probably true if the patient is beyond the developmental age (probably 6 years or older). However, if the same type of case is treated at a much earlier age, the prognosis may be better. Amblyopia of arrest, therefore, is not always a deterrent to treatment if the patient is very young; but if treatment is delayed until the child is older, the prognosis becomes worse.

The prognosis for a case of amblyopia of extinction is thought to be good, no matter at what age the treatment is given. The difference is that an older patient may require a more lengthy therapy program than a younger patient. Amblyopia of extinction is a condition in which vision has deteriorated because of suppression resulting from either strabismus or anisometropia. The vision that was once lost can usually be recovered through the re-educative process of vision therapy.

These concepts of Chavasse are not without dispute. Argument against them stems from the fact that many authorities have found that the results of amblyopic therapy do not always correspond to the level of visual acuity that is traditionally expected. It often happens that better acuity is achieved than was thought possible in cases of relatively early onset of amblyopia. This would seem to contradict the concept of amblyopia of arrest. However, if modern normative visual acuity levels expected for certain ages are properly matched with the time of onset, the concept of amblyopia of arrest is on solid ground. The apparent mismatch arose because of the old assumption that an infant's vision is poorer than it actually is. Chavasse thought that the acuity level of a 4-month-old child would normally be about 20/2500. Research has shown that this is not true and that infants have acuity much better than expected in the past. This may explain why treatment in cases of early onset is often successful. Perhaps the condition being treated is not that of amblyopia of arrest, but rather, one of amblyopia of extinction.

The presence of ARC is a very unfavorable factor in the prognosis of esotropia. Flom[1] reported that while ARC is highly unfavorable in cases of constant esotropia, it is less significant in cases of constant exotropia. The cure rates of Ludlam[5] were reported as 23% of esotropes with ARC, compared with 86% for esotropes with NRC. Exotropes with ARC had a cure rate of 62% as opposed to 89% with NRC. Etting[6] reported a cure rate of 10% of the esotropes with ARC, whereas it was 75% of the esotropes with NRC. The cure rate for exotropes with ARC was 50%. It appears that anomalous correspondence is a serious factor in cases of esotropia but less so in exotropia.

Lack of correspondence is considered extremely unfavorable. Current procedures offer no hope for a functional cure in the older child or adult who has a complete lack of correspondence. The best recommendation in such cases is either no treatment, or to make an attempt for a cosmetic cure.

In cases of *horror fusionis,* the usual recommendation is no treatment, i.e., the prognosis is poor. If the ARC can be broken, however, horror fusionis may not be a significantly adverse factor for functional cure. This is assuming the horror fusionis was produced by the ARC. (Refer to the discussion in Chapter 5.)

Accommodative infacility is not an unfavorable factor in strabismus; however, it frequently accompanies amblyopia with eccentric fixation. Accommodative flexibility training ("rock") is often used as part of amblyopia therapy, and considerable time may be required before both the fixation and accommodation are improved.

There are poor fusional vergences in strabismus. Sensory fusion must be attained so that disparity vergence can be established. When this is accomplished, fusional vergence ranges can often be increased by means of vision training. The prognosis for functional cure of strabismus, therefore, is not necessarily poor because of poor fusional vergences prior to vision therapy.

Other Factors

The time of onset, mode of onset, duration of strabismus, previous treatment, developmental history, and additional evaluative procedures all play important roles in determining the prognosis in any case of strabismus. The prognosis is better when the onset of amblyopia and/or strabismus is late than when it is early. A short duration is better than a long one, since immediate therapy helps the chance for cure. Furthermore, existing anomalies that were once successfully treated are often easy to eliminate by re-education. Also, developmental history that is normal can be considered favorable in many cases.

Testing for sensory fusion at the *centration point* is another important supplemental prognostic procedure. Plus-power lenses may be efficacious for getting the eyes to the ortho posture. The appropriate amount of plus-lens power and the centration point distance (where the visual axes cross) must be determined. For example, assume the esotropia is 15^Δ and the interpupillary distance is 60 mm. The centration point would be 40 cm from the patient. This is determined by calculating the lens power that will place the eyes in the ortho posture, from the formula:

$$\text{Diopters} = \frac{H}{IPD}$$

Angle II is the horizontal objective angle of deviation expressed in prism diopters, and IPD is the interpupillary distance expressed in centimeters. From the above example, if 15 is divided by 6, the answer is 2.50 (i.e., diopters). The distance at the centration point is the focal distance of the lenses ($100/2.50 = 40$cm). If 2.50 D lenses are worn, the patient is seeing at 40 cm as though at optical infinity. The horizontal deviation should, therefore, become ortho at the 40 cm test distance with the patient wearing the +2.50 D lenses. That being so, various sensory fusion tests can be given, e.g., Worth 4-dot and stereopsis testing.

The centration point calculation is theoretical in the sense that the visual system does not always work in a predictable mechanical manner. For example, in some cases of esotropia, plus-power lenses seem to have little or no immediate effect, and only upon prolonged wearing (e.g., 1 hour) may there be reduction of the deviation toward the centration point. Unfortunately, many stabismic patients (particularly those with ARC) adapt back to their original angle.

Cooperation is a vital factor in treatment when vision training methods are used. The patient must be perceptive and of reasonably good intellect in order to go through this form of therapy. This, along with genuine interest on the part of the patient, and parents in the case of a child patient, is extremely helpful. It may explain the irony of why a family history of strabismus is favorable. The parents may feel motivated to do something about their child's condition because of their familiarity with binocular anomalies.

The age of the patient is an important factor, often dictating what form of therapy the patient will receive. Vision training can best be done when the child is age six or older. Some patients as young as 4 years of age may cooperate, but it is rare to find sufficient cooperation for complex vision therapy procedures in those younger than 4 years.

Farpoint strabismus is commonly more difficult to cure than one at near. Convergence excess is typically easier to treat than divergence insufficiency. Similarly, convergence insufficiency (nearpoint exo problem) is less difficult to treat than divergence excess (farpoint exo problem).

Proper refractive care may prevent some of the binocular anomalies. In this regard, a history of good vision care can be considered favorable to the prognosis in many cases.

Cosmetic Cure of Strabismus

A fault of many reports in the literature is that no distinction is made between functional and cosmetic cure. Many ophthalmic surgeons label the patient "cured" just because the eyes "look straight." Studies purporting to give cosmetic cure rates are unreliable because this is a subjective value judgment with each reporter using his or her own criteria.

Certain cosmetic factors have a great effect on the appearance of the strabismic individual, e.g., interpupillary distance, lid shape, epicanthal folds, facial shape, and symmetry. Another important factor is angle kappa (technically angle lambda). For example, a negative angle kappa may make an individual with orthophoria appear to have esotropia. Similarly, cosmesis may be good in moderately large angles of strabismus. For instance, a 15^Δ esotrope with a positive angle kappa may appear to have no strabismus. Because of the various combinations of cosmetic factors affecting the appearance of the individual, there are no hard-and-fast rules relating the magnitude of strabismus to cosmesis. In the majority of cases, however, we find that if the strabismic angle is reduced to 10^Δ or less, the cosmesis is usually good. The esotrope may get by with a larger angle, such as 15^Δ or 20^Δ, before the deviation is noticeable. This is because most people have a positive angle kappa that masks the appearance of esotropia. Conversely, an exotropia of the same magnitude will probably be quite noticeable.

Hyperdeviations of 5^Δ or less are not noticeable. Deviations beyond 10^Δ may be unsightly and present a cosmetic problem for patients (and parents of young patients). On the other hand, cyclo deviations alone are not a cosmetic problem; however, they are usually associated with vertical and possibly, horizontal deviations.

When the goal is only for cosmetic acceptability and not for a functional cure, the most frequently used form of therapy is extraocular muscle surgery. Lenses are occasionally used for this purpose in the form of single-vision lenses for the correction of hyperopia. Plus additions (bifocals) generally serve no purpose in cases in which cosmesis is the sole concern. Minus adds for farpoint exotropia have been employed, although this procedure is not highly recommended because the cosmetic gain is only transitory. Nothing is achieved in the long run, since the cosmetic problem returns as soon as the individual relaxes accommodation, or if the overcorrection is removed. Minus lenses do play an important role, however, in certain cases of exotropia in which there is hope for a functional cure. Alignment of the visual axes helps promote sensory fusion.

Inverse prisms have been used for cosmetic improvement with limited success. The main problem is the thickness and weight factor of glass or plastic prisms. Fresnel prisms eliminate these drawbacks, but they introduce the problem of degraded visual acuity, and the occasional complaint of noticeable lines for the patient looking through the prisms. This becomes a significant problem with powers greater than 15^Δ. If, however, the prism is confined to the deviating eye, the complaint of blurred vision is usually removed. The patient wearing a Fresnel prism may also object to the appearance of the lines visible to someone looking at him or her. Thus, the use of inverse prism may become impractical because of its objectional appearance.

In strabismic deviations of moderate magnitude (criteria listed in Chapter 4) that are just beyond the limit of cosmetic acceptance, a combined method of direct and inverse prism application can be tried. This is illustrated in Figure 6-1 in which the right eye is esotropic (see Figure 6-1a). If a direct prism (base-out) is placed before the left eye, the dextroversion diminishes the esotropic appearance of the right eye (see Figure 6-1b). Inverse prism (base-in) is then placed before the right eye (see Figure 6-1c). Although there is probably no movement of the right eye because of suppression, the optical effect of the prism (image shifted toward the apex) further enhances the

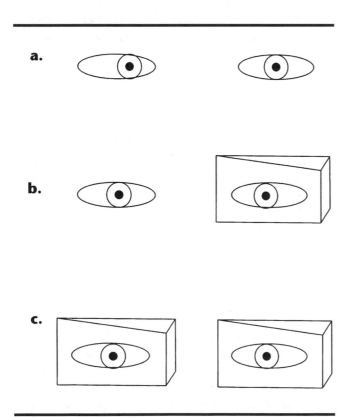

FIGURE 6-1—The use of prisms to improve cosmesis in an example of esotropia of the right eye: **(a)** Noticeable esotropia of right eye. **(b)** Base-out prism before the left eye causes the left eye to turn in and the right eye out (dextroversion equal to magnitude of prism). **(c)** Yoked prism with base-in before the right eye enhances cosmetic appearance because of the shifting of the palpebral aperture toward the apex of the prism.

salutory cosmetic results. The amount of prism power necessary in this procedure is usually about 40% of the magnitude of the strabismus. For example, an esotropic deviation of 20^Δ would require an 8-diopter prism before each eye (i.e., yoked prisms).

Patients may be taught the tactic of controlling head movements or using specified positions of gaze to minimize a cosmetically noticeable strabismus. This is applicable in cases of comitant as well as noncomitant strabismus. For example, suppose a patient with 20 prism diopters of comitant constant esotropia of the right eye wishes to appear to be orthophoric during a job interview. The effect of "straight eyes" may be accomplished by the individual making a small dextroversion, such as fixating on the interviewer's left ear, for example, rather than looking directly face-to-face. Such advice can be helpful to patients in their occupational and personal lives.

Heterophoria

The prognosis for improving existing visual skills in heterophoria is almost always good, providing the patient is cooperative and motivated. If a patient demonstrates outstanding motivation, that patient can be told the prognosis is "excellent." Such superlatives, however, should be used sparingly. Heterophoria therapy is usually effective in abating associated signs and symptoms (Table 6-5). In the sensory realm, stereopsis might be improved by means of vision training, lenses, or prisms. In the motor realm, vision training may help increase fusional vergence ranges, which may be necessary in cases of fixation disparity. Also, the use of prisms is applicable in cases of heterophoria, especially for patients with fixation disparity.

Of the four generally recognized types of vergence (tonic, accommodative, fusional, and proximal), most authorities believe tonic convergence is the least changeable as a result of training. Although there is some dispute over whether the basic deviation can be changed by means of training, we believe it remains approximately the same in the long run. On immediate testing, however, there

---

TABLE 6-5. *Signs and Symptoms Frequently Occurring in Heterophoria*

1. Blurring of vision at farpoint
2. Blurring of vision at nearpoint
3. Frowning or squinting of eyelids
4. Excessive blinking when reading
5. Covering or closing one eye during reading
6. Confusing, omitting or repeating words when reading
7. Sustaining nearpoint work with difficulty
8. Reading at a very slow rate
9. Losing place when reading a book
10. Burning, aching, itching, or tearing of eyes, or photophobia

---

may appear to be a difference following training. However, when there is prolonged occlusion (e.g., several hours), tonic convergence is usually found to be the same as it was before training.

As to accommodative vergence, Manas[15] reported an increase (by measuring the accommodative-convergence to accommodation ratio) with convergence training. Flom[16] also found a similar increase. However, upon retesting after about one year, the AC/A appeared to have decreased and approximated the original values.

There are numerous references regarding the trainability of fusional vergences. Costenbader[17] stated, "In general, the treatment of strabismus includes . . . improving fusion and the fusional vergences." Jones[18] wrote, "In regard to motor fusion, it is the aim of orthoptic treatment . . . to increase them sufficiently." This was in reference to fusional vergence ranges. Griffin[19] summarized research proving the efficacy of fusional (disparity) vergence training. In general, the prognosis for increasing fusional vergence is usually good. The easiest is fusional convergence followed by fusional divergence. Vertical fusional vergence is the next in difficulty to improve by means of training. In most cases torsional fusional vergence is even more difficult to treat successfully.

Excessive proximal convergence usually diminishes by familiarization with the testing environment that originally produced the increased vergence. This has occupational importance, e.g., controlling the tendency to overconverge the eyes when using binocular instruments such as a biomicroscope.

For all patients (strabismic, heterophoric, or orthophoric), testing and diagnosing deficiencies of other visual skills should be done. These skills include *saccades, pursuits, fixations, accommodation* (sufficiency, facility, stamina), and the status of *fixation disparity*. The prognosis is generally good for resolving problems in these skills by means of vision therapy.

MODES OF VISION THERAPY

Before a prognostic statement for either a functional or cosmetic cure is complete, the doctor must take into account the type of therapy to be administered in order to effect the desired results. An overview of approaches to vision therapy in cases of binocular anomalies is presented in this section (Figure 6-2). In cases with a poor prognosis, the doctor may recommend *no treatment* instead of vision therapy. Sometimes this is the wisest option for certain patients. (Refer to case examples in this chapter.)

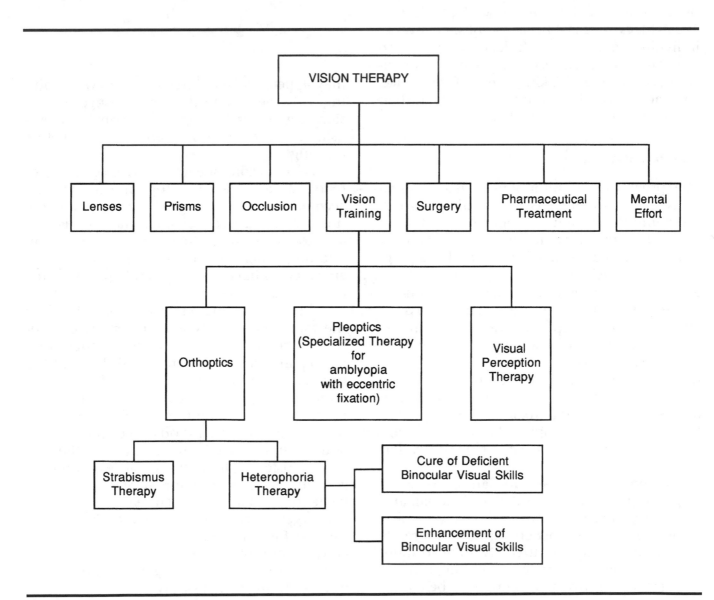

FIGURE 6-2—Classification of Vision Therapy

Lenses

The first consideration in the treatment of any binocular vision condition is full correction of the refractive error, since a defocused or distorted image to either eye (or possibly to both eyes) is an obstacle to fusion. Lens additions (plus and minus) are also used in the treatment of certain types of strabismus and heterophoria. Lens therapy is discussed in subsequent chapters.

Prisms

For more than 100 years prisms have been used to compensate the angle of strabismus. The primary limitation has been the amount that can be effectively incorporated into spectacle lenses. Prisms often become impractical due to weight and distortion when more than 10^Δ per lens is required. With the advent of Fresnel prisms, the limit has increased to 30^Δ per lens, which is usually sufficient since most strabismic deviations are less than 60^Δ in magnitude. However, Fresnel prisms seem, at best, only a temporary solution because of optical distortion, reduced visual acuity, and loss of contrast. Furthermore, compensating prisms do not help (but hinder) the cosmetic aspects of a strabismus, which exacerbates this major concern of most strabismic patients. Reverse (inverse) prisms, however, may be attempted to improve the cosmetic appearance in some strabismic cases. When a borderline cosmetic unilateral strabismus is present, small amounts of reverse prism can often mask its appearance. Reverse prisms have also been used to break the adaptations of suppression, ARC, and eccentric fixation in selected cases.

The use of compensating (relieving) prisms in cases of heterophoria has continued to grow in clinical practice, especially in cases of excessive heterophoria. If the angle of deviation does not adapt to the prism power (i.e., phoria increasing in magnitude), asthenopic complaints are usually resolved or lessened. Unfortunately, some patients show prism adaptation, which suggests that this is not a viable therapeutic option.

Occlusion

Occlusion (i.e., opaque patches or attenuating filters) is used in therapy for amblyopia (refer to Chapter 10), ARC (Chapter 11), suppression (Chapter 12), and comitant and noncomitant strabismus (Chapters 13 through 15). Prognostic considerations regarding occlusion are discussed in the above-mentioned chapters.

Vision Training

When more than lenses, prisms, and occlusion are necessary to achieve the desired results, vision training procedures may be the therapy of choice. Sometimes vision training is done without other forms of vision therapy, but other modes of treatment are often included in the vision training program. Vision training relative to binocular vision disorders historically has been called *orthoptics*, which etymologically means "straight sight." Orthoptic procedures are usually successful in breaking suppression, building ranges of fusional vergence, and improving the reflex aspects of ocular motility. For this reason, orthoptics has the greatest utility in cases of intermittent strabismus, heterophoria, and deficient ocular motor skills.

Many orthoptic procedures (including monocular regimens) are used in the treatment of amblyopia, but *pleoptics* is a specific type of training designed exclusively for amblyopia with eccentric fixation. The term pleoptics etymologically means "full sight." These procedures involve light stimulation techniques to diminish the influence of the eccentric fixation point in the amblyopic eye and enhance foveal fixation. In some cases of severe amblyopia of long duration, both pleoptic and orthoptic techniques are required to achieve a successful outcome, as well as an agressive patching (occlusion) program.

Visual perception therapy procedures for certain types of learning disabilities are not covered in this text. Perceptual training procedures are, however, occasionally used in therapy of amblyopia, e.g., figure-ground, visual discrimination, and closure.

Extraocular Muscle Surgery

The surgical form of binocular therapy may be necessary in certain cases when the angle of deviation is too large to be consistently and easily overcome by fusional effort, or when there is a significant noncomitant deviation. There are many differing procedures used by ophthalmologists in extraocular muscle surgery. Some basic principles, however, are accepted by most ophthalmic surgeons. Only those general approaches to correction of deviations of the visual axes are discussed. There is no intention to cover this subject in depth, but merely to discuss it briefly as one of the several alternatives for the treatment of binocular anomalies. There are many fine books for reference purposes covering the details of surgical procedures on extraocular muscles, and other anomalies affecting ocular motility. Particularly good references in this regard are publications by Hugonnier et al.,[20] Hurtt et al.,[21] Mein and Trimble,[22] Von Noorden,[23] and Dale.[24] In addition, several case reports are included in the treatment chapters of this book describing various surgical approaches.

General Approach

The general approach to extraocular muscle surgery is that the action of a particular muscle should be made either weaker or stronger. Examples of weakening procedures include recession, tenotomy, tenectomy, myotomy, and myectomy. When the muscle is *recessed,* the insertion is moved from the original site and transplanted to another location to produce less mechanical advantage (Figure 6-3). Another weakening procedure is tenotomy either marginal or free (i.e., disinsertion at the scleral attachment). In many varieties of controlled *tenectomies,* the tendon is appropriately cut for weakening the action of an overacting muscle. Either *myotomy* or *myectomy* is the term used when the muscle, rather than the tendon of the muscle, is altered.

Examples of strengthening procedures include resection, tucking, and advancement. *Resectioning* of a muscle or tendon changes the angle of deviation by shortening it (see Fig-

ure 6-3b). The method of *tucking* may involve the tendon or the muscle; it also effectively serves to shorten the muscle. *Advancement* of the insertion serves to strengthen the action of the muscle by giving it greater mechanical advantage.

Prism adaptation testing was introduced by Woodward and reported by Jampolsky.[25] Surgeons use this to estimate the amount of surgery required for alignment. The prism adaptation test (PAT) is also used to predict success (often when surgery is anticipated) in cases of esotropia. The testing procedure involves the application of base-out prism for the manifest eso deviation. The patient wears prisms for a period of time, usually an hour, while the clinician measures the angle of deviation at certain intervals of time, usually every 10 minutes. Jampolsky recommended giving the patient an overcorrection whereby the prism power is slightly stronger than the magnitude of the esotropia. For small deviations, an overcorrection of 5^Δ is recommended, and for larger deviations, a 10^Δ overcorrection. For example, suppose the patient has esotropia of 25^Δ. The patient is given 35^Δ base-out to wear for one hour. Fresnel prisms are more comfortable for the patient than glass or plastic clip-ons. The immediate measurement on the alternate cover test should show a 10^Δ exo movement. In many cases, the exo will become less in a very short time and, after about 10 minutes, the patient shows an eso movement on the cover test. In some cases, the eso deviation becomes larger. Assume that after an hour the alternate cover test shows a 20^Δ movement of the eyes. The eso deviation is now 35^Δ plus 20^Δ, or a total of 55^Δ. The angle of the deviation has more than doubled in magnitude as a result of the PAT.

Jampolsky felt that this indicates a poor prognosis for cure by surgery and probably by other means as well. If the deviation had remained the same or had increased only slightly, the prognosis would have been considered much better. As a rule, after wearing compensating prisms over a period of time the increase in the angle of deviation can probably be expected in more than half the cases of esotropia. In a study of 88 patients with esotropia, Aust

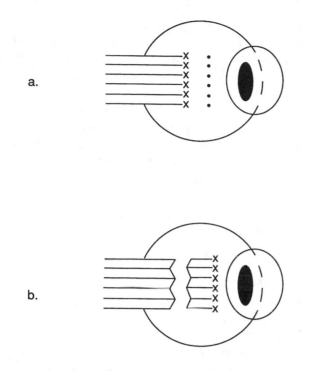

FIGURE 6-3—Schematic, highly diagramatic, of extraocular muscle surgery on a rectus muscle. (**a**) Recession as a weakening procedure. The insertion of the tendon is removed and reattached posteriorly in the globe. (**b**) Resecting as a strengthening procedure. The tendon or muscle is cut, a portion removed, and then it is rejoined.

and Welge-Lussen[26] found that 71.5% of the patients increased the angle of deviation over a period of five to nine days. ARC was thought to be more commonly associated with the increase than NRC.

Alpern and Hofstetter[27] reported a well documented case of esotropia in which the angle of deviation increased by the same amount as the power of the compensatory prisms. The strabismus was constant and unilateral of 14^Δ with the presence of ARC clearly established. A total of 18^Δ base-out was worn for five days. The rate of increase was rapid within the first three hours, with only a slight gradual increase for the next few days until tapering off to the maximum of 32^Δ (total increase of angle H of 18^Δ). After prisms were removed, angle H decreased rapidly within a few hours, but it took approximately one week before the strabismus was finally reduced to its original angle of 14^Δ.

Postar[28] investigated the use of the PAT for esotropic patients. He concluded that changes in the angle of deviation were related to the status of sensory fusion. The overconvergence reaction to the base-out prisms tended not to occur when sensory fusion was good, but the tendency was there when sensory fusion was poor. Postar advocated improving stereopsis early in the therapy program to keep the deviation from increasing when prisms are applied. He further concluded that the 1-hour testing time was too short, and a longer period of time should be allotted for evaluating the effects of prism adaptation.

In taking a different approach to prism adaptation testing, Carter found that heterophoric individuals with good binocularity and without symptoms showed the same magnitude as the original heterophoria before prisms were worn. Thus, a 5^Δ esophore, corrected with 5^Δ base-out, still showed 5^Δ of esophoria by cover test through the prisms that were worn for approximately 30 minutes. On the other hand, individuals who had heterophoria and asthenopia (possibly with fixation disparity) accepted compensatory prisms. Their symptoms were relieved and there was no prism adaptation effect.

From the previous discussions, it appears that prism compensation should be considered in cases of heterophoria with symptoms. In contradistinction, heterophoric patients without symptoms will likely increase the magnitude of deviation as a result of wearing compensatory prisms. In the case of esotropia, the deviation is likely to increase when the sensory fusion is poor, e.g., ARC and suppression. If, however, sensory fusion is good, the strabismic deviation is likely to stay the same or increase only slightly. On rare occasions, the basic deviation appears to be reduced in magnitude as a result of wearing prisms.

There is general agreement that when there is little or no increase (or occasionally a decrease) in the angle of strabismus, this type of result on the PAT is an indication of a good prognosis. However, there is not complete agreement as to the interpretation from the results of the PAT when the angle increases significantly. The majority opinion holds that the prognosis is unfavorable in these instances, but some clinicians believe there may be exceptions to the rule. Some cases result in a functional cure in spite of the dismal expectations derived from the PAT. This points out the need to be cautious when making a prognosis and not to place too much reliance on any one test.

Adjustable Suture Procedure

Jampolsky[29] pioneered the adjustable suture technique that allows a surgeon to refine the surgical result within 24 hours following the operation. Many surgeons find this procedure improves the long-term results, although some dispute this point. At least, the adjustable suture procedure helps avoid large overcorrections and undercorrections. The severed muscle tendon is not reattached tightly to the sclera during the operation. After the muscle is resected or recessed by the necessary amount, long sutures in the tendon are passed through the superficial sclera and secured externally with a slip knot. Under a local anesthetic, the final adjustment of alignment can be made the day of the operation or the next day while the patient is awake. Most adults and many school-age children can adequately tolerate the procedure. Using the cover test to check alignment, the surgeon loosens the slip knot and repositions the muscle insertion as needed. The loose ends of the sutures are pulled either to advance the insertion (a strengthening procedure) or pulled in the opposing direction to get more recession (a weakening procedure). The dissolvable sutures are then secured in position externally with surgeon's knots and the muscle tendon adheres permanently to the sclera during the healing process. This procedure can be used with any of the rectus muscles and the superior oblique tendon. Adjustable sutures are particularly appropriate when the outcome is not readily predictable (e.g., cases of previous unsuccessful surgery) or when the patient has fusion potential and precise alignment is critical to a successful outcome, as in cases of thyroid ophthalmopathy. Some strabismus surgeons use adjustable sutures in nearly every case of rectus muscle surgery.

Surgical Considerations

Most patients and parents are naturally apprehensive about undergoing strabismus surgery.

The doctor needs to give realistic information regarding the potential complications and what is involved with the procedure. This information usually relieves some anxiety. The patient should be encouraged to ask all the questions they wish during the preop visit. For medical–legal purposes, the surgeon should document in the patient's record the specific complications that were discussed. Not every possible complication, however, need be mentioned. According to Helveston,[30] preoperative informed consent requires a discussion of at least three possibilities: diplopia, loss of vision, and need of reoperation.

Diplopia is a common occurrence during the initial postoperative phase of healing depending on the age and sensory status of the patient. Most patients experience only transient diplopia that disappears within a week or so after the operation. Older patients tend to notice diplopia more often, as one might expect. If it is debilitating, the patient can wear a patch or be given a Fresnel prism in an attempt to achieve sensory fusion. Many patients will notice diplopia only if they consciously look for it in some extreme field of gaze, and this behavior should be discouraged. Concern is shown for diplopia that disrupts the normal course of daily activities.

An extremely rare, but serious complication of strabismus surgery is loss of vision. This devastating complication can be caused by perforation of the sclera and retina with a surgical instrument or needle. Loss of vision in this event occurs subsequent to retinal detachment, vitreous hemorrhage, cataract, glaucoma, optic nerve incision or transection, endophthalmitis, or other damage. Some patients have an unusually thin sclera making them vulnerable to this complication and, of course, there is the ever-present possibility of human error.

Patients usually want to know about the need for reoperation. They often ask whether the results are permanent, but in any case this issue needs to be discussed prior to surgery. The chance of additional operations at some future time depends primarily on the type and characteristics of the strabismus and the skill of the surgeon. The surgeon needs to discuss with the patient, his or her success rate in similar cases. In cases of congenital esotropia, Helveston[30] informs his patients that the motor alignment is considered acceptable by doctor and parents 90% of the time. They are also told that between 10% and 20% of children will need one or more additional surgical procedures months to years later for new problems such as secondary exotropia, overacting obliques, A or V pattern, dissociated vertical deviation, or recurrent esotropia even when alignment is perfect following the surgery.

Some other complications that can occur that may be discussed with patients are: (1) postoperative nausea and vomiting due to anesthesia and possibly, traction on the extraocular muscles; (2) acute allergic suture reaction can occur in about 10% of cases in which organic absorbable suture material is used; topical steroids are given in this case for 7 to 10 days; and (3) ptosis of the upper lid can occur after excessive recession of the superior rectus, or the lower lid may lag with large recession of the inferior rectus.

Besides learning about the potential complications of surgery, patients generally want to know about several other practical issues relative to the operation. In most cases, strabismus surgery is a 1 day "in-and-out" procedure. An overnight stay at the hospital is not usually required, except for general health considerations or when other surgical procedures are also being done besides the strabismus. The patient registers with the selected hospital and standard blood tests are completed. The anesthesiologist usually meets with the patient or parents immediately before the operation to check the patient and to ensure that the preop instructions from the hospital have been followed. The strabismus operation itself usually takes only about one hour, give or take 15 minutes. Besides a scrub nurse, some surgeons work with an assistant surgeon, although others do not. During the immediate postsurgical phase, many doctors bandage the operated eye for a short time, usually one day, to help prevent infection and to increase patient comfort due to photophobia. A topical wide-spectrum antibiotic is usually given for daily instillation for the first week to 10 days. Conjunctival injection usually disappears in a month or two. The frequency of postop visits varies widely depending on the case and the surgeon, but a typical schedule

might consist of one-day, one-week, and six-week postop examinations. After these visits, if no complications develop, the patient is then placed on a standard recall schedule or instructed to return to the referring doctor for comanagement (e.g., vision training) and shared responsibility relative to the strabismus.

Pharmacological Treatment

Although there have been numerous pharmaceutical agents used at one time or another for the treatment of binocular anomalies, those in use today are relatively few. Cycloplegics may be used for purposes of occlusion. Miotics for accommodative esotropia are sometimes used. The two more popular anticholinesterase drugs are diisopropyl fluorophosphate (DFP) and echothiophate iodide (Phospholine®). They greatly increase accommodation, without a significant increase in accommodative convergence. This results in a lower AC/A.

Abraham[31] pioneered the use of DFP to reduce esotropia. A report by Gellman[32] summarized the effectiveness of DFP by citing case reports in which the nearpoint eso deviation was reduced by the use of the drug. However, echothiophate iodide (Phospholine) has become the more popular of the two. It apparently causes fewer side effects (e.g., formation of iris cysts) than DFP. One effect that should always be avoided is the cardiovascular or respiratory failure that may happen when a drug of this type is combined with those used for general anesthesia. Bartlett and Jaanus[33] emphasized that Phospholine and DFP are very stable drugs and produce action of long duration. Manley[34] warned of the danger of giving general anesthesia in cases of surgery for esotropia when the patient has previously been taking one of these anticholinesterase drugs. If succinylcholine chloride is used prior to endotracheal intubation, there will be an overeffect if the patient has been taking anticholinesterase drugs. Cessation of respiration may result. A careful history should be taken to determine if any such drug was used several months prior to the scheduled time of extraocular muscle surgery.

The use of drugs to treat binocular anomalies appears to be somewhat limited and may be on the decline. At times, however, their use may be advantageous in the treatment of accommodative esotropia. They may be effective when the AC/A is high, in cases of significant hyperopia, and when wearing of lenses is not tolerable. Under most of these circumstances, it is feasible to prescribe bifocals; but in the case of infants and some children, drugs may be a means to reduce an eso deviation.

Botulinum Toxin

Chemodenervation using botulinum toxin A injections is another nonsurgical approach in vision therapy. Scott et al.[35] introduced this as a method for weakening extraocular muscle function, as though a surgical weakening procedure had been performed. The toxin prevents release of acetylcholine to produce paresis. McNear[36] emphasized the convenience of this method but questioned its overall effectiveness in strabismus therapy. Because the effect may be only temporary (although possibly lasting for several months) and side effects (e.g., ptosis, other muscles possibly being affected, and inducing possible hyper deviations) are fairly common, clinical trials are needed to evaluate its efficacy, compared with conventional strabismus surgery of comitant strabismus. Botulinum therapy has, however, been used effectively with increasing frequency for noncomitant strabismus, particularly to prevent contracture. It is also used for relieving symptoms of blepharospasm.

Other Approaches

The doctor must serve his or her patients as a counselor regarding visual health and welfare. Sometimes the best interest of the strabismic patient is served by doing nothing, except monitoring the condition for changes with time. For example, if the spectacle lens prescription is current, the deviation cosmetically and functionally stable, and the patient is satisfied with the status of the strabismus, then the doctor should not recommend treatment but rather describe the condition to the patient, its prognosis for long-term changes, and any other practical considerations. Sometimes patients

cannot follow through on a recommended vision therapy program for several reasons and prefer simply to live with the condition for the time being. The clinician has a duty to explain, in a sensitive manner, any consequences that may result from that decision and how best to manage the situation. The doctor must make recommendations with the best interest of the patient in mind rather than promote a particularly preferred mode of therapy.

The vision specialist must be sensitive to the need for referral when it arises. Many types of strabismus and other binocular vision conditions can be subtle indicators of active ocular or systemic disease. Patients should also be encouraged to seek a second opinion if any questions remain in the mind of the clinician or the patient. Occasionally, vision specialists examine patients whose binocular vision condition is of psychogenic origin, e.g., hysterical amblyopia, or esotropia following emotional trauma. The professional services of a psychologist or psychiatrist may be necessary for resolution of the condition.

Hypnosis is an alternative mode of therapy that has some applications within the field of binocular vision therapy. Kohn[37] stated that vision therapy lends itself ideally to hypnosis since it is "focused attention" that helps patients achieve functional cures. Hypnosis has been used to build motivation in patients for vision training as well as increasing acceptance of occlusion, spectacle lenses, surgery, and many procedures in vision training. Hypnosis can also be considered in cases of intractable diplopia.

When one mode of treatment is not adequate, others may be used. It is possible that any combination of these basic methods may be employed, and some cases require them all. The treatment portion of this book contains further discussion on their uses and various combinations in case studies.

CASE EXAMPLES

The previous discussions consisted of generalities regarding favorability of the various prognostic factors. This section presents 12 specific cases that illustrate typical diagnostic types having a prognosis for functional ranging from poor to good.

Some clinicians may disagree with our prognostic judgments because of differences in clinical experience. We tend to be slightly conservative, as conventional wisdom dictates. A surprisingly successful cure following therapy is never unappreciated by patients. The same cannot be said when therapeutic results do not match the expectations of patients.

Poor Prognosis

Case no. 1

The patient is 10 years old with a history of esotropia of the right eye since birth. The strabismus has been constant since then, although the magnitude is less now than in infancy. No previous treatment has been given. Further history reveals possible traumatic injury during delivery. Developmental history appears normal, except the child always has difficulty abducting the right eye. The refraction is:

> O.D. Plano 20/400 (6/120)
> O.S. Plano 20/20 (6/6)

The deviation is a noncomitant, constant, unilateral esotropia of the right eye of 15^Δ at far and near, with a normal AC/A (6/1), and good cosmesis. The associated conditions include lack of any fusion; deep amblyopia; nasal, unsteady, parafoveal, eccentric fixation; complete lack of correspondence; poor accommodative facility in the amblyopic eye; no motor fusion; and slightly noticeable facial asymmetries. Muscle testing indicates a complete paresis of the right lateral rectus. Cosmesis is not a concern to the patient or parents.

The basic esotropia of this 10-year-old patient is congenital. The prognosis for a functional cure by any or all means of therapy is poor. Flom's prognosis chart for a functional cure of the strabismus would indicate 0% chance of success (see Table 6-4).

It is also probable that the prognosis is poor for any significant change in the status of the amblyopia because the deviation has probably been unilateral since birth; therefore, it can be

speculated that the reduced visual acuity is due to amblyopia of arrest. The ultimate differential diagnosis would be made by treating the condition to find out if there is any improvement. If there is enhancement of visual acuity, the amount of improvement represents that portion of visual loss due to amblyopia of extinction. If there is no improvement, the presence of amblyopia of arrest is confirmed, assuming any organic cause of reduced visual acuity has been ruled out.

No treatment for the strabismus is recommended in this case if the cosmesis is acceptable to the patient. Because the deviation is not large, the appearance of the eyes is fairly good in the primary gaze; however, the esotropia may become noticeable on right gaze because of the right lateral rectus paresis. Cosmesis is acceptable otherwise.

Direct total occlusion should be recommended except when the patient cannot see well enough in school with the amblyopic eye. This should continue for 1 or 2 months to find out if there is any improvement. If visual acuity improves in the right eye, pleoptics to treat the eccentric fixation may be advised. If there is no change in visual acuity after that, further vision therapy is not indicated. The patient would then be advised to have a routine follow-up examination in one year.

Case no. 2

The patient is 9 years old with a history of constant esotropia since the age of 1 year. No previous treatment has been given. The patient has no complaints of diplopia. Refraction is:

> O.D. +2.50 −0.50 x 180   20/40 (6/12)
> O.S. Plano   20/20 (6/6)
> Vision at near was commensurate
> with that at far.

The deviation is a comitant, constant, alternating, esotropia, with the left eye being preferred. The deviation is 45^Δ at far and 35^Δ at near with the AC/A being low (2/1). Cosmesis is poor. The associated conditions include deep peripheral suppression; shallow amblyopia with unsteady central fixation;

probable HARC; horror fusionis; and no motor fusion or stereopsis.

This case can be described as divergence insufficiency esotropia because of the larger deviation at far. The prognosis for a functional cure by any or all means of therapy is poor. The Flom prognosis chart would indicate only a 10% chance for success (see Table 6-4). The prognosis, however, for a partial cure is poor to fair, meaning that the large manifest deviation could be converted into one that is small by means of surgery. This implies that peripheral fusion could possibly be developed and/or re-educated, thereby helping the patient hold the eyes relatively straight. The patient would technically be strabismic; but if motor ranges could be developed, the patient could function with at least some degree of binocularity. This would be a monofixation pattern. With a history of no previous treatment and a duration of 8 years of constant esotropia, there is little hope for anything beyond this expectation.

The shallow amblyopia is probably due to the anisometropia rather than the strabismus since the deviation is alternating and not unilateral. The prognosis for cosmetic cure by means of extraocular muscle surgery is fair to good. Prism adaptation testing would be useful in this case to predetermine whether the angle of deviation would be stable after the operation. The patient should be advised that several appointments are needed for further evaluation and that vision training will be tried on a short-term basis, approximately 5 weekly visits, to determine if there is any improvement in visual acuity. Correcting lenses should be worn during this time along with constant patching of the left eye in an attempt to improve the acuity of the right eye. After lenses and vision training have achieved the maximum results, surgery should be recommended for cosmetic and, hopefully, functional improvement. A contact lens for the right eye may be considered as an alternative to the spectacles at a later time.

Case no. 3

Case history reveals that the onset of esotropia for this 7-year-old patient was at about 3 months of age. Examination at age 4 years found a refractive error of +0.75 diopter sphere in each eye. Lenses of this power were prescribed at that time, but were worn only a few days before being rejected by the patient. Present refraction is plano and 20/20 in each eye.

The deviation is a comitant, constant, alternating (right eye dominant) esotropia of 15^Δ at far and 13^Δ at near. There is also a large double-dissociated hyper deviation (dissociated vertical deviation - DVD). The AC/A is normal and cosmesis is good because angle kappa is positive. There is HARC, shallow central suppression, and the patient has no demonstrable fusion range.

The prognosis for a functional cure by means of any or all methods of vision therapy is poor from our clinical experience. The Flom chart, however, would indicate a chance of cure as 20% to 30% (see Table 6-4). The reason for a poor prognosis in this case of infantile esotropia is that the onset was very early and of long duration. Also, the constant deviation and ARC are negative factors, and possibly the DVD. If treatment had been given soon after the onset of strabismus, perhaps there would have been a chance for bifoveal fusion.

Since there is no cosmetic problem, no treatment should be recommended. Furthermore, onset of amblyopia is unlikely to occur, considering the age of the patient and the fact that the strabismus is alternating. The patient should be advised to have a routine follow-up examination in one year.

Poor-to-Fair Prognosis

Case no. 4

The patient is 10 years old with a history of exotropia of the right eye that was intermittent, beginning at 7 months through 1 year of age. The strabismus has been constant since then. Direct patching was attempted for a few weeks at age 3, but only token occlusion was accomplished. No other treatment has been given since. Refraction is:

O.D. −1.00 − 1.00 X 180 20/100 (6/30)
O.S. Plano   20/20 (6/6)
Vision at near was commensurate
with that at far.

The deviation is a comitant, constant, unilateral exotropia of the right eye of 25^Δ at far and 15^Δ at near with a high AC/A (10/1). Cosmesis is poor due to the magnitude of the deviation and to a large positive angle kappa (+1.5 mm). The associated conditions include: deep peripheral suppression; deep amblyopia; unsteady, temporal, parafoveal eccentric fixation; HARC; and no evidence of motor fusion (i.e., lack of disparity vergence). No stereopsis response could be elicited.

This patient has divergence excess exotropia. The prognosis for a functional cure of the strabismus by means of therapy is poor to fair. The Flom chart would indicate a 30% chance for success (see Table 6-4). However, the prognosis for achieving a monofixation pattern is fair; and the chance of partially ameliorating the amblyopia is also fair, because of the history of intermittency. Some of the amblyopia may be of extinction rather than arrest. It is unlikely that 20/20 (6/6) vision will be attained, although some improvement can be expected.

Assuming the amblyopia can be effectively reduced, minus-lens overcorrection may be used initially in an attempt to align the visual axes. The high AC/A is useful for accomplishing this. The ARC is probably not as unfavorable as is the deep suppression in this case of exotropia. A surgical overcorrection (resulting in a small eso deviation) may be called for, both for functional as well as for insuring a good cosmetic result in the event vision training fails to effect a functional improvement or cure. It is hoped that some fusional (disparity) vergences can be developed, and the patient at least achieves gross stereopsis.

The patient should be advised that approximately 25 office appointments and intensive home training will be recommended. Surgery may also be needed and the patient being given postsurgical vision therapy.

If the parents and the patient do not elect vision training along with the possibility of surgery and are concerned only with cosmesis, an optical approach can be tried. A 10^Δ base-in prism can be worn over the dominant left eye. The left eye would then fixate 10^Δ to the left and the exotropic right eye would appear straighter, possibly within the cosmetic limit. If, however, cosmesis remains unacceptable, yoked prisms may be tried. In this case, 10^Δ base-out would be worn over the right eye in addition to the 10^Δ base-in over the left eye.

Case no. 5

The patient is a 5-year-old strabismic with a history of constant esotropia beginning at age 2 years. There is a history of strabismus in the family. No previous examination or treatment has been given. The present refraction is:

Dry retinoscopy:
O.D. +2.00 D. Sph. 20/40 (6/12)
O.S. +1.00 D. Sph. 20/20 (6/6)

Wet retinoscopy (1% cyclopentolate)
O.D. +2.50 D.S. (same VA)
O.S. +1.50 D.S. (same VA)

The deviation is a comitant, constant, unilateral esotropia of the right eye of 10^Δ at far and 20^Δ at near with a high AC/A. Cosmesis is good because of a large positive angle kappa (+1.5 mm). The associated conditions include: deep suppression; shallow amblyopia; nasal, inferior, unsteady, paramacular, eccentric fixation; and no fusional (disparity) vergence. Correspondence is normal, and there is no evidence of horror fusionis. Neither gross nor fine stereopsis could be elicited.

This patient has convergence excess esotropia. The prognosis for complete functional cure is poor to fair. The Flom chart would indicate a prognosis of 30% for success (see Table 6-4). However, the prognosis for a partial cure, whereby a monofixation pattern is to be achieved, is fair to good. The chief reason a complete cure (where there is exact bifoveal fixation) is difficult to achieve in this case is that there has been a duration of constant strabismus of 3 years.

There are many cases in which bifoveal fixation is difficult to regain after the patient has lost it for a relatively long time. This is particularly so in very young patients.

In this case, however, the prognosis for cure of amblyopia by means of constant occlusion, pleoptics, and other monocular training activities is good because of the patient's young age and relatively late onset of the amblyogenic strabismus.

The patient should be advised that bifocal spectacle lenses will be necessary and that approximately 25 weekly office training sessions, along with home training, are needed to develop peripheral fusion and good fusional vergence ranges. Since cosmesis is good and functional results can be expected without surgical intervention, there is probably no need for an operation in this case. However, prisms may be required during and after vision training.

Fair Prognosis

Case no. 6

The patient is 9 years old and has had a slightly noticeable esotropia of intermittent onset of the right eye since the age of three. The strabismus is occasionally observed by family members when the patient is looking far away. No previous treatment has been given. Refractive history is incomplete, but the patient was taken for an eye examination at age 5. No treatment was given then, and the advice was that the strabismus would "eventually go away." The present refraction is:

> Dry subjective:
> O.D. +1.00 D. Sph.   20/30 (6/9)
> O.S. +1.00 D. Sph.   20/20 (6/6)
>
> Wet subjective (1% cylopentolate):
> O.D. +1.50 D.S. (same VA)
> O.S. +1.50 D.S. (same VA)
>
> Vision at near was commensurate with that at far.

The deviation is a comitant, intermittent (constant at far and estimated 25% of the time at near), unilateral esotropia of the right eye of 15^Δ at far and 4^Δ at near. Cosmesis is good because of a positive angle kappa and a relatively wide IPD of 65 mm. The AC/A is low (2/1). Associated conditions include intermittent, deep, central suppression; shallow amblyopia; small (foveal off-center) nasal eccentric fixation; HARC (covariation at near), good second-degree motor fusion range. Some peripheral stereopsis was occasionally elicited at near.

This patient has a divergence insufficiency esotropia. The prognosis for functional cure by means of therapy is fair. The Flom prognosis chart would indicate a 50% chance for functional cure (see Table 6-4). Although there is deep central suppression, the factor of intermittency helps the prognosis immensely. The primary purpose of vision therapy in this case is to improve the presently existing visual skills that are in play at least some of the time at near distances. Binasal occlusion for farpoint seeing may be tried, as well as the possibility of base-out prisms, followed by antisuppression training and the development of adequate fusional divergence. A certain amount of training to improve monocular fixation and accommodative facility would be helpful prior to the binocular therapy regimen.

The prognosis must remain somewhat guarded because of the long duration of strabismus and lack of previous treatment. The patient should be advised of the need for spectacles, occlusion therapy, and approximately 30 weekly office appointments along with intensive home vision training. Surgery should be recommended only if absolutely required for functional results.

Fair-to-Good Prognosis

Case no. 7

The patient is 6 years old and has had an exotropic deviation of the left eye since the age of 4 years. Since then, the strabismus has been intermittent. No previous treatment has been given. The present refraction is:

> O.D. Plano   20/20(6/6)
> O.S. Plano   20/30 (6/9)
> Vision at near was commensurate with that at far.

The deviation is a comitant, intermittent, unilateral exotropia of the left eye of 20^Δ at far and 5^Δ at near with a high AC/A (12/1) and poor cosmesis. The appearance of the strabismus is very noticeable because of the intermittency and a positive angle kappa (+1.5 mm). The exotropia is estimated to be present 90% of the time at far and 10% at near. Associated conditions include deep peripheral suppression when the deviation is manifest; shallow amblyopia with unsteady central fixation; and covariation between HARC and NRC. An exo fixation disparity is detected when there is bifixation at the nearpoint with an associated exophoria of 4^Δ. Motor fusion (disparity vergence) ranges are very limited, being from 22^Δ BI to 18^Δ BI at far and from 8^Δ BI to 1^Δ BO at near.

This patient has divergence excess exotropia. The prognosis for a functional cure by means of lenses and vision training is *fair to good*. The Flom prognosis chart would indicate a 70% chance for success (see Table 6-4). This case is a classic example of divergence excess. The prognosis must be guarded because of the larger deviation at farpoint and the intense and extensive suppression when the deviation is manifest. ARC is not a significantly adverse factor with which to be concerned since normal correspondence predominates while there is fusion.

Monocular vision therapy should be done in conjunction with binocular sensory and motor fusion training in order to eliminate the amblyopia as quickly as possible. The patient should be advised that spectacles, probably bifocals, and approximately 25 weekly office visits and diligent home training are recommended.

Case no. 8

The patient is 8 years old with a history of exotropia since the age of 3 years. The onset was intermittent and has been so ever since. An examination was given at age 4 years. No significant refractive error was found, and lenses were not prescribed. There has been no other examination since that time. The present refractive error is:

> O.D. Plano 20/20 (6/6)
> O.S. Plano 20/20 (6/6)
> Vision at near was commensurate
> with that at far.

The deviation is a comitant, intermittent (25% of the time at far and 95% at near), unilateral exotropia of the right eye of 15^Δ at far and 25^Δ at near. Cosmesis is fair. The associated conditions include moderately deep peripheral

suppression when the deviation is manifest; covariation between HARC and NRC; a limited motor fusion range; and poor stereopsis.

This patient has convergence insufficiency exotropia. The prognosis for a functional cure by means of vision training is fair to good. The Flom prognosis chart would indicate 80% chance for success (see Table 6-4). Other supplemental testing, such as the prolonged occlusion test, could help make the prognosis more decisive. It would also be helpful to know the patient's stereoacuity, if that can be elicited at times when the patient is fusing.

Surgery is probably not called for in this case. All that may be required to cure this patient with convergence insufficiency is vision training that emphasizes antisuppression and fusional convergence training.

The patient should be advised to plan for 25 weekly vision therapy appointments and vigorous home training with the remote possibility of extraocular muscle surgery.

Case no. 9

The patient is 35 years old with a complaint of intermittent diplopia of sudden onset following trauma to the head in an automobile accident three weeks ago. This resulted in a mild paresis of the left superior oblique. Refractive history is unremarkable with the exception of a small myopic refractive error. Present prescription being worn is:

> O.D. −1.00 D. Sph. 20/20 (6/6)
> O.S. −1.00 D. Sph. 20/20 (6/6)
> Vision at near was commensurate
> with that at far.

The deviation is a noncomitant, intermittent, unilateral hypertropia of the left eye of 6^Δ at far and near. Also, there are deviations of $1°$ excyclo and 4^Δ of eso at far and 7^Δ at near. Cosmesis is good in the primary position and on levoversion, but the hyperdeviation is quite noticeable on dextroversion. The frequency of the manifest deviation is approximately 50% of the time in the primary position and 100% on dextroversion. There is a vertical fixation disparity and the associated phoria is 4^Δ left hyper, which is measurable only when patient is fusing.

Additional information would be helpful before the final prognosis is made; for example, stereoacuity and motor fusion ranges. Assuming these are relatively normal, the prognosis for this adult patient is fair to good for a functional cure by any means of therapy. There is a good chance of spontaneous remission of the left superior oblique paresis with the passing of time, approximately 6 months being allowed to determine whether the paresis will be resolved. The Flom chart is not applicable in this case but we believe the overall prognosis is fair to good.

Management of the noncomitancy should emphasize the prevention of extraocular muscle contractures. The patient should be advised to make follow-up appointments as necessary for evaluation and training involving occlusion, prisms, and fusional vergence improvement. Communication with other specialists, particularly the neurologist, should be maintained. The patient should be advised of the eventual possibility of extraocular muscle surgery, although the necessity for this seems unlikely.

Good Prognosis

Case no. 10

The patient is 7 years old with a history of esotropia since age 4 years. The onset was intermittent and has been so ever since. The patient was examined at age 5 with a small amount of hyperopia found in each eye, but no lens prescription was given. Diplopia is noticed occasionally during nearpoint tasks. Cycloplegic and manifest refraction results are:

> O.D. Plano 20/20 (6/6)
> O.S. Plano 20/20 (6/6)
> Vision at near was commensurate
> with that at far.

The deviation is a comitant, intermittent (10% of the time at far and 90% at near), unilateral esotropia of the right eye of 6^Δ at far and 16^Δ at near. Cosmesis is good. There is NRC. Associated conditions include shallow central suppression; eso fixation disparity (associated esophoria of 5^Δ at far but nearpoint findings

could not be attained); and a good motor fusion range. Stereoacuity with contoured targets was 120" of arc at far and 60" of arc at near when +2.00 D addition lenses were worn.

This patient has an accommodative esotropia of the high AC/A type. The prognosis for a functional cure by means of lenses (bifocals) and vision training is good. It would be 80% by the Flom prognosis chart (see Table 6-4). This is a classic case of convergence excess being caused by a high AC/A. The far deviation may be partially alleviated by incorporating base-out prism (less than 6^Δ) in the patient's spectacles. This together with bifocal additions will partially alleviate the deviation at near.

The prognosis must be slightly guarded because of the possible unacceptance of the spectacles by this 7-year-old child. Other than that, we believe the prognosis is theoretically good. As in other cases, treatment depends upon good motivation and cooperation. These factors must always be taken into account.

The patient should be advised to have 5 weekly office appointments for vision therapy after the bifocal spectacles have been dispensed. The patient will be taught to accept and properly use the spectacles. Some antisuppression training and a great deal of fusional vergence training is required. Fortunately, much of this can be done at home, assuming the patient and parents are motivated and cooperative.

Case no. 11

The patient is 8 years old with a history of intermittent exotropia at near that was first noticed at age 6 years. The frequency of the deviation has increased somewhat since then. No previous treatment has been given. Refraction is:

> O.D. −1.00 D. Sph. 20/20 (6/6)
> O.S. −0.25 D. Sph. 20/20 (6/6)
> Vision at near was commensurate
> with that at far.

The deviation is a comitant, intermittent (5% of the time at far and 40% at near), unilateral exotropia of the right eye of 8^Δ at far and 20^Δ at near. The AC/A is very low (1.2/1). Cosmesis is good with far fixation but noticeable at times with near face-to-face viewing. There is NRC. Associated conditions include: shallow central suppression when the deviation is manifest; fixation disparity (associated exophoria of 1^Δ at far and 5^Δ at near); and poor motor fusion ranges. Stereoacuity is approximately 60" arc at far and near, during fusion.

The prognosis for a functional cure by means of lenses and vision therapy is *good*. It would be 90% for success according to the Flom prognosis chart (see Table 6-4). This case of convergence insufficiency exotropia should be aided by the wearing of lenses that correct the myopic anisometropia. Also, fusional vergence ranges can most probably be expanded by means of vision training. The patient should be advised to make 10 weekly office appointments and plan on an intense home vision training program.

Case no. 12

The patient is a 22-year-old college student who is complaining of blurring of vision and asthenopia during prolonged reading. The refraction is:

> O.D. Plano 20/20 (6/6)
> O.S. Plano 20/20 (6/6)
> Vision at near was commensurate
> with that at far.

The deviation is a comitant, exophoria of 5^Δ at far and 10^Δ at near. The AC/A is normal, being 4/1. Motor fusion ranges are fair (vergences at far of 11^Δ BI to 4^Δ BO and nearpoint vergences of 16^Δ BI to 3^Δ BO). The nearpoint of convergence is 12 cm. Associated conditions include: accommodative infacility (able to clear only 3 cycles of ±1.00 D lenses in one minute), and an exo fixation disparity at near (associated exophoria of 2^Δ). Noncontoured (random dot) stereoacuity was 20" of arc at near. The only other abnormal clinical findings were low positive and negative relative accommodation (PRA and NRA, respectively).

The prognosis for a functional cure by means of vision therapy is good. Even though this is a case of heterophoria and not strabismus, the patient does not meet the criteria of Flom as being functionally cured because of the blurring of vision, discomfort, and the inadequate nearpoint of convergence. (Note that in cases of strabismus in which the patient is cured, the patient is then treated as in heterophoria therapy to effect a cure of any deficient binocular visual skills and, hopefully, to enhance all binocular visual skills.)

The patient should be advised to make 5 weekly office appointments for vision therapy and plan on home training for approximately 30 minutes per day during this time. Afterwards, 5 to 10 minutes per day of continued home training may be recommended, as a home maintenance program, until a progress evaluation in 4 months.

REFERENCES

1. Flom MC. The prognosis in strabismus. *Am J Optom Arch Am Acad Optom.* 1958;35:509-514.
2. Flom MC. Issues in the clinical management of binocular anomalies. In: Rosenbloom AA, Morgan MW, eds. *Principles and Practice of Pediatric Optometry.* Philadelphia: J. B. Lippincott; 1990:222.
3. Manley DR. *Symposium on Horizontal Ocular Deviations.* St Louis: CV Mosby Co; 1971:28.
4. Griffin JR, Lee JM. The Polaroid Mirror Method. *Optom Weekly.* 1970;61:28-29.
5. Ludlam WM. Orthoptic treatment of strabismus. *Am J Optom.* 1961;38:369-388.
6. Etting G. Visual training for strabismus: success ratio in private practice. *Optom Weekly.* 1973;64:23-26.
7. Taylor DM. *Congenital Esotropia: Management and Prognosis.* New York: Intercontinental Medical Book Corp; 1973:75-79.
8. Wybar K. The use of prisms in preoperative and postoperative treatment. In: Fells P, ed. *First Congress of the International Strabismological Association.* St Louis: CV Mosby Co; 1971:245.
9. Parks MM. The monofixation syndrome. In: *Symposium of Strabismus, Transactions of the New Orleans Academy of Ophthalmology.* St Louis: CV Mosby Co; 1971:150.
10. Winter J. *Clinical Management of Amblyopia.* Houston: University of Houston, College of Optometry; 1973:39.
11. Aust W. Results of occlusion therapy in concomitant strabismus. In: Fells P, ed. *First Congress of the International Strabismological Association.* St Louis: CV Mosby Co; 1971:163.
12. Goodier HM. Some Results of Occlusion in Cases of Noncentral Fixation. In: Mein J, ed. *Orthoptics.* Amsterdam: Excerpta Medica; 1972:369.
13. Kavner RS, Suchoff IB. *Pleoptics Handbook.* New York: Optometric Center of New York; 1969:18.
14. Chavasse FB. *Worth's Squint.* 7th ed. Philadelphia: Blakiston's Son and Co; 1939.

15. Manas L. The effect of vision training upon the ACA ratio. *Am J Optom.* 1958;35:428-437.
16. Flom MC. On the relationship between accommodation and accommodative convergence. *Am J Optom.* 1960;37:630-631.
17. Costenbader FD. Diagnosis and Clinical Significance of the Fusional Vergences. *Am Orthop J.* 1965;15:14-20.
18. Jones BA. Orthoptic handling of fusional vergences. *Am Orthop J.* 1965;15:21-29.
19. Griffin JR. Efficacy of vision therapy for nonstrabismic vergence anomalies. *Optom Vision Sci.* 1987;64:411-414.
20. Hugonnier R, Hugonnier S, Troutman S. *Strabismus, Heterophoria, Ocular Motor Paralysis.* St Louis: CV Mosby Co; 1969:595-664.
21. Hurtt J, Rasicovici A, Windsor CE. *Comprehensive Review of Orthoptics and Ocular Motility.* St Louis: CV Mosby Co; 1972:202-238.
22. Mein J, Trimble R. *Diagnosis and Management of Ocular Motility Disorders.* 2nd ed. Oxford: Blackwell Scientific Publications; 1991:166-195.
23. Von Noorden GK. *Binocular Vision and Ocular Motility.* 4th ed. St Louis: CV Mosby Co; 1990:479-536.
24. Dale RT. *Fundamentals of Ocular Motility and Strabismus.* New York: Grune & Stratton, 1982:340-81.
25. Jampolsky AJ. A simple approach to strabismus diagnosis. In: *Symposium on Strabismus, Trans New Orleans Acad Ophthalmol.* St Louis: CV Mosby Co; 1971:66-75.
26. Aust W, Welge-Lussen L. Preoperative and postoperative changes in the angle of squint following long-term, preoperative, prismatic compensation. In: Fells P, ed. *First Congress of the International Strabismological Association.* St Louis: CV Mosby Co; 1971:217.
27. Alpern MB, Hofstetter HW. The effect of prism on esotropia: a case report. *Am J Optom.* 1948;25:80-91.
28. Postar SH. Ophthalmic prism and extraocular muscle deviations: the effect of wearing compensatory prisms on the angle of deviation in cases of esotropia. Unpublished research. Ketchum Memorial Library: Southern California College of Optometry; 1972.
29. Jampolsky A. Adjustable strabismus surgical procedures. In: *Symposium on Strabismus: Transactions of the New Orleans Academy of Ophthalmology.* St Louis: CV Mosby Co; 1978:320-328.
30. Helveston EM. *Surgical Management of Strabismus: An atlas of strabismus surgery.* 4th ed. St Louis: CV Mosby Co; 1993:305-333.
31. Abraham SV. The use of miotics in the treatment of convergent strabismus and anisometropia. *Am J Ophthalmol.* 1949;32:233-240.
32. Gellman M. The use of miotics for the correction of hypermetropia and accommodative esotropia. *Am J Optom.* 1963;40:93-101.
33. Bartlett JD, Jaanus SD. *Ocular Pharmacology.* 2nd ed. Boston: Butterworth Publishers; 1989:125.
34. Manley DR. *Symposium on Horizontal Ocular Deviations.* St Louis: CV Mosby Co; 197:68.
35. Scott AB, Rosenbaum AL, Collins CC. Pharmacological weakening of the extraocular muscles. *Invest Ophthalmol Visual Sci.* 1973;2:924-929.
36. McNeer KW. An investigation of the clinical use of Botulinum Toxin A as a postoperative adjustment procedure in the therapy of strabismus. *J Ped Ophthalmol Strabismus.* 1990;27:3-9.
37. Kohn H. Clinical hypnosis as an adjunct in vision therapy. *Optom Monthly.* 1983;74:41-44.

Chapter 7 / Types of Strabismus

Accommodative Esotropia   211
   Characteristics of Refractive
      Accommodative Esotropia   212
   Management of Refractive
      Accommodative Esotropia   212
      Optical Treatment   212
      Other Approaches   213
   Characteristics of high AC/A
      Accommodative Esotropia   214
   Management of High AC/A
      Accommodative Esotropia   214
      Optical Treatment   214
      Vision Training   215
      Miotics   215
      Surgery   216
Infantile Esotropia   216
   Characteristics   216
   Management   219
      Optical Treatment   219
      Vision Training   219

Surgery   220
Primary Comitant Esotropia   220
   Characteristics   221
   Management   221
Primary Comitant Exotropia   221
   Characteristics   222
   Management   223
A and V Patterns   224
   Characteristics   224
   Management   225
Microtropia   226
   Characteristics   226
   Management   227
Cyclovertical Deviations   228
   Comitant Vertical Deviations   229
   Dissociated Vertical Deviations
      (DVD)   230
Sensory Strabismus   230
Consecutive Strabismus   230

Several types of strabismus occur in young patients during their early formative years. If the deviation is caused primarily by genetic factors or developmental anomalies in ocular motor control, it can be described as a developmental strabismus. This chapter discusses the clinical characteristics and management principles of common developmental deviations that are usually comitant. Paralytic strabismus and ocular motor restrictions, although they often occur during childhood or may be congenital, are covered in Chapter 8.

ACCOMMODATIVE ESOTROPIA

The two general types of accommodative esotropia that often require different optical treatment approaches are *refractive* (normal AC/A) and *nonrefractive* (high AC/A). There exists an accommodative component to most eso deviations that occurs during the early developmental years; in that sense, most cases of esotropia can be considered partially accommodative in etiology. Our discussion begins with the characteristics of accommodative esotropia and an

TABLE 7-1. *Characteristics of Accommodative Esotropia*

	Refractive Esotropia	High AC/A Esotropia
Mechanism	Uncorrected hyperopia Limited divergence	High AC/A Limited divergence
Onset	Most 2-3 years old	Most 2-3 years old
Refractive error	+4.75 DS	Presents at near +2.25 DS
Constancy	Usually intermittent	Often constant at near distances
Correspondence	Usually NRC	Usually NRC
Amblyopia	Rare	Rare
AC/A	Normal	High
Prognosis	Good with correction of hyperopia	Fair with plus-addition lenses and vision training

overview of management when the mechanism is primarily accommodative, causing excessive accommodative convergence.

Characteristics of Refractive Accommodative Esotropia

Both types of accommodative esotropia usually occur between the ages of 2 and 3 years. This happens concurrently with the development and increased use of accommodation; but the range of onset is broad, extending from infancy into young adulthood. The strabismus can become manifest with illness, excessive emotions, or eye fatigue. Refractive accommodative esotropia has the best-understood etiology of all the developmental types of strabismus. Moderate and high uncorrected hyperopia, usually between 2 and 6 diopters, forces the individual to accommodate sufficiently to attain clear retinal images. An average hyperopia of +4.75 D was reported for accommodative esotropes.[1] There is usually a normal AC/A, but excessive accommodation required to overcome the hyperopia evokes excessive convergence. If compensating fusional divergence is insufficient, a latent eso deviation becomes manifest. This is due to the combination of uncorrected hyperopia and inadequate fusional divergence ranges. The onset of accommodative esotropia is usually gradual and intermittent. Because of its intermittent nature, there is usually normal retinal correspondence (NRC)

and seldom any amblyopia. If the manifest deviation becomes constant at an early age, amblyopia, anomalous retinal correspondence (ARC), and/or a microtropic component can develop. Older children may complain of intermittent diplopia, blur, and eyestrain, particularly when performing near tasks. In some cases of high uncorrected hyperopia (e.g., more than 6 diopters), the eyes may remain straight much of the time when the individual is not using accommodation; however, the consequence may be bilateral amblyopia (i.e., isometropic amblyopia). Characteristics of accommodative esotropia (refractive and high AC/A types) are listed in Table 7-1.

Management of Refractive Accommodative Esotropia

Optical Treatment

With early treatment the prognosis is good for complete resolution of the strabismus, particularly if normal binocularity existed prior to the onset of the deviation. Usually all that is necessary is a prescription of lenses for the full optical correction of the uncorrected hyperopia (and any significant astigmatic component), as verified by cycloplegic refraction (Figure 7-1). The goal of optical treatment is not necessarily orthophoria. Some authorities recommend leaving the patient slightly esophoric so there is a continuing demand for fusional divergence.[2] If the patient's accommodation does not fully relax after wearing the prescription lenses for a few days and there is significant blurred distance vision, the doctor should also recommend accommodative rock training, or administer a cycloplegic drug, atropine if absolutely necessary. The purpose of which would be to reduce an accommodative spasm. Occasionally, even using these measures, the patient is still unable to relax accommodation sufficiently for the full ametropic correction. If the accommodative spasm persists for weeks, power of the plus lenses must be reduced accordingly.

Soft contact lenses have been particularly useful and acceptable to patients for alleviation of accommodative esotropia.[3] The optical properties of contact lenses may be beneficial compared with spectacle lenses. Slightly less accommodation is required to focus an image at near using plus contact lenses than with plus lens spectacles due to the difference in vertex distance. Grisham et al.[4] recently found that contact lenses were more effective than spectacle lenses in reducing residual angles of eso deviation (either phoria or tropia). Wearing of contact lenses also has resulted in better fusional control in cases of NRC.

With patients, under 1 year of age, retinoscopy should be repeated every 3 months due to frequent refractive changes during infancy. New lenses are indicated if there is a change of 1 diopter or more. Follow-up examinations should be done at least every 6 months in these children from ages 1 to 5 years old to ensure that the lens prescription is current and that fusional control of the deviation is maintained.

Other Approaches

Vision training is useful in many cases of accommodative esotropia if the child can cooperate. Patients who undergo vision training tend to maintain a good result longer than those who do not. If there is normal correspondence, the goals of vision training are to eliminate any amblyopia, break suppression, and build fusional divergence ranges with reflex control. (Refer to Chapter 13 for vision training techniques.) Often a patient who has com-

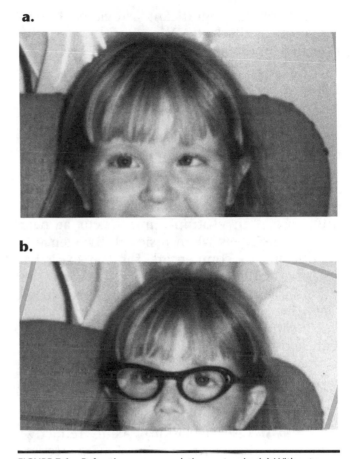

a.

b.

FIGURE 7-1—Refractive accommodative esotropia: **(a)** Without spectacle lens correction; **(b)** With lenses that fully correct the manifest deviation.

pleted vision therapy can remove the lenses for a period of time, such as for swimming or other sports and still maintain fusional control of the deviation.

The use of miotics or surgery in cases of refractive accommodative esotropia is strongly discouraged. Miotics are only a temporary solution at best and have many possible undesirable side effects. They should be tried only after complete optical treatment has failed to achieve alignment and fusional control.

In postsurgical cases of refractive esotropia, consecutive exotropia is a common finding when lenses are eventually worn for the hyperopia. Surgery may be indicated, however, in cases of partially accommodative esotropia in which remains a conspicuous residual strabismus after full correction of the refractive error.

Surgery for any significant associated hyper-deviation or marked A-V pattern may also be necessary and appropriate.

Characteristics of High AC/A Accommodative Esotropia

Accommodative esotropia may occur even when there is little or no hyperopia. This can be due to a high AC/A causing an excessive amount of accommodative convergence with a relatively small amount of accommodation. For this reason, an esotropia may occur at near fixation distances when fusional divergence is insufficient to compensate for the excessive accommodative convergence. This type of accommodative strabismus is also known as *convergence excess* esotropia in the Duane-White classification system. The main distinguishing feature of high AC/A accommodative esotropia is that the magnitude of the near deviation exceeds that at far. This is in contrast to refractive accommodative esotropia in which the near and far deviations are approximately equal (i.e., a *basic* eso deviation). As in refractive accommodative esotropia, high AC/A accom-

modative esotropia is usually intermittent with normal correspondence.

High AC/A accommodative esotropia is relatively independent of refractive error. High hyperopia is possible, but rare. Many patients, however, have minor amounts of hyperopia. In one series of patients with high AC/A accommodative esotropia, the average refractive error was +2.25 D.[1] This is about half the average amount of hyperopia found in refractive accommodative esotropia. There is, however, wide variability in refractive error, with some patients presenting with emmetropia and even myopia. In cases of moderately high hyperopia in combination with a high AC/A, treatment must address both causes of the deviation.

Management of High AC/A Accommodative Esotropia

Optical Treatment

It is usually necessary to correct any manifest hyperopia with lenses since the AC/A is high. Cycloplegic refraction should be done to reveal any latent hyperopia. In addition, the optimum bifocal lens power should be determined to promote fusion at the patient's nearpoint working distance. This amount is, of course, determined under noncycloplegic testing conditions. Plus lens additions are used for the patient's preferred working distance to determine empirically which power will best align the eyes. This technique utilizes, in effect, the measured AC/A (i.e., lens gradient method) to determine the optimum bifocal power. When prescribing bifocals for very young children, it is important to fit the bifocal line high, at midpupil, if it is to be utilized properly (Figure 7-2). For older children and adults, the segment height can be lowered slightly.

For older children and adults, bifocal contact lenses may be considered as an alternative to bifocal spectacles in the high AC/A type of accommodative esotropia. The added near power is useful in all fields of gaze, unlike spectacle bifocals, and many patients do not complain of the slight decrease in contrast inherent in the bifocal contact lens design.[4]

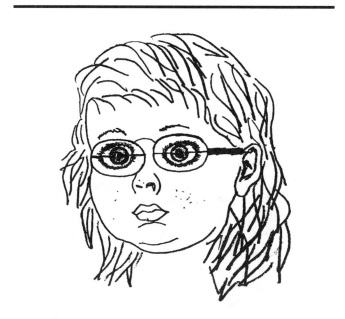

FIGURE 7-2—Proper segment height for a young child with high AC/A accommodative esotropia.

Vision Training

After the optimum bifocal correction has been prescribed to promote alignment at far and near, vision training is recommended to build a reserve of fusional vergence function. Vision therapy should be programmed to eliminate amblyopia and suppression and then develop and improve fusional divergence. Adequate fusional vergences serve to improve control of the deviation at all viewing distances; this is important since the deviation varies in magnitude from far to near. (Refer to Chapter 13 for vision training techniques.) Without adequate vision training, these patients tend to lose control of the deviation at near, and suppression can reoccur at near fixation distances. The higher the AC/A, the more a patient tends to lose control of the deviation with time.[5] We do not recommend combining miotic therapy with a vision training program. Although some clinicians may disagree, our experience indicates that vision training progress is erratic when miotics are used simultaneously. It is unclear why this is so, but results are better when one or the other is administered at a time.

Miotics

If the nearpoint deviation cannot be adequately controlled using bifocals and vision training, miotics may be considered as a treatment option. We believe that topical anticholinesterase drugs have been overused in the treatment of accommodative esotropia. They have significant side effects and do not offer a long-term solution; it seems prudent to try to control the near deviation by other means if possible. These pharmaceutical agents, however, may be effective initially to achieve temporary alignment when other methods have failed. Introduction of more conservative vision therapy methods for long-term management of the deviation can then be made. Common anticholinesterase eyedrops such as DFP (0.025% diisopropyl fluorophosphate ointment) and Phospholine Iodine (echothiophate iodide solution, 0.03%, 0.06%, or 0.125%) produce an accumulation of acetylcholine at the myoneural junction of the ciliary muscle. This results in a decrease in the innervation that is necessary for effective accommodation and, therefore, to a corresponding decrease of accommodative convergence. Vergence is effectively decoupled from accommodation so an increasing eso deviation at near does not occur with accommodative effort. An additional factor responsible for the reduction of accommodation and accommodative convergence is the miosis itself. The small pupils increase the depth of focus so that near objects can be seen clearly with much less accommodation than with normal-sized pupils. Of the two, DFP is the most effective with less systemic absorption. However, Phospholine Iodine (PI) is readily available in different concentrations and, therefore, has greater versatility in clinical management. DFP is often preferred for preschool children and PI for older children and adults. The miotic agent is given once a day, often at night, before sleep.

Clinicians need to be aware of the complications associated with the use of miotics (anticholinesterase agents), some of which are serious. The most hazardous complication occurs when a patient taking topical miotics is given a depolarizing muscle relaxant, such as succinylcholine, during general anesthesia. This can result in a prolonged, and even fatal, apnea. Consequently, patients taking a topical miotic should carry a card clearly identifying its use in case of emergency surgery. A patient should discontinue the use of miotics for at least six weeks before succinylcholine can be used safely. Another potentially fatal mistake is to ingest topical miotics orally. These agents need to be kept securely out of the reach of children. Death is caused by a cholinergic crisis resulting from blockage at motor end plates of the heart and lungs.

Serious systemic toxicity using miotics, although uncommon, has been reported as affecting the gastrointestinal system, such as nausea, abdominal discomfort, and diarrhea.[6] Manual depression of the lacrimal canaliculi during and after topical administration should prevent, or minimize, these systemic side effects.

The most common ocular side effect is the development of iris cysts at the pupillary margin occurring in approximately 50% of children taking Phospholine Iodide. The cysts can grow large enough to obscure vision, but these usually are reversible by discontinuing the use of the miotic. The development of such cysts can be minimized by instilling a drop of 2.5% or 10% phenylephrine (Neosynephrine) concurrently with the miotic. Iris cysts occur less often as a side effect with the administration of DFP than with PI.

Miotics cause other ocular side effects including ciliary spasm with browache, conjunctival injection, and iritis. These are usually transitory, but more serious complications can occur such as angle-closure glaucoma, retinal detachment, and anterior subcapsular cataracts (usually reversible in children). Because of these possible side effects, we recommend the initial use of optical and vision training procedures rather than miotics in most cases of high AC/A accommodative esotropia.

Surgery

An operation may be indicated if the AC/A is extremely high (e.g., $10^\Delta/1D$ or higher) or if the deviation at near is not adequately controlled by optical means and/or vision training. If the deviation occurs intermittently and infrequently at near, the operation should be deferred until age 5 or 6 years, at which time the patient is usually old enough to cooperate with pre- and post-surgical vision training. The conventional surgical procedure is a recession of both medial rectus muscles (e.g., 5 mm, each eye).[7] This procedure reduces the deviation more at near than at far. In cases of very large esotropic angles at near (e.g., over 45^Δ), other surgical procedures may also be required for adequate reduction of the eso deviation at near. If the patient has fairly good fusional abilities prior to surgery, the surgical results are usually good. In some surgical cases, however, the long-term result is a microtropia with peripheral fusion.[8]

INFANTILE ESOTROPIA

In the past, the term "congenital esotropia" was applied to those cases of primary comitant eso-

tropia that had an onset within the first 6 months of life. The term "congenital," however, means "existing from birth" and does not adequately describe most of the esotropia cases occurring at an early age that have many of the same clinical characteristics. The term "infantile esotropia" is preferable and connotes a period of onset from birth to 6 months. Nixon et al.[9] reported that only a fraction of cases of infantile esotropia are reliably observed to originate at birth. Furthermore, the eyes of a neonate are rarely aligned during the first week of life; the deviation is usually variable, sometimes aligned, and other times convergent or divergent. Normally, alignment and coordinated oculomotor control are not rudimentarily established until the age of 3 months.[9,10] Nevertheless, the specific age of onset in constant esotropia is fundamentally important in establishing the prognosis for treatment when the patient is first seen at a later time. The more time normal binocular vision has had to develop prior to a constant manifest deviation, the better is the prognosis for a cure of the strabismus.

The term "infantile esotropia" does have ambiguity since the etiology of the strabismus, often innervational, seems to be the same as in primary comitant esotropia. Von Noorden suggested that the primary etiology of infantile esotropia is either a delayed fusional vergence development or a primary defect of fusional vergence.[11] However, associated clinical features, e.g., DVD, inferior oblique overaction, and latent nystagmus tend to occur in infantile esotropia verses esotropia of later onset.

Characteristics

Approximately half of the infantile esotropic patients have hyperopic refractive errors of +2.00 D or greater.[12] Ingram,[13] however, reported a study of 1-year-old infants with infantile esotropia from a general pediatric practice with only 11% having hyperopia in this range. Although accommodation may be a factor in the etiology of infantile esotropia, most infantile esotropic cases are not exclusively accommodative. The angle of deviation is usually large (30^Δ or more), stable, comitant, and approximately the same magnitude at all distances (which indicates a normal AC/A). Characteristics of infantile esotropia are listed in Table 7-2.

Clinicians frequently observe crossed fixation in infantile esotropia. The child uses the right eye for targets in the left visual field and the left eye for objects in the right field. This crossed fixation behavior accounts for an apparent limitation of abduction of each eye that is often observed. It is difficult to test ocular rotations adequately in extreme fields of gaze in infants, particularly if they have developed the habit of crossed fixation. Repeat testing and observation may be needed to differentiate a true paresis from an apparent abduction limitation resulting from habitual crossed fixation. Observing abduction during the doll's head maneuver, left and right, may help make the distinction between a lateral rectus paresis and a pseudoparesis. The examiner holds the infant directly in front and makes eye contact while rotating the patient's head to the left and right. For example, the examiner should look for abduction of the patient's right eye as the head is rotated to the patient's left. If the right eye is seen to abduct, pseudoparesis is indicated. The unaffected eye should be patched for a few days to see if abduction rapidly develops in the other eye. If it does, then pseudoparesis is confirmed. If, however, there is a paresis, there will be little or no abduction.

Amblyopia is often associated with infantile esotropia if the child habitually fixates with only one eye. Two large clinical surveys of infantile esotropic children found amblyopia present in 35% and 41% of their samples respectively.[14,15] Established amblyopia at this early age, if not identified and treated early, will most likely become deep and unresponsive to subsequent therapy.

Vertical deviations are often associated with established infantile esotropia, but their etiologies are not well understood. One common condition is overaction of one or both inferior oblique muscles (Figure 7-3). The clinician may observe an increasing hyperdeviation of an eye as it moves nasally during versions. The other eye is similar as this inferior oblique overaction is usually bilateral. In one series of 408 infantile

TABLE 7-2. *Characteristics of Infantile Esotropia*

Mechanism	Innervational; familial tendency (genetic)
Onset	Birth to 6 months of age
Refractive error	About 50% have less than 2 D of hyperopia
Constancy	Usually constant angle >30$^\Delta$
Comitancy	Usually comitant
Eye laterality	Often either alternating or crossed fixation pattern
Correspondence	Usually ARC; some have lack of correspondence
Amblyopia	About 40% of cases
AC/A	Usually normal
Symptoms	Usually none except for cosmetic concerns
Long-term prognosis	Poor if treated past age 2 years Fair if treated before age 2 years
Long-term associations	Overacting inferior obliques, DVD, latent nystagmus

esotropes, overaction of the inferior obliques was found in 68% of the sample.[16] For unknown reasons, the condition is usually not present during the first year of age, but appears later in childhood.

Another little-understood associated condition with infantile esotropia is dissociated vertical deviation (DVD), which must be distinguished from bilateral overacting inferior obliques in young children. DVD is also referred to as "double hyper." On cover testing, either eye that is covered drifts up; when it is uncovered, a downward movement is observed, i.e., either eye is hyper on the cover test (Figure 7-4). This is opposite to the usual hyper-hypo relationship seen in most vertical deviations. One eye may show a larger hyper deviation than the other, which suggests there is an ordinary hyper deviation component that is obscured by the double hyper. In contrast to overacting inferior obliques, DVD is usually evident in all fields of gaze. The prevalence of DVD in infantile esotropia is high, ranging from 51% to 90% depending on the patient series.[16,17] The onset of DVD is usually after age 2 and it may occur years after successful surgical management of

a.

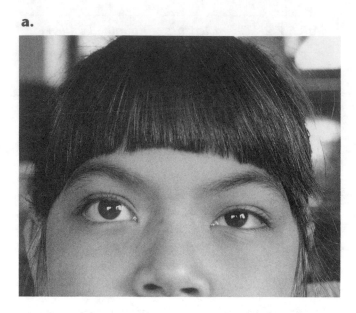

b.

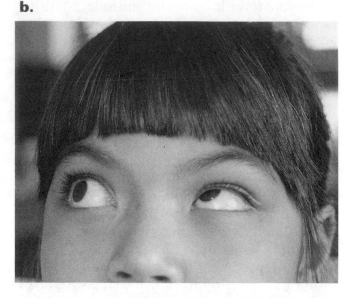

c.

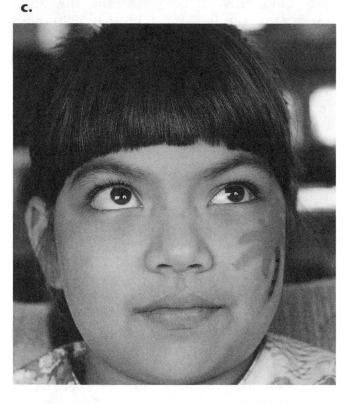

FIGURE 7-3—Overacting inferior oblique muscle: **(a)** primary gaze; **(b)** right gaze with large overaction of the left inferior oblique; **(c)** left gaze with small overaction of the right inferior oblique muscle.

the esotropia. It is advisable to discuss this possibility with the parents. If DVD should occur in the future, it would, at least, not come as a complete surprise. We have seen, however, cases of DVD in orthophoric (or nearly orthophoric) patients who have normal binocularlity in all other respects.

Another fairly common feature of infantile esotropia is nystagmus, both latent nystagmus and manifest nystagmus with a latent component. Reported prevalences range from 25% to 52% depending on the particular patient series.[16,17] Many nystagmus patients with esotropia have an abnormal head posture in an

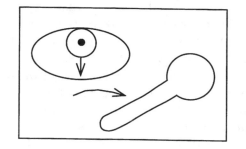 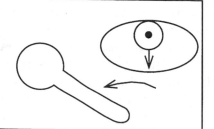

FIGURE 7-4—Dissociated vertical deviation as seen on the alternate cover test.

unconscious attempt to dampen the nystagmus. Lang[17] proposed that the reason nystagmus and DVD are associated with infantile esotropia is the presence of a midbrain lesion disrupting both vestibular and ocular motor control centers.

Management

A cardinal principle in the management of infantile esotropia is early intervention. Generally, the longer effective therapy is delayed, the worse is the long-term prognosis. (Refer to Chapter 6.) The ideal time to initiate vision therapy is at the onset of the condition. Prognosis for a functional cure of very early infantile esotropia approaches zero if treatment is delayed beyond the age of two years. Early treatment is not just important, it is essential. Another principle is frequent examinations of the child because the visual status can change dramatically and rapidly during the first few years of life. General principles of clinical management are as follows.

Optical Treatment

Full cycloplegic retinoscopic findings should be prescribed if there is a significant refractive error. Spectacle lenses are intended to correct any accommodative component of the deviation as well as any significant astigmatism or anisometropia. Prescription for even small amounts of hyperopia is warranted if the lenses are also intended to provide a platform on which to mount Fresnel prisms. The prism power should be equal to or greater than the amount of the residual deviation. Prism spectacles should be worn at least three hours daily in the attempt to provide normal binocular stimulation during the critical developmental period. This should be done before surgical intervention. Retinoscopy should be repeated at least in three-month intervals during the first two years of life since changes in refractive status can occur frequently and rapidly.

Vision Training

Vision training should begin with monocular occlusion. Even in cases of no amblyopia, patching ensures that it will not develop. Appropriate patching builds monocular fixation, prevents suppression and the development of ARC, while promoting abduction. Other than those times when the infant is wearing prism spectacles for binocular stimulation, constant patching should be used if there is constant esotropia. If the strabismus is intermittent, a rare occurrence in cases of infantile esotropia, patching should be done intermittently during those times the patient is likely to have a manifest deviation, e.g., fatigue in afternoons or evenings. Care must be taken to avoid occlusion amblyopia when patching a patient under the age of 5 years. Infants under 2 years should receive daily alternate patching even in cases of unilateral amblyopia. (Refer to Chapter 10 for discussion of occlusion.)

Parents and caregivers should be instructed on active stimulation of fixation and abduction of the child's strabismic eye. To build fixation and eye-hand coordination skills, small toys, candies, and objects can be offered to the child to touch while the dominant eye is patched. To stimulate abduction, interesting and desired objects can be slowly introduced into the child's restricted field of gaze. Unfortunately, many vision training techniques for building binocularity are not practical for children under two years of age. The goals of training procedures, however, are to establish equal and normal visual acuity, free alternation of the eyes (to prevent reoccurrence of amblyopia), and good ocular motility. The next step is eye alignment to promote development of normal binocular vision.

Surgery

If the residual angle of deviation after full correction of the refractive error is too large for practical management with prisms (greater than 20^Δ), surgery is necessary before the age of two years to have a reasonable chance for normal binocular vision. In a now classic study, Taylor[18] demonstrated the advantage of early surgical intervention. (Refer to discussion in Chapter 6.) Subsequent studies have also confirmed this advantage, but even so, the best results that can be expected in many cases appears to be peripheral, but not central, fusion. Often there remains a microtropia (monofixation syndrome), reduced stereopsis, and ARC. Nevertheless, there may be fairly good vergence ranges. Normal stereoacuity should not be expected in many cases of infantile esotropia.

Although there exists considerable disagreement among surgeons, there appears to be little advantage for a successful outcome in performing surgery before age 1. There is, also, some risk with general anesthesia. The patient should maintain a patching regimen until age 1 which seems, in our opinion, to be the optimum time for an operation if free alternation has been established by occlusion and monocular vision training procedures. Most authorities recommend that surgery be performed before 2 years of age, although von Noorden[19] reported some good results between ages 2 and 4 years. The recommended type of operation varies from one authority to another. Dale[2] recommended a recession-resection operation of the affected eye for deviations under 50^Δ even though this may result in mild noncomitancy. For deviations of 50^Δ

to 70^Δ, he recommended a three-muscle operation, recession-resection for one eye, and recession of the medial rectus of the other eye. For deviations 70^Δ to 90^Δ, four-muscle surgery may be necessary, i.e., a recession-resection for each eye. Von Noorden,[19] on the other hand, recommended an initial bimedial recession of varying amounts depending on the magnitude of the deviation; this is followed by, on another occasion, a resection of one or both lateral recti if needed. If one or both inferior obliques are found to be overacting, then von Noorden[19] combines myectomies of the affected muscles.

Botulinum injection into the medial recti is not recommended in cases of infantile esotropia for several reasons: frequent injections are needed under general anesthesia, transient vertical deviations and ptosis are common complications, and research has not demonstrated better results than conventional surgical techniques.[19]

PRIMARY COMITANT ESOTROPIA

Primary comitant esotropia (PCE) is also referred to as "acquired nonaccommodative esotropia." Under the Duane-White classification system, there are three subclasses: basic eso, convergence excess, and divergence insufficiency. This simplified classification is based on the farpoint deviation in relation to the AC/A. (See Chapter 3 in which this classification also applies to heterophoria.) The category of convergence excess was discussed in the above section on accommodative esotropia; only basic esotopia and divergence insufficiency esotropia are discussed here. Primary comitant esotropia (PCE) occurs in early childhood, as does infantile esotropia. The distinguishing feature of PCE, however, is a later onset of the manifest deviation, after 6 months of age but usually before age 6 years. Presumably, a child with PCE has had at least 6 months of normal binocular development with the neurologic architecture supporting normal binocular vision having matured to a considerable degree. Generally speaking, subsequent associated conditions such as suppression and amblyopia may be absent or only mild in severity. For example, ARC may or may not be present depending largely on the age of onset of a constant deviation. However, in cases of untreated infantile esotropia, it is almost always present.

Characteristics

The most important consideration of PCE is the age of onset (Table 7-3). The later the onset, the better is the prognosis. The onset is often gradual and the child passes through a period of intermittent esotropia before the strabismus becomes constant. The size of the deviation is usually between 20^Δ and 70^Δ, and the magnitude may slowly increase over time. Refractive error is often independent of the onset of the deviation since many cases have little or no ametropia. However, there can be a partially accommodative component to the strabismus that requires optical compensation. The cause of PCE is thought to be a developmental innervational anomaly, possibly a multifactorial genetic trait, but the specific pathogenic mechanism is unknown. There are a small number of PCE cases originating from a supranuclear tumor that may be life threatening.[20] In most tumor cases, however, the deviation is noncomitant and conspicuous. The clinician needs to be a very conscientious in cases of strabismus that develop early in life.

Most cases of PCE are basic eso (BE) deviations, which means they have a normal AC/A with the deviations at far and near being approximately equal. A common exception, however, is divergence insufficiency (DI) esotropia in which the AC/A is low; the near eso deviation is significantly less than at far. It is important for the clinician to distinguish DI from divergerence paralysis, which has serious neurological implications. Divergence paralysis originating from a midbrain lesion often presents with a greater eso deviation at far than at near, as in DI. However, the deviation is usually noncomitant initially, but may gradually evolve toward comitancy with time. This can complicate the differential diagnosis between divergence paralysis and DI. For this reason, clinicians should closely monitor all new patients presenting with characteristics of divergence insufficiency.

TABLE 7-3. *Characteristics of Primary Comitant Esotropia*

Mechanism	Innervational; familial tendency (possibly genetic)
Onset	6 months of age to 6 years; can be rapid or gradual.
Refractive error	Most have some hyperopia; wide variation, about 5% myopic
Constancy	Usually constant angle 20-70$^\Delta$. Initial stage may be intermittent
Comitancy	Comitant horizontally, many have an A or V pattern
Correspondence	Usually ARC if early onset and NRC if late onset.
Amblyopia	About 30% of cases
AC/A	Usually normal, some have low AC/A
Symptoms	Usually none
Prognosis	Good if NRC; Poor if ARC

Management

Prognosis is generally good in cases of PCE if there is early intervention with vision therapy (often including surgery). The later the onset of PCE, the better is the prognosis. Lang[21] reported that an onset of PCE after 1.5 years of age indicates a good prognosis after surgical alignment; many patients can develop good random dot stereopsis. If vision therapy is delayed, however, patients often develop amblyopia, ARC, suppression, increased magnitude of the esotropia, and other problems adversely affecting the prognosis for improvement later on.

The surgical approach in PCE usually relies on recession and resection procedures. Adjustable sutures are frequently used to fine-tune the surgical results, the day after the operation. Also, Botulinum toxin injections into the medial recti to weaken them are sometimes used in older children. (Detailed discussions of vision therapy for eso deviations are in Chapter 13.)

PRIMARY COMITANT EXOTROPIA

Under the Duane-White classification of primary comitant exotropia there are three sub-

TABLE 7-4. *Characteristics of Primary Comitant Exotropia*

Mechanism	Innervational; familial tendency; affects females 2:1
Onset	Birth to 8 years; usually gradual.
Refractive error	Wide variation; same as general population
Constancy	Usually intermittent; angle 20^Δ-70^Δ About 80% are intermittent, tends to become constant over time
Comitancy	Comitant horizontally, many have an A or V pattern
Correspondence	Usually NRC; ARC cases often covary with the intermittent deviation
Amblyopia	About 5% of cases
AC/A	Usually normal or low AC/A; about 10% have high AC/A.
Symptoms	Frequent photophobia, squinting (eyelids), or asthenopia
Long-term prognosis	Good if intermittent; poor if constant with ARC.

classes: basic exo, divergence excess, and convergence insufficiency. This simplified classification is based on the farpoint deviation in relation to the AC/A. (See Chapter 3 in which these classifications also apply to heterophoria.)

Characteristics

Primary comitant exotropia (PCX) has a similar etiology to that of primary comitant esotropia (PCE), an innervational anomaly probably of multifactorial genetic origin. Table 7-4 indicates some of the features of PCX. This condition is less prevalent than PCE (about 1/3) and reportedly occurs more frequently in females than males (2:3) for unknown reasons.[22,23] Unlike cases of esotropia, most exotropes are intermittent (approximately 80%) throughout life. Jampolsky[24] pointed out that the progression of exotropia is usually gradual, starting with an exophoria, then evolving to an intermittent strabismus, and a small portion becoming constant exotropes. He suggested that

suppression is the mechanism of decompensation from exophoria to exotropia. Evidence suggests that the onset of exotropia is often early in life, with approximately 40% occurring at birth.[25] Nevertheless, these congenital cases are not usually referred to as "infantile exotropia." This is because of the common intermittent nature of exotropia compared with constant esotropia. Also, the sequelae are also different in the two conditions.

Exotropia is more likely to manifest at a later age than esotropia. Late onset intermittent exotropia is often associated with illness, fatigue, and other precipitating factors such as alcohol intoxication, daydreaming, inattentiveness, and photophobic reactions. All these factors can disrupt fusional control of an exo deviation. Clinicians have traditionally associated exotropia with myopia. The implication was that myopia played some part in the etiology of exotropia. However, most studies indicate that the distribution of refractive error in exotropia resembles that in the general nonstrabismic population, and myopia does not appear to play any special role in its etiology.[26,27] Anisometropia, however, can hinder the control of exophoria and can be a precipitating factor.

The intermittent nature of exotropia causes some special problems. Constant strabismus of developmental origin rarely results in subjective complaints of asthenopia from patients, but patients with an intermittent deviation, even with deep suppression when strabismic, frequently experience symptoms. Many individuals with intermittent exotropia manifest their deviation mostly at distance and maintain fusion (with effort) at near. Besides the common symptoms associated with excessive heterophoria at near (i.e., tired eyes, sleepiness, eyestrain, intermittent blurring of vision, reading difficulties, and headaches), the intermittent exotrope seems unusually predisposed to photophobia. It is a common to observe an individual with intermittent exotropia close one eye or lapse into the deviation when stimulated by bright light (e.g., as when walking from inside a darkened theater into full sunlight). This "dazzle" effect disrupts fusional control of the latent exo deviation when fusional amplitudes are restricted whereas patients with adequate fusional amplitudes are not greatly affected in this manner.[28] The reason for this higher sensitivity of intermittent exotropes compared with other strabismics is unknown.

Intermittent exotropia also presents the examiner with some unique difficulties in establishing the correct diagnosis. The measured angles of deviation at far and near are often not the true angles of deviation. The distance deviation is often less when measured in a small narrow examination room compared with that found in the open environment. Burian and Smith[29] reported significantly larger exo deviations in 31 of 105 patients when measured at 30 meters (100 feet). For this reason, a questionable exotropic magnitude at far should be remeasured while the patient is outdoors or looks at a distant target through a window.

The measured deviation at near, where the exotropic patient is usually fusing, can also be erroneous. Many exotropes fusing at near present with a smaller measured nearpoint deviation than at far. Frequently, however, patching one eye for about 30 minutes results in an increased near deviation that equals the farpoint magnitude.[30] These patients have *simulated (pseudo) divergence excess.* We believe this is about as prevalent as *true divergence excess.* Any patient presenting with a larger exo deviation at far than at near should be patched to break down any spasm of fusional convergence that can mask the true magnitude of the deviation at near. The examiner must take care not to allow any binocular fusion before the nearpoint angle is remeasured. The cover paddle should be placed before the patient's occluded eye as the patch is removed. If the nearpoint deviation is not influenced by occlusion, the patient can be considered to have true divergence excess and treated accordingly. Another test used to identify simulated divergence excess is the gradient AC/A. The angle of deviation at near is remeasured with plus sphere lenses in place (+2.00 D recommended) to find the gradient AC/A. This gradient AC/A is then compared with the calculated AC/A based on the initial cover test findings for distance and near. If the calculated AC/A is high and the gradient AC/A is low, then the implication is simulated divergence excess. However, if the calculated and gradient AC/A prove to be

high, true divergence excess is implicated. For example, if the calculated AC/A is 10/1 and the measured gradient AC/A is 7/1, they both are considered to be high and the difference between them is as expected for the two different techniques. A true divergence excess is, therefore, indicated. However, if the calculated ACA is 10/1 and the gradient test measures 4/1, the difference between the two is relatively large; simulated divergence excess is indicated. Whenever simulated divergence excess is suspected, a prolonged cover test should be done; it is the definitive diagnostic procedure.

Another important clinical feature of intermittent exotropia is variable diagnostic findings, day to day and hour to hour. The amount of fusional vergence available to compensate for a deviation varies from time to time depending on the state of fatigue, alertness, and general health. Patients tend to lapse into their exotropic deviation when inattentive, day dreaming, or gazing at the ceiling or sky. The time of day of the visual examination can influence the measured clinical features of the condition. Early in the day the patient may present with exophoria with excellent stereopsis, whereas during late afternoon the same patient may have exotropia with deep suppression. For this reason it is often advisable to examine patients with intermittent strabismus late in the day for comparison with results found earlier in the day.

With time there is a tendency for intermittent exotropia to worsen; the condition is usually progressive. Von Noorden[31] followed 51 young patients with intermittent exotropia for an average of 3.5 years without treatment; 75% of the cases were found to worsen, often becoming a constant deviation. No change occurred in 9%, and 16% improved without therapy. The examiner needs to take this into consideration when making recommendations for treatment; we recommend early and aggressive treatment, especially with vision training, as soon as the condition is identified.

Management

Prognosis for recovery of binocular function in exotropia is good in patients who experience a long period of intermittency, compared with a child having a constant deviation from early childhood. Amblyopia is relatively rare in PCX unless there is significant anisometropia. Likewise, ARC is not a serious clinical problem since the angle of anomaly can covary with the magnitude and intermittency of the exo deviation. (Refer to the discussion of covariation of correspondence in Chapter 5.)

In our experience, if the angle of deviation in PCX is less than 20^{Δ} to 25^{Δ}, our preferred treatment option is vision training, provided the patient is mature enough to participate actively in the program. For larger deviations, we recommend beginning with a vision training approach, but expecting that surgery may be necessary to achieve comfortable alignment of the eyes at all distances and times of day. The surgical principles in PCX depend not only on the magnitude of the strabismus but also whether the deviation is basic exo, divergence excess, or convergence insufficiency. (See Chapter 14.)

A AND V PATTERNS

The terms "A and V patterns" are used to describe significant changes in the horizontal deviation, eso or exo, as the eyes move from up-gaze to the primary position to down-gaze. (See Figure 7-5.) A and V patterns are, therefore, a form of noncomitancy of the horizontal deviation. Specifically, an *A pattern* is present when there is an increased convergence (or less divergence) of the eyes in up-gaze and increased divergence in down-gaze. If a patient has an A pattern esotropia, the eso deviation increases in up-gaze and decreases in down-gaze; whereas in A pattern exotropia, there is decreasing exo deviation in up-gaze and increasing exo when looking down. Conversely, a *V pattern* is indicated when the visual axes diverge in up-gaze and converge in down-gaze. The V pattern esotropia increases in magnitude in down-gaze whereas a V pattern exotropia increases in up-gaze. These changes in the horizontal deviation with vertical gaze changes are clinically important because they significantly influence the diagnosis, prognosis, and management of strabismus.

Characteristics

An A or V pattern is diagnosed by comparing the alternate cover test results from the primary position to those found in the extreme up and down positions of gaze. By convention, an A pattern is indicated if the horizontal deviation changes 10^{Δ} or more between up and down gaze. However, a V pattern is indicated when there is 15^{Δ} or more change. This difference in criterion is because there is a physiological tendency for relative divergence in up-gaze, hence the larger criterion for V patterns. We recommend moving the patient's head back (chin up) for measurement in down-gaze and the head down (chin down) for measurement of angle H in up-gaze.

In addition to A and V patterns, some patients may show an X pattern in which divergence increases in up and down gazes, e.g., exotropia in both up and down gaze. This could possibly be due to overaction of inferior and superior oblique muscles to cause a combination of a V and an A pattern.[32]

There are widely varying estimates of the prevalence of A and V patterns depending on the source and diagnostic criteria. Prevalence is probably less than one-third of all strabismic patients.[33] The relative frequency of these patterns from most prevalent to least is as follows: (1) V-pattern esotropia (by far the most prevalent); (2) A-pattern esotropia; (3) V-pattern exotropia; and (4) A-pattern exotropia.[34] The V patterns occur about twice as often as A patterns, probably because esotropia is more prevalent than exotropia.

The etiology of A and V patterns is usually not paretic, but mechanical in nature. The principal factors seem to be overactions and underactions of the oblique and vertical recti muscles. For example, the most frequent cause of a V pattern esotropia is the underaction of one or both superior oblique muscle(s). In down-gaze the eso deviation is increased by the loss of abduction by the underacting superior obliques. In up-gaze the eso deviation is decreased by the relatively increased abduction by the normally acting or overacting inferior obliques. Anatomical abnormalities of the bony structure of the orbit and abnormal insertions

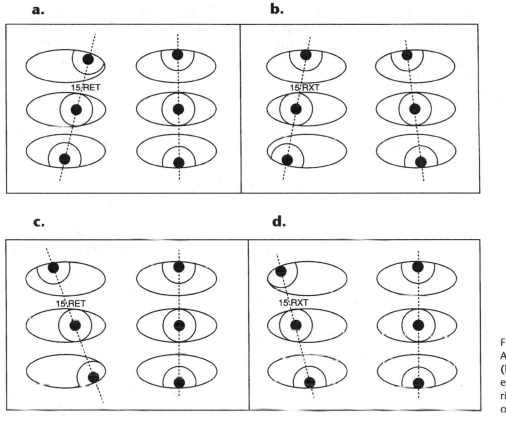

a.

b.

c.

d.

FIGURE 7-5—A and V patterns: **(a)** A-pattern in esotropia of the right eye. **(b)** A-pattern in exotropia of the right eye. **(c)** V-pattern in esotropia of the right eye. **(d)** V-pattern in exotropia of the right eye.

of muscle tendons have been cited also as etiological factors in producing A and V patterns.[35] A and V patterns are frequently associated with infantile strabismus, Duane retraction syndrome, Brown syndrome, acquired bilateral fourth nerve palsy, dysthyroid eye disease with inferior rectus muscle contracture, and orbital malformations found in Down syndrome.[36] On the sensory side, anomalous correspondence can occur in strabismic patients with A and V patterns; however, as the horizontal angle of deviation (H) changes in up and down gaze, the angle of anomaly may covary with it.

If a strabismic individual can achieve normal fusion in some field of gaze, the person usually adopts a head posture allowing fusion to occur. If a patient presents with habitual chin elevation or depression, A and V patterns should be suspected. For example, a V-pattern esotrope who can achieve fusion in up-gaze may present with a chin depression (mischievous appearance), and a V-pattern exotrope may show a chin elevation (snobbish appearance) since the deviation is reduced in down-gaze.

Management

Significant A and V patterns can often be treated surgically, usually either operating on the oblique muscles or transpositioning of the horizontal rectus muscles.[32] Surgical correction of an A or V pattern is indicated if the vertical noncomitancy contributes to excessive fusional demands or to unacceptable cosmesis in cases of horizontal strabismus. An esotropia with an A pattern that has no oblique involvement may be treated by recession of the medial recti and transposed above the original insertion, approximately a muscle-width. The specific surgical technique depends, of course, on the observed patterns of over- and underactions of the vertically acting muscles. For example, if there is also overaction of the superior obliques in an eso A pattern, weakening procedures for these obliques may be necessary. An underaction of the inferior obliques may also aggravate an A pattern and may require strengthening procedures. Esotropias with V patterns may require recession of both medial recti and downward displacement of the original insertion. Since underaction of the superior obliques will increase a V pattern, these may require strengthening procedures. Similarly, an overaction of the inferior obliques exacerbates a V pattern and may require weakening procedures. Exotropia with A pattern may require recession of both lateral recti with downward displacement of the insertions. If the eyes are exotropic with an A pattern due to an overaction of the superior obliques, weakening procedures for these may be required. Exotropias with V-pattern may be treated by recessing both lateral recti with an upward transposition of the insertions. If the inferior obliques are overacting, the exo deviation tends to increase on up gaze; these, therefore, may require weakening procedures.

Vision training is often helpful in cases where the patient has some fusional vergence ranges, particularly in exotropic cases that are intermittent. Where the exo deviation is small or moderate in the primary position, vision training has great value. However, in cases of large exo deviations with V-patterns, surgery may be necessary. Otherwise, when the person looks up to the sky or ceiling where there are minimal environmental contours to stimulate fusion, the exo deviation will likely be manifest.

MICROTROPIA

The definition of microtropia is disputed. Clinicians disagree on its characteristics. The terms microstrabismus, monofixation pattern (or syndrome), and subnormal binocular vision all refer to the same or similar conditions. Microtropia is our term of choice for the condition with the characteristics described in the following section.

Characteristics

We believe that manifest deviations must be 1^Δ or greater in magnitude to be classified as strabismus. A fixation disparity, however, is much less in magnitude, usually not exceeding 20 minutes of arc. (Refer to discussion of fixation disparity in Chapter 3.) Microtropia has been erroneously described, in our opinion, by some clinicians as an "unusually large fixation disparity." We prefer to use the term microtropia to describe a frequently seen condition that has most of the following characteristics shown in Table 7-5. There is a manifest deviation on the unilateral cover test from 1^Δ to about 8^Δ or 9^Δ. This angle may show some variability in magnitude. Besides the manifest deviation, there is often a latent deviation (a "phoric" component) seen on the alternate cover test. On the alternate cover test, one eye or the other is always being occluded which reveals the fusion free deviation. Clinically, the results of the unilateral cover are compared with the alternate cover tests. A larger magnitude is frequently seen on the alternate cover test indicating a "phoric" component to the strabismus. These microtropic patients usually show foveal suppression of the deviated eye. Nevertheless, fusional vergence ranges can be measured and are sometimes almost normally sufficient. Usually, but not necessarily, there is ARC that is harmonious relative to the strabismic component of the deviation. Similarly, there may or may not be amblyopia. Peripheral stereopsis is often present but central stereopsis is absent or greatly reduced, especially with random dot targets.

There are two major types of microtropia, primary and secondary. Primary microtropia is indicated if there is no prior history of a larger angle of strabismus. Etiology of this condition is unknown, but like primary comitant esotropia, there appears to be some genetic basis. Secondary microtropia is often the result of vision therapy and/or surgery for a larger angle of strabismus, particularly in cases of early onset. Other secondary causes may be aniseikonia, anisometropia, uncorrected vertical deviations, and foveal lesions.

Lang[36] reported that most cases are microesotropes, but there are exceptional cases of microhypertropia that usually result from surgical intervention of a large angle hypertropia.

TABLE 7-5. *Characteristics of Microtropia*	
Mechanism	Unknown, often secondary to surgery or vision training for an infantile or primary comitant esotropia.
Onset	From birth or the time of therapeutic intervention
Refractive	Probably no relationship
Deviation	1^Δ to 9^Δ strabismic component, usually has an additional phoric component. Eso deviations much more common than exo or hyper.
Constancy	Usually constant in all fields of gaze and fixation distances.
Comitancy	Usually comitant
Correspondence	Usually ARC relative to the strabismic component
Fusion	Peripheral fusion with some vergence ranges, some stereopsis, central suppression of the deviating eye
Amblyopia	Shallow amblyopia frequently present
Symptoms	Usually none
Prognosis	Poor for bifoveal fusion, usually a stable end-stage condition

Secondary microtropia is much more prevalent than primary microtropia.

There are specialized tests that help identify microtropia. The *unilateral neutralization* test gives a direct measure of the manifest deviation seen on the unilateral cover test. When there is a phoric component, the alternate cover test is no longer useful in measuring magnitude of the strabismic component. To measure this horizontal angle of strabismus objectively, the examiner must simultaneously occlude the dominant eye and place the correct amount of base-out prism before the deviated eye to neutralize any movement of the esotropic eye. Take, for example, a micro-esotropia of the right eye. The patient is instructed to look at a straight-ahead target while the clinician occludes the left eye. A

small outward movement of the right eye is observed and estimated to be 5^Δ. To measure this deviation, the doctor must simultaneously occlude the left eye and place the correct magnitude of base-out prism before the right eye to neutralize any movement of that eye (Figure 7-6). If 5^Δ base-out is placed before the right eye and there is no movement of that eye when the left is covered, then 5^Δ is the *measured magnitude*. If there is eccentric fixation, that must be taken into consideration to calculate the *true* strabismic deviation. (Refer to discussion in Chapter 4.)

Another useful test for determining the clinical characteristics of a microtropia is the *Bagolini striated lens test*. A transluminator light (or a penlight) is the fixation target. The typical response of a microtropic patient on this test is the report of the two lines crossing at the light but a small gap is seen in the line clued to the strabismic eye. The microtropic angle of deviation can be directly observed by using the unilateral cover test to verify the deviation. Perception of intersecting lines at the light suggests HARC, i.e., an angle *S* of zero in the presence of a strabismus. A gap in the line seen by the deviating eye indicates central suppression. HARC and deep central suppression are frequently seen in cases of microtropia. If there is any amblyopia, visuoscopy must be done to check for the presence and magnitude of eccentric fixation, since this can influence the interpretation of the cover test.

Management

Microtropia in adults does not generally require vision therapy. These patients are usually symptom free, with no cosmetic problems. In addition, they usually have rudimentary binocular vision with fairly good fusional vergence ranges and peripheral stereopsis (but not central). A small portion of adult microtropic patients, however, do have asthenopic symptoms related to the use of their eyes. Like the heterophoric patient having inadequate fusional vergence for visual comfort and efficiency, microtropic patients can also have inadequate vergence and accommodative skills for their visual requirements at school, work,

a.

b.

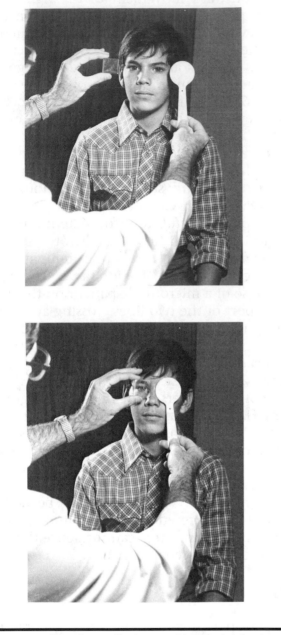

FIGURE 7-6—Unilateral neutralization test: (a) Preparing for the unilateral cover test for neutralization of an esotropic right eye with base-out prism; (b) Simultaneously covering the left eye with an occluder and the right eye with base-out prism. The prism power that equals the esotropic angle of the right eye neutralizes the angle of deviation so that eye movement does not occur.

and play. Prisms and added lenses do not seem to help in these symptomatic cases due, possibly, to prism adaptation. We have trained the visual skills of many of these patients, often with good results. Vergence ranges increased almost to normal levels; stereopsis increased slightly; and visual symptoms disappeared after a relatively short office and home training program, from 6 to 10 weeks in length. The microtropia still appeared on the unilateral cover test, but most patients were pleased with the outcome. Unfortunately, we have also seen some symptomatic microtropia cases where no form of vision therapy intervention relieved the symptoms. These patients had to avoid those visual activities that exacerbate the symptoms, which, in some cases, required a change in employment. In most symptomatic microtropic cases, we recommend vision training similar to that given in cases of heterophoria.

Some clinicians report curing microtropia in early childhood. Von Noorden[37] discussed three patients under age 5 years who had microtropia, anisometropia, and shallow amblyopia. These patients wore spectacle lenses for the anisometropia and the dominant eye was patched. The results included elimination of the microtropia, 20/20 (6/6) vision in each eye, and stereoacuity of 40 seconds of arc. It is possible that these patients were not actually microtropic but instead had anisometropic amblyopia with eccentric fixation (which von Noorden noted) in which the movement on the unilateral cover test reflected the eccentric fixation. Nevertheless, it seems prudent to treat any young patient with amblyopia, whether or not there is an associated microtropia, with patching and optical correction when required. Apparent spontaneous remission of microtropia in young children may be possible.[38]

CYCLOVERTICAL DEVIATIONS

Cyclovertical deviations involve either the oblique muscles or the vertical recti muscles. Vertically acting muscles have both vertical and cyclorotary actions in most positions of gaze. Therefore, innervational or mechanical abnormalities of these muscles usually results in both a vertical and a cyclo deviation. Hyper deviations are also prevalent among patients with horizontal strabismus; about 40% of all esotropes have a small vertical component.[39] Although vertical deviations are frequently found in combination with horizontal strabismus, they can occur as isolated abnormalities. Since vertical fusional vergence is relatively weak compared with fusional convergence or divergence, a small vertical deviation, of even 1^Δ or 2^Δ may cause disturbing symptoms of diplopia, intermittent blur, eyestrain, and nausea. Moreover, a small vertical component can be the primary obstacle to fusion in some cases of horizontal strabismus. Most cyclovertical deviations are noncomitant (see Chapters 8 and 15). The following discussion in this section, however, pertains to comitant vertical deviations.

Comitant Vertical Deviations

Isolated comitant vertical deviations greater than 10^Δ are rare. On the other hand, small comitant hyper deviations, as isolated conditions or associated with moderate or large angle horizontal deviations, are common. Large angles of vertical deviation (greater than 10^Δ) almost always show signs of noncomitancy, including those with paretic etiology and a subsequent "spread of comitancy." Amblyopia and ARC are less often associated with vertical deviations than with horizontal strabismus. The etiology of comitant vertical deviations presumably includes anatomic factors and abnormal innervation (Table 7-6).

The obvious conservative treatment for a comitant vertical deviation, either heterophoria or strabismus, is the prescription of vertical prism. Comitant vertical deviations 10^Δ or less can usually be successfully managed with spectacle prisms if the prism amount is split between the eyes and the frame does not have a large vertical dimension. Vertical prism corrections greater than 10^Δ may result in cosmetic problems due to the optical displacement of the eyes. Vision training is a second choice as a treatment option to increase vertical fusional ranges. However, vision training is often used in conjunction with prism therapy to help relieve symptoms.

Cosmetic hypertropia (and hypotropia) greater than 10^Δ often requires surgical manage-

TABLE 7-6. Characteristics of Comitant Vertical Deviations

Mechanism	Innervational, anatomical
Onset	From birth to about 3 years
Refractive	Probably no relationship
Deviation	Usually small angles 1^Δ to 10^Δ; often associated with moderate to large horizontal strabismus, eso or exo
Constancy	Can be intermittent or constant depending on magnitude and fusional status
Comitancy	Comitant; may be secondary to a spread of comitancy after a noncomitant deviation.
Correspondence	Often ARC if associated with a constant horizontal deviation; ARC less prevalent than in pure horizontal deviations
Amblyopia	Less than in horizontal strabismus
Symptoms	More often than in horizontal strabismus
Prognosis	Poor if ARC; good if NRC

ment. In patients with a combined horizontal and vertical strabismus, with the vertical component less than 12^Δ, surgical correction of the vertical deviation can often be accomplished by a vertical transposition (vertical offset) of the horizontal muscles. To correct a hyper deviation, for example, the insertions of the horizontal recti of the higher eye are lowered. This procedure is done in addition to the appropriate recession or resection procedure for the horizontal deviation. To correct for a hypotropia, the horizontal muscle insertions of the lower eye would be raised. Dale reported the correction is anywhere between 0.5^Δ and 1.0^Δ for each millimeter of offset surgery.[40] For vertical deviations of 12^Δ or greater, it is usually necessary to recess the appropriate vertical muscles. For example, if the patient has a comitant right hypertropia of 25^Δ, the superior rectus in the right eye and the inferior rectus in the left eye should each be recessed to obtain the best possible comitant result.

Dissociated Vertical Deviations (DVD)

These *double hyper* deviations are frequently, but not always, associated with infantile esotropia. (Refer to the discussion on DVD in this chapter under infantile esotropia.)

SENSORY STRABISMUS

A blind eye usually becomes a turned eye. When sensory fusion is lost, strabismus usually results. Severely reduced visual acuity in one or both eyes can be an insurmountable obstacle to sensory fusion. When the primary cause of a strabismus is loss of vision, then the term *sensory strabismus* is used to describe the condition. The causes of sensory strabismus are therefore as varied as the causes of blindness or severe low vision. Some of the common causes in early childhood include ocular trauma, congenital cataracts, optic atrophy or hypoplasia, congenital ptosis, and high anisometropia. The second most common presenting sign of retinoblastoma in infancy is, in fact, esotropia.[41] Sensory strabismus is usually comitant, but if the condition is of long standing, secondary contractures can occur causing restriction of the horizontal movements of the affected eye. When a patient presents with strabismus and reduced visual acuity in one eye, it is important to establish which condition preceded the other. If a strabismus is secondary to the acuity loss, sensory strabismus may be present? On the other hand, the acuity loss may be due to stabismic amblyopia, which has a good prognosis for recovery if early patching and vigorous therapy are initiated.

The direction of eye-turn in sensory strabismus appears to relate to the age of onset. In a series of 121 sensory strabismus cases, Sidkaro and von Noorden[42] observed that esotropia and exotropia were about equally distributed if the onset was within the first five years of life. However, if the sensory obstacle occurred later than age 5 years, exotropia predominated by a large margin. This is consistent with our clinical observations that if vision is lost in adulthood, an exotropia usually occurs, rather than esotropia. It is not clear why some patients become esotropic and others exotropic. Chavasse[43] speculated that there are various degrees of tonic convergence during early childhood resulting in either esotropia or exotropia, but during adulthood there may be less forceful tonic convergence, in which case exotropia would predominate.

In many cases of sensory strabismus, the very nature of the condition (e.g., optic atrophy) precludes the restoration of binocular vision. In some cases of congenital cataract or ptosis, early surgery and proper optical correction may offer some hope of recovering part or all of the visual loss. In most cases of sensory strabismus, however, therapy is directed toward improving the cosmetic aspects of the eye-turn. If the deviation is relatively small, spectacle prisms may be used to correct the appearance of the strabismus (as described in Chapter 6). For larger deviations, cosmetic extraocular surgery is usually advisable. The psychological consequences of having a conspicuous, unsightly, turned eye is usually worthwhile preventing, particularly for school aged children. The standard operation is a recession and resection procedure of the appropriate horizontal eye muscles of the deviated eye.[44] Surgical results in sensory strabismus are often unpredictable, but adjustable sutures provide a means of making postoperative corrections. Long-term surgical results are often not as stable as in cases where some form of binocular vision exists. The original deviation, or even a consecutive strabismus, can be the result over the years, requiring further operations to maintain acceptable cosmesis. The patient or parents need to be informed of this possibility.

CONSECUTIVE STRABISMUS

Consecutive strabismus refers to an eye-turn that changes from one direction to the opposite direction, e.g., when an exotropia becomes an esotropia following surgery. There are very few spontaneous cases reported that are independent of a specific event, such as eye surgery or ocular trauma. Consecutive esotropia occurs almost exclusively after surgical overcorrection of an exotropia.

A common surgical goal in management of exotropia is to leave the deviation slightly on the eso side of alignment, approximately 10^Δ eso, since there is a tendency for the eyes to diverge during the healing process. Occasionally, the overcorrection is excessive and a cosmetic esotropia is evident. When this occurs, these patients often complain of post-surgical diplopia. The reported prevalence of surgical overcorrections for exotropia varies, according to different authors, from 6% to 20%.[45,46] The immediate therapy for small angles of consecutive esotropia is simply to wait and see if the deviation resolves with the healing process. Many small overcorrections disappear with time, but larger deviations tend to increase. A large overcorrection with limitation of ocular motility on the day after surgery may require further immediate surgical management.[47] In most cases of overcorrection, another operation should not be performed until after 6 months, unless there is a significant degree of noncomitancy. Attempts to eliminate diplopia can be made with compensating Fresnel prisms or spectacle overcorrection using plus fogging lenses over the deviating eye.

The prevalence of consecutive exotropia is lower than consecutive esotropia, ranging from only 2% to 8% depending on the investigator.[48] Consecutive exotropia can arise spontaneously, although most are surgically induced. As a rule, consecutive exotropia decreases with time. Therefore, a wait and see policy is appropriate unless the deviation is extreme or complicated with a marked reduction of ocular motility. Six months is a reasonable waiting period. Attempts to align the eyes and eliminate diplopia with base-in prisms or minus lens overcorrection may prove beneficial. In cases where the AC/A is moderate to high, we suggest prescribing between 2 D and 4 D of minus lens overcorrection for young patients as a temporary (although periodic) measure to straighten the eyes. In cases where lens overcorrection is indicated, we also recommend accommodative facility training to prevent asthenopia.

REFERENCES

1. Parks MM. Abnormal accommodative convergence in squint. *Arch Ophthalmol.* 1958;59:364-380.
2. Dale RT. *Fundamentals of Ocular Motility and Strabismus.* New York: Grune & Stratton; 1982:193
3. Calcutt C. Contact lenses in accommodative esotropia therapy. *British Orthop J.* 1989;46:59-65.
4. Grisham JD, Gee C, Brott H, Burger D. Evaluation of bifocal contact lenses in the control of accommodative esotropia. OD Thesis, University of California School of Optometry, Library, 1992.
5. Ludwig IH, Parks MM, Getson PR, Kammerman LA. Rate of deterioration in accommodative esotropia correlated to the AC/A relationship. *J Ped Ophthalmol Strab.* 1988;25:8-12.
6. Amos DM. Pharmacologic management of strabismus. In: Bartlett JD, Jaanus SD, eds. *Clinical Ocular Pharmacology.* 2nd ed. Newton, Mass.: Butterworth-Heinemann; 1989:729.
7. Mein J, Trimble R. *Diagnosis and Management of Ocular Motility Disorders.* 2nd ed. London: Blackwell Scientific Publications; 1991:221.
8. Pratt-Johnson JA, Tillson G. The management of esotropia with high AC/A ratio. *J Pedriatric Ophthalmol Strab.* 1985; 22: 238-242.
9. Nixon RB, Helveston EM, Miller K, Archer SM, Ellis FD. Incidence of strabismus in neonates. *Am J Ophthalmol.* 1985; 100:798-801.
10. Friedrich D, deDecker W. Prospective study of the development of strabismus during the first 6 months of life. In: Lenk-Schafer M, ed. *Orthoptic Horizons: trans of the Sixth Intern Orthoptic Congress.* Harrogate (UK): 1987:LIPS 21.
11. Von Noorden GK, *Binocular Vision and Ocular Motility.* 4th ed. St. Louis: CV Mosby Co; 1990:293-294.
12. Costenbader FD, Infantile esotropia. *Trans Am Ophthal Soc.* 1961;59:397-429.
13. Ingram RM, Barr A. Changes in refraction between the ages of 1 and 3 1/2 years. *Br J Ophthalmol.* 1979; 63:339-342.
14. Von Noorden GK. Infantile esotropia: a continuing riddle. *Am Orthop J.* 1984 34:52-62.
15. Costenbader FD. Infantile esotropia. *Trans Am Ophthalmol Soc.* 1961;59:397-429.
16. Von Noorden GK. A reassessment of infantile esotropia, *Am J Ophthalmol.* 1988;105:1-10.
17. Lang J. Der kongenitale oder fruhkindliche strabismus. *Ophthalmologica.* 1967;154:201-208
18. Taylor DM. Congenital Esotropia. *Management and prognosis.* New York: Intercontinental Medical Book Corp; 1973.
19. Von Noorden GK, *Binocular Vision and Ocular Motility.* 4th ed. St Louis: CV Mosby Co; 1990, 301-305.
20. Williams AS, Hoyt CS. Acute comitant esotropia in children with brain tumors. *Arch Ophthamol.* 1989;107:376-378.
21. Lang J. Normosensorial late convergent strabismus. In: Campos E, ed. Transactions of the Fifth Meeting of the International Strabismological Association. St. Louis: CV Mosby Co; 1986: 536.
22. Graham PA. Epidemiology of strabismus. *Br J Ophthalmol.* 1974, 58:224-231.

23. Krzystkowa K, Pajakowa J. The sensorial state in divergent strabismus. In: Orthoptics, Proceedings of the Second International Orthoptics Congress. Amsterdam: Excerpta Medica Foundation, 1972:72.

24. Jampolsky A. Ocular deviations. *Int Ophthalmol Clin.* 1964;4:567-569.

25. Costenbader FD. The physiology and management of divergent strabismus. In: Allen JH, ed. *Strabismic Ophthalmic Symposium I.* St Louis: CV Mosby Co; 1950:353.

26. Gregersen E. The polymorphous exo patient. Analysis of 231 consecutive cases. *Acta Ophthalmol.* 1969;47:579-590.

27. Burian HM. Pathophysiology of exodeviations. In: Manley DR, ed. *Symposium on Horizontal Ocular Deviations.* St Louis: CV Mosby Co; 1971:119.

28. Wirtschafter JD, von Noorden GK. The effect of increasing luminance on exodeviations. *Invest Ophthalmol.* 1964;3:549-352.

29. Burian HM, Smith DR. Comparative measurement of exodeviations at twenty and one hundred feet. *Trans Am Ophthalmol Society.* 1971:69:188-192.

30. Scobee RG. *The Oculorotary Muscles.* 2nd ed. St Louis: CV Mosby Co; 1952:172.

31. Von Noorden GK. *Binocular Vision and Ocular Motility.* 4th ed. St Louis: CV Mosby Co; 1990:326.

32. Pratt-Johnson JA. Tillson G. *Management of Strabismus and Amblyopia: A Practical Guide.* New York: Thieme Medical Publishers, 1994:140-141.

33. Costenbader FD. Introduction. Symposium: the A and V patterns in strabismus. *Trans Am Acad Ophthalmol Otolaryngol.* 1964;68:354-374.

34. Breinin G. The physiopathology of the A and V patterns. Symposium: the A and V patterns in strabismus. *Trans Am Acad Ophthalmol Otolaryngol.* 1964;68:363.

35. Mein J, Trimble R. *Diagnosis and Management of Ocular Motility Disorders.* 2nd ed. Oxford: Blackwell Scientific; 1991:275-276.

36. Lang J. Lessons learned from microtropia. In: Moore S, Mein J, Stockbridge L, eds. *Orthoptics, Past, Present and Future.* Miami, Symposia Specialists; 1976: 183-190.

37. Von Noorden GK. *Binocular Vision and Ocular Motility.* 4th ed. St Louis: CV Mosby Co; 1990:313.

38. Keiner EC. Spontaneous recovery in microstrabismus. *Ophthalmologica.* 1978;177:280-283.

39. Scobee RG. Esotropia: incidence, etiology and results of therapy. *Am J Ophthalmol.* 1951;34:817-833.

40. Dale RT. *Fundamentals of Ocular Motility and Strabismus.* New York: Grune & Stratton; 1982:238.

41. Ellsworth RM. The practical management of retinoblastoma. *Trans Am Ophthalmol Soc.* 1969;78: 462-534.

42. Sidikaro Y, von Noorden GK. Observation in sensory heterotropia. *J Pediatr Ophthalmol Strabis.* 1982;19:12.

43. Chavasse FB. *Worth's Squint or the Binocular Reflexes and the Treatment of Strabismus.* 7th ed. London: Bailliere, Tindall, and Cox; 1931:519.

44. Von Noorden GK. *Binocular Vision and Ocular Motility.* 4th ed. St. Louis: CV Mosby Co; 1990:315.

45. Hardesty HH, Boynton JR, Keenan JP. Treatment of intermittent exotropia. *Arch Ophthalmol.* 1978;96: 268-274.

46. Dunlap EA. Overcorrections in horizontal strabismus surgery. In: *Symposium on Strabismus. Transaction of the New Orleans Academy of Ophthalmology.* St. Louis: CV Mosby Co; 1971:255.

47. Von Noorden GK. *Binocular Vision and Ocular Motility.* 4th ed. CV Mosby Co; 1990:335.

48. Von Noorden GK. *Binocular Vision and Ocular Motility.* 4th ed. St. Louis: CV Mosby Co; 1990:317

Chapter 8 / Other Oculomotor Disorders

Neurogenic Palsies   233
    General Considerations   233
    Sixth Cranial Nerve (Abducens)
        Palsy   235
    Mobius Syndrome   235
    Fourth Cranial Nerve (Trochlear)
        Palsy   235
    Third Cranial Nerve (Oculomotor)
        Palsy   236
Myogenic Palsies   238
    Myasthenia Gravis   238
    Dysthyroid Eye Disease   239
    Chronic Progressive External
        Ophthalmoplegia (CPEO)   241
Mechanical Restrictions of Ocular
    Movement   241
    Duane Retraction Syndrome   241
    Brown (Superior Oblique Tendon
        Sheath) Syndrome   242
    Fibrosis of the Extraocular Muscles   243
    Adherence Syndromes   244

Orbital Anomalies   244
Internuclear and Supranuclear
    Disorders   244
Internuclear Ophthalmoplegia
    (INO)   245
Supranuclear Horizontal Gaze Palsy   246
    Frontal Eye-Field Lesions   246
    Occipital and Parietal Cortical
        Lesions   246
    Brainstem Lesions   246
Supranuclear Vertical Gaze Palsy   246
    Parinaud Syndrome   247
    Progressive Supranuclear Palsy   247
    Parkinson's Disease   248
Nystagmus   248
    Physiologic Nystagmus   249
    Voluntary Nystagmus   249
    Congenital Nystagmus   250
    Nystagmus Blockage Syndrome   252
    Latent Nystagmus   256
    Rare Types of Nystagmus   256

Neurological and muscular diseases affecting efficiency of binocular vision are discussed in terms of clinical diagnosis and management

NEUROGENIC PALSIES

General Considerations

Noncomitant strabismus is considered neurogenic palsy if it results from damage to one or more of the three cranial nerves subserving ocular motility. In the global sense, palsy refers to either a paresis or paralysis. If the nerve damage is complete and no innervation flows to the affected eye muscle, the strabismus is said to be *paralytic*. If disruption of innervation is partial, as is often the case, the term *paretic* is used. Paresis can be of any degree, from mild to severe, depending on the extent of the muscle's dysfunction. In cases of recent paresis or paralysis, the angle of deviation varies in amount in different fields of gaze. Also, the deviation varies depending on which eye is fixating. The *primary deviation* refers to the magnitude of strabismus when the unaffected eye is fixating; the *secondary deviation* is measured when the affected eye is fixating. In palsy of recent onset, the secondary deviation is larger than the primary deviation due to Hering's Law of Equal Innervation (discussion in Chapter 4).

Some of many possible causes of neurogenic palsies that result in strabismus are: direct trauma to the oculomotor nucleus or anywhere along the course of the nerve, inflammations, myasthenia gravis, multiple sclerosis, brain stem or neuronal tumors, and vascular disorders (e.g., aneurysms, hypertension, atherosclerosis, bleeding from diabetes). Table 8-1 lists the frequency of etiologic factors found by Rush and Younge.[1] The recent onset of diplopia associated with noncomitant strabismus at any age is a harbinger of active disease or injury. When this occurs, careful medical evaluation and management are indicated.

Patients with paretic strabismus often adopt an abnormal head posture, allowing them to maintain fusion in the least affected field of gaze. The head is usually turned in the direction of the action field of the affected muscle. (Refer to discussion in Chapter 4.) Some patients with noncomitant neurogenic strabismus turn their heads in the opposite direction to that expected to increase the separation of the diplopic images so that one of the images may be more easily suppressed or ignored. The same strategy may apply when some patients choose to fixate with the affected eye. The larger secondary deviation has increased separation of the double images.

Congenital torticollis of the head can arise from a structural deformity of the cervical vertebrae or the sternocleidomastoid muscle. This rare condition is easily differentiated from ocular torticollis (caused by extraocular muscle

TABLE 8-2. *Differential Diagnosis of Paretic Strabismus and Developmental Strabismus*

	Paretic Strabismus	Developmental Strabismus
Mode on Onset	Usually sudden	Usually gradual or shortly after birth
Age of Onset	Any age	Between birth and about age 6 years
Diplopia	Common	Uncommon
Comitancy	Noncomitant, but can become comitant with time	Comitant; A or V pattern may be present
Head Posture	Usually abnormal	Usually normal
Amblyopia	Rare, only if early onset	Common
Correspondence	Usually NRC	ARC common
Trauma, Neurologic or Systemic Disease	Common	Uncommon

palsy) by direct questioning of the patient or parents or testing for a restricted range of head movement.

Recent diplopia, noncomitancy, and abnormal head posture are clinical features that distinguish acquired neurogenic palsy from developmental comitant strabismus. Table 8-2 lists differential diagnostic features.

In paretic strabismus, it is important to distinguish between a strabismus of recent origin, possibly due to active pathology, and a benign noncomitant deviation of long duration. Clinical features more commonly associated with deviations of recent origin are disturbing symptoms (e.g., diplopia, nausea, vertigo) and signs of abnormal head posture. These problems diminish or disappear when an eye is occluded. The later the onset of the deviation, the more likely is the complaint of diplopia.

In congenital or old cases of paretic strabismus, the clinician may find suppression, muscle contractures, and abnormal head posture.

TABLE 8-1. *Etiological Frequency of Oculomotor Palsy[1] (shown in percentages)*

Causes	N VI	N IV	N III
Vascular	18	19	21
Head trauma	17	32	15
Other known causes	18	8	15
Tumors	15	4	12
Aneurysm	4	2	14
Unknown causes	27	36	23

Old childhood photographs may reveal a head tilt pattern of long-standing. In congenital cases, the pathological condition causing the deviation is usually inactive; however, if a patient reports sudden onset of diplopia, even when the deviation appears to be comitant, it is advisable to suspect active pathology until proven otherwise.

Sixth Cranial Nerve (Abducens) Palsy

The most prevalent noncomitant deviation is acquired sixth nerve paresis. Congenital sixth nerve palsy is rare and the cause is often difficult to determine. Perinatal trauma is one possible cause. The causes of acquired sixth nerve palsy are numerous. In older patients, the cause is often vascular in nature (e.g., ischemic infarction). In patients under age 40, one frequent cause is multiple sclerosis. When a vascular lesion is in the brain stem, the damage usually involves other nuclear centers as well, with obvious clinical manifestations such as facial hemiplegia (damage to the fifth or seventh nucleus). Frequent causes are closed head trauma or a blow to the side of the head where the sixth nerve is particularly vulnerable.

If a sixth nerve palsy occurs during visual immaturity, suppression, amblyopia, or even ARC can develop. In older patients, diplopia is usually reported. The deviation and diplopia increases in the field of gaze of the involved lateral rectus. A compensatory head turn is made in the direction of the action field of the affected eye. If the paresis is severe, the duction (monocular) may be limited in the involved field of gaze and, generally, an abnormal version (binocular) movement is even more noticeable (because of increasing magnitude of the deviation) than the abnormal monocular duction. Management of noncomitancy is discussed in Chapter 15.

Mobius Syndrome

One special condition involving bilateral sixth nerve palsy is Mobius syndrome. This congenital condition was once thought to be caused by a bilateral palsy of the abducens (VI) and facial (VII) nerves since patients were found to have an esotropia (a bilateral inability to abduct the eyes) and a bilateral facial palsy (facial diplegia). Glaser[2], however, noted that the etiology is usually much more complex, and little understood, because of the many other associated conditions. Besides limited abduction and facial palsy, these children are found to have variable disorders in several body systems including an almost total lack of facial musculature; decreased bulk (atrophy) of one side of the tongue; mild to moderate mental retardation; congenital heart defects; limb and chest deformities; hearing, speech, and swallowing difficulties; and other manifestations.[3]

Ocular treatment usually involves correcting any significant refractive error and giving vision therapy for amblyopia if present. These patients should be encouraged to adopt a crossed-fixation pattern, if they have not already done so, since abduction is limited. Surgical correction of the esotropia in the primary position might be attempted, but the results are frequently unsatisfactory.

Fourth Cranial Nerve (Trochlear) Palsy

The fourth cranial nerves emerge dorsally from the medullary velum and quickly decussate. This anatomical relationship, places these nerves in a vulnerable position. Traumatic closed-head injury from a frontal blow is one of the main causes of superior oblique palsy, unilateral or bilateral. Even minor head injuries can result in nerve damage. The causes of fourth nerve palsies are numerous. Frequently the etiology is vascular. The nutrient vessels to the nerve, the vasa nervorum, can be occluded causing an ischemic infarction and death of the nerve. Damage can also occur when blood leaks from vessels as a result of diabetes. In cases of unexplained nerve involvement, a glucose tolerance test is appropriate. Herpes zoster is another potential etiologic factor.

The most prominent sign of a recent superior oblique palsy is a hypertropia in the primary position that increases in downgaze and with convergence. Also in primary position, there is an excyclodeviation and often a small eso deviation. In the case of weakness of the left superior oblique, for example, the compensatory head turn would be a right head tilt, a right face turn, and chin depression. (Refer to the discussion on abnormal head posture in Chapter 4.) Even if spread of comitancy, a positive Bielschowsky head-tilt test, in which the left hypertropia increases on left head tilt, is an indication that the underlying disorder is an underacting left superior oblique muscle, possibly due to a left fourth nerve palsy.

Patients with a fourth nerve palsy who choose to fixate with the paretic eye demonstrate the *falling eye* syndrome (more correctly sign). When the patient fixates with the affected eye particularly in adduction, excessive innervation to the superior oblique is necessary to maintain fixation. Because of Hering's Law, the yoked contralateral inferior rectus overacts, making that eye appear to "drop."

Von Noorden et al.[4] reported that 21% of traumatic fourth nerve palsies in a large clinical series were bilateral. Other authors have reported even higher proportions of bilateral superior oblique involvement.[5] Severity of the paresis is often asymmetric (one eye higher than the other) which can mask the bilateral nature of the condition. One distinguishing feature of bilateral involvement is finding a right hypertropia on left gaze and left hypertropia on right gaze. Another differential observation is a positive Bielschowsky head-tilt test on either right or left tilt. For example, in a case of bilateral involvement in which the patient presents with a right hypertropia in the primary position, the right hypertropia increases on right tilt; on left tilt, a left hypertropia manifests and increases. Another diagnostic indication of bilateral trochlear palsy—a particularly sensitive one—is the patient's observation of a double excyclo tilt on a double Maddox rod test.

Third Cranial Nerve (Oculomotor) Palsy

Fortunately, congenital third nerve palsies are rare. The full syndrome includes: (1) exotropia due to medial rectus involvement; (2) hypo-tropia due to weakness of the superior rectus and inferior oblique; (3) limited depression in abduction due to inferior rectus weakness; (4) ptosis of the affected eye due to levator involvement; and (5) possible dilation and fixed pupil that does not react to direct or consensual light stimulation. If the fourth and sixth cranial nerves are uninvolved, the affected eye can be seen to abduct and intort with attempted depression (Table 8-3).

In cases of congenital third nerve palsy, there is often aberrant regeneration of the nerve (the so-called *misdirection syndrome*). Aberrant regeneration can consist of any of several features, all of which are not necessarily present in a given patient:[6]

1. Pseudo-Graefe sign—elevation of the upper lid on attempted downgaze.
2. Widening of the lids on adduction and narrowing on abduction.
3. A dilated, fixed pupil that does not react to direct or consensual light stimulation but that does react slightly on convergence or on adduction. This has been called the pseudo-Argyll Robertson pupil.
4. Retraction and adduction of the eye on attempted upgaze.

TABLE 8-3. *Features of Oculomotor Palsy (N III)*

1. Exotropia due to involvement of the medial rectus.
2. Hypotropia due to involvement of the superior rectus and inferior oblique.
3. Ptosis due to involvement of levator palpebrae.
4. Limited depression in abduction due to involvement of the inferior rectus.
5. Chin elevation in bilateral cases due to limited elevation and bilateral ptosis.
6. In some cases, dilated fixed pupil of the affected eye(s). These cases are referred to as internal ophthalmoplegia. Cases in which the pupils are normal are called external ophthalmoplegia.
7. Aberrant regeneration of the N III in congenital cases can cause several unusual effects: Jaw-wink reflex, widening of lids on depression, and retraction of eye on attempted elevation.

Aberrant regeneration is thought to be due to axional regrowth after a compression injury to the third nerve, such that may occur during childbirth. New axons that are misdirected innervate inappropriate muscles, resulting in the paradoxical ocular movements and pupillary reactions characteristic of this syndrome.

Acquired third nerve palsy is a fairly common neurologic condition. Depending on the site of the lesion, the entire nerve (resulting in the characteristic signs described above under congenital third nerve palsy) or only a particular division or isolated root of the nerve can be damaged. Isolated palsies of various extraocular muscles supplied by the third cranial nerve occur less commonly than a more generalized condition. Any degree of paresis can be present. Deficiencies in elevation, depression and adduction, along with ptosis, occur in various combinations with or without pupillary involvement. When there is extraocular muscle weakness along with pupillary involvement, the condition is called *internal ophthalmoplegia. External ophthalmoplegia* is, however, indicated when extraocular muscle weakness exists without pupillary involvement.

Isolated superior rectus palsy is usually congenital. When the uninvolved eye fixates in the primary position, a hypotropia of the affected eye is seen. The hypotropic deviation increases maximally when the patient moves the affected eye into the field of action of the superior rectus, the superior temporal field. Since most cases are congenital, the patients do not usually complain of symptoms. The recommended surgical procedure for an isolated superior rectus palsy consists of an appropriate amount of inferior rectus recession and superior rectus resection in the involved eye. A 4 mm recession of the inferior rectus, by itself, may give up to 15^{Δ} of vertical correction in the primary position.[7] A recess-resect operation of the same amount may provide as much as 40^{Δ} of vertical correction.

Isolated medial rectus, inferior rectus, and inferior oblique muscle palsies are extremely rare. These three muscles are all innervated by the inferior division of the third nerve so damage to that root tends to involve all three. However, isolated palsies do occur occasionally

for inexplicable reasons. In isolated medial rectus palsy, a noncomitant exotropia is seen along with limited adduction. The corrective surgical procedure is usually a recess-resect operation of the horizontal muscles in the affected eye. The extremely rare isolated inferior rectus palsy can be congenital or acquired. When it is acquired, the cause is usually head trauma, e.g., a blow-out fracture to the orbital floor. In the primary position, a hypertropia of the affected eye is found. An incyclo deviation of the involved eye is expected. If there is no restriction of the superior rectus as revealed by the forced duction test, a small hypertropia can usually be corrected surgically by a resection of the affected inferior rectus. However, if a superior rectus restriction is found, it must be recessed as well. In large deviations, a combined recession of the superior rectus and a resection of the inferior rectus can correct up to 40^{Δ} of vertical deviation in the primary position.

An isolated inferior oblique palsy is also extremely rare and can be either congenital or acquired. A hypotropia and incyclotropia is seen if the patient fixates with the nonparetic eye. The vertical deviation in the primary position, however, is generally not as large as in cases of isolated superior rectus or superior oblique palsy. If the patient chooses to fixate with the paretic eye (as in some acquired conditions where the paretic eye has been the dominant sighting eye), a hypertropia of the noninvolved eye is found. As the patient moves the paretic eye into adduction, the contralateral hypertropia increases greatly. This observation is called the *rising eye* syndrome (more correctly sign). A recommended surgical procedure for an isolated inferior oblique palsy is to recess the contralateral superior rectus and resect the contralateral inferior rectus. This procedure gives greater comitancy when the paretic eye is adducted.

Double elevator palsy can be either congenital or acquired. All patients described as having double elevator palsy must demonstrate an inability to elevate the affected eye from any horizontal position—primary, adduction, or abduction. Some patients present with a chin elevation indicating that they can fuse in downgaze. Visual acuity is usually good in each eye. Patients often report diplopia with fixation in the primary position. Other congenital cases show a hypotropia of the affected eye, a pseudoptosis due to the hypotropia, and deep amblyopia.

At one time double elevator palsy was thought to be caused by weakness of both the superior rectus and inferior oblique of the affected eye, but the anatomy of the third nerve casts doubt on this explanation. Within the third nerve nucleus complex, innervation for these two muscles arises from disparate locations. Since the superior rectus is innervated by the superior division of the nerve and the inferior oblique by the inferior division, it is difficult to explain the neurological basis for double elevator palsy. One possible explanation is that the initial deviation is an isolated palsy of the superior rectus and, with time, there is involvement of the inferior oblique. The features that distinguish the double elevator palsy then become evident. A second explanation suggests that the condition is not a palsy at all but a restriction. In one study, three-fourths of the patients thought to have double elevator palsy were found to have restriction in upgaze on the forced duction test.[8] It appears that an apparent congenital double elevator palsy can be caused by either a weakness or a restriction.

If there truly is a weakness of elevation, the *Knapp procedure* has proven effective in correcting the hypotropia in the primary position. The medial and lateral rectus muscles of the paretic eye are transposed to a position toward the insertion of the superior rectus. If the elevation limitation is caused by a restriction, the surgical intervention is directed to releasing the restriction. The procedure in such cases often involves a recession of the inferior rectus and the inferior conjunctiva.

MYOGENIC PALSIES

Myasthenia Gravis

Myasthenia gravis is a chronic progressive disease characterized by skeletal muscle weakness and fatigue, and has a predilection for the muscles of mastication, swallowing, facial expression, and, particularly, lid and ocular motility (Table 8-4). Ptosis and diplopia often occur as the first signs of the condition, especially in adults. Ocular muscle involvement eventually occurs in 90% of all myasthenia patients and accounts for 75% of initial complaints.[9] The deviation can mimic any ocular motor palsy. In this sense, it is the "great pretender." The onset can happen at any age, but the disease usually becomes manifest between the ages of 20 and 40, affecting women more often than men. Infantile forms are rarely encountered, but the course of the condition in infants and children differs from that in adults, children showing a wider range of muscular involvement. The condition characteristically is variable, marked by periods of exacerbation and remission. Muscle function may change within minutes, hours, or weeks.[10]

Myasthenia gravis is a skeletal muscle autoimmune disorder distinguished by a reduction of the available postsynaptic acetylcholine receptor sites on the end-plates at myoneural junctions. The anti-acetylcholine receptor antibody is present in about 80% of patients with the generalized disease and in about 50% of patients with myasthenia restricted to ocular muscles.[11] Diagnosis of myasthenia gravis is based on demonstration of easy muscular fatigability and its rapid relief by systemic administration of an anticholinesterase agent such as edrophonium chloride (Tensilon).

TABLE 8-4. *Features of Myasthenia Gravis*

1. Unilateral, but usually bilateral, ptosis that is variable and subject to fatigue. Often the first sign.
2. In 90% of cases, there is an oculomotor or strabismic deviation that can mimic any single or combined muscle palsy including supra and internuclear palsies. In this sense, it is the "great pretender."
3. More frequent in females than males, particularly in ages 20 to 40 years.
4. Frequently affects the muscles of mastication, swallowing, and facial expression.

Treatment of myasthenia gravis falls within the purview of a neurologist. Systemic anticholinesterase medications are given to treat the disease, but these are rarely successful in completely controlling ptosis and diplopia. In the purely ocular form of the disease, the administration of corticosteroids (e.g., prednisone) on an alternate-day schedule has yielded remarkably good results, approaching 90% to 100%.[12] Due to the variable nature of the condition, prism therapy is usually unsuccessful; the clinician often resorts to occluding one eye to relieve diplopia. Even though myasthenia gravis may mimic any single or combined extraocular muscle palsy, including supranuclear and intranuclear ophthalmoplegia, eye muscle surgery is generally not indicated unless the deviation is stable over a long period of observation. A ptosis crutch fitted to a frame to eliminate the drooping lid or lids is occasionally beneficial. Thus, the ocular manifestations of the disease are often managed on a symptomatic basis.

Dysthyroid Eye Disease

The association of hyperthyroidism and eye disease has been known for two centuries. In 1835 Graves[13] described the eye signs of a hyperthyroid female patient in detail, particularly exophthalmos (proptosis). His name became attached to the condition when exophthalmos is present. Graves' ophthalmopathy can appear at any time during the course of hyperthyroidism with its elevated levels of thyroid hormone. Systemic symptoms include nervousness, irritability, emotional lability, sweating, palpitations, difficulty breathing, fatigue, weight loss, increased appetite, leg swelling, and increased bowel movements. Commonly associated signs are goiter (enlarged thyroid), tachycardia, skin changes with abnormal pigmentation, and tremor.[14] Thyroid eye disease in children and adolescents is uncommon; the condition occurs most commonly in females, 30 to 50 years old. The overall female-to-male ratio in systemic hyperthyroidism is 4:1; however, in thyroid eye disease, the ratio is less, approximately 2.5:1.[15] At the time of diagnosis, the eye symptoms and signs associated with hyperthyroidism occur in

20% to 40% of patients. Most patient present with the systemic symptoms. However, about 20% initially seek ophthalmologic or optometric care due to the ocular manifestations without prior identification of systemic hyperthyroidism.[16] Graves' disease is an autoimmune disorder, although its etiology and pathology are not precisely understood. The goals of laboratory studies are to demonstrate either systemic hyperthyroidism or altered immune response to thyroid-related antigens, or both. Char[17] recommended the diagnostic laboratory test for thyroidtoxicosis that determines the serum thyroid-stimulating hormone (TSH) level, which is abnormally low in this disease.

Proptosis of the eyes is a common sign associated with Graves' ophthalmopathy. Bilateral exophthalmometer readings over 22 mm or a difference between the eyes of 2 mm or more is regarded by most clinicians to be suggestive of orbital pathology. The average amount of proptosis in Graves' disease is not large, about 3 mm compared with controls.[18] There is usually some proptosis asymmetry. The lids are usually retracted in cases of Graves' disease and the sclera shows superiorly and inferiorly (i.e., Dalrymple's sign). Lid retraction associated with proptosis is so specific to Graves' disease that it is used as the primary clinical indicator of the condition. Day[19] noted this finding in 94% of his series of 200 cases. In proptosis of nonthyroid origin, patients usually do not have eyelid retraction, although exceptions do occur. Due to the lid retraction, the patient may have the appearance of staring or being startled. Infrequent and incomplete blinking often occur. On downgaze, the upper lids usually lag, exposing sclera superiorly (i.e., von Graefe sign). Exophthalmos is not always pathognomonic of thyroid eye disease. Many other conditions, (e.g., high myopia, steroid use, Cushing's syndrome) result in proptosis or a pseudoproptosis. The combination, however, of bilateral exophthalmos, lid retraction, stare, and an enlarged thyroid are virtually pathognomonic of Graves' disease.[20]

Proptosis in Graves' disease is caused by extraocular muscle enlargement. The muscles are usually enlarged 2 to 5 times their normal size due to fatty infiltrates, lymphocytes, macrophages, mast cells, and interstitial edema.[21,22] The increased muscle size is not due to the muscles fibers themselves, which histologically appear normal, but is due to inflammatory infiltrates, cells, and edema. Orbital connective tissue and extraocular muscle antibodies have been detected in the serum of patients with Graves' ophthalmopathy.[23] The immunologic mechanism of involvement is not well understood. Because of the enlarged muscles, there is a resistance to retropulsion (pressing the eye back into the orbits). The most common extraocular muscles involved in thyroid eye disease, in order of frequency, are the inferior recti (80% of patients), medial recti (44%), superior recti, and lateral recti.[24] Oblique muscles are rarely involved. Inferior rectus involvement results in a tethering of the eye, restricting movement in upgaze. In this case, the forced duction test is positive for a restrictive myopathy of elevation. Patients often complain of diplopia in upgaze and eventually, the primary position. In fact, the most common cause of spontaneous diplopia in middle-aged or older patients is Graves' disease.[25] Increased IOP can occur due to the pressure of the muscle against the eye on attempted upgaze. Some investigators believe that a 4 mm increase in IOP between inferior and superior gaze is highly suggestive of restrictive myopathy. Gamblin et al.[26] observed that all patients with long-standing thyroid exophthalmos had increased IOP and in 68% without measurable proptosis in the primary position. There is CT or ultrasound evidence for orbital involvement in almost all patients and clinical evidence of bilateral eye involvement in 80% to 90% of the cases of hyperthyroidism.[27,28] Even cases in which the condition appears unilateral, CT scans usually show enlarged extraocular muscles.[29]

Char[30] proposed an abbreviated classification system for the progressive eye changes found in Graves' disease (Table 8-5). The first two categories have minimal eye involvement; the others represent more serious eye findings. Soft-tissue involvement, class 2, refers to symptoms of excessive lacrimation, sandy sensation, retrobulbar discomfort, and photophobia, but not diplopia. There can be injection of conjunctiva and lid edema. Corneal involvement, class 5, refers to varying degrees of exposure keratitis

TABLE 8-5. *Classification of Ocular Changes in Graves' Disease*[30]

Class	Definition
0	No signs or symptoms
1	Only signs (upper eyelid retraction and stare with or without eyelid lag or proptosis); no symptoms
2	Soft-tissue involvement (symptoms and signs)
3	Proptosis
4	Extraocular muscle involvement
5	Corneal involvement
6	Sight loss (optic nerve involvement)

due to the proptosis and lagophthalmos. Loss of sight, class 6, is usually caused by compression of the optic nerve at the apex of the orbit by the enlarged extraocular muscles.

Almost 90% of patients who develop the eye signs of Graves' disease undergo spontaneous remission of most signs and symptoms within 3 years of systemic treatment.[31] Lid retraction and lag on downgaze usually resolves when hyperthyroidism is brought under control. Similarly, many patients with extraocular muscle involvement improve. Many ophthalmic problems, like exposure keratitis, should be monitored and conservatively treated during the course of systemic treatment. Systemic treatment of Graves' disease includes radiation of the thyroid, steroids, diuretics, and immunologic medication. If the patient's restrictive ocular motility does not respond sufficiently to systemic treatment, ocular muscle surgery is usually indicated. Similarly, if the proptosis does not diminish, the patient may benefit from orbital decompression surgery.

Several therapy approaches are available in the management of thyroid myopathy, but each has its limitations. The extraocular muscles are usually inflamed, enlarged, and are fibrotic late in the disease. Most patients have either simple hypotropia or hypotropia combined with esotropia. Some patients assume an elevated chin posture because of the restriction of motility in upgaze. Each of these factors needs to be considered in the choice of therapy options. Initially, the patient's response to medical treatment (antithyroid medication, corticosteroids, and immunosuppressive drugs) is evaluated. In cases of diplopia, prisms are often found to be helpful unless the deviation is over 10$^\Delta$. Since the deviation is usually noncomitant, prism spectacles need to be designed for specific uses at far and near. Presbyopic Graves' patients generally do better with single-vision glasses than with bifocals. If the magnitude of the deviation is variable, Fresnel prisms are practical during this phase, since the prism power can be changed easily. Muscle surgery should not be considered until the deviation is stable for 4 to 6 months. When muscle surgery is indicated, and it usually is following orbital decompression, it is advisable for the surgeon to use adjustable sutures along with a large recession of the restricted muscle. The adjustable sutures give the surgeon the opportunity to fine-tune the residual deviation the day after the operation. The success rate of muscle surgery in correcting diplopia with a single operation is reported in 50% to 65% of patients.[32,33] Single binocular vision over a wide range of gaze is, however, an unrealistic expectation in most cases of Graves' ophthalmopathy, but the combination of surgery and prisms usually eliminates diplopia in the primary position and at the reading angle. Lid surgery for long-standing lid retraction or other lid abnormalities should be undertaken as the last step following orbital and muscle surgery.

Chronic Progressive External Ophthalmoplegia (CPEO)

Chronic progressive external ophthalmoplegia is a rare ocular myopathy that affects the extraocular muscles, levator palpebrae, orbicularis, and occasionally other facial muscles, especially those used in mastication.[34] CPEO is also referred to as ocular myopathy of von Graefe. The first presenting sign is often bilateral ptosis that does not improve with the administration of anticholinesterase agents, unlike the ptosis found in myasthenia gravis. There is usually a slowly progressive loss of ocular motility affecting elevation more than in other fields of gaze. In extreme cases, motility is lost in all fields of gaze and the eyes appear "frozen" in place. The onset is usually before 30 years of age and may occur during early childhood. The condition appears to be genetic in origin, affecting males and females equally.

Treatment is based on the patient's symptoms. A ptosis crutch may be required to relieve the drooping lids. Prism therapy and surgical alignment of the eyes may be necessary to eliminate diplopia in some patients, often with satisfactory results.

MECHANICAL RESTRICTIONS OF OCULAR MOVEMENT

Noncomitancy may be caused by restriction of extraocular muscles. Several causes are discussed in this section.

Duane Retraction Syndrome

Although Duane was not the first to identify this syndrome, in 1905 he rigorously analyzed a series of 54 cases, and his name subsequently became attached to the condition. The retraction syndrome is a fairly common congenital anomaly that has been reported in infants as young as 1 day old.[35] It has been found in monozygotic twins, indicating a genetic basis.[36] There appears to be an autosomal dominant pattern, but many cases are sporadic. The retraction syndrome has an unexplained predilection for the left eye (3:1) and seems to occur more often in females, although some recent evidence casts doubt on this observation.[37] Approximately 20% are bilateral in nature.

The clinical characteristics in its classic form are as follows:

1. A marked limitation or absence of abduction, often associated with widening of the lids on attempted abduction.
2. A mild to moderate limitation of adduction, often associated with an upshoot or downshoot of the eye on adduction.
3. Retraction of the globe on adduction with narrowing of the lids.

4. Esotropia of the affected eye in the primary position, frequently greater at far than at near. Exotropia and non-strabismus are less often seen.
5. Often a head turn in the direction of the affected eye is needed to achieve limited range of binocular fusion.
6. Poor gross convergence (remote NPC).

There are several etiologic factors that combine to account for the features of the retraction syndrome. Electromyographic studies indicate a misdirected innervational pattern. On attempted abduction the lateral rectus is often electrically silent. In some cases the sixth nerve and nucleus have been absent.[38] In addition, it was found that several small branches of the inferior division of the third nerve entered the lateral rectus. With adduction, innervation flows to both the medial and the lateral rectus simultaneously, although the medial rectus receives the greater proportion. This anomalous innervation pattern causes co-contraction of both horizontal muscles. Co-contraction results in retraction of the globe, partial limitation of adduction, and narrowing of the palpebral fissures. The evidence that Duane retraction syndrome is a mechanical restriction comes from the result of the forced duction test. All cases show some physical limitation to passive movement of the globe and most show marked limitation. Fibrosis of the lateral rectus has been confirmed by biopsy in many cases. It is possible, however, that the mechanical restriction is secondary to the anomalous innervation pattern.

Significant variations from the classic form of Duane retraction syndrome have been reported by many authors. Huber[39] suggested the following classification that describes three principal types:

1. Duane I: Marked reduction or absence of abduction, mildly defective adduction, retraction on adduction with lid narrowing. This is the classic and most prevalent form.
2. Duane II: Marked reduction or absence of adduction, mildly defective abduc-

tion, retraction on abduction with lid narrowing. This is sometimes called the inverse Duane.
3. Duane III: Marked limitation of both abduction and adduction, retraction of the globe with narrowing of the lids on adduction. This is the rarest form of the three.

The majority of patients having Duane retraction syndrome are asymptomatic. Many have a restricted range of binocular fusion and learn to turn their head habitually to pick up fixation rather than turn their eyes. When strabismus is present, suppression is usually deep, preventing visual complaints or diplopia. In those few cases that do present with complaints related to fusional control of the deviation, vision therapy can be attempted to build fusional reserves. (See Chapter 15 for a description of such a case.) Surgical intervention is usually considered only to reduce a cosmetically disfiguring strabismus or head turn and not necessarily to increase ocular motility or fusion ranges. When surgery is indicated, simple procedures are generally recommended, mainly medial or lateral rectus recessions.

Brown (Superior Oblique Tendon Sheath) Syndrome

The predominate feature of Brown syndrome is reduced or absent elevation on adduction.[40] Restriction is the same degree on versions (binocular) or ductions (monocular). There also may be some limitation of elevation in the primary position and even on abduction in some cases. The condition usually affects only one eye, either left or right; however, we have seen several bilateral cases. Many patients maintain normal binocular vision in the primary position, but many have hypotropia, esotropia, or exotropia of the affected eye. Brown syndrome is a congenital anomaly with familial occurrence. Mirror reversal (i.e., opposite eye affected) was reported in monozygotic twins.[41]

Clinical characteristics of Brown syndrome are as follows:

1. Absence or marked limitation of elevation on adduction.
2. Normal or near normal elevation in the primary position and on abduction.
3. Depression of the affected eye (hypotropia) may occur on versions (nasalward position of the eye).
4. Usually widening of palpebral fissure on adduction.
5. Divergence in upgaze; usually a "V" pattern, with or without a strabismus in the primary position.
6. Restriction to passive elevation on adduction with the forced duction test.

Several etiologies have been found in Brown syndrome. Brown first described the superior oblique tendon sheath as fixed to and terminating at the pulley. If the sheath is short and fixed at the pulley and the tendon insertion, it becomes a physical barrier to adduction of the eye. On adduction, the globe slips under the stretched sheath and in some cases there is an audible "click." The sheath prevents elevation on adduction. Other cases have been reported in which the tendon itself fails to slip through the pulley and restricts ocular motility in the same manner as described above. Some individuals with Brown syndrome have had spontaneous recoveries. There is a sudden release of the restriction, the tendon moves normally through the pulley and full motility is found. It is interesting to note that more cases of Brown syndrome are found in children, suggesting that many cases do spontaneously resolve. Other less-prevalent etiologies include anomaly of the superior oblique muscle, paradoxical innervation analogous to the findings in Duane retraction syndrome, surgically induced restrictions, and restriction secondary to paralysis of the inferior oblique muscle.[42]

Many patients with Brown syndrome have normal binocular vision in the primary position, no visual complaints, and have learned to move their head rather than the eyes to the affected field of gaze. Surgery is not recommended unless there is a significant strabismus, usually hypotropia, in the primary position, or the patient has adopted a cosmetically unacceptable head turn. Brown advocated dissecting and stripping the sheath while leaving the tendon intact. Although his cure rate was only 20%, some improvement was reported in 50% of the cases.[40] Von Noorden[42] recommended performing a complete tenectomy of the superior oblique muscle, which dramatically improves the restriction. This, however, creates a weakness in inferior-nasal ductions. Further surgery is often required. Patients should be carefully selected before an operation in cases of Brown syndrome.

Fibrosis of the Extraocular Muscles

Generalized fibrosis syndrome is usually an autosomal dominant anomaly in which all the extraocular muscles, including the levator, are fibrotic. Both eyes are tethered downward and the patient elevates the chin to fixate. A bilateral ptosis is usually evident. Surgical treatment is often unsatisfactory. One surgical approach is to recess both inferior rectus muscles and perform bilateral frontalis suspensions to correct the ptosis. There is a danger of causing exposure keratitis, which if it occurs would require further surgical intervention.

Strabismus fixus is a rare congenital condition in which one or both eyes are tethered in an extreme position of gaze, usually convergent and exceeding 100[Δ]. This anomaly is cosmetically less acceptable than the generalized fibrosis syndrome in most cases. The eyes are firmly fixed in position, which is easily confirmed by the forced duction test. The patient must assume an extreme head turn to fixate with the preferred eye, since one eye is chosen over the other by habit. This anomaly is congenital and thought to be due to fibrosis of the medial rectus muscles. The condition is treated surgically, hopefully at an early age, by an extensive recession of the medial recti and the overlying conjunctiva. The eyes are anchored in a slightly abducted position and maximum resection of the lateral recti may help hold the eyes in a central position. Even though ocular motility after surgery remains very limited, cosmetic and functional improvement may be considerable.

Adherence Syndromes

Johnson[43] described two very rare restriction anomalies called adherence syndromes. They are usually acquired, often introduced by previous eye surgery; however, a few congenital cases have been reported. In the *lateral adherence syndrome,* the muscle sheaths of the lateral rectus and the inferior oblique are joined by abnormal fascial tissue attachments. This produces a limitation of movement in the field of action of the lateral rectus (i.e., abduction). The forced duction test reveals a lateral restriction to passive rotation of the eye. In the *superior adherence syndrome,* there is abnormal adherence between the superior rectus muscle sheath and the superior oblique tendon that produces a limitation of movement in the field of action of the superior rectus. Diagnosis is often established during surgery, using the forced duction test. Treatment for these adherence syndromes requires loosening the adhesions by forcefully rotating the globe after detaching the lateral or superior rectus.

Orbital Anomalies

A *blow-out fracture* of the orbit may occur as a result of blunt trauma to the soft tissues of the eye, for instance when an eye is hit with a tennis ball or a fist, or the face hits the dashboard in a car accident. A fracture usually occurs in the anterior and nasal orbital floor where the bone is thinnest and most vulnerable to impact forces. The maxillary and ethmoid sinuses can be involved. (A *blow-in fracture* is also possible in this area from trauma to the infraorbital rim; the maxillary sinus can buckle and rupture through to the floor of the orbit.)[44] Marked limitation of eye movements (elevation and depression), diplopia, and enophthalmos are common consequences. In many blow-out fractures, internal eye damage may be absent because the fracture itself helps to cushion the blow. Of course, after an injury, the eyes need to be thoroughly inspected for macular edema, retinal detachment, hemorrhage, ocular motor palsies, and other possible problems.

Depending on the size of the fracture, orbital contents can prolapse into the maxillary sinus. Orbital fat, fascia, the inferior rectus, and the inferior oblique can all become entrapped, thereby severely limiting eye movement, often elevation and sometimes depression. Hypotropia may be present in the primary position. A small crack in the orbital floor can incarcerate some orbital tissue, thus causing diplopia and other symptoms. After a recent blow-out fracture, the most conspicuous clinical manifestations are swelling and ecchymosis of the lids and periorbital soft tissue. Initially this swelling may cause a proptosis of the eye, but later, as the swelling subsides in 4 to 6 weeks, the loss of orbital fat may cause an enophthalmos. Radiological investigation and CT scans of the orbit can provide evidence about whether an initial restriction of eye movement is due to local swelling or hemorrhage or to the entrapment of orbital contents.

In cases when diplopia and ocular motor restriction persists past the initial healing phase, herniated orbital tissue needs to be extracted surgically from the bone fracture, and then the fracture repaired. Von Noorden[45] does not recommend surgery for patients with orbital floor fractures who initially have no diplopia or in whom diplopia disappears within 2 weeks after injury. It is important to remember that diplopia after orbital fracture is not necessarily caused by entrapment of orbital tissue; associated extraocular muscle and cranial nerve palsy are common.[46] Surgical repair of the orbital floor is indicated when the forced duction test shows a mechanical restriction of elevation and a CT scan reveals entrapped tissue in the fracture.

INTERNUCLEAR AND SUPRANUCLEAR DISORDERS

Lesions between the nuclei of the third, fourth, and sixth cranial nerves are discussed as well as lesions above these nuclei.

Internuclear Ophthalmoplegia (INO)

A lesion in the medial longitudinal fasciculus (MLF) blocks information from the pontine gaze center and the sixth nerve nucleus to the contralateral third nerve nucleus. A lesion in this long internuclear pathway produces a characteristic set of clinical manifestations known as *internuclear ophthalmoplegia* (INO) (Table 8-6). The patient presents with deficient or absent adduction of the eye on the affected side on attempted version. In the subtle form, the adduction defect may be apparent only as a mild decrease in the velocity of adducting saccades. There is abduction nystagmus of the eye opposite the lesion on attempted version. The nystagmus may be present in the abducting eye only, or in both eyes, with the abducting eye having a larger amplitude of nystagmus. The dissociated or asymmetric horizontal nystagmus in these patients appears to be a secondary compensatory response to the weakness of adduction and not caused directly by the central defect.[47] INO is named for the side of the MLF lesion, which is indicated by the eye with deficient adduction on conjugate gaze. For example, a left INO is indicated when the left eye lacks adduction and the right eye shows abduction nystagmus on attempted right gaze. In bilateral cases, there is usually abduction nystagmus of both eyes on lateral gaze associated with little or no adduction of either eye. INO can be distinguished from an isolated medial rectus palsy, which also results in a loss of adduction, by the associated abduction nystagmus on lateral gaze.

The saccadic, pursuit, and vestibulo-ocular systems are all affected; however, gross convergence is usually intact. This is seen in the most prevalent type, Cogan's posterior INO, due to a pontine level lesion of the MLF.[48] A unique feature in pontine INO is that the medial rectus contracts in response to a convergence stimulus, but does not in response to a version stimulus. INO produced by a midbrain lesion, however, is usually bilateral with a reduction or absence of gross convergence (Cogan's anterior INO).[48]

TABLE 8-6. Features of Internuclear Ophthalmoplegia (INO)

1. Adduction defect of one or both eyes on attempted horizontal versions.
2. Abduction nystagmus on horizontal versions.
3. Gross convergence is intact in most cases of posterior lesions of MLF (pons and medulla). Gross convergence is absent in anterior lesions of MLF (midbrain).
4. Vertical nystagmus on upgaze is frequently seen.
5. Usually no strabismus present in the primary position, but esotropia or exotropia is seen in a few cases.

There is often a coarse vertical nystagmus on upgaze of both eyes in unilateral and bilateral cases. Most patients with INO have no strabismus in the primary position, unlike a medial rectus paresis. Occasionally, a horizontal strabismus is found superimposed on an INO due to specific involvement of the respective nuclei, i.e., an exotropia associated with a lesion of the medial rectus component of the oculomotor nucleus (NIII) or an esotropia due to abducens nucleus (NVI) or nerve damage.

There are two primary etiologies of INO. Bilateral INO in a young adult is most often caused by multiple sclerosis, a demyelinating disease; INO in patients older than 50 years is frequently caused by a vascular lesions (e.g., an infarction). When multiple sclerosis is the cause, there are often other presenting symptoms such as decreased bladder control, limb weakness, unusual parasthesia sensations, or optic neuritis. Unilateral presentation almost always indicates an infarct (occlusion) of a small branch of the basilar artery and is often accompanied by vertigo and other brain stem symptoms.[49] Other rare causes of INO have been reported; these include brain stem and fourth ventricular tumors, hydrocephalus, infections (including those associated with AIDS), pernicious anemia, head trauma, and drug intoxications (e.g., narcotics, tricyclic antidepressants, lithium, barbiturates, and other psychoactive drugs).[50]

Treatment options of INO are, unfortunately, limited. Ocular complaints are managed on a symptomatic basis. Patients usually do not present with a strabismus in the primary position and therefore do not complain of diplopia except on lateral gaze. They compensate by turning their head for lateral fixation, rather than turning their eyes. Comfortable reading and safe driving, however, may require patching an eye—either total or partial occlusion. There may be some spontaneous or slow recovery of function with healing if the cause is of vascular origin. Patients with multiple sclerosis frequently have periods of remission and recovery of some motor functions during the course of the disease. Unfortunately, there is no treatment for multiple sclerosis to date that has proven effective in the long term.

Supranuclear Horizontal Gaze Palsy

Frontal Eye-Field Lesions

The two most common causes of lesions in the frontal cortex (Brodmann's area 8) are acute cerebrovascular accident (stroke) and head trauma. The frontal eye fields initiate voluntary saccadic eye movements, so a lesion on one side results in a conjugate turning of the eyes (and usually the head) toward the side of the lesion; the contralateral area 8 has unopposed action. If the lesion is isolated and the patient is sufficiently conscious, pursuit eye movements can be demonstrated on either side. Since the vestibular pathway is intact, the eyes can move into the field opposite the lesion using the doll's head maneuver. Eventually, this gaze palsy may partially resolve, possibly due to other systems generating saccades, e.g., the superior colliculus.[51]

Occipital and Parietal Cortical Lesions

An extensive lesion in the parieto-occipital lobe secondary to a vascular accident or tumor is the most likely cause of a gaze-dependent disorder of pursuit eye movements. The patient is unable to follow a moving target smoothly, but uses a series of small saccadic steps for tracking. These saccadic steps are re-

ferred to as "cog wheel" pursuits. To a lesser degree, smooth pursuit tracking reduces in old age in many people, but the loss is usually symmetric in direction. The smooth pursuit phase of OKN is similarly affected when the stripes are rotated in the direction of the lesion, but it should be normal when the stripe rotation is reversed, i.e., toward the opposite side of the lesion. The associated and definitive clinical sign of this pathological condition is homonymous hemianopsia. Lesions located solely in the occipital region result in a visual field cut, often without pursuit abnormalities; lesions in the parietal region, however, often produce visual agnosia so that interpretation of the visual image's meaning is defective, i.e., apperceptive agnosia. Patients having parieto-occipital lesions initially require management by a neuro-ophthalmologist, but they usually can be followed subsequently by the primary eye care doctor.

Brainstem Lesions

Brainstem lesions affect the descending fibers in the brain stem from the cortical areas subserving pursuit and saccadic eye movements to the defuse lateral gaze centers in the pons, specifically, the paramedial pontine reticular formation (PPRF). Stroke is the most likely cause of lesions in the rostral brain stem whereas lesions at a lower level in the pons, involving the PPRF, can arise from several sources, e.g., vascular, demyelinating disease, and tumors.[52] If these descending fibers are interrupted, both pursuits and saccades are deficient or absent on the side of the "deprived" lateral gaze center. If a lateral gaze center itself is damaged, vestibular-ocular responses can also be affected since the PPRF is the beginning of the final common pathway to the horizontal oculomotor nuclei. Consequently, if a patient presents with a complete unilateral gaze palsy for all eye movements, the most likely cause is a lesion in the pons involving the lateral gaze center.

Supranuclear Vertical Gaze Palsy

Isolated lesions producing vertical gaze palsy are rare. Bilateral upgaze deficits have been reported in the literature more often than downgaze palsies. The reported cases usually involve vascular lesions or metastases in portions of the MLF connecting the fourth and third nerve complex or connections with the superior colliculus.[53] Most cases of vertical gaze palsy involve generalized neurologic syndromes in which the gaze palsy is merely one, but possibly the first, of many expressions of the disease process.

Parinaud Syndrome

Often the first sign of Parinaud syndrome is upgaze saccadic dysfunction. Initially the patient finds that making upgaze eye movements requires much effort; the eyes may swing back and forth in a serpentine movement when attempting elevation. With elevation effort, both eyes often converge while simultaneously retracting into the orbits. Many later have convergence-retraction nystagmus with oscillopsia. The nystagmoid movements can be exaggerated by rotating OKN stripes downward, thus requiring upward saccades. Convergence-retraction nystagmus on vertical OKN testing is a common sign in Parinaud syndrome. Other common signs include dilated pupils that are unresponsive to light, anisocoria, light-near dissociation (i.e., pupil constriction to a near stimulus but not to light), and papilledema. Table 8-7 lists signs of Parinaud syndrome. The sluggish pupillary light response and nystagmus are indicators that the upgaze restriction is not orbital in nature, as it is in Graves' disease. High resolution CT scanning and MRI are usually helpful in the differential diagnosis. Parinaud syndrome usually indicates a neuro-ophthalmologic emergency.

Parinaud syndrome can be congenital or acquired. It is also referred to as sylvian aqueduct syndrome and dorsal midbrain syndrome indicating its etiology. Parinaud syndrome is frequently caused by sylvian aqueductal stenosis (i.e., a restriction of cerebral spinal fluid that flows between the third and fourth ventricles) resulting in hydrocephalus and papilledema. Some other causes are tumors of the pineal gland or in the region of the aqueduct or superior colliculus, neurosyphilis, mul-

TABLE 8-7. *Ocular Signs of Parinaud Syndrome (dorsal midbrain syndrome)*

Common:
1. Deficiency or loss of saccades in upgaze.
2. Sluggish or tonic dilated pupils.
3. Light-near dissociation; good constriction at near.
4. Convergence-retraction nystagmus with oscillopsia (increased by rotating OKN stripes downward).
5. Papilledema.

Less common:
1. Disturbances of downgaze saccades.
2. Skew deviation.
3. Lid retraction (Collier's sign)
4. Fourth nerve palsy (Troclear palsy).
5. Loss of upgaze pursuits.

tiple sclerosis, trauma, and stroke.[53] In cases of sylvian aqueductal stenosis, signs and symptoms are usually relieved by surgical insertion of a shunt to promote the flow of cerebral spinal fluid. Although tumors in this area are often inoperable, they frequently respond well to radiation therapy. The long-term survival rate for these patients is generally good.[54]

Progressive Supranuclear Palsy

Progressive supranuclear palsy is a generic category for a number of rare degenerative diseases with similar features that affect pursuit and saccadic eye movements, the best known of which is Steele-Richardson syndrome. These patients are typically seen in the sixth or seventh decades of life complaining of the inability to move their eyes into downgaze. The ophthalmoplegia progresses to loss of voluntary upgaze saccades, loss of horizontal saccades, and finally, loss of pursuit eye movements. The oculomotor deficits are often compounded by a stiff neck. Vestibular ocular reflexes are usually intact, but severe neck rigidity may make their demonstration difficult. As the disease progresses, patients may develop strabismus and diplopia, lost of facial expression, and dementia. These patients usually have a progressive downhill course and die 8 to 10 years after the

TABLE 8-8. Ocular Signs of Parkinson's Disease

1. Hypometric saccades in all field of gaze, but initially in upgaze.
2. Saccadic "cogwheel" pursuits
3. Lid apraxia (difficulty in opening)
4. Decreased blinking
5. Sporadic oculogyric crisis

onset of signs. Ocular complaints are treated symptomatically. Yoked base-down prisms may be helpful for tasks in downgaze, e.g., reading and eating. Prisms or occlusion may be necessary to bring relief from diplopia.

Parkinson's Disease

Parkinson's disease is fairly common (0.1% to 1% of the population) and has conspicuous systemic and ocular manifestations. It usually occurs with old age. The condition stems from a depletion of the neurotransmitter dopamine secondary to the death of nerve cells in the substantia nigra, a basal ganglion nucleus of the upper brain stem. The specific causes of nerve cell death are many: carbon monoxide poisoning, viral infections, arteriosclerosis, syphilis, tumors, and it may even be part of the normal aging process in some people. Parkinsonian patients lose control of muscular activity. They tremble at rest and have trouble with fine-motor coordination. There is often muscular rigidity, stiffness, and slowing of movements. In advanced cases, balance, posture, and walking are affected; patients often adopt a hurried shuffling gait. Physical articulation of speech becomes difficult and facial expression flattens. Early in the course of the disease, conjugate saccadic eye movements become hypometric in all fields of gaze, but upgaze is usually affected initially (Table 8-8). Jerky "cogwheel" pursuits are seen. Patients may also have difficulty opening their eyes (i.e., lid apraxia) and the rate of blinking decreases. Complaints of diplopia are often associated with convergence weakness and a developing convergence insufficiency. Later in the course of this slow degenerative

condition, the eyes may periodically go into oculogyric crisis where they are locked in an extreme field of gaze for a few minutes up to a few hours.

There is no known cure for Parkinson's disease. Drug therapies have not proven successful as yet. Treatment is therefore symptomatic and directed toward support and comfort. There are often unpredictable periods of remission when systemic and ocular signs diminish; but overall, the condition is progressive. Patients are often directed toward psychological support groups to help them adjust emotionally to the limitations of their condition.

NYSTAGMUS

The appearance of nystagmus in early childhood or later in life causes considerable distress for patients, family, and friends. Its presence is usually interpreted as a sign of serious visual dysfunction or possibly brain damage. Nystagmus (i.e., the involuntary rhythmic oscillations of one or both eyes) may indeed be the presenting sign of either a pathologic afferent visual pathway lesion or a disorder in ocular motor control. Thirteen percent of cerebral palsy patients have nystagmus among many other visual disorders.[55] Approximately 10% to 15% of visually impaired school-aged children have nystagmus. Nystagmus can be conceptualized as a disorder of the mechanisms that keep fixation stable.[56]

Nystagmus, affecting about 0.4% of the general population,[57] is not a disease entity as such; it is a sign of an underlying disorder. The clinician should attempt to describe the condition as either congenital or acquired and determine the general category of etiology, e.g., genetic, traumatic, toxic, metabolic error, developmental, or visual deprivation. This discussion focuses on the most prevalent types of nystagmus: physiologic, voluntary, congenital, and latent nystagmus. Rarer types, which may be harbingers of active neurologic disease, are presented in Table 8-16 for the purpose of differential diagnosis.

Many clinical observations in the routine vision examination are complicated by the

TABLE 8-9. *Clinically Relevant Characteristics of Nystagmus*

Characteristic	Observations
Global observations	General posture, head position (turns or tilts), facial asymmetries
Type of nystagmus	Pendular, jerk, or mixed
Direction	Horizontal, vertical, torsional, or combination
Amplitude	Small (> 2 degrees), moderate (2 degrees to 10 degrees), large (>10 degrees)
Frequency	Slow (1/2 Hz), moderate (1/2-2 Hz), fast (>2 Hz)
Constancy	Constantly present, intermittent, periodic
Conjugacy	Conjugate (eyes move in same direction), disjunctive (eyes move independently)
Symmetry	Symmetrical, asymmetrical, monocular
Latent component	Increase of nystagmus with occlusion of one eye
Field of gaze changes	Null point, dampening, or increase of nystagmus in any field of gaze, or with convergence

presence of nystagmus. The patient's inability to maintain steady fixation affects the accuracy of keratometry, retinoscopy, subjective refraction, cover test, the internal and external health inspection, and other measurements. For this reason, the clinician needs to exercise skill, patience, and persistence in clinical evaluation. The gross observation of nystagmus is necessary in all fields of gaze and at far and nearpoint distances, since many types of nystagmus show significant variation in these respects. When observing the characteristics of nystagmus, magnification is often useful (e.g., loop, +20 D BIO lens, or slit lamp). Table 8-9 presents characteristics of nystagmus that are clinically relevant for differential diagnosis.

Physiologic Nystagmus

When a person is very tired, it is not unusual for a jerk nystagmus to develop in extreme positions of gaze (Table 8-10). This is a normal type of nystagmus and of no particular consequence; it disappears after a good sleep. The oscillations are of small amplitude, conjugate, rapid, and may be unequal in each eye. It is present only at the extremes of horizontal and, occasionally, of vertical gaze. Since the condition is related to fatigue, it is usually intermit-

tent, but if sustained, it must be distinguished from pathological types of nystagmus. A reasonable clinical guideline is to regard fine conjugate jerk nystagmus, detected beyond 30° of gaze or beyond the range of binocular vision, as physiologic unless there is a good reason to suspect otherwise.[58] Alcohol intoxication causes physiologic nystagmus to decompensate and the nystagmus becomes abnormal on moderate lateral shifts of gaze. This is used in law enforcement as one of the indications of a suspect driving under the influence of alcohol.

Voluntary Nystagmus

Voluntary nystagmus might be more properly called "voluntary flutter" because it is not a true nystagmus. It is a series of rapidly alternating saccades usually initiated willfully with a convergence movement and represents nothing more than a "trick" with the eyes (Table 8-11).[59] This voluntary flutter is accompanied by oscillopsia and is quite fatiguing. It can only be sustained for a short period of time, 30 seconds or less. Approximately 5% to 8% of the population can demonstrate voluntary nystagmus and this ability seems to run in families.[60] It is unlikely that preschool children would discover this ability, but occasionally an older child has

TABLE 8-10. *Characteristics of Physiologic Nystagmus*

Type	Jerk; conjugate
Direction	Usually horizontal; fast phase of jerk is toward side of gaze
Constancy	Occasional, usually when tired
Frequency	Rapid
Amplitude	Small, may be unequal in each eye
Field of gaze	Occurs in extreme horizontal fields of gaze beyond 30°, occasionally in vertical gaze
Latent component	Can occur in extreme field of gaze where binocular vision is broken
Symptoms	None
Associated conditions	None
Etiology	Specific mechanism unknown but seems to be caused by extreme general fatigue
Comments	This common condition is relieved with rest or sleep; no other therapy recommended

TABLE 8-11. *Characteristics of Voluntary Nystagmus*

Type	Pendular saccades; conjugate
Direction	Horizontal
Constancy	Occasional, dependent upon conscious effort, cannot be sustained for more than 30 seconds at a time
Frequency	Very rapid oscillations, 3-43 Hz
Amplitude	Usually small, 2° or 3°
Field of gaze	Usually initiated by a convergence eye movement, probably accommodative convergence
Latent component	None
Symptoms	Oscillopsia, may be associated with malingering symptoms (e.g., blurred vision)
Associated conditions	None
Etiology	Not a true nystagmus, back and forth saccades without an intersaccadic interval, ability to do it may be hereditary
Comments	This is a "trick" of the eyes that is quite fatiguing, so the oscillation bursts are of short duration, prevalence is about 8%; may be associated with malingering behavior in school-aged children

used this eye maneuver as part of malingering behavior, an emotional episode, or a hysteric reaction. Ciuffreda[61] has demonstrated that voluntary nystagmus can be part of a spasm of the near reflex if a patient voluntarily crosses the eyes. The clinician can usually distinguish voluntary nystagmus by its distinctive features. The oscillations appear pendular (specifically "Sawtooth"), conjugate, horizontal, rapid (3 to 43 Hz), usually small amplitude, and are of short duration due to their fatiguing nature. The rapid oscillations of spasmus nutans might be confused with voluntary nystagmus, except

that spasmus nutans presents in infancy but not in school-aged children. Furthermore, it is much more sustained. Voluntary nystagmus, therefore, should be easily recognized.

Congenital Nystagmus

The most common type of nystagmus is congenital nystagmus, apparently affecting males twice as frequently as females.[62] It is notoriously variable, but fortunately, for the sake of differential diagnosis, certain clinical features are quite characteristic and distinguish it from

TABLE 8-12. *Characteristics of Congenital (infantile) Nystagmus*

Type	Pendular and/or jerk; conjugate
Direction	Usually horizontal, rotary, rarely vertical; fast phase of jerk is toward size of gaze
Constancy	Usually constant, but can become quiet occasionally
Frequency	Variable, increases with peripheral gaze
Amplitude	Variable, increases with peripheral gaze and effort
Field of gaze	Often dampens with convergence and 10° to 15° to one side (null point)
Latent component	Usually present, nystagmus increases in amplitude and frequency with occlusion of either eye
Symptoms	Most have reduced acuity to varying degrees, many have cosmetic concerns, head turns, rhythmic head movements
Associated conditions	Esotropia often found, amblyopia, moderate to high astigmatism, head shaking, 40% have defective VOR and OKN, paradoxical response to OKN seen occasionally
Etiology	Congenital, specific mechanism unknown, can be afferent or efferent pathway lesions, often hereditary pattern (sex-linked, autosomal dominant, and others), efferent type often assumed to be a defect in the pursuit system at the level of the brain stem
Comments	Condition improves with age; often acuity and cosmesis can be improved at any age with spectacles, contact lenses, prisms, vision training, or auditory biofeedback

other forms of nystagmus (Table 8-12). It is present at birth or shortly thereafter, and for this reason it is sometimes referred to as infantile nystagmus. The oscillations can be solely jerk (the most prevalent pattern), solely pendular, or a combination of the two. The oscillations can convert from one waveform to another spontaneously or may do so in different fields of gaze. If the waveform pattern is jerk, then the fast phase most often occurs in the direction of gaze.[63] Amplitude and frequency can vary from moment to moment and, on occasion, the eyes may become "quiet." The amplitude usually increases in some field of gaze and, for this reason, a patient may habitually assume a head turn or head tilt to dampen the nystagmus as much as possible. The position of gaze in which the eyes are quiet is known as the null region. The nystagmus is often accentuated by active fixation, attention, or anxiety and possibly diminished by convergence and purposeful lid closure.[64] It usually presents as conjugate and horizontal, but occasionally clinicians see vertical and torsional waveforms or some combination of these. When the nystagmus is horizontal, it usually remains horizontal even on up and downgaze.

The condition is rarely associated with oscillopsia even though the eyes may be in constant motion, but one may find head nodding or shaking.

The specific neuropathology resulting in congenital nystagmus is not well understood in most cases, but the clinical conditions causing it can be broadly classified into afferent and efferent groups. Afferent congenital nystagmus is associated with poor visual acuity. Congenital optic nerve atrophy or hypoplasia, congenital cataracts, ocular albinism, achromatopsia, and aniridia are all diseases of the eye or the *afferent* visual pathway that can result in congenital nystagmus. Visual acuity reduction is usually profound and the prognosis for improvement poor. In these cases, approximately 40% of all congenital nystagmus cases, the etiology is usually obvious on clinical examination. The majority of cases, about 60%, are considered to be *efferent* due to some disorder of the ocular motor systems. A disorder or lesion of the pursuit system at the level of the brain stem is suspected by some authorities.[56] Lo[65] reported computed tomographic abnormalities in 50% of congenital nystagmus patients. Magnetic resonance image (MRI)

TABLE 8-13. *Characteristics of Spasmus Nutans*

Type	Pendular, often the eyes are asymmetric in amplitude
Direction	Usually horizontal, can be rotary or vertical
Constancy	Constant or intermittent
Frequency	Fast, 6-11 Hz
Amplitude	Small, about 2°, often eyes are asymmetric, some cases may appear monocular because of asymmetry
Field of gaze	Present in all fields, but variable with gaze
Latent component	None
Symptoms	Usually head nodding or wobbling; abnormal head position (tilt or chin depression) in 50% of cases
Associated conditions	Usually none, benign condition, occasionally esotropia or amblyopia, a rare association with gliomas
Etiology	Mechanism unknown, may be hereditary
Comments	Onset not at birth, but usually develops in first year, often lasts 1 or 2 years, then disappears with no lasting consequences; no treatment is indicated; computed tomography scan recommended to screen for gliomas

scanning may identify an even higher percentage in the future. There is often a hereditary pattern of involvement, but some members may have one waveform (e.g., jerk) and some another (e.g., pendular). In most efferent cases, the etiology is idiopathic. Patients with efferent congenital nystagmus usually have better visual acuity than those with afferent types.

The incidence of strabismus in congenital nystagmus is high, 40% to 50%.[66] The eye-turn is usually esotropic; however, exotropias and hypertropias are frequently found. The strabismus may be difficult to identify due to the pattern of nystagmoid movements, so it is possible that the incidence of strabismus is actually underestimated. The etiology of a strabismus can be completely independent of that causing the nystagmus, but most often the two conditions appear to be part of the underlying problem affecting the visual system. One controversial view is that most cases of esotropia associated with congenital nystagmus are secondary to the nystagmus and originate as an attempt to stabilize the eyes. This condition is known as nystagmus blockage syndrome.

Congenital (infantile) nystagmus must be differentiated from other types of nystagmus that occur very early in life, such as spasmus nutans. The diagnosis is apparent if the nystagmus is associated with an obvious afferent lesion (e.g., albinism, congenital cataracts, optic atrophy), but efferent etiologies can present the clinician with a diagnostic challenge. In summary, the most distinctive feature of congenital nystagmus, besides its early onset, is its variability. Congenital nystagmus, although often constantly presents, can vary in frequency, amplitude, and type, and alternate between pendular and jerk. There is usually a latent component. There may be a family history revealing a genetic condition. Spasmus nutans is an altogether different type of nystagmus and has a later onset than congenital nystagmus. (See Table 8-13.) It is characterized by high frequency, small amplitude oscillations that are often intermittent and asymmetric when comparing each eye (Table 8-13). For further information on differential diagnosis, refer to an extensive review by Grisham.[67]

Nystagmus Blockage Syndrome

A less-well-known form of congenital jerk nystagmus is associated with esotropia. The amplitude of nystagmus is reduced or absent when the fixating eye is converged (adducted). It is thought that by holding the fixating eye in

TABLE 8-14. *Characteristics of Latent Nystagmus*

Type	Jerk, conjugate
Direction	Horizontal
Constancy	Occasional, occurs on occlusion of either eye
Frequency	Variable
Amplitude	Variable
Field of gaze	Decreases in gaze toward covered eye; increases toward uncovered eye
Latent component	Manifest only under monocular conditions
Symptoms	Usually none since it is a latent condition
Associated conditions	Usually associated with one or more of the following conditions: congenital nystagmus, esotropia, amblyopia, disassociated vertical deviation (DVD), retrolental fibroplasia (RLF), occasionally occurs as an isolated condition
Etiology	Congenital condition, mechanism unknown, disturbed cortical binocularity, monocular OKN asymmetry, abnormal localization, and proprioception, monocular reduction of illumination
Comments	Fairly common, complicates the assessment of strabismus and ocular motility, no treatment indicated

TABLE 8-15. *Characteristics of Vestibular Nystagmus*

	Central	Peripheral
Type	Jerk, conjugate	Jerk, conjugate
Direction	Often purely horizontal, vertical, or torsional	Usually mixed, never just vertical
Constancy	Constant	Intermittent, recurrent
Frequency	Increases with gaze toward fast phase, decreases or reverses to slow phase	Increase with gaze toward fast phase, decreases or reverses to slow phase
Amplitude	Increases with gaze toward fast phase, visual fixation tends not to reduce nystagmus	Increases with gaze toward fast phase, fixation tends to reduce nystagmus
Field of gaze	See above	See above "Amplitude"
Latent component	Reduced by covering an eye if cerebellar disease; increased if vestibular disease	None
Symptoms	Mild vertigo, nausea, variable oscillopsia	Severe vertigo, nausea, persistent oscillopsia
Associated conditions	Deafness and tinnitus rare; usually other neurologic signs	Deafness and tinnitus frequent
Etiology	Damage to vestibular nucleus or connections in brain stem or cerebellum (e.g., neuromas, demyelination)	Damage to labyrinth-vestibular nerve (e.g., vascular, demyelination, neoplastic)
Comments	Caloric testing useful; signs can mimic peripheral disease clinically	Caloric testing useful; signs do not mimic central disease; higher prevalence than central type

adduction to "block" the nystagmus, the hypertonicity of the medial rectus eventually results in esotropia. The mechanism is not fully understood, but this association of congenital nystagmus and esotropia is known as *nystagmus blockage syndrome.* Often there is an accommodative element to the strabismus as well. The syndrome has these main features: (1) The onset is in infancy. Jerk nystagmus precedes the onset of a variable esotropia that may be alter-

TABLE 8-16. *Rare Types of Nystagmus*

	Periodic Alternating Nystagmus (PAN)	See saw Nystagmus	Gaze Paretic Nystagmus	Muscle Paretic Nystagmus	Upbeat Nystagmus	Downbeat Nystagmus
Type	Jerk usually acquired, can be congenital	Pendular, eyes move in opposite vertical directions	Jerk conjugate and equal between eyes	Jerk, fast phase toward the affected field more in affected eye	Jerk	Jerk
Direction	Beats to left, then to right in 3 minute cycles	Conjugate torsional oscillations with disjunctive vertical movements	Horizontal but sometimes has torsional component	Horizontal or vertical in direction of the affected muscle	Vertical, slow phase downward	Vertical, slow phase upward
Constancy	Constant with pauses as it changes direction	Intermittent, transient	Constant	Constant or intermittent depending on lesion	Periodic, usually in primary and upgaze	Intermittent, periodic, depends upon head and body posture
Frequency	Fast, variable	Slow, 1 Hz or less	Variable	Varies with gaze, increasing in affected field	Variable, fast	Variable fast, increases with head hanging, and convergence
Amplitude	Variable	Variable, usually small	Usually small, sometimes large	Variable	Types: large amplitude increases in upgaze; small, increase in downgaze	Small, maximum when eyes turned laterally and slightly down
Field of gaze	Increases in extreme horizontal gaze	Torsional movement in all fields but "see-saw" in up, down, and primary	Increased amplitude in affected field of gaze	Increased amplitude in affected field of gaze	Not present in all fields of gaze, see above ("Amplitude")	Most prominent when looking down and laterally, not present in all fields
Latent component	None	None	None	None	None	None

	Symptoms	Associated neurologic signs or conditions	Etiology	Comments
	Oscillopsia	Smooth pursuit usually is impaired, gaze evoked and down beat nystagmus may accompany multiple sclerosis, syphilis, head trauma	Multiple sclerosis, hydrocephalus	Compressions at foramen magnum level (Arnold-Chiari malformation), encephalitis, alcohol, spinocerebellar lesions, magnesium deficiency
	Infrequent oscillopsia	Associated with paretic strabismus, sometimes ophthalmoplegia	Posterior fossa disease	May be congenital or acquired, reports of improvement using base-out prisms in spectacles and drug therapy: clonazepam
	Often associated with diplopia if of recent onset	Due to single muscle weakness, paresis, myasthenia gravis	Lesion in frontal gaze center or brain stem projections or pontine gaze centers	Types: (1) lesion in anterior vermis of cerebellum or medulla; (2) intrinsic medullary disease or structural deformity
	Inability to hold eye in the affected field of gaze	Same in the two eyes, fairly prevalent form of nystagmus	Cerebellar disease, especially flocculus lesions, one type related to vestibular disease	These drugs may increase the nystagmus: barbiturates, phenothaizide, dilantin
	Decreased visual acuity, occasionally bitemporal hemianopsia field defect	Bitemporal hemianopsia, septo-optic dysplasia, seen in some comatose patients following severe brain stem injury	Sellar or parasellar tumor disease of the mesodiencephalic junction, trauma, or vascular disease	Rare, usually acquired, congenital type has been seen, the intorting eye rises and the extorting eye falls in acquired cases, congenital opposite
	Oscillopsia, impaired visual acuity, alternating head turn may occur	Asymmetric between the two eyes, which distinguishes it from gaze paretic type, little or no nystagmus in the unaffected eye	Vestibulocerebellum or craniocervical disorder, multiple sclerosis, trauma, intoxication, encephalitis, vascular disease	Acquired PAN treated successfully with Baclofen, may continue during sleep, can occur as a side effect of some anticonvulsive drugs

nating or unilateral. Amblyopia is common; other infants appear to cross fixate so that amblyopia is prevented. (2) There is an abnormal head posture in which the head is turned toward the adducted fixating eye, i.e., there is a left head turn if the left eye is the fixating eye. (3) The fixating eye remains adducted with occlusion of the fellow eye. The condition can, therefore, initially simulate a paralysis of the lateral rectus. With further testing, abduction can usually be demonstrated, indicating a pseudoparalysis of abduction. (4) On adduction of the fixating eye, the nystagmus is reduced or absent, but nystagmus intensity increases as the fixating eye moves toward the primary position and into abduction. Generally speaking, the treatment of nystagmus and esotropia in nystagmus blockage syndrome is more difficult than management of either condition independently. Surgery is often necessary to compensate for both the head turn and the strabismus.

Latent Nystagmus

A conjugate, jerk nystagmus evoked by occlusion of one eye is a latent nystagmus (Table 8-14). It is often associated with strabismus, particularly congenital esotropia, double hypertropia (DVD), and amblyopia.[68] This is a congenital condition that might occur independently of other visual conditions; however, a latent component to congenital nystagmus is often seen, and a jerk pattern can be superimposed upon a pendular waveform. The jerk pattern of latent nystagmus is characterized by a fast phase in the direction of the fixating eye and by the increase of nystagmus amplitude on temporal gaze. Visual acuity is better with both eyes open than with either eye occluded. No specific therapy is indicated since the condition is only manifest with monocular occlusion.

Rare Types of Nystagmus

There are many types of nystagmus that can present at any age due to acquired pathologic factors, e.g., developmental anomalies, trauma, drug toxicity, vascular accidents, and endocrine imbalances. Fortunately, most of these conditions are extremely rare, but the incidence increases during old age. Table 8-15 lists characteristics of vestibular nystagmus, and Table 8-16 lists the clinical characteristics of several other rare conditions. As a rule, the clinician should be quite familiar with the previously described common types of nystagmus. If a nystagmus case does not fall naturally into one of the common diagnostic categories, refer to Table 8-15 and Table 8-16 in an attempt to establish the probable diagnosis. It seems prudent that all patients having nystagmus, except for physiologic and voluntary nystagmus, should be examined by a neurologist or neuro-ophthalmologist.

REFERENCES

1. Rush JA, Younge BR. Paralysis of cranial nerves III, IV, and VI: causes and prognosis in 1,000 cases. *Arch Ophthalmol.* 1981;99:76-79.
2. Glaser JS. *Neuro-ophthalmology.* 2nd ed. Philadelphia: Lippincott; 1990:424-425.
3. Wishnick MM, Nelson LB, Huppert L, Reich EW. Mobius syndrome and limb abnormalities with dominant inheritance. *Ophthalmic Paediatrics and Genetics.* 1983;2:77-81.
4. Von Noorden GK, Murray E, Wong SY. Superior oblique paralysis. A review of 270 cases. *Arch Ophthalmol.* 1986;104:1771-1776.
5. Neetens A, Janssens M. The superior oblique: a challenging extraocular muscle. *Doc Ophthalmol.* 1979;46:295-303.
6. Dale RT. *Fundamentals of Ocular Motility and Strabismus.* New York: Grune & Stratton; 1982:294.
7. Jampolsky A. Vertical strabismus surgery. In: *Symposium on Strabismus.* St. Louis: CV Mosby; 1971:366.
8. Metz H. Double levator palsy. *Arch Ophthalmol.* 1979;97:901-903.
9. Osserman KE. Ocular myasthenia gravis. *Invest Ophthalmol.* 1967;6:277-287.
10. Glaser, JS. *Neuro-ophthalmology.* 2nd ed. Philadelphia: Lippincott; 1990:392.
11. Soliven BC, Lange DJ, Penn AS. Seronegative myasthenia gravis. *Neurology.* 1988;38:514.
12. Burde RM, Savino PJ, Trobe JD. Clinical decisions. In: *Neuro-ophthalmology.* 2nd ed. St. Louis: CV Mosby Co; 1992:246.
13. Graves RJ. Newly observed affection of the thyroid gland in females. *London Med Surg J.* 1835;7:516-520.
14. Char DH. *Thyroid Eye Disease.* 2nd ed. New York: Churchill Livingstone; 1990:7.

15. Jacobson DH, Gorman CA. Endocrine ophthalmopathy: current ideas concerning etiology, pathogenesis and treatment. *Endocr Rev.* 1984;5:200-220.

16. Gorman CA. Temporal relationship between onset of Graves' ophthalmopathy and diagnosis of thyrotoxicosis. *Mayo Clin Proc.* 1983;58:515-519.

17. Char DH. *Thyroid Eye Disease.* 2nd ed. New York: Churchill Livingstone, 1990:22.

18. Jamamoto K, Itoh K, Yoshida S, Saito K, Sakamoto Y, Matsuda A, Saito T, Kuzuya T. A quantitative analysis of orbital soft tissue in Graves' disease based on B-mode untrasonography. *Endocrinol Jpn.* 1979; 26: 255-261.

19. Day RM. Ocular manifestations of thyroid disease: current concepts. *Trans Am Ophthalmol Soc.* 1959;57: 572-601.

20. Char DH. *Thyroid Eye Disease.* 2nd ed. New York: Churchill Livingstone; 1990:37.

21. Kroll HA, Kuwabara T. Dysthyroid ocular myopathy. *Arch Ophthalmol.* 1966;76:244-257.

22. Daicker B. The histological substrate of the extraocular muscle thickening seen in dysthroid orbitopathy. *Klin Monatsby Augenheilk.* 1979; 174:843-847.

23. Kendall-Taylor P, Perros P. Circulating retrobulbar antibodies in Graves' ophthalmopathy. *Acta Endocrinol.* 1989;121(suppl 2):31-37.

24. Scott WE, Thalacker JA. Diagnosis and treatment of thyroid myopathy. *Ophthalmology.* 1981;88:493-498.

25. Char DH. Thyroid Eye Disease. 2nd ed. New York: Churchill Livingstone; 1990:118.

26. Gamblin GT, Harper DG, Galentine P, Buck DR, Chernow B, Eil C. Prevalence of increased intraocular pressure in Graves' disease-Evidence of frequent subclinical ophthalmopathy. *N Engl J Med.* 1983;308: 420-424.

27. Grove AS Jr. Evaluation of exophthalmos. *N Engl J Med.* 1975;292:1005-1013.

28. Dallow RL. Evaluation of unilateral exophthalmos with ultrasonography: analysis of 258 consecutive cases. *Laryngoscope.* 1975;85:1905-1918.

29. Enzmann DR, Donaldson SS, Kriss JP. Appearance of Graves' disease on orbital computer tomography. *J Comput Assist Topnogr.* 1979;3:815-819.

30. Char DH. *Thyroid Eye Disease.* 2nd ed. New York: Churchill Livingstone; 1990:42.

31. Char DH. *Thyroid Eye Disease.* 2nd ed. New York: Churchill Livingstone; 1990:123.

32. Dyer JA. Ocular muscle surgery in Graves' disease. *Trans Am Ophthalmol Soc.* 1978;76:125-139.

33. Evans D, Kennerdell JS. Extraocular muscle surgery for dysthyroid myopathy. *Am J Ophthalmol.* 1983;95:767-771.

34. Kiloh LG, Nevin S. Progresive dystrophy of the external ocular muscles (ocular myopathy). *Brain.* 1951;74:115.

35. Archer SM, Sondhi N, Helveston EM. Strabismus in infancy. *Ophthalmology.* 1989; 96:133-137.

36. Meldorn E, Kommerell G. Inherited Duane's syndrome: mirror-like localization of oculomotor disturbance in monozygotic twins. *J Pediatr Ophthalmol Strabismus.* 1979;16:152-155.

37. Tredici TD, von Noorden GK. Are anisometropia and amblyopia common in Duane's syndrome? *J Pediatr Ophthalmol Strabismus.* 1985; 22:23-25.

38. Hotchkiss MG, Miller NR, Clark AW, Green WR. Bilateral Duane's retraction syndrome. A clinicopathologic case report. *Arch Ophthalmol.* 1980; 98: 870-874.

39. Huber A. Electrophysiology of the retraction syndrome. *Br J Ophthalmol.* 1974; 58:293-300.

40. Brown HW. Congenital structural muscle anomalies. In Allen JH. ed. *Strabismus ophthalmic symposium I.* St. Louis: CV Mosby Co; 1950:205.

41. Katz NN, Whitmore PV, Beauchamp GR. Brown's syndrome in twins. *J Pediatr Ophthalmol Strabis.* 1981;18:32-34.

42. Von Noorden GK. *Binocular Vision and Ocular Motility.* 4th ed. St. Louis: CV Mosby Co; 1990:406-407.

43. Johnson LV. Adherence syndrome: pseudoparalysis of the lateral or superior rectus muscles. *Arch Ophthalmol.* 1950; 44:870-878.

44. Raflo GT. Blow-in and blow-out fractures of the orbit: clinical correlations and proposed mechanisms. *Ophthalmol Surg.* 1984;15:114-119.

45. Von Noorden GK. *Binocular Vision and Ocular Motility.* 4th ed. St. Louis: CV Mosby Co; 1990:417.

46. Wojno, TH. The incidence of extraocular muscle and cranial nerve palsy in orbital floor blow-out fractures. *Ophthalmology.* 1987;94:682-685.

47. Von Noorden GK. *Binocular Vision and Ocular Motility.* 4th ed. St. Louis: CV Mosby Co; 1990:389.

48. Cogan DC. *Neurology of the Ocular Muscles.* 2nd ed. Springfield: Charles C Thomas; 1956:87.

49. Cogan DC. *Neurology of the Ocular Muscles.* 2nd ed. Springfield: Charles C Thomas; 1956:89.

50. Leigh RJ, Zee DS. *The Neurology of Eye Movements.* 2nd ed. *Contemporary Neurology Series.* Philadelphia: FA Davis Co; 1991:432.

51. Mein J, Trimble, R. *Diagnosis and Management of Ocular Motility Disorders.* 2nd ed. Oxford: Blackwell Scientific; 1991:369.

52. Mein J, Trimble, R. *Diagnosis and Management of Ocular Motility Disorders.* 2nd ed. Oxford: Blackwell Scientific; 1991:370.

53. Burde RM, Savino PJ, Trobe JD. *Clinical Decisions in Neuro-ophthalmology.* 2nd ed. St. Louis: CV Mosby Co; 1992:214-215.

54. Beck RW, Smith CH. *Neuro-Ophthalmology: A Problem-Oriented Approach.* Boston: Little, Brown; 1988: 179-182.

55. Scheiman MM. Optometric finding in children with cerebral palsy. *Amer J Optom Physiol Optics.* 1984;61: 321-323.

56. Leigh RJ, Zee DS. *The Neurology of Eye Movements.* Philadelphia: FA Davis Co, 1983:194.

57. Anderson JR. Latent nystagmus and alternating hyperphoria. *Brit J Ophthal.* 1954;38:217-231.

58. Lavin PJM. Nystagmus. In: Walsh TJ. *Neuro-Ophthalmology: Clinical Signs and Symptoms.* 2nd ed. Philadelphia: Lea & Febiger, 1985:427.

59. Stark L, Shults WT, Ciuffreda KJ, Hoyt WF, Kenyon RV, Ochs AL. Voluntary nystagmus is saccadic: Evidence from motor and sensory mechanisms. In: *Proceedings of the Joint Automatic Control Conference.* Pittsburgh: Instrument Society of America; 1977:1410-1414.

60. Zahn JR. Incidence and characteristics of voluntary nystagmus. *J Neurol Neurosurg Psychiatr.* 1978;41: 617-623.

61. Ciuffreda KJ. Voluntary nystagmus: new findings and clinical implications. *Amer J Optom Physiol Optics.* 1980;57:795-800.
62. Anderson JR. Cases and treatment of congenital eccentric nystagmus. *Brit J Ophthal.* 1953;37:267-281.
63. Nelson LB, Wagner RS, Harley RD. Congenital nystagmus surgery. *Internat Ophthal Clinic.* 1985;25: 133-138.
64. Shibasaki H, Yamashita Y, Motomura S. Suppression of congenital nystagmus. *J Neurol Neurosurg Psychiatry.* 1978;41:1078.
65. Lo C. Brain-computed tomographic evaluation of noncomitant strabismus and congenital nystagmus. In: Henkind P, ed. *ACTA, 24th Intern Congress of Ophthal.* vol 2. Philadelphia: Lippincott; 1982: 924-928.
66. Mallett RFJ. The treatment of congenital idiopathic nystagmus by intermittent photic stimulation. *Ophthalmol Physiol Optics,* 1983;3:341-356.
67. Grisham D. Management of nystagmus in young children. In: Scheiman MM, ed. *Problems in Optometry: Pediatric Optometry.* Philadelphia: Lippincott; 1990;2;3:496-527.
68. Harley RD. Pediatric neuro-ophthalmology. In: *Pediatric Ophthalmology.* 2nd ed. Philadelphia: WB Saunders Co, 1983:803.

PART TWO

TREATMENT

Chapter 9 / Philosophies and Principles of Binocular Vision Therapy

Philosophies   261
   Javal and the French School   261
   Worth and the English School   263
   Optometric Vision Therapy   264
Principles   265
   Sequence of Vision Therapy   265
   General Vergence Training
     Methods   267
     Sliding Vergence Training   268
     Step Vergence Training   268

Tromboning Vergence Training   269
Jump Vergence Training   269
Isometric Vergence Training   269
Office Training versus Home
   Training   270
Open Environment versus Instrument
   Training   271
Patient Motivation   271
Monitoring Training Progress   273
Retainer Home Training   274

PHILOSOPHIES

Throughout antiquity there have been many attempts to cure strabismus, since it is a disfiguring condition. The ancient Egyptians recommended exotic ointments such as ground tortoise brain and oriental spices rubbed into the eyes. The classical Greeks prescribed exercise and physical conditioning for relief of eyestrain. In medieval Europe, where strabismus was associated with the "evil eye" and witchcraft, hats with colored tassels were worn in an attempt to straighten the wandering eye. In sixteenth century Germany and France, stabismics wore "squint masks" with eyeholes that were positioned in such a way as to make full-field vision impossible only when the eyes were actually aligned. Although squint masks were unattractive, this procedure may have been the first effective vision therapy technique for intermittent strabismus. The masks provided patients with a visual feedback system, which let them know when the eye was straight and when it was not, so a conscious effort could be made to hold the eye in alignment. Binocular vision therapy principles and techniques evolved out of the attempt to cure strabismus and were later applied to many other binocular anomalies, with significant success. This chapter presents the philosophical foundations for binocular vision therapy, its efficacy with various binocular anomalies, and current principles guiding its clinical application.

Javal and the French School

Louis Emile Javal (1839-1907), a French ophthalmologist and professor at the Sorbonne in Paris, is considered the "father of orthoptics." Orthoptics is a traditional term, literally meaning "straight eyes;" it refers to a training process for eliminating strabismus and other binocular vision or oculomotor anomalies. Javal's work was unique among eye doctors, past and present, in the time he devoted to each patient and the detail of his observations. His father, an esotrope, underwent one of the early operations for strabismus with the sad outcome of a large consecutive exotropia. Javal did not want the same fate to befall his younger sister,

---

> **TABLE 9-1.** *Philosophical Approaches to Binocular Vision Training*
>
> **Javal and the French School**
>
> - Orthoptics developed as an alternative to extraocular muscle surgery in cases of strabismus.
> - Correction of ametropia with lenses.
> - Emphasis on antisuppression techniques.
> - Introduction of free-space, centration-point training.
>
> **Worth and the English School**
>
> - Theory of faulty faculty of fusion as an etiology of strabismus.
> - Development of amblyoscope for sensory-motor fusion training.
> - Importance of pre- and post-surgical vision training.
> - Emphasis on early vision therapy intervention.
>
> **Optometric Vision Therapy**
>
> - Adopting the concepts of Javal, Worth, Maddox, and other medical authors, optometrists have significantly expanded the scientific literature on the nature of binocular vision, its disorders, and management.
> - Emphasis on optical management of binocular conditions using prisms and adds.
> - Development of many open-environment training techniques.
> - Emphasis on training for efficient binocular skills and achieving visual comfort in cases of minimal binocular dysfunction, strabismus, and other conditions.

Sophie, who also had an esotropia. As an alternative to surgery, he devised a series of sensory and motor fusion exercises to straighten the eyes. An excellent summary of the functional training procedures for strabismus used by Javal can be found in a book by Revell.[1] Javal's first step was to equalize the vision in each eye by means of spectacles for refractive error. He then eliminated amblyopia by occlusion, an idea he probably found in the published works of the French naturalist Buffon.[1] Even after amblyopia had been cured, occlusion was continued to treat suppression, which was his important personal contribution.

Javal's recognition of the role of suppression in strabismus is one of the great strides in the field of binocular vision therapy. He used stereoscopes for antisuppression training by modifying stereograms with suppression clues. Brewster stereoscopes were used for small deviations; Wheatstone stereoscopes were used for larger angles of strabismus. Training began with large peripheral targets that were gradually made smaller as progress was made in breaking suppression. Javal advocated free-space training at the crossing point of the visual axes (i.e., the centration point) in cases of esotropia. The purpose was to create fusion at that point by using a flame as a target and an awareness of diplopia by placing an object either in front or in back of the fixation target (i.e., physiological diplopia). Vergence ranges along the midline were developed by moving the fixation target back and forth while the patient monitored suppression via physiological diplopia. Bar reading was then used for breaking central suppression. Javal believed that treatment could be expected to take as long as the duration of strabismus, and many of his cases took three to five years to effect a cure. Javal's remarkable success in many cases, including his sister's, established the practice of orthoptics. Table 9-1 summarizes philosophic approaches to strabismus therapy.

Notable among those practitioners following the teachings of Javal were Remy and Cantonnet. Remy is known for refining Javal's methods of antisuppression training and for the development of the Remy separator (used for divergence training in eso deviations). Cantonnet introduced the concept of "mental effort," and antisuppression methods included the hole-in-hand, adaptation of the Wheatstone stereoscope (as a home training device), and the effective use of anaglyphic targets.[2]

Mental effort is an important factor in the therapy of strabismus.[3] It may aid the esotrope in making divergence movements. A way to instruct the patient to do this is to have the patient imagine looking at a distant object above the horizon. In a similar manner, the exotrope should try to visualize fixating an object nearby in a downward position of gaze.

"Mental effort" represents a mental attitude in which the patient actively attempts to hold the suppression clues in perception and a fused binocular image. Vision training is not a passive process, like wearing a patch or a compensating prism; patients are expected to exert a mental effort at all times. With repetition, this mental effort to fuse becomes automatic and reflexive, which is a primary vision training goal.

Worth and the English School

The concept that strabismus is caused by poor sensory fusion is largely attributed to an English ophthalmologist, Claude Worth (1869-1936).[4] He wrote, "Thus the essential cause of squint is a defect of the fusion faculty." He contended that binocular vision was either developed in the early plastic years or not at all. Worth thought the "fusion faculty" necessary for binocular vision normally reached full development before the end of the sixth year of life and that any attempt to train the fusion sense after that time was futile. According to this philosophy, it is wise to begin fusion training as soon as possible in cases of strabismus. In stressing the importance of early detection and treatment of strabismus, Worth stated, "Of the cases of squint in which efficient treatment is carried out from the first appearance of the deviation, only a small proportion will ever need operation." He believed in treating children 3 to 5 years old and sometimes younger, providing they were cooperative. He trained the fusion sense by using the amblyoscope, which he invented for that purpose. The idea behind fusion training was that good sensory fusion creates a "desire for binocular vision." Worth wrote, "In children under 3 years of age, this treatment is apt to be rather difficult, though I have succeeded in many cases. After 5 years of age the fusion training takes longer, and a much less powerful desire for binocular vision is obtained." Worth conceded that some older patients who had strabismus for a long time could achieve binocularity as a result of the deviation being corrected. He stuck to the contention, however, that the apparently new development of fusion was not really new, but was present before the deviation became manifest although it was originally too weak to prevent the deviation from becoming manifest. The concept of re-education of fusion is still generally accepted today.

Worth thought that a faulty "faculty of fusion" was sometimes congenital. Today this is recognized as a genetic possibility in many cases of infantile esotropia in which there is lack of retinal correspondence. Even some non-strabismic individuals are missing a particular class of cortical disparity detectors for stereopsis, probably a genetic defect.[5]

Worth's philosophy was elaborated by Chavasse,[6] who stressed that the development of binocular vision was dependent on reflexes that require both time and usage. Chavasse, however, did not accept the concept of a faulty fusion faculty, but rather, he believed that the mechanism for fusion is present at birth, even in congenital strabismics. In order for the binocular reflexes to develop normally, it was extremely important for the infant to have the opportunity for early single binocular vision. Worth believed that most strabismics had an inherently weak or absent "fusion faculty," whereas Chavasse maintained that strabismus was caused by "obstacles to fusion," sensory, motor or central. Lyle and Bridgeman[7] presented a modified outline of these obstacles (Table 9-2). Both Worth and Chavasse were in accord to the extent that any hindrance to fusion should be eliminated and treated as quickly and early as possible.

Chavasse emphasized the need to eliminate obstacles by means other than orthoptics, namely optical and surgical procedures. As a result, many of his followers became disinterested in the functional training approach to strabismus. This negative influence notwithstanding, the overall influence of Chavasse can be considered positive. His great contributions were in the area of the developmental aspects of binocular vision. In terms of treatment, Chavasse emphasized the optical-surgical approach and Worth emphasized sensory-motor fusion training. We believe these two approaches are complementary in the full scope of strabismus vision therapy. The Worth-Chavasse model of binocular development and treatment is applicable today. An amalgamation

TABLE 9-2. *Obstacles in the Reflex Paths for Development of Binocular Vision (from Lyle and Bridgeman)*[7]

A. Sensory Obstacles
1. Dioptric obstacles
a. Uncorrected errors of refraction
b. Opacities of the media
2. Prolonged uniocular activity
a. Unilateral ptosis
b. Occlusion for one reason or another (e.g., injury)
3. Retinoneural obstacles (lesions in the visual pathways)
B. Motor Obstacles
1. Abnormalities of the orbit and adnexa (e.g., tumor that is space taking)
2. Conditions affecting one or more of the extrinsic ocular muscles
a. Congenital abnormalities (e.g., faulty insertion of a muscle)
b. Injury, particularly to lateral rectus in birth trauma
c. Contractures in cases of paresis
d. Disease of the muscle itself
3. Conditions affecting the central nervous system
a. Congenital absence of the oculomotor nerves or their supranuclear pathways
b. Head injury
c. Inflammation (e.g., encephalitis)
d. Supranuclear lesions
4. Decompensation of an extrinsic ocular muscle imbalance
C. Central obstacles
1. Psychogenic
2. Hyper or hypo excitability of the central nervous system
3. Central uniocular inhibition
4. Inability of the infant to learn

of the French and English schools of thought gradually evolved into what has become the standard philosophy of orthoptics.

Ernest Maddox (1863-1933), an English ophthalmologist, incorporated both the surgical and orthoptic treatment of strabismus. He developed several binocular testing and training instruments, including the cheiroscope, and trained his daughter, Mary Maddox, as a vision therapist.[8] Together, they founded one of the first orthoptic clinics that offered both pre- and post-surgical vision training. Mary Maddox became the first president of the British Orthoptics Association, a paraprofessional society of orthoptists who assist ophthalmologists in the management of strabismus. To this day, small paraprofessional groups of orthoptists are found in most English-speaking countries, including the United States. Many of them publish annual journals on the diagnosis and treatment of strabismus by surgical and nonsurgical methods.

Optometric Vision Therapy

At the beginning of the twentieth century in America, optometrists were concerned almost exclusively with clarity of eyesight. They determined the refractive error and prescribed lenses that eliminated blurred vision. In the 1920s, Charles Sheard, a biophysicist at Ohio State University, College of Optometry, designed a 19-point vision examination and binocular case analysis procedures, using phorometry measurements.[9,10] His concepts regarding binocular vision were in harmony with the scientific tradition of Helmholtz, Donders, Javal, Worth, and Chavasse. Sheard's contributions set the stage within academic optometry for the conceptual framework and the measurement of the "zone of clear, single, *comfortable,* binocular vision." Optometrists' interest centered on the evaluation and management of nonstrabismic binocular anomalies. They realized that vision problems and symptoms of many patients stemmed from deficient binocular skills. The vision training procedures of Javal, Worth, and Maddox were elaborated, modified, and applied to anomalies of vergence and accommodation in cases of heterophoria, as well as to strabismus. The later scientific works of Fry,[11,12] Morgan,[13,14] and Hoffstetter,[15,16] largely completed in the 1940s, substantially formed the basis for modern evaluation and management of accommodative-vergence anomalies. Ogle's work on fixation disparity,[17,18] in the 1950s and 1960s, added an important complimentary dimension. Since the 1930s, clinicians like Brock and

Vodnoy designed many open-environment training instruments and techniques to improve accommodative and vergence skills. This continuous scientific tradition, reaching back to the 19th century, has become known as classical optometric case analysis and management.

During the 1930s, A.M. Skeffington, a practicing American optometrist, founded a postgraduate education organization, the Optometric Extension Program (OEP). Skeffington promoted a "holistic" concept of vision and its development that emphasized how environmental demands might cause visual disorders (abnormal adaptations) and modify human behavior. A lasting influence of Skeffington's ideas and the OEP perspective within optometry is the concern for *vision efficiency and enhancement.* Optometrists now routinely measure how accommodation, vergence, and other visual skills affect performance over time. Developmental vision training (which includes procedures to improve visual, perceptual, and motor skills) and sports vision training follow in this "holistic" clinical tradition.

Binocular vision training evolved within the "medical model" of vision care. Developing within ophthalmology as a rehabilitative training technique for strabismus, orthoptics has a lot in common with physical therapy for general neuromuscular disorders or conditions. Vision training techniques were designed initially to reeducate and restore binocular vision with strabismics. This approach remains valid and beneficial for many patients, but optometry has taken binocular vision training several steps further. The term "vision therapy" is optometric in origin and refers to an overall program, usually including vision training besides other approaches (e.g., optics, surgery, hygiene, etc.), to remediate or enhance visual skills, not just binocular skills. When vision therapy is done to remediate binocular vision, the specific term indicating this activity would be binocular vision therapy or its synonym, orthoptics.

Approximately one in seven optometric patients, in our experience, has signs or symptoms of deficient binocular vision. Their primary care eye examination reveals no strabismus, disease, or other condition requiring medical or surgical treatment. These patients simply have a mismatch of their particular binocular vision physiology and their vision demands at school, work, or play. They experience visual discomfort, task inefficiency, and/or task avoidance and can be said to have minimal binocular dysfunctions. Exophoria, hyperphoria, reduced vergences, and hyperopia have all been found to occur more frequently among poor readers.[19] We believe that the primary care optometrist has the responsibility to identify these problems and manage them with optics and/or vision training. The therapeutic goals are binocular visual comfort and efficiency. This type of therapy is sometimes used for rehabilitation and other times for enhancing vision efficiency. Binocular enhancement training, per se, is a specialized form of physical education or conditioning. In this respect, it falls within the professional spectrum of health care activities, i.e., the primary care model. Modern day health care involves both concepts of rehabilitation, when necessary, and preventive "holistic" health conditioning. Primary care optometrists who provide vision therapy services utilize both these perspectives.

PRINCIPLES

Several principles of vision therapy apply generally to the practical implementation of a training program designed to remediate binocular vision. This section discusses these important principles and therapy options available to the clinician.

Sequence of Vision Therapy

One of Javal's first principles of binocular vision therapy in cases of strabismus is to address sensory obstacles before dealing with motor deficits. In a general sequence of implementing therapy for strabismics and heterophoria cases, any significant refractive error should be corrected optically. The results of both cycloplegic and noncycloplegic refractions should be evaluated to determine the optimum lens prescription for the patient. We want to emphasize that

TABLE 9-3. *General Sequence of Vision Therapy for Strabismus.*

- Ametropia correction; prisms and added lenses, if normal fusion can be achieved.
- Amblyopia therapy, visual acuity to at least 20/60 (6/18).
- ARC therapy, if prognosis for its elimination is favorable.
- Antisuppression therapy, if NRC, to establish diplopia awareness.
- Sensory-motor fusion enhancement, if NRC, for good stereopsis and fusional vergence ranges.
- Surgical procedures to reduce the angle of deviation to within the range of reflex fusional vergence, if necessary.
- Development of good oculomotor and binocular efficiency skills.
- Maintenance home exercises and periodic progress checkups.

correcting even small amounts of refractive error (e.g., 0.50 D of astigmatism or anisometropia; +1.00 D of hyperopia) can help patients maintain a higher level of binocular vision in many cases. At this point it is also appropriate to consider the effect of prescribing prisms and lens adds in reducing and controlling the deviation. The clinician should determine whether normal fusion can be immediately established using optics at some position in space. The prognosis for a functional cure significantly improves if fusion can be obtained, so the extra effort is often justified. Table 9-3 lists the general sequence of vision therapy for strabismus.

Amblyopia, eccentric fixation, deficient fixations, saccades, pursuits, and accommodation problems are all conditions that require early intervention in the general sequence of vision therapy. Monocular training predominates at this stage in the management of strabismus. Nearly all practitioners insist that attempts should be made to reduce amblyopia significantly before the binocular phase of training is started.[20] However, the degree of importance placed on the monocular phase of training varies from one practitioner to another. Some believe that all monocular motor responses should be improved to their maximum before binocular techniques are introduced; others, however, prefer to implement binocular along with monocular procedures. In this respect, we are not rigid in our therapeutic approach. We recommend an attempt initially be made to improve monocular fixation skills and the acuity of the amblyopic eye to the 20/60 (6/18) level or better. If progress becomes stalled at a poorer acuity level, we consider introducing binocular techniques earlier, particularly in anisometropic patients, in an attempt to continue momentum in the vision therapy program. When some progress is made, monocular techniques can be reintroduced. (See Chapter 10 for a complete discussion of amblyopia therapy.)

Once acuity has been improved to at least the 20/60 (6/18) level, the state of correspondence becomes the immediate concern. If normal "retinal" correspondence (NRC) exists, the practitioner can proceed to deal with suppression, which is the next step in the sequence. However, if the patient has anomalous "retinal" correspondence (ARC), a major decision needs to be made at this point. In many cases of strabismus of early onset, ARC can be an insurmountable obstacle to establishing normal binocular fusion and bifoveal fixation. Patients who show horror fusionis on the amblyoscope have a poor prognosis for developing good binocular vision with vision therapy. Also, if a patient has ARC on all tests (e.g., afterimages, amblyoscope, and Bagolini lenses), the prognosis for its elimination with vision therapy is poor. In such cases, we often do not recommend binocular training. The large investment of time, effort, and expense is often not justified by the hoped-for results. There is also the possibility of causing intractable diplopia in some cases.

If the strabismic patient with poor prognosis had amblyopia that was either partially or totally eliminated, techniques are now used to prevent regression of acuity and fixation skills. A monovision prescription (spectacles or contact lenses) may also be prescribed to promote alternate fixation. (Refer to discussion on optical penalization in Chapter 10.) Occasional direct occlusion may be recommended to maintain good results. If the strabismus is borderline cosmetically, reverse prisms may be prescribed to create the appearance of straight eyes. In cases of a large angle of deviation, we often refer the patient to a skilled strabismus surgeon in the hope of achieving a cosmetically acceptable result. Postsurgically, these patients are closely monitored for changes in the deviation or a reoccurrence of amblyopia.

On the other hand, if there are indications that ARC can be eliminated with vision therapy, we prefer to attempt a functional cure of the strabismus, which also means there will be a cosmetic cure. Certain patients respond well to ARC therapy, e.g., small-angle comitant esotrope (using the divergence training technique in the major amblyoscope), most comitant exotropes, and most other esotropes with lightly embedded ARC. (Refer to Chapter 11 for a discussion of ARC therapy indicators and techniques.)

The next step in the sequence of strabismus management is antisuppression training. When a patient has gone through ARC therapy, usually relatively little suppression remains. ARC is a form of binocular vision, an antidiplopia mechanism; relatively little suppression is necessary. Techniques used to remediate ARC are also powerful antisuppression methods; so by the time NRC is firmly established, central suppression usually has been eliminated. However, most strabismic patients having NRC as part of their original diagnosis have developed suppression to prevent diplopia. These patients as well as those who have gone through monocular amblyopia therapy usually require an aggressive attack on suppression to re-establish sensory and motor fusion. Antisuppression techniques were an important part of Javal's therapeutic approach to strabismus and amblyopia, and they remain so today. At this stage, an attempt is made to establish both physiological and pathological diplopia as an intermediate goal in the training sequence. (See Chapter 12 for a discussion of antisuppression procedures.)

The next step is referred to as sensory and motor fusion enhancement. (Sensory refers to the integrative functions of image singleness and stereopsis.) This step involves maximally increasing the fusional vergence ranges, both convergence and divergence, without suppression. At this point the strabismic patient may be aligned in the open environment using prism and lens add combinations, if possible, so that training instruments such as Vectograms or Tranaglyphs can be applied at the centration point. If alignment is not achieved, detailed second-degree or third-degree targets are placed at the angle of deviation using instruments, such as an amblyoscope, a Brewster stereoscope, and a Mirror Stereoscope. Fusional vergence ranges are increased using a variety of targets and techniques with an emphasis on breaking any suppression that occurs within the range of fusional vergence. Third-degree targets are used to build the awareness of stereopsis as well as to provide a further stimulus to maintain and increase fusional vergence ranges. At this point in the therapy sequence a decision regarding the need for extraocular muscle surgery must be made and acted on. The decision depends on whether sufficient sensory fusion and fusional vergences have been achieved. If they have not, surgery may be indicated. Sensory and motor fusion should be maximally increased prior to the operation. (See Chapter 13 for information on eso deviations and Chapter 14 for exo deviation.)

The final step in the management of strabismus is an integrative step referred to as vision efficiency training. All the oculomotor and binocular skills the patient has developed during the therapy program are finally enhanced, refined, and integrated. Speed, accuracy, and stamina of all oculomotor and binocular skills are developed to the highest degree to prevent or reduce the possibility of regression. (See Chapter 16 for a discussion on vision efficiency training.)

General Vergence Training Methods

Deficient fusional vergence responses are a characteristic feature in many binocular vision disorders. Strabismus results when there is insufficient fusional vergence to compensate for a deviation due to tonic and/or accommo-

---

TABLE 9-4. Vergence Training Methods

Vergence Training Method	Accommodative Demand	Vergence Demand	Vergence Response Process	Principal Training Goals for Increasing:
Sliding	Nonchanging	Continuous	Tonic	Vergence Ranges Smoothness Accuracy
Stepping	Nonchanging	Discontinuous	Phasic	Speed Vergence Ranges Stamina
Tromboning	Changing	Continuous	Tonic	Near-far range Smoothness Stamina
Jumping	Changing	Discontinuous	Phasic	Speed Near-far range Stamina
Isometrically Bifixating	Nonchanging	Stationary	Tonic	Vergence Ranges Stamina

---

dative vergence. Asthenopia occurs in many cases of heterophoria when fusional vergence is significantly stressed. Therefore, one of the principal goals in most vision therapy programs is to expand the range and quality of fusional vergence responses. To accomplish this, five modes of training fusional vergence are commonly used (Table 9-4). For a particular patient, some methods may be more appropriate and efficacious to apply than others at various stages in the vision training program. However, we recommend that each method be used at some point for the sake of generalization of skills, if for no other reason.

Sliding Vergence Training

Sliding vergence occurs when second- or third-degree fusion targets are set at a particular accommodative demand and slowly disparated in a continuous manner. The most common example of this method is the measurement of fusional vergence ranges with Risley prisms. Blur, break, and recovery points are routinely recorded. This testing method becomes a training technique when the patient is instructed to make a conscious effort to hold the targets single and clear for as long as possible with repetition. The speed of vergence tracking is not usually the goal, but effort is directed to increasing the horizontal or vertical vergence ranges as well as the smoothness and accuracy of vergence responses. The amblyoscope and Mirror Stereoscope are particularly suited to this mode of training in cases of strabismus; split Vectograms and Tranaglyphs are often used in heterophoric cases. The training targets typically contain suppression controls. If suppression occurs during the procedure, disparation is temporarily stopped and suppression is broken before proceeding. The patient's best vergence ranges are recorded at the end of each day's training session to monitor progress.

Step Vergence Training

Step vergence refers to the phasic introduction of a vergence stimulus in which the stimulus to accommodation is fixed. A common example is the use of loose prisms. The patient's attention is directed to a target at a particular viewing distance. A loose prism of an appropriate amount is placed before an eye. The patient may temporarily see a double image and makes a conscious effort to fuse the images quickly into one. As soon as the images are joined, the prism is removed or a larger step is introduced. In this case, the primary goal is to increase the speed of step vergence responses. The patient usually counts and records the number of steps completed within an assigned time interval (e.g., 1 or 2 minutes).

Additional goals can be established to increase the size of the step responses and to increase stamina by extending the training time. Another common training instrument, the Brewster stereoscope, has many stereograms with step demands of various sizes and suppression controls built into the target design. Step vergence training can be quite effective and efficient because of a rigorous time frame for the exercise and the direct stimulation of the dynamic components of fusional vergence; these are response latency, velocity, and amplitude.

Tromboning Vergence Training

Tromboning is a colloquial term that refers to a method of vision training in which the stimuli to both vergence and accommodation are continuously changing. A push-up exercise with a pencil is a common example. The patient attempts to track a pencil smoothly, moving from arm's length to the binocular nearpoint of accommodation (NPA) and convergence (NPC) and back again to arm's length. The primary goal is to increase the near-far bifixation range for clearness or singleness with the particular target or instrument assigned by the therapist. The patient records the best daily NPA and NPC achieved during the training session. Speed of vergence tracking can be an auxiliary goal, although it usually is not; increasing smoothness and stamina, however, are. For patients with eso deviations, tromboning targets on a Brewster stereoscope is particularly challenging. Paradoxically, as the accommodative stimulus increases, so does the stimulus to fusional divergence. Tromboning techniques can be conveniently done with most handheld vergence targets (e.g., eccentric circles, red-green circles, and Minivectograms). Tromboning is a popular method of vergence training with many primary eye care doctors.

Jump Vergence Training

Jump vergence (sometime incorrectly referred to as jump ductions and occasionally confused with step vergence) is another popular method of vergence training. Jump vergence occurs when a patient alternates fixation between two vergence targets placed at two different distances in space. The stimuli to both accommodation and vergence change in a phasic manner. For example, the patient can be asked to alternate fixation as quickly as possible between a television screen at far and a pencil tip positioned at approximately the patient's NPC. The patient counts the number of cycles completed during a commercial break in a program and attempts to increase that number with practice. Physiological diplopia can be used as a control on suppression. Besides speed, the goals include increasing the near-far amplitude of the jump and building stamina. Jump vergences can be used with many vision training instruments and most handheld targets.

Isometric Vergence Training

Isometric exercise occurs when the tension in a muscle increases without physical shortening of the muscle. This can be done with extraocular muscles by increasing a stationary, tonic load on the fusional vergence system using prisms, added lenses, or fusion targets with BI or BO demands. For example, base-out Fresnel prisms can be applied to the spectacle lenses of an exophoric patient and worn daily for a prescribed period. In this way, the demand on fusional convergence is increased. Similarly, a minus-add or a base-in clip-over can be prescribed for an esophoric patient to wear during the morning hours, to increase fusional divergence. Another example would be to require an esotropic patient to hold a maximally diverged position on an amblyoscope using fused third-degree targets for 5 minutes at a time. Experiments by Vaegan[21] have shown that isometric vergence exercises of this type result in large and sustained increases in vergence ranges after a short training time. Although effective, this mode of vergence training must be carefully monitored by the therapist because a patient may experience intolerable symptoms or the demand may prove to be too large to maintain bifixation. Besides increasing vergence ranges, isometric exercise is effective in building stamina.

Each method of vergence training has a logical application with particular types of vergence dysfunctions. These will be described in subsequent chapters, but usually all five modes can and should be utilized, in our opinion, at some point within a sequence of training procedures. Generally speaking, we believe a training program should emphasize the phasic methods of step and jump vergence. Daum[22] found that phasic techniques expanded convergence and divergence ranges more effectively than did the tonic methods of tromboning and sliding vergence. We believe there is value in utilizing all five methods of vergence training, if possible, to promote the generalization and permanence of the training effect. Even though conscious effort is used to improve vergence skills, the permanence of results requires training at a reflexive level of functioning. Certainly, vision training builds conditioned reflexes through repetition. Sufficient repetition is fundamental to acquiring motor skills in athletics, physical therapy, or vision therapy. We also think that generalization of vergence training is an important means of extending the training effect to the required reflexive level.

Office Training versus Home Training

Most vision training programs for strabismic and heterophoric conditions involve some combination of home training and office training visits, but practitioners vary greatly in the relative emphasis of the two. We have no strong recommendations in this regard since there are so many variables involved; however, it may be helpful to review some of the important considerations. The more severe the condition, the greater is the need for office training visits. Office visits directly supervised by the doctor or vision therapist are usually more effective, efficient, and motivating than unsupervised home training sessions. This principle applies to patients of all ages. Moreover, when a particular in-office procedure proves too difficult or ineffective, it can be changed immediately to a more effective one. Most patients with strabismus and amblyopia make better progress with frequent office training visits, ideally two or three times per week, supplemented by home training.

We have found that most cases of heterophoria, accommodative dysfunction, and minimal binocular disorders can be successfully managed on a home training basis when supplemented with weekly in-office visits. The patient must be mature enough and sufficiently motivated to complete at least five home sessions per week, although seven sessions per week is the stated goal. Consistent and frequent repetition produces the best results. If the patient is 6 years old or younger, office visits (two or more times per week) are often needed for effective treatment, despite good parental involvement at home. School-aged children routinely need direct adult supervision, usually that of a parent. In some cases, a friend, relative, or paid tutor can be substituted. The home training supervisor (the "coach") needs to attend at least some office visits to receive proper instructions from the doctor or vision therapist and directly observe the techniques in process. The home supervisor must be capable of effective supportive communication with the child to maintain a high level of motivation and compliance. In older children who do not have sufficient self-discipline or effective adult supervision in the home, relatively frequent office visits are required to achieve a successful vision training outcome.

For a home training program, we usually assign three different training techniques each week. Patients tend to get bored with only one or two procedures, and overwhelmed or confused when more than three are given. At least one technique should be changed each week to add variety, build motivation, and promote generalization of the learned skills. Initially in a training program, fairly easy training procedures should be assigned so the patient will experience some early successes. The patient must demonstrate the ability to perform each technique correctly to the doctor's or vision therapist's satisfaction before it is assigned for home use. In our clinics, printed instruction sheets for each exercise are given out to help patients remember the proper way to perform each technique.

We require a minimum commitment of 30 minutes per day of active training during the home therapy program. In this way, each technique is practiced at least 10 minutes each day. In the case of vergence dysfunction, it is preferable and more effective to conduct two or three short training sessions at different times each day rather than assigning one long daily session.[23] Some patients, due to favorable schedules and good motivation, can find and commit more than 30 minutes each day to active vision therapy. This commitment is of course desirable and to be encouraged. We have had some strabismic patients who routinely completed 2 hours of active vision training each day for a 3-month period. We feel this level of time commitment from the patient should be voluntary and not demanded by the doctor. Before initiating a home-based vision therapy program, the patient needs to review his or her weekly schedule realistically and to commit the required amount of time to the program. If a realistic appraisal reveals that regular home training sessions will be difficult to achieve due to unavoidable circumstances, then 2 or 3 hour in-office training program conducted each week may offer a better solution.

Open Environment versus Instrument Training

Whenever possible, the practitioner should assign open environment training procedures rather than instrument training. Closed-box type instruments, such as the amblyoscope, Brewster stereoscope, and cheiroscope, have some inherent disadvantages. They often stimulate spurious accommodative and vergence responses. Also, visual skills learned inside an instrument do not always transfer well to the open environment. For example, it is preferable and more effective to train an exotropic patient to fuse at near fixation distances using gross convergence techniques rather than working on vergence ranges around the angle of deviation in an amblyoscope. However, an amblyoscope or Brewster stereoscope has its

place in many vision therapy programs. These instruments are particularly effective in establishing NRC in cases of ARC, breaking suppression, and building fusional vergence ranges. Vision training for esotropes and amblyopes often involves the use of an amblyoscope or other box-type instruments, but most other binocular vision cases can be managed more efficiently using open-environment instruments and techniques (e.g., television trainers, Vectograms, Tranaglyphs, and prism flippers).

Patient Motivation

Proper patient motivation is indispensable to success in a vision training program. Without a real desire for success, patient compliance with vision training procedures falters and fails. For many adults, particularly for those who are well-educated, simply knowing that they can overcome their binocular deficiency or ameliorate their visual symptoms is motivation enough to comply. Nevertheless, some adult patients who would otherwise qualify for a binocular cure with vision training may not want to make the prerequisite effort or cannot find enough time in their busy schedule. Everything that can be done with lenses and prisms should be done for these patients. The doctor simply explains the condition and the treatment options to the patient, makes appropriate recommendations, and then gives the patient time to make a considered decision.

Preschool and elementary school children usually comply with vision therapy procedures to please their parents or doctor. The doctor's rapport with the child in vision training is critical for success. When working with a child in a vision training program, it is wise for the doctor to spend time and energy building a relationship characterized by respect, caring, personal knowledge, and fun. Each doctor, as an individual, has a unique way of establishing rapport with children. Table 9-5 lists some recommendations in this regard.

A critical skill in building motivation is effective communication. In the case of children, the doctor needs to remember he or she is talking with a child, not a small adult. The language used needs to be age appropriate.

TABLE 9-5. Ways to Build Rapport with a Child in a Vision Training Program

- Design a child's corner in the patient's waiting area equipped with a table, chairs, games, coloring books, and reading books.
- Take a personal interest in the child as a unique individual. Ask about interests, hobbies, pets, games, likes, and dislikes. Write these in the record and refer to these on future occasions.
- Modify the training activities to reflect the child's individuality.
- Post the name and a photo of each child in vision training on a conspicuous bulletin board.
- Ask the child to make a drawing or painting that can be posted on the bulletin board.

Vision training techniques and instructions should be matched to the patient's cognitive level and understanding. For example, chiastopic fusion in the open environment is usually an unrealistic procedure for a child under age 7 who is in Piaget's preoperational stage of cognitive development,[24] but a 3-dot convergence card can usually be mastered at this stage. The goals of each technique must be clearly stated and understood by the patient. We find that if goals are put within a time frame, the technique is often more effective. For example, the goal of a jump vergence procedure (e.g., looking from a wall clock to a favorite small toy placed just beyond the nearpoint of convergence) might be to count the number of jumps completed in 1 minute. A minimum of seven 1-minute sets are to be completed and recorded each day with the goal of increasing the number of jumps (per set). A printed instruction sheet is given to the parent to ensure that the technique is done correctly at home. The vision therapist must also be responsive to the patient's complaints and expressions of frustration. Often simply listening and acknowledging a patient's complaint sufficiently encourages continued effort. Other times, instruments, techniques, or applications of procedures need to be changed.

Another important topic to complete this discussion on building motivation in children

is the use of rewards. Ideally, the vision training activity itself should be reward enough. The child should want to do the task or exercise because it is challenging, rewarding, and enjoyable. Unfortunately, many children find some vision training techniques too challenging, boring, or unpleasant. The doctor's goal should be to use rewards so the child's attitude approaches the ideal. One good place to start is to try to incorporate the child's enjoyable activities into the training program. In cases of strabismus, every attempt should be made with optics and active training to get the patient fusing at least part of the time in the open environment. If the patient is heterophoric, so much the better. To build accommodative and vergence skills, the training targets become the television, a favorite toy, an exciting story or comic book, or a computer game. Appropriate powers for flipper lenses and prisms can be used with these targets while the child engages in a desired activity. As it happens, many games and fun activities can be effectively used for amblyopia therapy while the child is occluding the dominant eye. (See Chapter 10 for a description of amblyopia therapy techniques.) The clinician should look for opportunities to incorporate the child's prized activities, interests, and games into the training program.

When standard orthoptic instruments and targets are utilized, boredom can be lessened by putting the technique into a time frame, as discussed above, and by using a pointer stick to touch targets. Varying techniques or instruments frequently is important because variety remains the proverbial "spice of life." Also, verbal rewards, tokens, or prizes are often underutilized motivational techniques of parents, teachers, employers, and vision therapists. Most adults work for interest, money, goods, services, acknowledgment, and other expressions of appreciation. Children similarly need reinforcers when they perform demanding and sometimes unpleasant tasks.

Many types of rewards can be used as reinforcers to shape a child's behavior, attitudes, and learning skills. This point was made repeatedly in psychological research of the 1960s and 1970s on learning theories.[25] Some general conclusions were made that may be applicable to vision training. Learning any new skill seems to progress most rapidly and effectively when the desired response is rewarded immediately, frequently, and regularly. Initially, little steps in the correct direction are reinforced; later, larger steps toward improvement are rewarded. As skills, behaviors, and attitudes are shaped and correctly learned, the most effective reinforcement schedule of rewards seems to be intermittent and variable.[26] The vision therapist may want to apply these Skinnerian concepts in a concerted way if the child seems to be losing interest, slacking in effort, or making slow progress during the training program. Table 9-6 lists several rewards children have responded to that have resulted in heightened motivation in a vision therapy program. Giving children rewards for doing vision therapy should not be considered a bribe. Children often find vision training difficult and demanding. Instead, a parent or vision therapist should reward a child's effort, endurance, and self discipline.

A number of computer-based vision training programs are commercially available. Three popular systems are Computer Orthoptics, the Opti-mum System, and the Bernell System (see Appendix F for addresses). These programs are designed to break suppression, increase fusional vergence ranges and facility, improve accommodative skills, train oculomotor skills, and also enhance certain perceptual skills. The training tasks are often structured in an interactive game format for which children seem to have a natural affinity. Some parents believe that computer games have become a national obsession. Although the addictive quality of these games may be some parent's nightmare, computer vision training just may be the vision therapist's dream come true. In our clinics, we have successfully used computer vision training with children as a highly prized reward for home training compliance and after other difficult in-office procedures. The enormous potential of computer vision training is being realized.

In summary, we believe that a vision therapist can be successful in building a patient's motivation to participate fully in a vision therapy program through the means of building

TABLE 9-6. *Rewards for Children in Vision Training Programs*

- Use immediate rewards to shape behavior: stickers, beads, small toys, marbles, peanuts, raisins, cereal.
- Videotape the child doing training to show afterwards as a reward.
- Show the child a magic trick once a week. After faithfully completing home training, give the child the trick and show how it is done.
- Allow a child, who has participated well in an in-office vision training session, to pick a prize from the treasure chest and take another prize for a friend if home training was completed.
- Let the child earn coupons for desired minor items: ice cream, hamburger, toy, book, a movie, etc.
- Have the parents agree to purchase some desired major item (e.g., skates, a wagon, or a bicycle) for the child at the end of the training program provided enough credits have been built up. The child earns the prize by collecting 50 tokens, for example, during the program. A token is given when the therapist wants to reward the child's behavior.
- Post a progress chart on a wall. One popular version is a trip through the solar system in which the child gets a prize each time his/her "rocket ship lands on a planet."
- Present a Certificate of Completion, generated on a computer, with the child's name, suitable for framing, of course.

rapport, effective communication, and the judicious use of rewards.

Monitoring Training Progress

An important principle of vision therapy is providing the patient with feedback regarding the status of his or her visual condition and training progress at every stage of the program. Most of the targets used in vision training have means to monitor sensory and motor fusion status, e.g., checks for suppression and stereopsis. Afterimage or Haidinger brush foveal tags are examples of visual feedback indicators for fixation accuracy. Buzzing devices provide auditory feedback for correct or incorrect responses. For example, the Franzbrau Coordinator and the Wayne Talking Pen are auditory feedback instruments used in the development of eye-hand coordination. Furthermore, some of the new computerized vision training programs have incorporated auditory as well as visual feedback indicators. Pointer sticks are often used with many training procedures to provide tactile-kinesthetic feedback, e.g., placing toothpicks in a soda straw in amblyopia therapy. Continuous feedback to the patient is fundamental for effective vision training.

The doctor must receive accurate and frequent information about the patient's home training progress. With in-office training, the doctor or therapist is present to observe the patient's performance, but monitoring home training must take a different form (Table 9-7). At each office visit, the doctor or therapist must carefully question the patient about symptoms, complaints, compliance with prescribed therapy, performance, and any difficulty experienced. The patient should return with a completed home training recording sheet of each day's progress, and review it with the therapist. The patient should also demonstrate each of the techniques used at home the previous week, so the therapist can make suggestions and corrections to improve performance. We want to emphasize this point. Some doctors prescribe home training procedures, assuming the patient fully understands each, and then schedules the patient for a progress visit in a month. In most cases, this is a recipe for failure and patient frustration. Careful and frequent monitoring of a patient's progress is the only way to ensure effective home vision training. The patient's motivation level should also be assessed at each office visit. Motivational support for the patient and the home training coach, if there is one, should be sincerely offered in a professional manner. Two or three appropriate clinical tests, depending on the patient's diagnosis, should be regularly monitored by the doctor for independent evaluation of therapy progress. The remainder of the office visit can be spent performing directly supervised training procedures that are not feasible at home and teaching the patient new home training techniques. An in-office monitoring and/or training visit usually takes between 45 minutes to 1 hour to complete. The patient may

---

TABLE 9-7. *Objectives for In-office Monitoring of a Home Vision Training Program*

- Review weekly home training progress, performance, difficulties, symptoms, questions, and compliance.
- Directly observe the patient performing the assigned home training procedures and give advice.
- Give motivational support to the patient and home training coach, if there is one.
- Evaluate progress in the training program using both standardized and informal testing, and modify the program accordingly.
- Thoroughly instruct the patient (and "coach" or helper at home) in new home procedures for the following week.

---

not be required to perform the home training exercises that day if effective in-office training is done and home training compliance has been satisfactory.

Retainer Home Training

The last principle we want to discuss here is the need to prescribe some means for the trained patient to monitor any regression of the learned skills. The literature indicates that in most cases of heterophoria and vergence insufficiency, one can expect to see little clinically significant regression if the patient has been sufficiently trained to meet high release criteria.[27,28,29] (Specific release criteria for each condition are in accordance with criteria in Chapter 2 and discussed in subsequent chapters.) If a patient is released from therapy before all the criteria have been satisfactorily achieved, regression can occur within the period of a year or two.[28] In cases of amblyopia and strabismus, some regression may be expected over time. For these reasons, all patients should be given at least one home training technique and monitored periodically for regression. If regression of skills is observed, the patient can implement one or two prescribed home training procedures, 20 minutes per day, for 1 week or so, as needed. If the previously achieved level of performance is not met within a week, or easily maintained thereafter, the patient should return to the doctor for additional vision therapy. When the doctor suspects that regression is inevitable, retainer exercises can be prescribed on a reduced but regular schedule, indefinitely.

There are many other important principles of vision therapy that will be discussed in subsequent chapters focusing on specific binocular conditions. Specific examples of the principles discussed in this chapter are found in the chapters on therapeutic management.

REFERENCES

1. Revell MJ. *Strabismus: A History of Orthoptic Techniques.* London: Barrie & Jenkins; 1971:15-23.
2. Cantonnet A, Filliozat J. *Strabismus- Its Re-education: The Physiology and Pathology of Binocular Vision.* London: M Wiseman and Co; 1934.
3. Gibson HW. *Textbook of Orthoptics.* London: Hatton Press Ltd, 1955:289-290.
4. Worth C. *Squint- Its Causes, Pathology, and Treatment.* Philadelphia: P Blakiston's Son and Co; 1921.
5. Richards W. Anomalous stereoscopic depth perception. *J Opt Soc Am.* 1971;61:410-414.
6. Chavasse FB. *Worth's Squint, the Binocular Reflexes and the Treatment of Strabismus.* 7th ed. Philadelphia: P Blakiston's Sons and Co; 1939.
7. Lyle TK, Bridgeman GJ. *Worth and Chavasse's Squint- The Binocular Reflexes and the Treatment of Strabismus.* 9th ed. London: Bailliere, Tindall and Cox; 1959.
8. Duke Elder S. *Ocular Motility and Strabismus in System of Ophthalmology.* vol vi. London: Henry Kimpton; 1973:245.
9. Sheard C. *Dynamic Ocular Tests.* Columbus: Lawrence Press; 1917.
10. Sheard C. Zones of ocular comfort. *Trans Am Acad Optom.* 1928;3:113-129.
11. Fry GA. An experimental analysis of the accommodation-convergence relation. *Trans Arch Am Acad Optom.* 1937;14:402-414.
12. Fry GA. Further experiments on the accommodation-convergence relationship. *Trans Am Acad Optom.* 1938;12:65-74.
13. Morgan MW. Accommodation and its relationship to convergence. *Am J Optom Arch Acad Optom.* 1944;183-195.
14. Morgan MW. Analysis of clinical data. *Am J Optom Arch Am Acad Optom.* 1944;21:477-491.
15. Hofstetter HW. Zone of clear single binocular vision. *Am J Optom Arch Am Acad Optom.* 1945;22:301-333; 361-384.
16. Hofstetter HW. Orthoptics specification by a graphical method. *Am J Optom Arch Am Acad Optom.* 1949;26:439-444.
17. Ogle KN. *Research in Binocular Vision.* Philadelphia: Saunders; 1950.
18. Ogle KN, Martens TG, Dyer JA. *Oculomotor Imbalance in Binocular Vision and Fixation Disparity.* Philadelphia: Lea & Febiger; 1967.
19. Grisham JD, Simons H. Perspectives on Reading Disabilities In: Rosenbloom A, Morgan M, eds. Pediatric Optometry. Philadelphia: Lippincott; 1990:518-559.
20. Ciuffreda KJ, Levi DM, Selenow A. *Amblyopia: Basic and Clinical Aspects.* Newton, Mass.: Butterworth-Heinemann,; 1991:411-493.
21. Vaegan. Con and divergence show large and sustained improvement after short isometric exercise. *Am J Optom Physiol Opt.* 1979;56:23-33.
22. Daum KM. A comparison of the results of tonic and phasic vergence training. *Am J Optom Physiol Optics.* 1983;60:769-775.
23. Daum KM. The course and effect of visual training on the vergence system. *Am J Optom Physiol Opt.* 1982;59:223-227.
24. Wilson JAR, Robeck MC, Michael WB. Psychological Foundation of Learning and Teaching. New York McGraw-Hill Book Co, 1974.
25. Klausmeier HJ, Ripple RE. *Learning and Human Abilities: Educational Psychology.* 3rd ed. New York: Harper & Row; 1971.
26. Hershey GL, Lugo JO. *Living Psychology: An Experimental Approach.* London: Macmillan Co; 1970.
27. Grisham JD, Bowman MC, Owyang LA, Chan CL. Vergence orthoptics: validity and persistence of the training effect. *Optom Vision Sci.* 1991;68:441-451.
28. Pantano F. Orthoptic treatment of convergence insufficiency: a two year follow-up report. *Am Orthopt J.* 1982;32:73-80.
29. Griffin JR, Bui K, Ko C. *Durability of vision therapy.* Ketchum Library, Southern California College of Optometry, Fullerton, 1991. Thesis.

Chapter 10 / Therapy for Amblyopia

Management of Refractive Error   278
Occlusion Procedures   280
   Direct Occlusion   280
   Preventing Occlusion Amblyopia   282
   Types of Occluders   282
   Motivation and Patching
     Management   283
   Patching Progress   284
   Efficacy of Occlusion and Amblyopia
     Therapy   284
   Penalization   286
     Penalization Methods   286
     Penalization Management   288
     Efficacy of Penalization   289
   Red Filter Therapy and Occlusion   290
   Prism Therapy and Occlusion   290
   Short Term Occlusion   291
Monocular Fixation Training   292
   Fixation and Ocular Motility Activities
     (Without Foveal Tag)   292
   Eye-Hand Coordination
     Techniques   292
     Tracing and Drawing T10.1   293
     Throwing and Hitting Games
       T10.2   293
     Video Game Tracking T10.3   293
     Swinging Ball Training T10.4   294
     Tracking with Auditory Feedback
       T10.5   295
     Visual Tracing T10.6   295
     Ann Arbor Tracking T10.7   295
   Resolution Techniques   297
     Hart Charts T10.8   297
     Counting Small Objects T10.9   298
     Reading for Resolution T10.10   299
     Tachistoscopic Training
       T10.11   299

     Monocular Telescope T10.12   299
Foveal Tag Techniques   300
   Preparation for Haidinger Brush
     Training   300
   Preparation for Afterimage Transfer
     Training   300
   Foveal Tag Training   301
     Basic Central Fixation Training
       T10.13   301
     Steadiness of Fixation Training
       T10.14   301
     Saccadic Movements with Tag
       T10.15   302
     Foveal Localization (Fast Pointing)
       T10.16   303
     Pursuits with Tag T10.17   303
     Resolution Practice with Tag
       T10.18   304
Pleoptics   305
   Bangerter's Method   305
   Cüppers' Method   306
   Efficacy of Pleoptics   307
   Practical Pleoptic Techniques   308
     Vodnoy Afterimage Technique
       T10.19   308
     Cüppers Home Pleoptics T10.20   309
Binocular Therapy for Amblyopia   309
   Anomalous Correspondence
     Considerations   310
   Suppression and Amblyopia   310
   Antisuppression Techniques for
     Amblyopia Therapy   310
     Red Filter and Red Print T10.21   311
     Visual Tracking with a Brewster
       Stereoscope T10.22   311
     Bar Reading and Tracking
       T10.23   312

Recommendations for Binocular Training 312

Progress in Amblyopia Therapy 313

Case Examples 314

Case no. 1: Adult Anisometropic Amblyopia 314

Case no. 2: Anisometropic and Strabismic Amblyopia 319

This discussion of amblyopia therapy presupposes that an accurate differential diagnosis has been established and that the patient's visual acuity loss is not caused by psychogenic, structural or pathological processes. (See Chapter 5 regarding amblyopia diagnosis.) The patients we are concerned with here have primarily a functional type of amblyopia (i.e., isoametropic, anisometropic, strabismic, or image degradation amblyopia) and have a realistic chance for either improvement or cure with vision therapy.

Besides *optical correction,* the most commonly used therapeutic method for amblyopia is *direct occlusion.* Many cases are managed successfully using only these two "passive" therapy options. "Active" vision therapy is often recommended to speed up the rehabilitation process and to increase the chance of success. Some of the intermediate vision training goals include: (1) training steady central fixation; (2) building accurate pursuit and saccadic eye movements; (3) increasing the amplitude and facility of accommodation; (4) breaking suppression and building sensory and motor fusion; and (5) improving visual acuity to normal or near normal levels. If the patient with functional amblyopia does not respond to the use of optics, occlusion, and conventional vision training, then pleoptic techniques and other special procedures may be tried in a last attempt for visual rehabilitation. This chapter discusses the use of amblyopia remedial methods in sequence, their advantages and disadvantages, their efficacy, and will address several important issues in the overall implementation of amblyopia therapy. Table 10-1 lists the general sequence of amblyopia therapy and training objectives; this sequence serves as the organizational structure for our discussion. Specific training techniques are numbered for easy reference (T10.1 to T10.23) as they are introduced.

MANAGEMENT OF REFRACTIVE ERROR

Correction of any significant refractive error, particularly anisometropia and astigmatism, is fundamental to effect a cure of functional amblyopia. The patient's refractive error is often an important factor, if not the most important, in the etiology of amblyopia. Successful, efficient, and enduring visual rehabilitation requires the elimination of all amblyogenic

---

TABLE 10-1. Sequence of Amblyopia Therapy

1. Correct the full refractive error
2. Occlusion therapy
3. Eye-hand coordination training
4. Visual resolution training
5. Active vision training to establish steady central fixation with foveal tag procedures.
   a. Train central fixation
   b. Train steady fixation
   c. Train saccadic accuracy
   d. Train foveal localization
   e. Train pursuit accuracy
6. Auxiliary therapy for eccentric fixation (if necessary): pleoptics, red filter, and inverse prism
7. Active vision training of accommodation
8. Establish normal binocular vision (if possible and prudent)
   a. Break suppression
   b. Train monocular fixation and resolution of the amblyopic eye under binocular conditions
   c. Extend the range of sensory and motor fusion to the maximum degree
   d. Surgery for strabismus (if necessary)
9. Prescribe appropriate maintenance procedures (e.g., periodic occlusion, retainer home training, monovision lenses)
10. Periodic office visits to monitor for regression and provide follow-up management

factors. Even small amounts of refractive error (e.g., 0.50 D of anisometropia and astigmatism) can be significant in some cases. The clinician should remember there is often a latent component to hyperopia that may need to be revealed with cycloplegia. We believe the importance of correcting the full refractive error cannot be overemphasized. If a patient continually refuses to wear a needed optical correction or demonstrates persistent noncompliance, the clinician is forced to dismiss the patient from amblyopia therapy and reschedule only when cooperation can be fully enlisted.

Many practitioners find that frequent changes in the lens prescription may be necessary for the amblyopic eye for various reasons.[1] Objective cycloplegic refractive techniques are usually required that may lack sufficient accuracy depending on the skills of the clinician and other factors. The refraction may not be precisely on the visual axis due to a strabismus or eccentric fixation. Also, in younger children, the actual refractive error may change over short time periods. Therefore, clinicians should frequently recheck and refine an amblyopic patient's refractive correction, possibly once a month in some cases. As visual acuity improves, subjective refractive techniques can become more refined for an exact lens prescription. Patients or parents need to understand that several lens changes may be necessary as part of a vision therapy program for amblyopia.

Some clinicians are conservative when prescribing for the full amount of hyperopia, astigmatism, and anisometropia. They anticipate that the patient may not adapt easily to the new prescription lenses. They reduce the optical correction by some amount based on their experience or previous training. In managing binocular vision cases in general, and amblyopes in particular, we believe this approach is not usually warranted. Since the amblyopic eye is usually suppressed to some degree, adaptation symptoms to a new optical correction are often less severe compared with patients having good binocular vision. Nevertheless, forewarning the patient of potential adaptation symptoms can provide the motivation to endure some temporary discomfort, if it occurs. The initial steps of amblyopia therapy usually involve occlusion, in addition to full optical correction; binocular

adaptation complaints are therefore not immediate problems. We have seen many mildly amblyopic patients, particularly in cases of isoametropic and meridional amblyopia, achieve a complete functional cure, with 20/20 (6/6) visual acuity, by simply wearing the full spectacle correction over a period of a few months without the necessity of occlusion or active training. Pickwell[2] reported curing 7 of 14 anisometropic amblyopes (8 years of age on average) merely by prescribing the full lens correction. Amblyopia is often abated, even in adults, as a result of clear retinal imagery. For these reasons, we recommend immediate and full optical correction of any significant refractive error in both the normal and the amblyopic eye.

In many cases of moderate or marked anisometropia, the clinician should consider correcting the refractive error with contact lenses. Contact lenses have several advantages over spectacles. The patient may be more likely to wear the prescription lenses. Children frequently object to wearing glasses in general, but in addition, the anisometropic patient usually notices no immediate benefit in acuity with the glasses since he relies on the visual acuity of the least ametropic eye. Contact lenses are cosmetically more acceptable; and cosmesis is good since the eyes are not differentially magnified to an observer. Also, there is no induced prism effect with the contact lenses since the optical centers of the lenses remain relatively centered with eye movements (e.g., vertical prismatic effects are induced in spectacle lenses of unequal power in upward and downward positions of gaze). Contact lenses for hyperopia should also be seriously considered in cases of strabismic amblyopia, particularly if there is a large accommodative component to an esotropia. (The vertex distance with spectacles causes greater accommodation demand.) The disadvantages of contact lens wear, however, must be weighed against these advantages. Prisms cannot be effectively used with contact lenses and may be necessary in the overall management of strabismic amblyopes. The handling requirements, lens care responsibilities, expense, and psychological adjustment to wearing contact lenses can all become overriding contraindications in some cases. Since there are frequent lens changes in cases of amblyopia (particularly children), we often pre-

---

TABLE 10-2. Classification of Occlusion Variables

A. According to area of visual field occluded:
  1. Total (one eye completely monocular)
  2. Partial (only a portion of visual field of either or both eyes occluded)
B. According to the effect on light transmission:
  1. Opaque
    a. Bandage (adhesive) patch
    b. Tie-on patch
    c. Clip-on patch
  2. Attenuating (partial light transmission)
    a. Neutral density filters
    b. Crossed polarizing filters
    c. Colored filters
    d. Translucent lenses (frosted or etched)
    e. Blurring (spectacle lens, contact lens, drugs)
C. According to wearing time:
  1. Constant (full time)
  2. Intermittent (part time)
D. According to which eye is occluded.
  1. Direct (patching the better eye)
  2. Indirect (patching the amblyopic eye)
  3. Alternate (switching the patch from one eye to the other in a prescribed manner)

---

fer initially to correct the refractive error with spectacles. After a stable refraction is found and visual acuity has sufficiently improved in the amblyopic eye, contact lens wear may be recommended for long-term management. If, however, a patient resists wearing spectacle lenses after repeated attempts, then contact lens wearing necessarily becomes the preferred option.

OCCLUSION PROCEDURES

There are several variables involved in the management of occlusion therapy for amblyopia. Many forms of occlusion have been recommended to remediate amblyopia (Table 10-2 and Figure 10-1). Patching of the dominant eye is called *direct occlusion* and patching of the amblyopic eye is referred to as *inverse occlusion*. Occlusion can be total or partial; *total* usually means that the entire visual field is blocked out (e.g., bandage occluder or a pirate patch), whereas *partial* occlusion means that only part of the visual field is occluded (e.g., a sector occluder). An occluder can be opaque (blocking out all light) or *translucent*, to degrade form vision. Each type of occlusion has its own clinical merits and disadvantages.

Direct Occlusion

The oldest and most popular therapy for amblyopia is direct, opaque, total occlusion, e.g., patching of the good eye with a bandage. In 1743, De Buffon, a French naturalist, stretched gauze over a ring of whale bone to make an occluder for the dominant eye.[3] Such direct occlusion forces the patient to use the amblyopic eye (the "lazy" eye), perhaps for the first time for some amblyopic individuals (Figure 10-2). Assuming significant refractive error of the amblyopic eye has been corrected with lenses, direct occlusion has several beneficial physiologic effects: (1) The patient is forced to practice monocular oculomotor skills of fixation, pursuits, saccades, and accommodation. (2) The faulty localization associated with eccentric fixation is broken down through practicing correct eye-hand coordination. (3) Proper sensory stimulation of the amblyopic eye is achieved and allows for the development of cortical receptive field

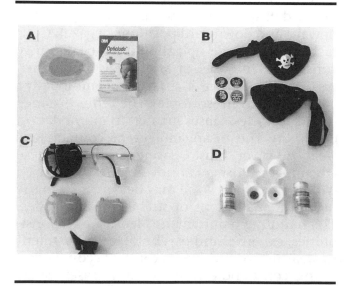

FIGURE 10-1—Examples of occluders: (a) bandage patch; (b) tie-on patch; (c) clip-on patch; (d) opaque contact lens.

organization, i.e., young children who neuro-logically have sensory plasticity. (4) Patching tends to break down the pattern of suppression associated with both anisometropic and strabismic amblyopia. (5) In cases of strabismic amblyopia, occlusion prevents the development or reinforcement of anomalous "retinal" correspondence (ARC).

There is general agreement about prescribing full-time direct occlusion for the infant and preschooler who has constant strabismus. In cases of anisometropia without strabismus, or only intermittent strabismus, part-time (3 to 6 hours per day), opaque, direct occlusion is usually recommended along with full-time spectacle correction of any significant refractive error when the amblyopic acuity is 20/100 (6/30) or better. This part-time schedule of occlusion promotes development of monocular skills of the amblyopic eye and still allows for development of normal binocularity when the patch is removed. Patients with deep amblyopia (worse than 20/100) usually require relatively long periods of daily occlusion. Most individuals during infancy develop normal acuity in the amblyopic eye within 1 or 2 months following this schedule, but preschool children may take longer, 2 to 4 months. Long-term, constant wear of the spectacles to correct anisometropia is required in all cases to prevent the reoccurrence of amblyopia. If, however, a young child has constant strabismus, with or without anisometropia, initial occlusion should be constant, total, and opaque. The clinical guideline is: If there is constant strabismus at all distances, constantly patch. Care must be taken, however, to avoid occlusion amblyopia (discussed in the next section).

If the amblyopic patient is over age 6, we recommend the traditional method of direct, opaque occlusion as the initial choice for therapy. Also with adult amblyopes, direct occlusion is the most effective single therapeutic choice. Typically, the more time each day the patient wears the patch directly, the quicker is visual acuity improvement. When a child attends school or an adult drives a car and works for a living, the practical requirements of these activities for adequate vision unfortunately limit the occlusion schedule. It must be remembered that an amblyopic patient with

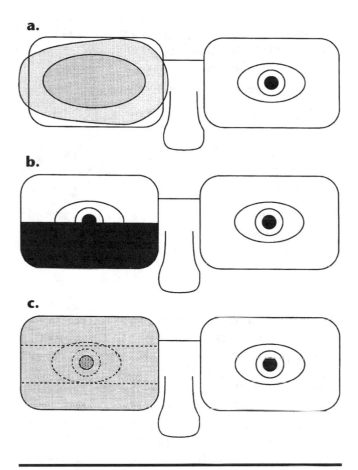

FIGURE 10-2—Occlusion of an eye. (a) Total occlusion with a tan-colored bandage patch worn over the eye but behind the spectacle lens. (b) Partial occlusion with an opaque tape on the inferior portion of the spectacle lens. (c) Attenuating occluder as achieved with strips of translucent tape.

20/200 (6/60) acuity who is patched directly can be considered legally blind. When normal visual acuity is a practical necessity, the patient is allowed to wear the patch inversely during those times. As a result, the overall treatment time will take longer, but this may be a necessary compromise. For students and working adults, it is often expedient to postpone amblyopia therapy until vacation time when direct patching can be intensively undertaken. On vacation, the patient with deep amblyopia stays at home, wears a constant, direct bandage occluder, and does intensive active vision therapy to speed acuity improvement. Many times the visual acuity improves rapidly to moderate or mild levels so that further direct patching at school or in the work place is no longer debilitating. In cases of anisometropic amblyopia, in which some binocular vision exposure is desir-

TABLE 10-3. *Constant Patching Schedule to Prevent Occlusion Amblyopia (Amblyopia Due to Constant Strabismus)*

AGE	Days Direct	Days Inverse
1 year or less	1	1
2 years	2	1
3 years	3	1
4 years	4	1
5 years	5	1
6 years	6	1
7 years or older	constant	0

able, the patient should try to coordinate activities that require good acuity with the binocular vision period (during which the patch is not worn). It is important to have all patients commit to following a specifically agreed on patching schedule before occlusion therapy is initiated. If the patient cannot realistically find the necessary time in the daily schedule for patching, then treatment should be delayed to another time or, unfortunately, forsaken.

Preventing Occlusion Amblyopia

When a clinician prescribes constant, total, opaque occlusion for a patient 6 years old or younger, it must be remembered that the acuity may deteriorate in the patched eye. With infants, the acuity of the nonamblyopic eye that is patched can fall almost as fast as the acuity rises in the unpatched amblyopic eye.[4] In strabismic amblyopia, constant total patching is the most efficient and effective therapy, but the patch needs to be worn alternately, some days direct (on the nonamblyopic eye), and other days inverse (on the amblyopic eye). The ratio of direct versus indirect occlusion should vary depending on the child's age. We recommend using a wearing schedule for constant, direct, opaque occlusion based on the number of days corresponding to the child's age followed by one day of inverse occlusion (Table 10-3). For an infant 1 year old or younger, the patch would be alternated on a daily basis. (Note: In cases of constant infantile

strabismus, we also recommend the use of Fresnel prism glasses worn part-time to promote the possible development of binocular vision.) According to this patching schedule, a 3-year-old amblyopic child would be given 3 consecutive days of direct occlusion and 1 day of inverse. Patients older than 6 years typically do not develop occlusion amblyopia with constant direct patching no matter how long the patch is worn, but the clinician should monitor visual acuity in both the nonamblyopic and the amblyopic eye in all patients undergoing occlusion therapy, regardless of age. If occlusion amblyopia does develop during the course of patching therapy, the ratio of direct to inverse occlusion should be reversed to restore visual acuity.

Part-time direct patching is done in cases of anisometropic amblyopia or intermittent strabismus, 3 to 6 hours per day, depending on depth of the amblyopia.

Types of Occluders

The type of occluder chosen for a particular amblyopic patient depends on a number of factors (Table 10-4). The bandage occluder and tie-on patch are opaque and totally exclude light. Most clinicians prefer these occluders in the hope that a vigorous patching program will bring rapid therapeutic results. The bandage patch conveniently fits under spectacle lenses. This occluder is taken off at night and changed daily. At night, a moisturizing cream (e.g., Nivea ointment) can be applied to the skin around the eye to prevent or reduce irritation from the adhesive. Many patients prefer to wear a less cosmetically obvious patch and cooperate better using a clip-on or translucent occluder. Our preference, however, in most cases of amblyopia is to utilize a bandage occluder, full or part time, depending on the case. Adults may choose to wear the tie-on patch since, lacking adhesive, it is more comfortable and many come in designer colors. A contact lens occluder is our next preference if the child persists in resisting bandage occlusion. If neither of these alternatives is acceptable, penalization methods should be considered. Children who resist bandage occlusion often look around a tie-on, clip-on, or translucent occluder, thus compromising the therapy program.

TABLE 10-4. *Types of Occluders*

Types	Features	Advantages	Disadvantages
Bandage	Opticlude Elastoplast (opaque)	Total occlusion, convenient, effective, child & adult sizes	Some allergic reactions to adhesive, sometimes unacceptable cosmesis
Tie-on	Pirate patch elastic patch	Total occlusion	Loose, moveable, difficult to wear with spectacles
Clip-on	Clips on to plastic frames, sizes 32 to 50	Partial occlusion can be given	Children peek around the occluder. It can be too easily removed by the child.
Translucent	Magic Tape, nail polish, frosted lens, optical blur	Degrades form resolution of nonamblyopic eye, fusion, acceptable cosmesis	Children tend to peek around lens
Filters	Neutral density	Breaks suppression, allows some fusion	Effective visual acuity improvement uncertain
Contact lens	Opaque soft lens	Convenient, effective, acceptable cosmesis	Difficult for children to handle, requires cleaning, expensive

When peripheral fusion needs to be preserved, as in most cases of anisometropia or intermittent strabismus, the doctor can prescribe a frosted lens or the optical blur method of penalization. The dominant eye's image is degraded sufficiently to change fixation preference to the amblyopic eye without completely disassociating the eyes, thus minimizing disruption of binocular vision.

The amount of part-time opaque occlusion recommended for anisometropic amblyopia is based on the depth of amblyopia and the extent of normal binocular vision. Deep anisometropic amblyopia (20/200 or worse) with deep suppression and little binocular vision may initially require full-time occlusion. If the amblyopia is moderate, e.g., 20/100 (6/30) and peripheral fusion with stereopsis exists, then 3 to 6 hours a day of direct occlusion may be appropriate.

Motivation and Patching Management

When an amblyope wears a patch, it is not regarded as fun. If the visual acuity is 20/100 (6/30) or worse, the patient often feels visually disabled. For a child, it is a good idea to build the patient's confidence before the patch is worn. The patient should first be able to demonstrate proficiency in gross motor tasks. Otherwise, he will experience frustration and will most certainly reject being occluded. Parents and teachers should not allow the child to participate in potentially dangerous activities while being directly occluded. Children usually cooperate with patching to please the parents, and occasionally the doctor; it is important for all involved adults to give praise, support, and even rewards for compliance. Adults usually require rewards of some kind in exchange for hard, unpleasant work; the child's efforts also need to be acknowledged.

Many elementary school children are embarrassed to wear a patch because of questions and comments from their peers. We have found it helpful for the child to practice answering questions about the patch in the doctor's office before confronting them on the playground.

Sally: "Johnny, why do you wear that patch?"

Johnny: "The patch is going to make my other eye super strong so I can see really well with it. The doctor says only I can wear it."

It may also be helpful for the teacher to discuss the patch with the class if this is done in a positive way. Johnny's patch may provide a good opportunity for the teacher to talk about the eyes and the "wonders of vision."

Teenagers vary considerably in their compliance with patching. Some are very mature and make a personal choice to improve their vision regardless of comments of their peers. Others are absolutely terrified of "looking funny." In these cases, a contact lens occluder may be the only realistic alternative to enlist cooperation with vision therapy. Another alternative that can be proposed to self-conscious patients is to initiate the patching program during vacation time when peer interactions may be more controlled.

Patching Progress

In most cases of functional amblyopia, there is an initial rapid increase in visual acuity and improved fixation pattern of the amblyopic eye in response to conventional direct occlusion. Most improvement occurs during the first 3 months. In a study of 350 amblyopic children, Oliver et al.[5] reported an average increase of about 4 lines of visual acuity on Snellen charts during the initial 3 months of direct occlusion. About one additional line of improvement occurred in the next 3 months and only marginal increases accrued thereafter. After a patient starts following the occlusion schedule, regular office visits are indicated to monitor progress, build motivation, and coordinate active vision training procedures that shorten the total therapy time. We suggest weekly office visits initially to make sure the occlusion and vision training are correctly applied and effective. If a plateau in acuity or fixation pattern occurs for 4 weeks, we suggest changing the thrust of the therapy. If the patient develops steady eccentric fixation, the clinician may consider switching to inverse occlusion, applying different active therapy procedures (e.g., afterimage transfer techniques), applying pleoptics, using red filter techniques, monocular prism methods, or a monocular telescope. (These procedures are explained later in this chapter.)

If, however, there is no progress in visual acuity or the fixation pattern after the 2 or 3 weeks of occlusion with full patient compliance, the clinician should suspect amblyopia either of arrested development or possible pathologic etiology. In such cases, prognosis needs to be modified accordingly. However, if there has been a significant improvement after 1 or 2 weeks of patching, both the patient and clinician should be encouraged; the successful therapy approach should be continued until maximum improvement occurs.

Efficacy of Occlusion and Amblyopia Therapy

As a therapeutic procedure, patching an eye is easy, economical, and requires only minimal doctor involvement. For more than 200 years, direct occlusion has been, and remains, the standard treatment for amblyopia. According to an extensive literature review by Garzia[6] the success rates (i.e., achieving 20/40 visual acuity) range from 40% to 80% with noncompliance of patching being a significant reason for failure.

The literature is insufficient to evaluate the relative success rates with the different types of amblyopia. The depth of the acuity deficit and amount of eccentric fixation are probably more important factors than the type of amblyopia. We can, however, make some generalities. Meridional and low to moderate isometropic amblyopia are perhaps the easiest cases because the amblyopia is usually mild, 20/60 or better.[7,8] These patients often respond successfully over time simply by correcting the refractive error. Anisometropic amblyopia often improves quickly with full correction of the refractive error, occlusion, and antisuppression training, if there is no eccentric fixation. Kutschke et al.[9] recently reported an 82% success rate (using the 20/40 or better acuity criterion) for their clinical series of 124 anisometropic amblyopic patients. They found that myopic and compound myopic astigmatic anisometropic patients had the poorer visual outcomes. Strabismic amblyopia of long standing is frequently more difficult to treat, in part, because eccentric fixation is usually well established. Generally, when strabismus and anisometropia coexist as amblyogenic factors, the prognosis is even worse. The most difficult amblyopic patients to cure are those who have suffered deprivation amblyopia during early childhood due to a major sensory obstacle, e.g., congenital cataract or ptosis. Prognosis in such cases is guarded. It is important to emphasize that even though 20/30 acuity or better in an amblyopic eye is a good clinical goal, patients often appreciate making any progress in visual acuity.

In an excellent review paper, Birnbaum et al.[10] demonstrated that the age of treatment was not as important a factor in determining success in amblyopia therapy as once was thought. They analyzed 23 studies with a total sample size of over 1000 amblyopic patients of all ages. The overall success rates for adult treatment compared favorably with those for children. Using a success criterion of 20/30 visual acuity, there was no significant difference among four age groupings. Children under 7 years and older patients (16 years and above) both had a success rate of about 40%. Using the success criterion of 4 lines of improvement on a Snellen chart, the children were more successful, 57% versus 42%. The point is that 42% is not a bad success rate for amblyopia treatment for adults. Two comprehensive recent studies, a large survey of 368 amblyopic patients,[11] and a detailed analysis of 19 older anisometropic amblyopes,[12] are consistent with the conclusions of Birnbaum et al.[10] Age of treatment seems only a minor factor in the success rate for amblyopia remediation. Clinicians should no longer be surprised to hear about adult amblyopes who regain vision due to active vision therapy. Also, amblyopia is sometimes abated by an acquired loss of acuity in the nonamblyopic eye, e.g., from a developing cataract[13] (the cataract acts as an occluder). (Refer to Chapter 5 for discussions on age of onset of amblyopia, duration, and age of treatment as to prognosis for cure.)

Although the overall success rate does not change much with age, the length of treatment does increase; older patients generally take longer to achieve best results. In most cases of functional amblyopia, visual acuity can be improved at any age, but the physiologic changes occur more slowly with advancing age. The public suffers from much misinformation about amblyopia. It is still commonly believed that amblyopia cannot be treated successfully past age 5 or 6 years. It is more than a coincidence that the rate of patient compliance with

patching decreases significantly when the child enters school, presumably due to the lack of direct parental supervision. Oliver et al.[5] found that compliance with patching decreased from 72% among preschool children to 47% for children ages 8 to 12 years old. Most vision therapists know from experience that it is more difficult to enlist compliance for patching from school-aged children compared with preschoolers or adults. The most important barriers to successful amblyopia therapy past age 5 years are more psychological and managerial than physiologic.[14] Clinicians need to continue making the recommendation for preschool treatment of amblyopia primarily because it can be done with more acceptance and will help in establishing normal binocular vision; however, they should also emphasize that many patients with amblyopia can be treated successfully at any age.

Active vision training to remediate amblyopia and eccentric fixation is an important and effective adjunct therapy to occlusion, which alone is a passive form of therapy. There are several detailed case reports in the literature of patients who, unsuccessful with direct occlusion, responded successfully with active training.[1,12,15,16,17] Generally speaking, the reported success rate in studies that augmented occlusion therapy with active therapy (e.g., visual tracking, foveal tag, and antisuppression techniques) are usually higher (70% or better) than those using occlusion alone.[18,19,20,21,22,23] One study by François and James[23] directly compared results of one group of amblyopes using only occlusion (N100) with another group (N100) treated with occlusion and active vision training. The final success rates were the same, but the vision training group took significantly less time. Another comparative study by Leyman[21] of 62 amblyopes reported a success rate of 72% for occlusion alone, 50% for pleoptics alone, and 93% for combination group of occlusion and monocular and binocular vision training. One reason for the higher success rate when vision training augments optical correction and occlusion is that the overall treatment time is reduced by as much as 50%.[22,23] Patient compliance with patching tends to diminish over time, so anything that can be done to speed progress promotes the best overall outcome. We strongly recommend that, in addition to occlusion, amblyopic patients be given at least some of the vision training techniques described later in this chapter.

Besides acuity improvement, additional benefits of amblyopia therapy include increases in stereopsis in about half of anisometropic patients[24,25] and improvement in monocular and binocular contrast sensitivity in all types of amblyopia.[26]

Penalization

One alternative to standard total occlusion when a child refuses to wear a patch is some form of penalization. Penalization refers to the use of drugs or optical means to blur the preferred eye to favor the use of the amblyopic eye. A few clinicians prefer penalization to bandage occluders during the initial stage of amblyopia therapy, but most do not consider using these techniques until conventional total occlusion procedures have been tried and failed. However, penalization becomes the preferred treatment option when there is latent nystagmus, intermittent strabismus, or an allergic reaction to the bandage adhesive.

Penalization Methods

Each penalization method has a place in the management of some amblyopic patients. Generally speaking, these techniques are utilized more often in strabismic amblyopia than in anisometropic cases, with the exception of far penalization, which has been used with both types if normal fusion is the goal.

Penalization without Spectacles   When a child is totally uncooperative with either conventional occlusion or spectacle wear, pharmaceutical penalization provides the practitioner with an effective but somewhat risky alternative. Atropine (1% drops or salve) is instilled in the nonamblyopic eye once a day, and a miotic (e.g., 0.025% DFP, 0.06% Echothiophate Iodide, or 1% pilocarpine drops, bid) is used in the amblyopic eye. There is some pain associated with instillation of miotics, so some clini-

cians recommend applying the ointment or drops when a young child is asleep or at bedtime. The cycloplegic effect of the atropine prevents the patient from focusing for nearpoint objects with the nonamblyopic eye whereas the miotic pupil increases the depth of field of the amblyopic eye. Like a pinhole camera, the amblyopic eye has a clear image for objects at most distances. Spectacle correction of the refractive error, therefore, may not always be necessary using this method. The clinician does need to monitor closely the patient for drug side effects, particularly with this method, because of their common occurrence with the protracted use of miotics (e.g., iris cysts, brow pain, headaches, conjunctival irritation, anterior subcapsular cataract). The maximum increase of acuity in the amblyopic eye usually occurs between 3 to 6 months of drug therapy depending primarily on the patient's age and depth of amblyopia. Significant improvement of acuity has been reported in over 75% of patients irrespective of age.[27]

Near Penalization   This technique is often preferred to the others for patients with deep strabismic amblyopia. Atropine drops or salve (1%) is instilled in the nonamblyopic eye once a day. The spectacle correction for the dominant eye is worn to give good far acuity and prevent occlusion amblyopia. A single vision +3.00 D add is prescribed in addition to the refractive correction for the amblyopic eye (Figure 10-3). The effect of this add is to promote clear vision and fixation with the amblyopic eye for all nearpoint viewing distances and to blur far distances sufficiently to force alternation to the dominant eye for farpoint viewing, thus preventing occlusion amblyopia. The goal is to get alternate fixation, but the child must wear the eye glasses to get the maximum benefit from the technique. Near visual acuity needs to be monitored during near penalization to make sure the amblyopic eye has better acuity than the atropinized eye and is, in fact, being used for nearpoint fixation. If it is not, total penalization (see next section) should be considered. Maximum acuity improvement usually occurs between 1 and 6 months after initiating near penalization.

Total Penalization   Total penalization is a type of direct graded occlusion. Both far and near form vision are degraded, but light perception is still permitted. This method is used only with high hyperopic patients with strabismic amblyopia. Total penalization is achieved by atropinization of the nonamblyopic eye and given only a plano lens; however, full optical correction for distance is given to the amblyopic eye. Consequently, the amblyopic eye fixates objects at both far and near (Figure 10-4). It is prudent to use this technique only with children aged 6 years or older to avoid the possibility of inducing occlusion amblyopia.

Distance Penalization   If an uncooperative amblyopic patient has anisometropia or intermittent strabismus and fairly good binocular vision is preserved, penalization at far is the method of choice. The method works best when amblyopic reduction in visual acuity is mild to moderate, 20/100 or better (Figure 10-5). Atropine (1% drops or salve) is instilled daily in the nonamblyopic eye and a +3.00 D single vision add is also placed before that eye. The nonamblyopic eye is therefore fogged for viewing at far and is in focus only for targets at about 33 cm. Also, it cannot focus for very near distances because of cycloplegia. Nothing is done to the amblyopic eye except correction of any significant refractive error, so the patient can focus an image with that eye at all distances. The amblyopic eye will therefore be used primarily for viewing distant objects if its visual acuity exceeds that of the fogged dominant eye. Binocular vision is possible at 33 cm since both eyes are in focus for that working distance. If there is suppression, active antisuppression training techniques (e.g., polarized or anaglyphic reading bars) are recommended to promote fusion at 33 cm.

Optical Penalization   In cases of strabismic amblyopia that have been cured or almost cured, but the strabismus remains, a form of optical penalization may help to maintain the good visual acuity results. Some patients need to maintain an alternate fixation pattern indefinitely to prevent acuity regression. This can be achieved by a program of periodic direct occlu-

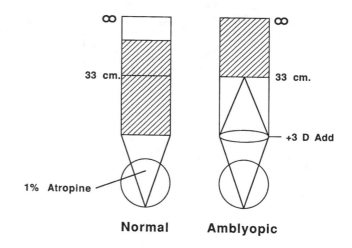

FIGURE 10-3—Near penalization with cycloplegia.

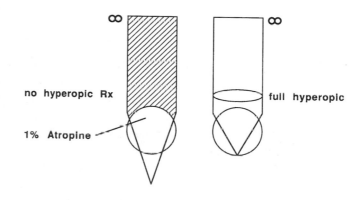

FIGURE 10-4—Total penalization with cycloplegia that is used with highly hyperopic amblyopes.

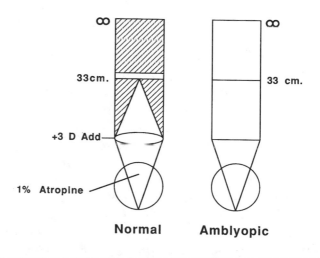

FIGURE 10-5—Farpoint and very near distance penalization of the nonamblyopic eye with cycloplegia and a plus-lens. Only a small depth of field is available to the left eye (at the 33 cm distance) with nearer objects being blurred because of paralysis of accommodation and farther objects being blurred that are beyond the focal distance of the lens.

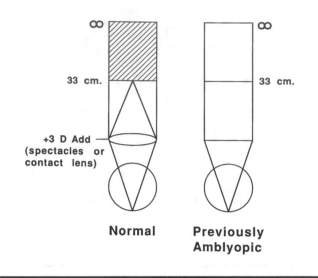

FIGURE 10-6—Farpoint optical penalization with plus lens.

sion, but optical penalization is often a preferred solution by both the patient and the parents. If a +3.00 D single vision spectacle add or contact lens is placed before an eye, that eye will most likely be used for nearpoint fixation and the other eye for viewing far targets. The addition lens is usually placed before the nonamblyopic eye to give preference for its use at near fixation distances, while the amblyopic eye will more likely be used for far viewing (Figure 10-6). This represents a monovision approach to promote habitual alternate fixation. Contact lens monovision corrections have been well accepted by many presbyopic contact lens wearers with normal binocular vision (85% in one study),[28] and this technique holds much promise for the long-term management and prevention of amblyopia in children.

Von Noorden and Attiah[29] reported good results preventing the reoccurrence of amblyopia in young children using alternating optical penalization. Most of their patients, aged 8 years or younger, had cures for amblyopia, but after surgery had eso microtropia. They prescribed two pairs of spectacles for used on alternate days. One pair had a +3.00 D overcorrection for the right eye, and the other pair had the same overcorrection in the left lens. If there was a significant refractive error, this was prescribed for both eyes in addition to the overcorrection. The 16 patients wore these glasses on

alternate days for 1 to 4 years depending on the child's age. All patients maintained 20/50 acuity or better in the formerly amblyopic eye. The investigators recommended maintaining this regimen of optical penalization until the age of 6 to 8 years old until the visual system is fairly mature. They observed that the reoccurrence of amblyopia is possible as late as the early teenage years in some cases. Therefore, all young patients should be monitored frequently for regression and, if it occurs, optical penalization and/or a short course of direct patching can be reinstated.

Penalization Management

Since atropine can have serious side effects in some individuals, clinicians who utilize penalization as an occlusion option must be vigilant in screening patients for signs and symptoms of overdose. Table 10-5 lists systemic and ocular signs and symptoms of atropine overdose that clinicians must be aware of. This is not a trivial concern. There are six reported deaths of children, ages 3 years and younger, in the literature due to topical application of atropine drops.[30] These children did, however, have some CNS abnormality or were sickly, so extra caution is appropriate in these cases.

It must be remembered that young children can develop occlusion amblyopia in the atropinized eye; von Noorden[31] reported three such cases in children aged 2 years or younger. Total penalization is a form of visual deprivation. A patient can form the habit of not fixating with the normal eye. A child must be carefully monitored weekly, or at least every 2 weeks, to ensure that alternate fixation is actually occurring with penalization.

Optical penalization can be an alternative to conventional occlusion in cases of mild amblyopia, 20/70 or better acuity in the amblyopic eye. It seems particularly appropriate in cases of patching noncompliance or in cases in which a monovision correction is needed to maintain good acuity in each eye. Repka et al.[32] demonstrated the effectiveness of this technique in their patient series of 34 anisometropic or strabismic amblyopes. They found that the plus-power addition required to make the patient switch fixation to the amblyopic eye ranged from +0.75 D to 2.00 D with an average of +1.25 D. This is considerably less plus than used by von Noorden and Attiah.[29] For patient acceptance, it is desirable to use the minimum amount of additional plus-power to create alternate distance-near fixation, while still ensuring that the patient does indeed fixate with the amblyopic eye. Repka et al.[32] recommended using a distant vectographic acuity chart to determine the effective minimum amount of plus addition. Patients are tested while wearing their best farpoint spectacle correction and crossed-polarizing (vectographic) filters. As the patient reads letters on a farpoint vectographic chart, plus-power lenses are added to the nonamblyopic eye in +0.25 D steps until the patient can switch fixation to the amblyopic eye (as indicated by reading letters clued to that eye). The lowest amount of plus addition needed to switch far fixation consistently to the amblyopic eye is then prescribed over the CAMP (corrected ametropia with most plus) lens correction. Either spectacle lenses or contact lenses can be used for optical penalization, whichever is more clinically appropriate.

Efficacy of Penalization

Generally, penalization techniques are an effective alternative to conventional direct total occlusion for treating amblyopia and preserving good acuity. Von Noorden and Milam[33] reported a series of 17 mildly amblyopic patients (all but one had an initial acuity of 20/100 or better) who did not accept conventional occlusion therapy for some reason. Ten patients, ages 2 through 12 years, improved two lines of acuity or more in the amblyopic eye and none showed any deterioration of vision in the nonamblyopic eye. They also reported that another group of 13 patients who had improved using conventional occlusion and penalization had prevented the reoccurrence of amblyopia in all but three cases.

Ron and Nawratzki[34] demonstrated impressive results using various penalization techniques for strabismic amblyopia with 38 children between 6 and 12 years, most of

TABLE 10-5. *Signs and Symptoms of Atropine Overdose*
Systemic:
Thirst
Ataxia
Fever
Sleepiness or insomnia
Dryness of skin, mouth, and throat
Red, flushed skin of the face and neck
Restlessness, irritability, or delirium
Tachychardia- rapid and weak pulse
Urinary retention
Ocular:
Allergic conjunctivitis, keratitis
Contact dermatitis of lids
Decreased lacrimation
Increased intraocular pressure
Photophobia

whom had moderate to marked amblyopia. The average duration of treatment was 10 months. After a 2-year follow-up period, they reported good acuities, 20/40 or better, in 74% of these patients with 50% achieving this level in cases of marked amblyopia. These results are even better than they found by conventional opaque occlusion in young children. They thought standard occlusion may be less effective due to unobserved peeking or occasional removal of the patch. They maintained close monitoring of penalization to ensure that the amblyopic eye was being properly stimulated.

The largest patient series reported to date is that of Repka and Ray,[35] which also had a very positive outcome. There were 166 strabismic and anisometropic amblyopic children (1 through 12 years old) who underwent penalization for at least 3 months. Optical penalization was used in 87 cases showing an average improvement from 20/38 to 20/28. In an additional 79 patients with atropine penalization, the acuity improved on average from 20/61 to 20/40. The percentage of patients who improved in visual acuity with optical penalization was 77%; and with atropine penalization, 76%, respectively. In the atropine group, a variation of near penalization was applied. The full hyperopic correction was given and atropine drops were instilled daily in the dominant eye. The amblyopic eye fixated near targets without the benefit of a plus-lens add. They reported no cases of occlusion amblyopia in either group.

Red Filter Therapy and Occlusion

When occlusion procedures do not produce the desired increase in visual acuity or if unsteady eccentric fixation becomes steady and eccentric, red filter therapy may be considered as an alternative technique to promote foveal fixation. We do not recommend utilizing this technique initially because most patients find the technique cosmetically unacceptable and will not cooperate for more than a few hours a day. The technique requires the patient to wear a total occluder on the nonamblyopic eye while a red filter is worn on the amblyopic eye. A Kodak gelatin Wratten filter No. 92, which excludes wavelengths shorter than 640 nanometers, was advocated by Brinker and Katz.[36] Unfortunately, this material is brittle and dissolves easily in water destroying its optical quality. Less expensive red transparent vinyl or a regular ruby Kodaloid filter can be used effectively.[37] The red filter is applied to the surface of a spectacle lens and the dominant eye is totally patched with a bandage occluder. The theory why a red filter promotes foveal fixation is that the fovea has a higher proportion of red sensitive cones compared with eccentric points. The fovea is, therefore, favored for fixation. Burian and von Noorden[38] found this technique effective is some amblyopic cases. The fixation pattern of the amblyopic eye should be closely monitored by visuoscopy and may require 1 to 3 months of treatment to be effective.[37] When the red filter is removed, the patient should immediately continue constant direct occlusion to reinforce the new foveal fixation pattern, if it has been established.

Prism Therapy and Occlusion

Another method of treating intractable steady eccentric fixation is the use of inverse prism and direct occlusion, either opaque or graded. Pigassou and Toulouse[39] recommended applying an inverse prism before the amblyopic eye, while the nonamblyopic eye is totally occluded with an opaque patch. Also using inverse prism, Rubin[40] recommended using graded direct occlusion with sufficient neutral density filters to reduce the visual acuity of the nonamblyopic eye by at least two lines below that of the amblyopic eye.

The hypothetical rationale behind using inverse prism in this monocular technique is to shift the principal visual direction from the eccentric point to the fovea. In the case of nasal eccentric fixation of the right eye, wearing a base-in prism causes the right eye to abduct (Figure 10-7). This turning outward of the eye puts the fovea in the "straight-ahead" or true primary position. The patient has a new opportunity to establish the oculocentric direction at the fovea since the old directionalization pattern is disrupted by the prism. The recommended amount of prism power slightly exceeds the amount of eccentric fixation, e.g., 6^Δ BI for 5^Δ steady nasal EF. In less prevalent cases of temporal eccentric fixation, the prism (Fresnel or clip-over) is applied base-out.

Several other versions of prism therapy for eccentric fixation have been suggested by various authors,[41] with and without penalization, but there is little evidence supporting their efficacy over conventional direct occlusion. For this reason, we suggest prism therapy be tried only if standard patching has not been successful and the patient has either steady eccentric fixation or unsteady eccentric fixation where the fixation pattern does not include the fovea.

Prism therapy is essentially a passive technique, but monocular fixation activities, such as eye-hand coordination exercises or after-image transfer and fast pointing, can be added for the purpose of associating the straight-ahead position with the true spatial location of the target (see Figure 10-7d). The exact true location of the fixation target is verified by the

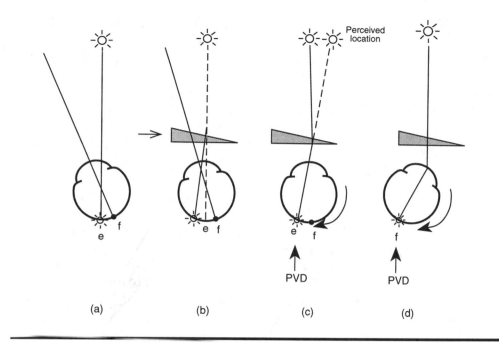

FIGURE 10-7—Inverse prism in case of nasal eccentric fixation of the right eye with the left eye being occluded. (a) The image of the penlight falls on point *e;* (b) a base-in prism is placed before the right eye to project the image of the penlight onto a point that is nasal to point *e;* (c) the right eye picks up fixation with point *e* as the patient wears the base-in prism for several weeks. The principal visual direction, however, remains at point *e.* There is now a disruption between the habitual eccentric eye position and the straight ahead perception for eye-hand coordination; (d) the eye further adducts so that the image of the penlight falls on the fovea, as a result of prolonged wearing of the reversed prism and fast pointing exercises. The principal visual direction is at the fovea.

tactual-kinesthetic sense when the patient touches the target with a finger or a pointer.

Short Term Occlusion

In the late 1970s, the introduction of the CAM stimulator therapy for amblyopia generated excitement since its use often seemed to result in quick improvement of visual acuity.[42] This rotating device consisted of seven high-contrast, square wave spatial frequency gratings presenting an acuity range from 20/20 to 20/200. Each grating is viewed monocularly with the amblyopic eye and rotated at the rate of 1 revolution per minute in ascending order, i.e., from low to high spatial frequencies. The total training time per session takes only 7 minutes. Snellen visual acuity was reported to increase about two lines on average after only a few sessions. However, controlled studies that followed the initial positive clinical reports indicated that the same level of improvement could be achieved by viewing uniform gray fields or merely by direct patching for 7 minutes per day.[43] The rotating gratings proved incidental and inconsequential. The acuity improvement is apparently due to a rapid learning curve for fixation with an amblyopic eye when that eye is initially forced to fixate with

direct occlusion. Some of the studies also had the patient practice eye-hand coordination activities while viewing the CAM stimulator through a transparent overlay. These CAM studies have made clinicians aware that significant improvement in visual acuity is possible in many cases of amblyopia with minimal patching and emphasis on eye-hand training techniques. Griffin et al. provided an example by reporting successful results with minimal patching and monocular vision training in a case of anisometropic amblyopia.[44] In summary, some patching is better than no patching, yet we must add that rigorous patching is often needed for the best therapeutic outcome. Good reviews of the literature on the CAM therapy can be found by Garzia[6] and Ciuffreda et al.[45]

There are certain cases of amblyopia in which *short-term occlusion* seems both appropriate and effective, if it is combined with active vision training. If a child or adult with mild to moderate amblyopia finds patching in public unacceptable, successful results may still be possible if direct patching is done as the patient participates in 1 to 2 hours per day of vigorous vision training. Several patient series have demonstrated positive results with this approach, although the cure rate is not quite as high as that found in studies utilizing full time

TABLE 10-6. *Amblyopia Training Activities*

Playing board games
Playing card games: Concentration, Canasta, etc.
Coloring in O's or vowels in books and magazines*
Coloring in coloring books*
Reading comic books
Working on craft projects: small materials
Solving crossword puzzles*
Connecting dot-to-dot patterns*
Drawing: houses, faces, cars, etc.
Hammering nails
Playing jacks*
Solving jigsaw puzzles
Playing with Lego and other blocks
Playing marbles
Solving mazes
Building models from kits: boats, cars, etc.
Working on pegboard activities
Using visual perceptual materials: Frostig, Rosner*
Playing pick-up sticks
Reading any printed materials*
Playing Scrabble®
Sorting cards and objects
Sewing clothes
Shooting games (target practice)
Stringing beads
Throwing or hitting games* (e.g., baseball, darts)
Playing with Tinker Toys®
Putting toothpicks in straw
Tracing*
Playing video and computer games*

*Authors' 10 best picks.

occlusion.[2,22,46,47] These good results are probably due more to the effect of the active vision therapy than only to short term occlusion.

MONOCULAR FIXATION TRAINING

The goals of monocular fixation and motility training with the amblyopic eye are to enhance these visual skills through conscious patient effort and performance feedback. Direct patching alone forces the patient to practice a certain level of oculomotor skills, but amblyopic patients when patched, frequently do not attempt as many critical seeing and eye-hand coordination activities as they could possibly perform. These monocular training techniques provide the patient with challenging activities that increase the speed of improvement of visual acuity. Fortunately, many of these activities are enjoyable for patients of all ages; training compliance is usually not a problem. Table 10-6 lists activities that we have found entertaining and effective. These games and activities can conveniently be done at home with a minimum of supervision. We usually ask our vision therapy patients to devote 30 minutes per day to home training; but when patients engage in many of these interesting activities, the home training time often extends past this recommendation.

The clinician needs to monitor the patient's progress closely during occlusion and active training. Patients who have eccentric fixation, steady or unsteady, may stabilize fixation on the eccentric point rather than moving fixation toward or to the fovea. In the rare case in which stable eccentric fixation occurs, patching is temporarily switched to inverse occlusion, rather than direct. Active fixation training is then given using foveal tag techniques and pleoptic therapy (described subsequently). Fortunately, most patients progress well without the need for foveal tag procedures and/or formal pleoptics.

Fixation and Ocular Motility Activities (Without Foveal Tag)

The number of monocular fixation and motility activities for the amblyopic eye that has therapeutic value is limited only by the clinician's imagination. The following materials and activities represent procedures we have found to be particularly interesting and effective with patients. At all times during this phase of training, the patient should have any significant refractive error optically corrected and should wear an occluder over the nonamblyopic eye.

Eye-Hand Coordination Techniques

The following techniques require a high level of accurate eye-hand coordination. The patient's goal is to become equally skilled in the activities using each eye to guide performance. Ideally, visual skills of the amblyopic eye should eventually be improved to equal those of the dominant eye.

Tracing and Drawing T10.1

Tracing and drawing activities are some of the easiest and most effective home techniques to improve eye-hand coordination, visual tracking, and visual acuity of the amblyopic eye. Pictures from any source can be used, e.g., comics, newspapers, magazines. If the amblyopia is deep (marked), simple pictures with bold lines should be selected. If the amblyopia is shallow (mild), then fine lines and a lot of detail are appropriate. Thin translucent tracing paper is placed over the picture and the patient traces it as quickly as possible using sharp colored pencils. The completed tracing is compared with the original picture and corrections should be made. Speed and accuracy are important goals.

Another home activity involves drawing a figure (such as an outline of a hand) and making as many internal and/or external concentric copies of that figure as possible. Each concentric figure should be drawn as close to the last as can be resolved with the amblyopic eye. If the drawing is done with colored pencils, the result is often quite stunning. Precision and detail are desirable. The patient should bring in all drawings and tracings for inspection by the therapist. Progress in eye-hand coordination is evident.

Connect-the-dots books provide excellent eye-hand coordination challenges to the amblyopic patient. The task requires accurate fixation, visual search, and tracking. Dot-to-dot games are available in most toy stores or bookstores.

Throwing and Hitting Games T10.2

To the delight of children and the chagrin of parents, throwing and hitting games are particularly suited for the development of accurate foveal fixation and spatial localization. The nonamblyopic eye is occluded during training activities. The accuracy of the outcome is immediately apparent to all (i.e., good visual feedback). There is constant motivation to improve performance by adopting compensating strategies. The reflexive eye-hand movements involved in the game are also thought to promote foveal localization. Some of the more popular activities include basketball, baseball batting and catching, ping pong, magnetic darts, beanbag toss, tennis, badminton, and marbles. With proper precautions, amblyopic children and adults should be encouraged to participate in these games as part of their direct occlusion program. This makes occlusion easier to accept psychologically.

Electronic fixation instruments are often used in developmental and sports vision training (Figure 10-8). In one mode, lights flash on in a random pattern and the patient hits an adjacent button to turn off each light. Speed and accuracy are monitored by the instrument. Since the activity develops reflexive eye-hand coordination, it is ideally suited for training proper localization with the amblyopic eye.

Video Game Tracking T10.3

Video and computer games are now omnipresent and they are conveniently available in many homes. Because of the addictive quality of some electronic games, many parents have to limit the amount of time their children spend on this activity. Amblyopic children, however, should be encouraged to practice various shooting, chasing, and other eye-hand coordination games using only the amblyopic eye since the game score gives immediate feedback as to the player's skill level. The patient should try to match his/her skill level using the amblyopic eye with that of the nonamblyopic eye and record the daily high score for inspection during the office visits. Requesting 30 minutes or 1 hour a day for these active visual tracking activities is usually considered by the patient a privilege rather than a burden. Shippman[20] reported good results with a clinical series of amblyopic children, ages 4 through 10 years, using video games as the orthoptic treatment. Fifteen of 19 patients who were unsuccessful using direct patching alone showed substantial improvements in visual acuity once home video games were introduced for an average training period of 9 weeks.

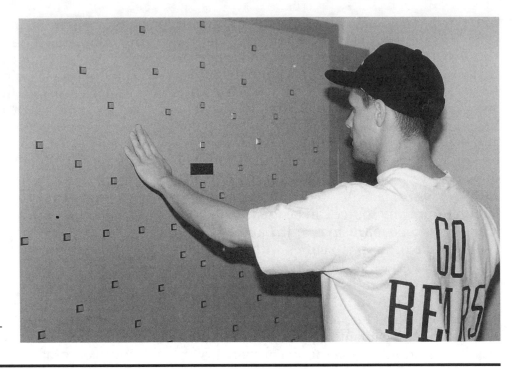

FIGURE 10-8—DynaVision 2000 electronic fixation instrument.

Several prepackaged vision training computer programs are commercially available. Two systems we have found to be effective with amblyopic patients in particular are Optimum and Computer Orthoptics. Each of these programs has screens and activities involving eye-hand coordination and visual tracking, usually in a game format. A doctor specializing in vision therapy should find these recommended systems useful in clinical practice.

Swinging Ball Training T10.4
A practical method of home training for improving smooth pursuits, accommodative facility, eye-hand coordination, and perceptual skills of directionality is the use of a bat and a Marsden ball (Figure 10-9). A rubber ball with letters drawn on it is suspended by a string from the ceiling. If an eye hook is used to suspend the ball and the string is tethered to a side wall, the ball can be easily raised and lowered as needed. The bat may be colored in various segments. Often four colors are preferred on each end of the bat symmetrically arranged, e.g., the end segments are red, the next are green, etc. While the dominant eye is occluded, one task is for the patient to hold the stick with two

hands and hit the ball with identical segments on the left side and on the right. The patient attempts to established a regular pattern for at least 20 hits. Using the end segments of the stick is, of course, the most difficult. Some therapists include a general balance requirement as the training progresses. The child is required to stand on one leg or on a balance board while hitting the ball. Children usually enjoy these activities and are willing to train for relatively long periods of time.

Visual tracking, with or without an afterimage tag, is also quite effective using a Marsden ball. Swinging the ball with letters drawn on it in a fore and aft circular pattern provides an accommodative as well as a pursuit tracking stimulus. The goal in this case is to keep the letters clear at all times as the arc of the excursion is increased. Simply swinging the ball in the horizontal plane with the patient standing perpendicular to the swing gives a periodic, predictable, smooth pursuit stimulus for the patient to follow. If the patient lies on the floor beneath the ball, a circular pursuit tracking pattern is demanded. These smooth pursuit techniques are particularly effective if an afterimage tag is used for visual feedback of tracking accuracy.

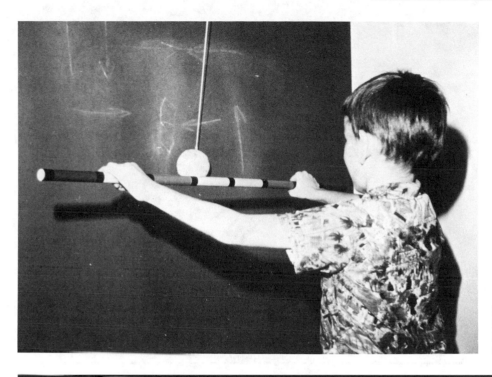

FIGURE 10-9—Bat and Marsden ball for laterality and directionality training combined with occlusion of the nonamblyopic eye.

Tracking with Auditory Feedback T10.5

The Franzbrau Coordinator and Wayne Perceptuomotor Pen are coordination devices that give auditory feedback (e.g., buzzing sound) when inaccurate manual tracking or pointing occurs (Figure 10-10). With the nonamblyopic eye patched, the patient attempts to trace curved line figures. For dot targets, the patient does fast-pointing. Many training tasks stimulate accurate fixation, pursuits, saccades, and eye-hand coordination. We have found T10.5 techniques most effective when timing each task so the patient can work on both speed and accuracy.

Visual Tracing T10.6

Visual Tracing by Groffman is an excellent method to build the visual skills of an amblyopic eye. The patient looks at a series of intersecting lines, each of which is connected to a letter on one end and a number on the other. The purpose is to match the number with the appropriate letter as the amblyopic eye sights along a line and follows it to its end. Workbooks with answer keys for monitoring progress are available from Mast/Keystone. Initially, the patient may require a pointer stick to help keep his/her

eye on the line, but as speed and accuracy develop, only visual tracking is needed. Besides recording the correct answers, the patient should also record the completion time for each task. We have discovered that some children enjoy making their own line mazes. An example of work of a 9-year-old patient is shown in Figure 10-11. The child feels a sense of pride in the designs he has made. A key is made up, and the patient can administer the test to siblings or friends who do not always fare too well on some of the more elaborate patterns. This sometimes provides a much needed ego boost to the amblyopic child who wears a patch. Groffman's visual tracing patterns are also available on the Computer Orthoptics system for in-office reinforcement of this skill.

Ann Arbor Tracking T10.7

Ann Arbor Publishers market some printed materials, the Ann Arbor Tracking Program (formerly referred to as "Michigan Tracking"). We have found these materials to be both motivational and effective in training saccadic eye movements, among other functions. The basic task is to find and circle a key sequence of letters, numbers, words, or symbols in a large,

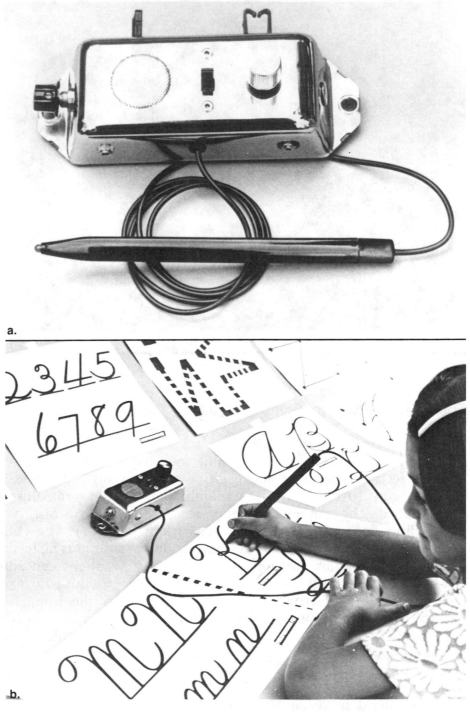

FIGURE 10-10—The Perceptuomotor Pen (also called the "Talking Pen") (a) The apparatus; (b) Example of its use in vision therapy. Photo courtesy of Wayne Engineering.

seemingly random, set of such. The exercise is timed and progress can be charted. The most useful workbooks for training amblyopic patients include *Letter Tracking* (Figure 10-12), *Symbol Tracking,* and *Word Tracking.* For adults, the Limericks Word Tracking is entertaining. Some of these workbooks are printed in red ink, which is very helpful in breaking suppression and training visual tracking with the amblyopic eye under binocular conditions. (These procedures will be discussed later in this chapter.) Ann Arbor Publishers also distribute two perceptual activity workbooks, which can be quite challenging for the amblyopic patient.

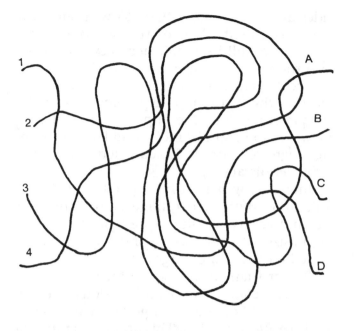

FIGURE 10-11—Sample visual tracing exercise, drawn first by the patient and later following the lines visually with the amblyopic eye.

Resolution Techniques

As is true in the nonamblyopic eye, the amblyopic eye can resolve and identify details best with foveal fixation.[51] In the case of amblyopia, the peak foveal acuity is often reduced and oculomotor and localization skills are deficient. The patient can be taught to use the peak area of the amblyopic eye for fixation by requiring the patient to search for and identify threshold letters or targets. These targets will only be recognized if there is foveal fixation. Most fixation techniques described previously can add the resolution requirement by using the appropriate threshold target size. This is an important step in the remediation of amblyopia and eccentric fixation. The following techniques are particularly suited for resolution training and can be introduced at any stage in the vision therapy program.

Hart Charts T10.8

Hart Charts are often used in the training of accommodative facility because the task involves discriminating and identifying letters in sequence from two charts, one at far and the

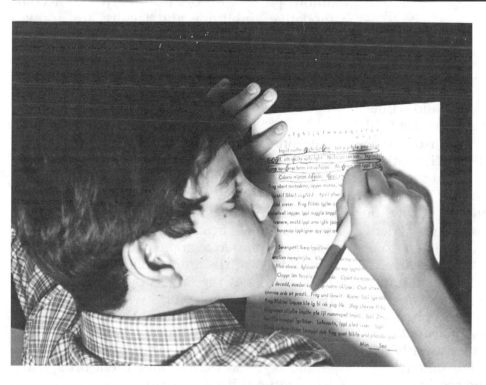

FIGURE 10-12—Ann Arbor tracking. The patient is instructed to make saccades to find each sequential letter of the alphabet but is to follow the pencil tip in a continuous motion. When performance is assured, the nonamblyopic eye is patched during the procedure.

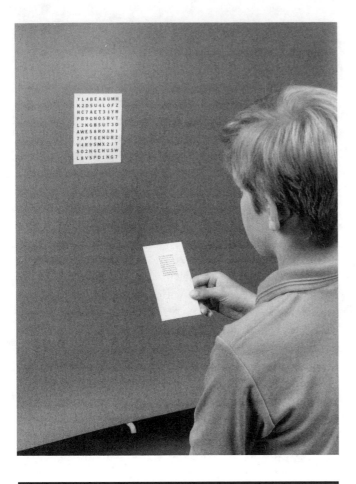

FIGURE 10-13—Hart Chart technique for near and far fixations (photo courtesy of Bernell Corp.).

other at near. (Refer to Chapter 16 for further discussion.) However, the task is also ideal for training saccadic eye movements and visual search with amblyopic patients. Two identical charts of different size are set up in different locations in a room (Figure 10-13). The patient alternately fixates the same letters in sequence on the charts as rapidly as possible. The therapist assigns an appropriate number of rows or columns to complete in a set based on patient observation. A single set should take 1 to 2 minutes before a short rest is allowed. A sufficient number of sets is assigned to fill at least a 10-minute time interval for this particular exercise. As the patient improves, the horizontal separation of the charts is increased. The patient should be reminded to use only eye movements for saccadic eye movements, no head movements. Realistically speaking, sac-

cades are rarely greater than 15 without some head movement,[48] but for the purpose of this exercise, to build saccadic accuracy and speed with the amblyopic eye, the saccadic demands can be larger. The distance from the targets controls the resolution requirement. Initially the patient would use suprathreshold letters (viewing at nearer distances) and later, as training progressed, threshold acuity letters (viewing at farther distances).

Introducing a near-far separation (e.g., 40 cm and 3 m) of the two targets also stimulates accommodative facility. Speed of focusing is emphasized. In this case, a smaller Hart Chart is used for the nearer target.

Rather than relying solely on Hart Charts, some clinicians photocopy various clinical nearpoint charts and enlarge them for use in home fixation training. This provides a range of letter sizes so that resolution practice can be conveniently added to the task. We suggest an emphasis on accommodative training when central fixation exists. The accommodative system responds optimally when foveal fixation is used and responsivity falls off quickly with eccentricity of fixation.[49,50] However, just because central fixation has been achieved in an amblyopic eye, it does not follow that accommodative amplitude and facility are normal. Usually this is not the case. Accommodative training is often needed to improve both amplitude and facility. (Refer to Chapter 16 for accommodative training techniques that can also be used in cases of amblyopia.)

Counting Small Objects T10.9

This technique requires resolution and sorting skills. As with all the other techniques in this section, the nonamblyopic eye is totally occluded. Small objects, such as multicolored candies, small beads, and colored dots on a paper, are chosen to approximate the threshold acuity level of the amblyopic eye. The patient is asked to sort the targets by some parameter (e.g., size, shape, color). A pointer stick or tweezers can be used to sort the objects. In the case of dots, the patient can draw dots of various sizes or colors on a paper. The training task would be to sort and count them on a visual basis without hand support.

Reading for Resolution T10.10

Reading recreational material using the amblyopic eye alone should be encouraged for as much time as is practical. The material (e.g., comic book, magazine, newspaper) is held at a threshold distance from the patient while the patient reads for meaning and enjoyment. The reading period should be at least 5 minutes for elementary school children and 10 minutes for older children and adults. The goals are to improve the threshold acuity (read the material at farther distances or progress from large print to small) and to increase the reading time or rate (higher efficiency). This procedure can be fatiguing and frustrating. This is because people ordinarily read print three times larger than their threshold size for optimum reading performance.[52]

A second reading technique is similar to word tracking in the Ann Arbor Tracking Program. The patient uses personally selected reading material and circles key words (e.g., the, is, are, she, he, if, etc.) or letters as they appear in the text. Again, the material is held at a threshold distance. The patient attempts each day to increase the number of key words or letters identified and circled within a prescribed time interval (5 or 10 minutes).

Tachistoscopic Training T10.11

A tachistoscope is a projection device that flashes targets (letters, numbers, words) at rapid rates of exposure, 1/10 second or faster. The patient does not have sufficient time to make a saccadic eye movement. The device is usually used by educators to increase the span of recognition of poor readers, but this technique has applicability with amblyopic patients also. This technique is usually applied as an office procedure because of the special equipment required. Using only the amblyopic eye, the patient attempts to improve the speed and span of recognition and resolution. Targets can be presented at a threshold size appropriate for the distance. Many educational supply companies market tachistoscopes, including an inexpensive home training model with a spring loaded mechanism.

A similar technique is using flash cards with words or pictures of objects. The therapist shows the patient a brief exposure of the flash card and the patient attempts to resolve and identify the word or picture with the amblyopic eye. The cards are initially shown at suprathreshold acuity levels and, as training progresses, at threshold. The goal is to increase both the speed of recognition and visual acuity.

Monocular Telescope T10.12

When some patients with eccentric fixation view letters or objects with the amblyopic eye through a 4X telescope, there is improvement in the fixation pattern and in visual acuity, more than expected on the basis of the magnification factor alone.[53] For example, a patient presents with 20/120 in the amblyopic eye (MAR = 6 minutes). With a 4X telescope, one would expect the patient to read the 20/30 line (MAR = 1.5, i.e., 1/4 of 6). The patient, however, may read the 20/20 line with the telescope, suggesting improved fixation. It is not known why fixation improves for some patients with a telescope, but one thought is that magnification and, particularly, the restricted field of gaze in some way disrupts the habitual fixation pattern and promotes foveal fixation. The magnified letters are also more isolated; single letter acuity is generally better than whole line acuity in amblyopia. Ciuffreda et al.[53] caution the clinician about relying on the magnification factor for prognostic purposed. They believe, however, that the use of a telescope has some merit in the treatment of amblyopia with eccentric fixation.

If visual acuity through a telescope does improve with a particular patient on initial testing, then prescribing a variable focus telescope for therapy should be considered. The most popular powers are 2.5X and 4X. We tend to keep this technique in reserve and recommend its use only if progress in vision therapy appears to be stalled using other methods. The therapy technique is simply to view distant objects, words, or television with the telescope for about 30 minutes a day for 1 to 2 months. An afterimage tag can be incorporated effectively with this method also. The improved fixation pattern and acuity becomes habitual in some cases and transfers to natural seeing conditions.

FOVEAL TAG TECHNIQUES

Foveal tag techniques for rehabilitating fixation and eye motility are among the most effective vision training procedures available to the primary eye care doctor, but their effectiveness still requires the support of occlusion or penalization. Several clinicians describe the afterimage transfer technique, in particular, as a valuable procedure for both in-office and home training.[54-56] We recommend utilizing foveal tag techniques as a standard part of therapy for eccentric fixation (EF). This method ensures that the fovea is being used correctly for fixation and motility. The tag is an entopic projection of the fovea in free space that provides the patient with visual feedback as to where the fovea is directed. If the patient attempts to make a saccadic eye movement with the amblyopic eye to a small target and has an undershoot, the patient becomes immediately aware of the error. The patient can then develop corrective saccadic and fixation strategies that become habitual with time and repetition. It must be remembered that when patients with EF fixate a target, they believe and feel that they are looking straight at it. The oculocentric direction of the amblyopic eye is associated with the eccentric point, not the fovea. Therefore, when the patient accurately fixates a target with the foveal tag, he feels he must look off to the side of the target. Foveal fixation "feels" abnormal to the eccentric fixator. Not only is localization abnormal, but usually all the oculomotor functions of an amblyopic eye are deficient to some degree. Patients feel that they cannot control their fixation or eye movements accurately, which is true. The therapist frequently needs to reassure most patients that with occlusion and active participation in amblyopia therapy, they will significantly improve their eye movement skills and visual acuity. In this respect, vision therapy is much like physical therapy.

Patient cooperation and honestly in reporting observations are critical to the success of these techniques. In our experience, most children, aged 8 years and older, can usually cooperate fully with these techniques. Some precocious 5-year-olds can also participate adequately.

Preparation for Haidinger Brush Training

Initially, the amblyopic patient is shown the Haidinger Brush (HB) with the normal eye for the purpose of identification. (See Chapter 5 for a description of HB testing.) The density of the cobalt filter is adjusted to maximize its vivid perception; filters can be added to the screen of the Macular Integrity Tester-Trainer (MITT). The patient wears CAMP lenses (if any ametropia) and sits approximately 40 cm from the MITT. With the dominant eye occluded, the patient fixates a suprathreshold letter with the amblyopic eye and locates the position of the HB on the screen. The therapist asks the patient to use a pointer stick to indicate the exact position of the HB. The patient and therapist are now ready to use any or all of the training techniques discussed subsequently in this section.

Preparation for Afterimage Transfer Training

An inexpensive electronic camera flash attachment can be easily modified for use in binocular assessment and training. For clinical purposes, a good afterimage (AI) is a thin streak with a small gap in the middle. The face of the flasher is masked off with opaque tape in the manner illustrated in Figure 5-40. The modified flasher is held vertically about 40 cm from the patient whose amblyopic eye is occluded. The patient fixates the center of the gap in the masked line with the nonamblyopic eye as the therapist triggers the flash. The occluder is then switched from the amblyopic to the nonamblyopic eye so the patient can see a transferred projection of the afterimage with the amblyopic eye. The AI can best be perceived and maintained if a light source directed to the nonamblyopic eye (from the side and behind the occluder) is constantly flashing on and off; blinking also helps. The AI usually persists for about 3 minutes and then the procedure is repeated.

In cases of strabismus with ARC, it is important to check that the AI has transferred to the fovea of the amblyopic eye rather than to an extrafoveal eccentric point. The alignment of the transferred AI for the amblyopic eye can be verified by having the patient simultaneously locate the position of the HB on the MITT. If the gap of the AI is coincident with the center of the HB, the transfer has been successful and on the fovea. However, if misalignment of the two exists, the AI has transferred incorrectly. Wick[57] recommends the patient physically hold the amblyopic eye closed with his/her fingers while the AI is applied to the dominant eye. He found that the AI is more likely to transfer to the fovea of the amblyopic eye if this is done, although it does not happen in every case. The reason for correct transfer of the afterimage is unknown, but we speculate that increased dissociation (less natural) between the two eyes, with fingers holding the eye closed, may elicit the innate NRC localization. In cases of strabismic amblyopia, it is prudent to check with HB testing to see if the AI has, in fact, transferred correctly. Once the therapist is assured of correct AI transfer, training of fixation and motility with this tag can proceed.

Foveal Tag Training

The following tagging techniques are hierarchically sequenced from our clinical experience. They can, however, be mixed during a therapy session based on the needs and responses of a particular patient.

Basic Central Fixation Training T10.13
The goal of this technique is to establish the rudimentary ability to move the foveal tag rapidly to a target of regard. Later, the goal is for reflexive responses. Initially, a guide target (e.g., pointer stick) is used to achieve central fixation. The goal is for the patient to achieve foveal fixation quickly without a guide target.

HB   If a patient with EF has difficulty moving the amblyopic eye to align the HB with a suprathreshold target, the therapist can use a pointer stick to guide fixation. The patient fixates the tip of the pointer stick with the EF point. The therapist moves the pointer as the patient tracks it to a position where the HB is centered on the target. On repeated trials, the pointer is

moved faster to achieve centricity of foveal fixation. Eventually, the patient should be able to make the fixation movement unguided. At this stage the patient does not necessarily "feel" he is looking directly at the target when the foveal tag is aligned. The patient may also find it difficult to hold the tag on the target for any length of time.

AI   With the dominant eye occluded, the patient is instructed to move the transferred AI directly to a suprathreshold letter or real object at any distance in the room. If difficulty is encountered, a guide object is held by the therapist and moved to the proper location to align the AI with the object of regard. The patient fixates the guide object with the EF point. Speed and accuracy of aligning the tag with the target of regard are developed by repetition. With practice, the patient should be able to achieve alignment quickly without a guide object.

Steadiness of Fixation Training T10.14
The goal of this technique is to develop steady central fixation. In most cases of amblyopia, with or without eccentric fixation, the fixation pattern is unsteady to some degree. Initially, there is little control of unsteadiness, but using this technique the patient can usually reduce the amplitude of unsteadiness in small steps. Visuoscopy can be used as an independent test to monitor progress. A clinical goal can be to improve the degree of steadiness with the amblyopic eye to that found with the nonamblyopic eye. Most cases take 10 or more training sessions to accomplish this goal, but there is large individual variation.

HB   The beginning slide is the one with five letters, each being inside a circle (Figure 10-14). The patient places the HB on one letter and notes the amplitude of unsteadiness of fixation. The patient moves closer or farther from the screen until the range of unsteadiness falls mostly within the circle and then the patient maintains that distance for training. The patient then makes a "mental effort" to hold the HB within the circle for a 20-second count. The patient counts aloud. When the center of the HB moves outside the circle, he stops counting.

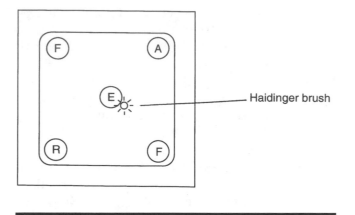

FIGURE 10-14—Slide of the MITT for use with the Haidinger brush for development of steady and central fixation.

The count is started again as the patient attempts to achieve this intermediate goal of 20 seconds of improved steadiness. When that is achieved, the patient moves farther back from the screen, establishes a new training distance, and begins again. When the circle slide is mastered, an acuity chart slide is substituted and the performance criterion becomes maintaining the HB on variously sized letters. The final goal is to maintain steady fixation on threshold letters.

AI With the AI transfer tag, the patient should note the position of the AI gap with respect to the boundary of the fixation target. Real objects can be placed around the room at various distances; golf balls or toys are often convenient targets. The patient attempts to hold the AI tag on each for the count of 20 seconds as a criterion. As the training progresses, smaller objects and greater distances are used. The goal is to maintain steady fixation on threshold letters or objects at all distances.

Saccadic Movements with Tag T10.15

Inaccurate saccades are usually found with amblyopia. The foveal tag allows the patient to be aware of these saccadic errors so corrective strategies can be learned. The goal of this technique is to build fast, accurate, single saccades from one threshold target to another. As a rule,

each timed set should take from 1 to 2 minutes of active effort followed by a short rest period.

HB With the circle slide in place, the therapist notes the time it takes the patient to fixate all five targets sequentially. When the HB is successfully centered on each target in sequence, the patient indicates this by saying "now." The therapist times the patient on both predictable and unpredictable target sequences. As training progresses, threshold letters (achieved by varying the distance) are presented and more targets are added to the routine. The goal is improved speed, since inaccuracies tend to reduce the completion time.

AI A number of objects or printed acuity charts (5 initially) are placed about the room separated by varying distances from each other and from the patient. Young children respond best to small toys as targets, whereas older children and adults can use Hart Charts. A specific letter on each chart becomes the fixation target so there is visual search requirement in a complex field. When the foveal tag is successfully placed on each target in sequence, the patient indicates this by saying "now" or counts the number of targets successfully fixated. The patient is timed on a sequence of predictable and unpredictable targets and with progress, longer sequences are added. If a desk clock is available for home training, some patients prefer to count the number of targets sequentially fixated within an assigned time, e.g., 2 minutes. The clock can be one of the fixation targets. A clinical goal is to maximize the number of fixations within a time period using targets that are almost threshold.

Another variation of this technique is to introduce a saccadic stimulus by a prism placed before the amblyopic eye while the patient fixates a particular target. The prism shifts the perceived image in the direction of the prism apex. The patient attempts to realign the AI on a target as quickly and accurately as possible. The prism amount and base orientation are varied to introduce new stimuli. Again, the number of the patient's correct responses is timed.

Foveal Localization (Fast Pointing) T10.16 Cüppers[58] believed that the cause of eccentric fixation was a shift of oculocentric direction to an extrafoveal point that occurred secondarily to the development of ARC. This idea may or may not be correct. Further research may answer this question, but successful treatment of EF requires a shift of the "straight ahead" locus back to where it belongs, the fovea. Remediation of oculocentric direction starts by demonstrating the monocular aiming error to the patient. This demonstration can be done by means of eye-hand coordination feedback. The goal is to establish central foveal spatial localization in the amblyopic eye, at least under monocular conditions.

Since there are no significant differences between the HB and AI foveal tag techniques, a generalized technique will be described. The technique involves fast pointing and adjusting to the result. The patient holds a pointer stick in a spear-like throwing position. A fast eye movement is made to the target. The patient checks to see if the foveal tag is directly on the target and makes the appropriate adjustment. With no hesitation, the patient "hurls" the pointer to the target without letting the pointer leave his hand. At the end of the thrust, no correctional hand movements are allowed. The patient, and the therapist, note the outcome, a "hit" or a "miss." Slow studied movements are not accepted during this procedure. We want automatic hits. The eccentrically fixating patient often misses in a particular direction and appropriate adjustment must be made. The therapist emphasizes verbally that the foveal tag position is the new "straight ahead" position. This provides motivation toward the goal. The patient adjusts the sighting on subsequent attempts; the error is compensated for and the patient's hit rate increases. With increasing proficiency, smaller targets are introduced and a remarkable effect occurs; the oculocentric direction shifts to the fovea. It is not known whether the physiologic process is gradual or instantaneous, or what mechanism is responsible. It can happen with occlusion alone, but vision training facilitates the shift in monocular localization. Fast pointing procedures hold the patient's interest; we find it effective if the

amblyopic patient advances to this level. The optimum technique is to combine T10.15 with T10.16. For each fixation target where the foveal tag is aligned, the patient attempts fast pointing. The clinical goal is to increase the hit rate at a reflex level when using threshold letters or objects.

Pursuits with Tag T10.17
Patient's typically enjoy pursuit training, particularly with an AI tag. It represents a competitive race. The amblyopic eye must keep up with, but not beat the moving target. This may be one that is moved by the therapist's hand. Initially, many amblyopic patients track a moving target with a series of saccades, similar to the pattern found during infancy. The goal is smoothness and accuracy of tracking. The foveal tag gives the visual feedback the patient needs to judge successful performance. The physiological development of pursuits is not sufficiently understood to describe how people inhibit saccades during pursuits. With visual experience and training, however, the amblyopic eye can improve pursuit skills.

HB The therapist moves a pointer stick slowly across the screen of the MITT as the patient attempts to keep the center of the brush on the tip of the stick. The patient attempts to join the HB "propeller" with the stick. The therapist adjusts the speed and predictability of the pointer movement to the skill level of the patient. The patient indicates inaccurate performance by simply saying "off." The therapist adjusts the target speed to a 75% success level, or more, judged by the time on target. The clinical goal is the maximum speed attainable at the 75% accurate tracking level depending on the choice of criterion by the therapist.

AI Tracking with the AI is much more fun for the patient because the technique can be performed in the open environment. Many moving targets are available depending on the inventiveness of the therapist and the patient. Some kids at an aggressive stage prefer to track with a pretend "laser beam" and others with a so-called "magic wand." The AI remains in per-

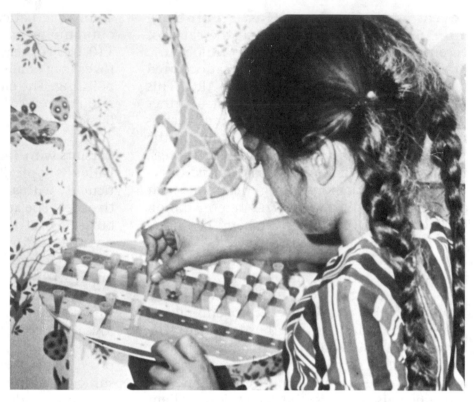

FIGURE 10-15—Rotating pegboard for eye-hand coordination training during direct occlusion. An afterimage can be used for feedback to the patient.

ception only about 3 minutes. This is the time require mnt for the tracking exercise. The patient should indicate when inaccuracy occurs and the speed of target movement should be adjusted to at least a 75% response time on target. The goal is to maximize the speed of accurate smooth pursuits. Target size is not an important variable. Rotators are particularly suited for this exercise (see Figures 2-14 and 10-15). The patient attempts to maintain the AI tag on a particular detail of the pegboard target, starting at the center and working toward the periphery of rotation. Later, the patient tries to place golf tees in the moving board. We particularly recommend the pegboard rotator because the task requires smooth pursuits, proper localization, and eye-hand coordination. The therapist should stop the exercise temporarily when the patient's success rate falls below 50%, either when placing or removing the golf tees. The AI foveal tag can also be effectively used with many other pursuit targets such as a swinging Marsden ball.

Resolution Practice with Tag T10.18

The goal of this technique is to increase the resolution and identification acuity of the amblyopic eye to its maximum. At all stages in fixation training the patient should attempt to resolve threshold letters and object detail. Visual acuity peaks at the fovea in the amblyopic eye.[51] Even though that peak may not be as high as in the nonamblyopic eye, when the target is on the fovea, resolution is best. The amblyopic patient who habitually does not use the fovea for fixation should practice foveal resolution so foveal fixation becomes reflexive. The peak acuity at the fovea can become another clue for the patient to establish central fixation. Increased resolution and identification acuity develop with motoric improvements in centricity, steadiness, and accuracy of fixation. Further improvement in acuity apparently occurs through some sensory adaptation mechanism and tuning of the receptive field organization, but this component is neither well understood nor documented in the literature.

The resolution practice technique is the same using either the HB or AI foveal tag. When the patient aligns the tag with a suprathreshold or threshold letter, the patient attempts to identify it quickly. The patient counts the number of identifications made in a particular time period, 1 or 2 minutes, and with subsequent trials attempts to increase the rate. This procedure works well at home using the AI tag where various magazines, books, newspapers, and comic books of interest to the patient are available. For the sake of efficient training, the therapist can supply Hart Charts or other printed materials and test the patient to establish the proper threshold training distance.

PLEOPTICS

Pleoptics is a form of amblyopia therapy quite popular during the 1950s and 1960s, but has since lost much of its attraction. One major appeal of this method was the use of inverse rather than direct occlusion. Patients patched the amblyopic eye for 1 or 2 months prior to active vision training with pleoptic instruments and during subsequent therapy. Inverse patching was intended to break the habitual pattern of eccentric fixation and suppression that the patient had established. Consequently, amblyopic patients could go about their lives basically unencumbered by poor vision. The disadvantages associated with pleoptics therapy, however, resulted in the current practice by most practitioners of avoiding its use altogether or reserving pleoptics techniques for intractable cases. Pleoptics techniques are time-intensive for the doctor and patient. These procedures require expensive instruments and necessitate pupillary dilation each session. Overall, they appear no more effective than direct patching alone. However, patients who have not responded well to direct occlusion frequently do make progress using pleoptics methods.

Bangerter's Method

In 1953 in Switzerland, Bangerter introduced the term "pleoptics," which means "complete sight" in its Greek derivation.[59] Bangerter had been using his bleaching and light stimulating method to treat amblyopia and eccentric fixation during the 1940s.[60] He believed that eccentric fixation is caused by a depression of foveal acuity to a level below peripheral retinal loci. The decreased visual acuity results from a deep suppression scotoma in the strabismic or anisometropic eye. In an attempt to see more distinctly when the normal eye is occluded, the amblyopic patient selects an eccentric point or area for fixation. Subsequent research[51] has not supported Bangerter's hypothesis on the etiology of EF. His therapy methods, however, have produced some important results and inspired the development of other active amblyopia therapy techniques. The emphasis of his remediation technique is to stimulate the development of the foveal light sense and visual acuity.

Bangerter designed the Pleoptophor that can accurately stimulate the fovea with light (Figure 10-16). The technique is intended to develop the suppressed light sense of a deeply amblyopic eye. The therapy procedure consists of two phases, the *bleaching* phase and the *stimulating* phase. These require dilation of the amblyopic eye as do most pleoptic methods. During the bleaching phase in the Pleoptophore, a macular "shield" is placed over the fovea of the amblyopic eye so that the eccentric point is bleached out with high intensity light while the fovea is spared. The clinician directly views the fovea's position and the macular shield during the bleaching (dazzling) phase to ensure this result is effectively achieved. Thus, the peripheral retina including the eccentric point is dazzled (i.e., relatively desensitized). Next, an annulus with a clear center is rotated into position over the fovea during the stimulation phase. The foveal area is then stimulated with 50 to 100 brief flashes of a small spotlight. The patient is instructed to perceive the light and look at it directly. After repeated series of bleaching and stimulating phases over several weeks, the patient is directly occluded and practices fixation exercises using the amblyopic eye. As the light sense develops, Bangerter introduced several other techniques and instruments he designed involving eye-hand coordination with auditory feedback (Acoustic Localizer), the crowding phenomenon (Separator), a spiral

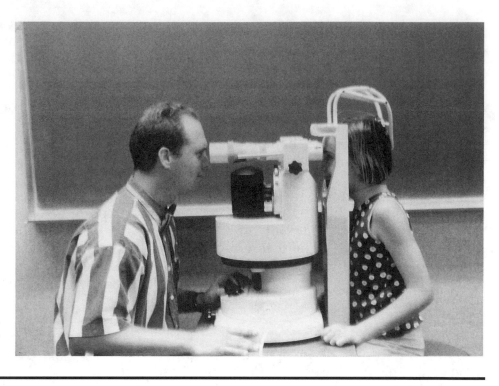

FIGURE 10-16—Child being treated for eccentric fixation with the Pleoptophor of Bangerter.

rotator (Centrophore), and the use of slide projection to build visual recognition of objects and memory (Mnemoscope).[61] These specific instruments are no longer manufactured, yet the principles are incorporated in various instruments currently available. (See section on monocular fixation training.)

Cüppers' Method

In 1956 in Germany, Cüppers took pleoptics methods a step further. He believed that the primary reason for eccentric fixation in an amblyopic eye is a shift of "straight ahead" localization away from the fovea. The individual fixates with an eccentric point (or area) because he feels he is looking straight at the target with that extrafoveal point. Cüppers thought the monocular shift in localization occurred secondarily to the development of ARC in strabismus cases. In anomalous correspondence, there is an eccentric point or area in the strabismic eye that corresponds in visual direction to the fovea of the dominant eye. He believed this point (or area) also represents the "straight ahead" direction under monocular conditions, i.e., oculocentric zero.[62]

Cüppers developed the Euthyscope by modifying an ophthalmoscope so the clinician could bleach an eye while sparing the fovea. In this respect, the technique is similar to Bangerter's method on the Pleoptophor. Euthyscopes are not currently being manufactured. However, a black spot can be painted on the center of a reticule of a direct ophthalmoscope to convert it into an euthyscope. The amblyopic eye is dilated and the nonamblyopic eye is occluded. The peripheral retina, including the eccentric fixation point, is dazzled as the clinician directly monitors alignment of the foveal shield (black spot) on the fovea. After dazzling, however, the patient monocularly views the negative afterimage of the foveal shield in free space on a wall of the vision therapy room (Figure 10-17). The patient is then instructed to center the afterimage on acuity letters or small objects and to identify them. The eventual training goal is for the patient to center the afterimage reflexively on small letters with the sense of "straight ahead" being associated with the fovea. Cüppers also advocated eye-hand coordination training, Haidinger brush procedures, and other vision therapy techniques to achieve this goal.[62]

a.

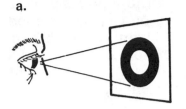

b.

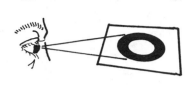

c.

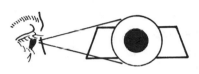

d.

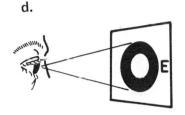

e.

f.

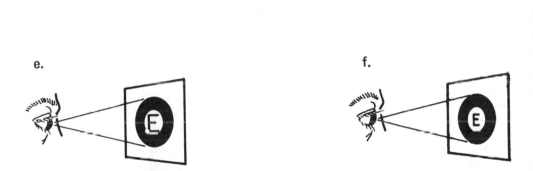

FIGURE 10-17—Euthyscopic afterimage advocated by Cüppers for eccentric fixation therapy. (a) Negative afterimage (black doughnut); (b) Afterimage with psychological characteristics of a real object; (c) Positive afterimage (white doughnut) that violates the psychological characteristics of a real object; (d) Nasal eccentric fixation of the right eye; (e) Central fixation; (f) Central fixation using a small letter as a fixation target.

Efficacy of Pleoptics

Availability of pleoptics instruments is limited. However, several large medical and optometric centers, and a handful of private practitioners, maintain these instruments and conduct remediation programs. Generally, pleoptics is not recommended by most authorities unless a patient has a large magnitude of EF (4^Δ or more) and has not responded well to conventional occlusion and training. This clinical guideline is supported by two excellent reviews of the extensive literature regarding the efficacy of pleoptics therapy, Garzia[6] and Ciuffreda et al.[63]

Overall, pleoptic therapy utilizing indirect occlusion has not proven any more effective than direct occlusion. Garzia[6] correctly pointed out, however, that pleoptic therapy was generally used with older patients and in cases with poorer acuity and larger amounts of EF. Furthermore, Ciuffreda et al.[63] tabulated the results of eight large patient series in which pleoptic therapy was successful in cases of amblyopia that did not respond to standard occlusion therapy. Among these studies, which included many adults, the success rate (i.e., 20/40 or better) varied from 38% to 100% with a weighted average of 52% for patients with eccentric

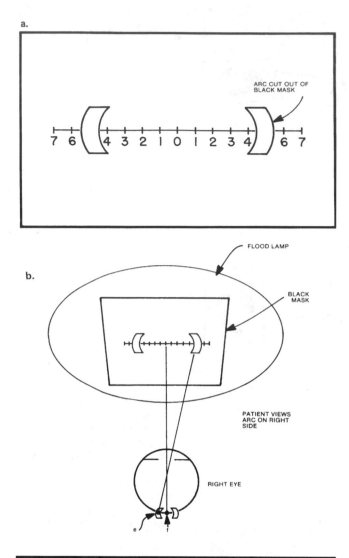

FIGURE 10-18—Method of Vodnoy in cases of eccentric fixation. (a) The opaque mask held before a flood lamp with arcs cut out for viewing by the right eye with nasal eccentric fixation; (b) drawing showing the fovea being protected while point *e* is dazzled by the arc on the right side of the mask.

fixation. These are impressive results for intractable cases of all ages and, in our opinion, justify the extra effort associated with pleoptics. If referral sources for pleoptic therapy are not available, we suggest using the custom-made pleoptics instruments and vision training methods described in the next section.

Practical Pleoptic Techniques

Two practical pleoptic techniques can be used for in-office or for home training in cases with steady or fairly steady EF. The important aspects of the techniques, based on Cüppers method, are to bleach out the EF point, preserving the functional integrity of the fovea, and to provide a foveal tag for active fixation training with objects in the open environment.

Vodnoy Afterimage Technique T10.19

Vodnoy[64] introduced a novel home training procedure to produce afterimages in the proper position when treating eccentric fixation. The EF point (point *e*) is dazzled and the position of the fovea is identified for proper fixation training. The patient's eccentric fixation must first be determined accurately by some means, such as by visuoscopy or Haidinger brush testing. When this is done, an afterimage is produced by putting an opaque mask in front of a bright frosted flood lamp, e.g., 100 watts (Figure 10-18). A pair of arcs is cut out of the mask so that the distance from the center of the arcs to the center of the mask is the same as that between point *e* and the fovea. (Convert prism diopters into mm at a 40 cm viewing distance by using the rule that each 4 mm represents a prism diopter.) For example, assume the right eye has steady nasal EF of 5^Δ. While occluding the nonamblyopic left eye, the patient is instructed to fixate steadily at the illuminated arc 20 mm to the right for 30 seconds. The arc dazzles point *e,* and the arc on the left side of the mask dazzles a temporal extrafoveal point the same distance away from the fovea. This gives the patient the advantage of having a bracket as a negative afterimage with the center positioned at the fovea. In normal room illumination, the patient is instructed to put these brackets around any target the therapist indicates, e.g., a Haidinger brush to confirm proper alignment of the brackets, Snellen letters of various sizes for resolution practice, or any real object for fixation training in free space. If the fixation target is a flashing light, the fovea is being stimulated in a manner recommended by Bangerter. Since the position of the fovea has been tagged, all the techniques described in the section on afterimage transfer can be effectively carried out. In this case, however, there is the additional advantage of having bleached out the eccentric point so it does not interfere with proper localization of targets.

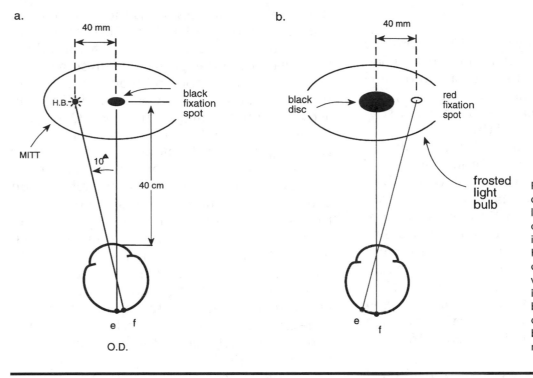

FIGURE 10-19—Use of a black disc taped on a frosted flood lamp for home training in cases of eccentric fixation. (a) Angle E is first determined by means of Haidinger brush testing; (b) The disk is used to protect the fovea while the extrafoveal area including point "e" is dazzled. The amblyopic eye must fixate in a direction opposite to the HB, but by an amount equal to the magnitude of angle E.

Cüppers Home Pleoptics T10.20

Another easy way to create a direct afterimage and use Cüppers' methods for in-office or home training in cases of steady or almost steady EF was described by Priestley et al.[65] We recommend the following materials: (1) a 100 watt frosted lamp; (2) a 2 cm round black disc cut from electrical tape and placed at the center of the lamp, and (3) a small red fixation spot also cut from tape (Figure 10-19). The magnitude of EF is measured and the distance between point e and the fovea relative to a 40 cm viewing distance is determined by calculation. Suppose the patient's right eye has 10^Δ steady nasal EF. To protect the fovea during bleaching, the patient necessarily has to fixate 40 mm to the right from the center of the black shield. The red fixation spot is placed in this position by direct measurement. The patient fixates the red spot with the amblyopic eye as steadily as possible for 30 seconds during the bleaching phase. An important point to remember is that this technique is of no value, and may actually hinder therapy, unless the center of the fovea is protected. The doctor must monitor the amount of eccentric fixation accurately and frequently (e.g., weekly) to ensure the effectiveness of this method. Continuing with direct occlusion, the patient perceives the negative afterimage of the shield, the center of which represents the position of the fovea in free space. The previously described afterimage training techniques can be used for about 3 minutes before the afterimage fades. If desired, a blinking background light helps to extend the perception of the afterimage to about 5 minutes. Repeated cycles of bleaching and training are done during each in-office therapy session. Wick[66,67] described a similar home pleoptics method, but he used a strobe flash to generate the afterimage more quickly.

BINOCULAR THERAPY FOR AMBLYOPIA

Both antidiplopia mechanisms of anomalous "retinal" correspondence (ARC) and suppression must be considered when binocular training procedures are introduced in amblyopia therapy.

ARC Considerations

In most cases of amblyopia with a constant strabismus and ARC, it does not make good sense to switch from monocular amblyopia therapy to binocular training. Frequently the prognosis for functional cure of constant strabismus and ARC is poor and the excessive training may not be worth the effort to achieve a possibly higher quality of binocular vision. ARC, it must be remembered, is a form of binocular vision in which there is rudimentary peripheral fusion and sometimes gross stereopsis, but not central fusion. In such cases, it seems appropriate to settle for a cure or improvement of the strabismic amblyopia. The follow-up goal would be to maintain the improved acuity in the amblyopic eye over time. Periodic occlusion of the nonamblyopic eye for a few hours each month may be all that is necessary for this purpose. Better yet, if the patient can practice alternate fixation, using each eye for fixation at different distances (e.g., with optical penalization), the good training results can usually be maintained without patching.

In cases of comitant strabismus with unharmonious or paradoxical ARC or a large noncomitant deviation (even with NRC), there is the possibility that intensive binocular training can result in intractable diplopia. Even treating the amblyopia alone, in these cases, is slightly risky for creating diplopia since patching has an antisuppression effect. Care should be taken to monitor the patient for diplopia as a result of patching; however, shortly after monocular amblyopia therapy, the patient usually begins to suppress again. In our opinion, it is inadvisable to initiate an intense binocular training program in certain cases because of the risk of intractable diplopia.

When there is NRC as in cases of anisometropic or meridional amblyopia or intermittent strabismic amblyopia, binocular training is effective and very helpful in improving both the amblyopia and developing normal sensory and motor integration of the images.

Suppression and Amblyopia

An amblyopic eye generally has deep foveal suppression as a fundamental characteristic of the condition. Suppression is thought to play a role in the etiology of amblyopia. Therefore, an important therapeutic goal in cases in which binocular vision is expected to be restored, particularly anisometropic amblyopia, is the elimination of suppression through occlusion and active vision training techniques. One commonly seen benefit of antisuppression therapy is an improvement in monocular visual acuity of the amblyopic eye. For this reason, many clinicians prefer to introduce antisuppression and sensory and motor fusion techniques when the visual acuity of the amblyopic eye improves to within a practical binocular range, 20/80 (6/24) or better. Other clinicians wait until 20/40 (6/12) acuity is achieved before introducing these techniques. There is no consensus in the literature as to when is the optimum time to emphasize antisuppression techniques, so the choice is properly left to the clinician's discretion in a particular case. If progress stalls in a remediation program of occlusion and active monocular training for 4 weeks or more and the amblyopic acuity is 20/100 (6/30) or better, we suggest switching the emphasis of the training to antisuppression techniques to see if further gains are possible. In many cases, this change is enough to achieve progress again.

Antisuppression Techniques for Amblyopia Therapy

The most effective antisuppression method for a particular patient depends on the type of amblyopia (strabismic or anisometropic), visual acuity level, and depth and extent of suppression. More discussion of specific antisuppression techniques can be found in Chapter 12, so here we will identify only a few that we have found effective particularly with amblyopic patients.

When suppression is deep and extensive, vigorous binocular light stimulation may be necessary to establish the rudiments of binocular vision. Strong light stimuli for breaking deep suppression can be introduced by: 1) the use of rapid alternate flashing, e.g., Allen Translid Binocular Interaction (TBI) method, 2) red lens with vertical prism method, and 3) flashing fusion targets in an amblyoscope with the illumination gradient favoring the amblyopic eye.

(Refer to Chapter 12.) Most cases, however, do not require these intensities of light stimulation. Standard orthoptic instruments and techniques can usually break suppression and build fusional vergence ranges simultaneously. We often use mirror stereoscopes, Brewster stereoscopes, Tranaglyphs, Brock string and beads, Minivectograms, and television trainers. At some point in fusion training of an amblyopic patient with the potential for normal fusion, practically all antisuppression methods are applicable and can be used for variety to build motivation. We recommend using the three antisuppression techniques described below for amblyopic patients because they improve other needed tracking and resolution skills besides breaking suppression. These techniques are particularly appropriate for anisometropic amblyopic amblyopes in which there is normal fusion potential.

Red Filter and Red Print T10.21

Many of the Ann Arbor Tracking Program workbooks are printed in red ink, which makes them appropriate for antisuppression training. A red filter or lens is placed in front of the nonamblyopic eye. (Red-green filter glasses also work well.) The contours of the workbook itself provide the binocular fusion clue since they can be seen by both eyes. Yet, the red print can be seen only with the amblyopic eye, if there is no suppression. (The red-filtered eye sees "red on red" with no figure-ground contrast, the red print is invisible through the red filter.) With suppression, the print is either absent or fades in and out of perception. When suppression occurs, the patient breaks through the suppression response by blinking, moving closer to the workbook, or waving a red pointer stick in the field of view. Tasks in the Ann Arbor Tracking program can be timed to inspire improvement. This visual tracking task is lead by the amblyopic eye under binocular viewing conditions, so monocular tracking skills are improved while suppression is being broken. This procedure is effective for amblyopia therapy and is suitable for home training.

An additional technique is simply to have the patient trace or draw detailed pictures with a red pencil while wearing a red lens over the nonamblyopic eye. Accuracy and speed of

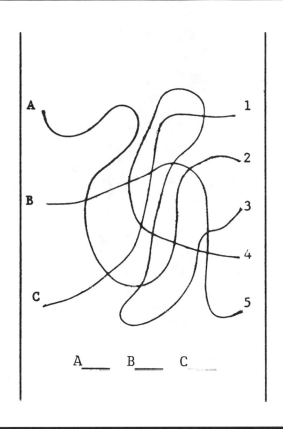

FIGURE 10-20—Example of a Groffman Visual Tracing pad for a Brewster stereoscope.

drawing should increase as suppression decreases.

Visual Tracking with a Brewster Stereoscope T10.22

Groffman Tracings booklets are designed with the figure printed in a middle panel with two blank panels flanking each side. This design allows the booklet to be used on a Brewster stereoscope so that one eye sees the printed figure and the other eye views the pencil while tracing the figure (Figure 10-20). In this manner, the Brewster stereoscope is converted into a cheiroscope for antisuppression training with kinesthetic as well as visual feedback. We recommend initially that the printed figure be viewed with the nonamblyopic eye so that the pencil tip is seen by the amblyopic eye. The patient is instructed to trace the figure only when the figure and the pencil tip are seen at the same time. If the pencil tip disappears, the patient can wiggle the pencil to break suppression. When the patient completes the tracing

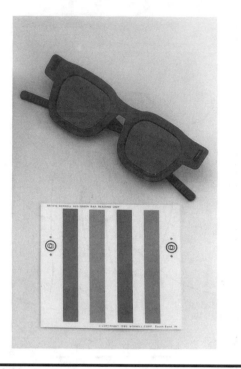

FIGURE 10-21—Bar Reading strips for antisuppression training (photo courtesy of Bernell Corp.).

task with the amblyopic eye, the figure is shifted so that it is now seen with the amblyopic eye. This is more difficult since visual tracking of the printed figure is without "hand support." Speed and accuracy of suppression-free tracings are the training goals for either eye viewing the printed target.

Bar Reading and Tracking T10.23

Filtered reading bars come as either polarized or red-green strips. The bars are vertically oriented strips of filter material interspaced with clear areas (Figure 10-21). The patient wears the corresponding filters for the selected system over appropriate spectacle or contact lenses. A reading bar can be placed over any reading material having threshold or suprathreshold acuity letters for the amblyopic eye. The patient should be able to read across a line of print when suppression is absent. Suppression is indicated if controls (e.g., red and green strips) for right or left eye appear black when the print underneath disappears from view. To break the suppression response, the patient should temporarily stop reading,

rapidly blink either or both eyes, move closer to the material, touch it, or increase the luminance on the page. Reading is resumed when the print reappears and the patient makes a "mental effort" to maintain it in view. The training goal is to achieve suppression-free reading for a 10-minute period using print almost to threshold size for the amblyopic eye. In this way, the patient can practice fixation and resolution with the amblyopic eye while breaking suppression.

A challenging combination of amblyopia training techniques is to add a reading bar with the Ann Arbor Tracking Program workbooks. Rather than circling the key letters or words, the patient counts the number of key items in a passage while the visual tracking performance is timed and recorded. This can also be done with ordinary print. For example, the patient can count the number of times a certain designated word appears in a newspaper article.

Recommendations for Binocular Training

In cases of NRC, in which gross suppression and monocular tracking under binocular conditions have improved, various sensory and motor fusion techniques can be introduced to establish optimum binocular skills. All inaccuracies in pursuits, saccades, and accommodation need not be eliminated before initiating further binocular training. Ideally, the patient should have achieved at least 20/40 (6/12) full chart acuity, no gross suppression, some degree of stereopsis, and basic monocular tracking skills before binocular vision training proceeds further. Once these goals have been achieved, the emphasis of the training program changes to new goals depending on the case: (1) establishing and reinforcing NRC if there is ARC and treatment is deemed advisable (see Chapter 11); (2) eliminating foveal suppression (Chapter 12) and building fusional vergence ranges and reflex responses (Chapters 13, 14, and 16); or (3) if strabismus remains, reducing the angle of deviation by surgical or optical means. Regardless of which direction subsequent therapy takes, the patient should be given maintenance procedures and periodic monitoring to prevent regression of the improved visual acuity of the amblyopic eye.

PROGRESS IN AMBLYOPIA THERAPY

We agree with Caloroso and Rouse[68] that a short diagnostic reassessment during vision therapy should be conducted at least every 4 weeks. Initially, we schedule patients for office visits on a weekly basis. The ideal acuity test to monitor progress in amblyopia therapy is the psychometric S-Chart, but if this test is not available, then a variety of Snellen Charts should be used to prevent memorization. Full chart, line, and single letter acuity thresholds should all be assessed periodically. The fixation pattern is usually monitored by visuoscopy. The refractive status also needs rechecking periodically since the ametropic correction sometimes needs refinement during the course of therapy.

Within week 1 or 2 of patching and vision training, the acuity of the amblyopic eye typically shows some increase. Further improvements may occur in steps in which there is an extended plateau at a particular acuity level. Changes in acuity and improvement in the patient's fixation pattern often are directly related, but not necessarily so. Sometimes the fixation pattern becomes more central without a corresponding improvement in acuity until a few weeks later. If there is no improvement in the fixation pattern or visual acuity during a 1-month period, we change the approach and introduce new techniques. For example, if a plateau occurs with direct patching and monocular viewing games in a case of anisometropic amblyopia, one might introduce binocular techniques even if the amblyopic acuity has not improved to the 20/80 (6/24) to 20/40 (6/12) levels as previously suggested. If the patient has a stabilized eccentric fixation point, however, indirect patching and in-office pleoptics may be an appropriate change. Therapy is continued as long as some improvement occurs during a 1-month interval. When there is no significant improvement for 2 months, despite the patient's best efforts, the maximum visual potential of the amblyopic eye has probably been reached. The remaining deficit can be considered to be amblyopia of arrested development and further improvement is unlikely.

In all cases of amblyopia therapy, the final step is to prevent its reoccurrence. The full optical correction of any significant refractive error must be worn indefinitely, at least for young children. Patients need to be aware of and accept this fact from the outset. If binocular vision has been rehabilitated, as is possible in most cases of anisometropic and isometropic amblyopia, maintenance home exercises are assigned. Periodic occlusion is usually unnecessary, but it is an effective way to prevent regression of visual acuity. We prefer to assign an antisuppression activity for 30 minutes, once a week, such as a reading bar or TV trainer. If the patient notes suppression returning or visual acuity regressing, an office visit is indicated so the doctor can prescribe an appropriate rehabilitation schedule and training techniques. In our experience, the reinforcement schedule of 30 minutes once a week is adequate in most cases, but some patients do require a more frequent and intensive maintenance program.

If strabismus persists after vision therapy, maintenance of good acuity in the formerly amblyopic eye requires that eye to be used periodically for fixation. The patient might simply patch the dominant eye for 30 minutes, once a week while reading, watching television, or engaging in other visual activities. Another approach would be to utilize optical penalization with spectacles or contact lenses on a regular basis as described previously. The doctor must be convinced, however, that the patient does, in fact, switch fixation in response to optical blur. In this way, one eye would be used for fixation at far and the other for nearpoint viewing, thus ensuring the visual integrity of each.

After the patient is dismissed from a completed vision therapy program for amblyopia, we prefer to schedule progress visits for 3 and 6 months and then, if all goes well, on a regular yearly basis.

CASE EXAMPLES

Case no. 1 Adult Anisometropic Amblyopia[69]

Abstract:

A 34-year-old female presented with a hyperopic anisometropic amblyopic eye that was legally blind with best lens correction. There was eccentric fixation, suppression and no measurable stereopsis. An occlusion and vision training program of 4 months duration resulted in central steady fixation, 20/40 visual acuity, and almost normal stereopsis.

Case History:

Mrs. Z, a 34-year-old homemaker, presented with the complaint of a "lazy" left eye originating in early childhood. She had no other visual complaints or symptoms. As a Venezuelan national, Mrs. Z followed her husband to the United States where he was completing a Ph.D. program. She had not previously received any treatment for her eye condition. In Venezuela during elementary school, she had been told that she had amblyopia, which was an incurable condition at her age, but she now wanted a second opinion about that poor prognosis. There was a family history of hyperopia on her mother's side, but to her knowledge no member had strabismus or amblyopia. She felt in excellent physical health, which was confirmed by a medical examination 6 months previously. Her schedule allowed considerable free time, which she enjoyed. She had the time, resources, and commitment to pursue amblyopia therapy.

Clinical Data:

VA at 6 m without Rx.

OD: 20/20 (Snellen) (6/6)

OS: 20/400 (6/120)

VA at 40 cm without Rx.

OD: .4 M (20/20 reduced Snellen)

OS: 2 M

External examination: and pupil reflexes normal.

Internal examination: Normal OU

Extraocular movements: (gross inspection) steady fixation OD, slightly unsteady fixation OS, no restrictions of monocular movements, but poor pursuits and saccades OS, no strabismus seen in 9 fields of gaze (Hirschberg). Near-point of convergence: 12 cm break, 17 cm recovery.

Cover test: Unilateral at 6 m: occasional eso flick of left eye

Alternate at 6 m: orthophoria with occasional eso flick of left eye

Unilateral at 40 cm: occasional eso flick of left eye

Alternate at 20 cm: orthophoria with occasional eso flick of left eye

Stereopsis (none Stereo Fly Test), suppression OS

Keratometry: OD: 44.50@ 180/45.00 @ 90
OS: 44.50@ 180/45.50 @ 90

Retinoscopy (dry) : OD: +0.75 DS
OS: +4.00 −0.50 axis 180

Retinoscopy (1% Cyclogyl) OD: +1.00 DS
OS: +4.25 DS

Subjective (dry): OD: +0.75 DS 20/20
OS: +4.00 DS 20/200

Phorometry: suppression OS, no data taken far or near.

Amplitude of accom.: OD: 7 D
OS: poor response

Accommodative facility: Normal OD. Poor response OS.

Visuoscope: OD: steady central fixation
OS: 4^Δ unsteady nasal and 1^Δ superior fixation with $\pm2^\Delta$ unsteadiness. Oculocentric direction associated with eccentric point OS.

Haidinger Brush: OD: steady central fixation. OS: no brush seen.

Fields: full by Tangent screen OD, OS. (Used tape to indicate the center of the field OS)

Amsler Grid: Normal OD, indistinct OS

Color Vision: (Farnsworth panel D-15)
OD: Normal OS: Normal

Tonometry: OD: 15 mm Hg OS: 14 mm Hg

Impressions and Diagnosis:

Mrs. Z can be described as having hyperopic, anisometropic, deep, amblyopia and nasal unsteady eccentric fixation of the left eye. There does not appear to be a strabismus, though it is possible that she has a small microtropia. There is deep suppression of the left eye and no stereopsis was elicited. Ophthalmoscopy, fields, tonometry, and color vision were all within normal limits, so the eyes appeared healthy. The visual loss of the left eye is probably not due to an organic cause. She apparently had substantial uncorrected hyperopic anisometropia during early childhood that resulted in a lack of development of high frequency resolution channels and poor fixation reflexes for that eye. The eccentric fixation is larger than is found in many anisometropic patients, but the amount does not totally account for the acuity reduction. Using the criterion of MAR = EF$^\Delta$+1, the acuity reduction predicted from 4$^\Delta$ of EF would be about 20/100. The Worth-Chavasse model of amblyopia would suggest that this patient would have acuity loss both from lack of development (arrest) and active suppression (extinction), but the proportion of each is unknown.

The prognosis for a complete functional cure of the amblyopia was guarded due to the large amount of unsteady EF that does not reach the fovea, the low presenting acuity, the unknown onset of anisometropia, and the late age of treatment. The age that treatment is initiated is an important factor in establishing the prognosis. Generally the earlier the treatment, the faster and better are the results. The patient explained that having an essentially blind eye had always disturbed her and she hoped that she could recover some vision. There had never been any therapeutic attempt in her case. If progress could be made, some improvement in acuity would be evident within a few weeks. There would be little risk or inconvenience to the patient in the attempt. A therapy program was recommended that included constant patching (initially) and a course of active training, 30 minutes per day,

lasting approximately 3 to 6 months, depending on the results. Mrs. Z enthusiastically accepted these conditions of treatment.

Many clinicians recommend part-time total direct patching, not full time, in cases of anisometropic amblyopia so binocularity is preserved. Since the corrected acuity was so reduced in this case and we wanted to learn quickly if any improvement was possible, we chose to attempt almost constant, total, direct occlusion. There seemed to be only minimal binocularity with full optical correction initially. Another approach would be constant inverse occlusion initially for several weeks and then inverse patching supplemented by pleoptics therapy, but we kept this option in reserve for reasons of expense and convenience.

Vision Training Plan

Mrs. Z decided to attempt therapy. The subjective refraction lenses were prescribed in the form of spectacles. The advantages and disadvantages of contact lenses were discussed, but she felt most comfortable with wearing glasses. Her spectacle correction is also consistent with Knapp's Law to reduce potential aniseikonia since the anisometropia is axial rather than refractive.

An Elastoplast occluder was worn on the right eye under the glasses during all waking hours except when she required good acuity as when driving or reading. She removed the occluder at these times, but continued to wear her glasses, so there was some limited binocular stimulation.

The overall sequential training goals were to: (1) establish steady central fixation and foveal localization OS; (2) build accurate accommodative, pursuit, and saccadic eye movements OS; (3) improve visual acuity in the amblyopic eye to the maximum level possible and; (4) to break suppression, develop stereopsis, and enhance sensory and motor fusion.

Monocular Fixation Training

Two or three techniques were given for home training each day. Although 30 minutes of training was the minimum expectation, we recommended that each exercise be done at a different time during the day. One technique was usually changed at each weekly office visit for the sake of variety as well as for therapy reasons. The following techniques were assigned:

1. *Afterimage transfer (AI) fixation training.* The location of the left eye's fovea was tagged with a transferred afterimage and various types of fixation activities were given. A circuit breaker was place in an incandescent lamp to provide a flashing background light. This helped to maintain the transferred AI in perception for 3 to 5 minutes before the AI had to be renewed. After the AI was generated, the nonamblyopic eye was occluded with a tie on patch. The following techniques were introduced in the order listed:

A. *Steadiness of fixation:* Using only the tagged amblyopic eye, she was instructed to place and steadily hold the afterimage on a large target (e.g., book) for a certain amount of time (e.g., 30 seconds). She initially found this difficult to do since the AI kept moving off to her left, but with practice she learned to hold the AI on the target for increasing intervals. Smaller and more demanding targets were then introduced (e.g., a small clock, circles of various sizes, figurines, thimbles, etc.).

B. *Accuracy and speed of fixation:* Mrs. Z set up five objects on a table. Using only the tagged amblyopic eye, she fixated each target in turn as rapidly as she could and counted the number of objects fixated within a 1-minute interval. At least seven 1-minute intervals were assigned each day at home, but she would usually complete many more than the required minimum. The number of objects within 1 minute increased slowly over the first month of training. She noted that the fixations were becoming more accurate; initially many saccades were needed to align the AI with each target, but later the eye moved quickly to the target without intervening stops.

2. *Foveal tag and fast pointing.* The transferred afterimage was used as a foveal tag for home training. After about a month of training, she could perceive the Haidinger brush with the amblyopic eye and this was also used for office training. Mrs. Z initially reported that she had to look off to the side to place the tag on the target, which seemed unnatural. She frequently past-pointed, but after about 5 weeks of training, it seemed natural to align the AI on a target and fast pointing was usually accurate.

3. *Marsden ball training with and without afterimage transfer.* Smooth tracking, accommodation facility, eye-hand coordination, and accurate fixation were all emphasized at various times. As her skills increased, amplitude and speed were increased and other orientations were introduced besides horizontal and vertical swings. By 2 months, she could track with good accuracy on large amplitude diagonals and rotations for intervals of 3 minutes.

4. *Hart Charts fixations and accommodative jumps.* This was the last technique introduced during the monocular phase of the training. Acuity and fixation skills had improved with the amblyopic eye. Suprathreshold and threshold letters were used to build fixation accuracy, saccadic speed, and accommodative facility of the amblyopic eye. For example, for accommodative rock training, a Hart chart was placed at a distance where the letters were just readable and a nearpoint chart was used at a distance where the letters could be resolved. Initially, an AI tagged the location of the amblyopic fovea. The patient slowly and alternately fixated letters on the two cards and timed herself for one line of letters. More lines were added as speed increased. As acuity increased, more demanding distances were introduced.

Binocular Training

After 2 months of monocular training and nearly full-time patching, visual acuity had improved to 20/80 by Snellen and S-chart. There was about 2^{Δ} nasal, unsteady, eccentric fixation, but the fovea was included in the unsteadiness. Direct total occlusion was reduced to 6 hours per day and the emphasis of the training shifted to breaking suppression and building sensory and motor fusion, although monocular exercises were still included in the program. The initial emphasis during the binocular phase was to break suppression, then to build suppression-free vergence ranges. Binocular accommodative techniques were introduced to integrate accommodative and vergence skills. Stereopsis awareness and discrimination was emphasized near the end of the program to complete the binocular phase. Specific binocular techniques included the following:

1. *Antisuppression: polarized TV trainer, polarized reading bar, string and beads, Vectograms, Tranaglyphs, and cheiroscopic drawings.* For example, the TV trainer was particularly effective and well accepted by the patient. Initially, she would have to sit about 1 meter from the television set to hold both images in perception for 80% of the time. When the amblyopic eye's image would fade, she would blink or lean forward toward the set to renew the image, then she would make a conscious effort to hold the image there for as long as possible. When 100% success occurred at a particular distance, Mrs. Z would move back about 50 cm and start the process again. When she was successful from across the room, prisms were introduced to stress her vergence and she again started at a close viewing distance. She liked to watch news and used the TV trainer for at least 30 minutes each day.

2. *Convergence and divergence: Vectograms, eccentric circles, red-green circles, loose prisms, and binocular flippers.* For example, the Chicago Skyline, #7 Vectogram, was used for home training for step-vergences in both directions. The skyline was placed at 3^Δ BI so the airplane would be at 3^Δ BO. This amplitude was within the fusional capacity of the patient. She was instructed to alternate her fixation and fuse each target, in turn, noting the suppression clues and to time herself for 20 cycles. She was to increase her speed of fusion to a maximum level, then to increase the prism demand by 1^Δ in both directions. She recorded the vergence setting of the targets and her best time each day. If suppression occurred, she was to break it by blinking before continuing the exercise. She increased her step vergences to 10^Δ BI and BO using this technique.

3. *Gross convergence: string and beads, pencil pushups, jump vergences.* For example, a push-up technique was using with the string and beads to build the smoothness of convergence training and the nearpoint of convergence. She held one end to her nose and tied the other end of the string to an object, e.g., door knob. She moved a bead slowly and smoothly and tracked it from arm's length to her NPC while holding the percept of the strings crossing at the bead. If a physiological diplopic clue of one string disappeared, she stopped to blink or jiggle the bead to renew the suppressed image before continuing. She would work on this of 2 minutes at a time, then rest her eyes a short time before continuing. Usually four sets of 2 minutes each were completed. The best NPC each day, the number of sets completed, and the number of times suppression occurred were recorded on the home training recording sheet.

4. *Accommodation: accommodative tracking, binocular flippers, jump focus.* For example, when visual acuity had improved to almost 20/40, Mrs. Z was asked to read a magazine for 10 minutes using a polarized reading bar while she tromboned the reading material from arm's length to her nearpoint of accommodation. The goal was to keep the print clear at all times over her range of accommodation without suppression, thus building smooth and accurate accommodation.

5. *Stereopsis: Vectograms, stereograms.* For example, stereopsis awareness was emphasized using Vectogram #5, the Spirangle, with clues for each of the letters on the spiral. The instructions were first to move her eyes around the spiral rapidly to maximize the overall depth percept, then to identify the stereo relief precisely in each particular letter. Stereo awareness was trained at various vergence demands to enhance her discrimination skills.

Additional monocular fixation, saccadic and pursuit exercises included "Michigan" tracking, Groffman tracing, dot-to-dot patterns, and threshold reading. Mrs. Z maintained excellent compliance throughout the vision therapy program and often exceeded the minimum training time expected each day.

Summary of Results

After 3 weeks of direct patching and active training there was substantial improvement in acuity and fixation skills. The S-chart acuity measured 20/120 consistently and the eccentric fixation appeared to have reduced to 3^Δ nasal unsteady combined with 1^Δ inferior. Mrs. Z subjectively noted the improvement in vision and the improved control of her fixation pattern. She found that direct patching was not a major inconvenience when she was at home, but she removed it for driving, shopping and other activities requiring precise vision. She estimated she wore the patch 10 to 12 hours per day. Each week she was tested for muscle balance (far and near) and no decompensation was noted. Gross stereopsis of approximately 3000 seconds of arc was found on the Stereo Fly. The basic thrust of therapy (the aggressive direct occlusion), and monocular fixation training, was continued.

After 2 months of therapy, 20/80 was consistently found and the eccentric fixation measured 2^Δ nasal with the unsteadiness excursion including the fovea. Mrs. Z faithfully complied with the patching and active therapy program and was gratified by the improvement. Stereopsis of 400 seconds of arc was found on the Stereo Fly test. The thrust of the therapy was changed to building binocular vision—intensive antisuppression activities, fusional vergence, stereopsis discrimination tasks, and fixation exercises while monitoring suppression clues. Mrs. Z welcomed the changes since several new instruments and procedures added variety to her home training. Direct patching was reduced to 6 hours per day to allow for more binocular stimulation.

There was slow progress with a few plateau periods over the next 2 months of active training. The acuity increased to 20/40 by Snellen (full chart and line acuity) and by S-chart. Central, steady fixation of the left eye was achieved and appeared similar to that of the right by visuoscopy. A suppression-free range of fusional vergence became normal (Chapter 2). Stereopsis slowly increased and stabilized at 70 seconds of arc. After 4 months of vision therapy, relevant data measured as follows:

VA at 6 m without Rx.

OD: 20/20

OS: 20/40

VA at 40 cm without Rx.

OD: .4 M

OS: .6 M

Ocular motility: steady fixation monocularly and binocularly, accurate pursuits and saccades, no strabismus seen in 9 fields of gaze, nearpoint of convergence 6 cm, and recovery 9 cm.

Cover test:	Unilateral at 6 m: no movement
	Alternate at 6 m: 1^Δ exophoria
	Unilateral at 40 cm: no movement
	Alternate at 20 cm: 2^Δ exophoria
Stereopsis:	70 seconds of arc (Stereo Fly Test)
Retinoscopy:	OD: +0.75
	OS: +4.25 − 0.50 X 180
Subjective (dry):	OD: +0.75 DS 20/20
	OS: +4.00 − 0.25 X 175 20/40 (Snellen full chart & S-chart)
Phorometry:	Phoria at far: 1^Δ exo, base-out: 9/16/9, base-in x/6/3

Phoria at near: 3^Δ exo, base-out 15/23/10, base-in 16/20/12

NRA +2.00 D, PRA −1.75 D

Amplitude of accommodation: OD 7 D, OS 7D

Visuoscopy and Haidinger brush testing:

OD: steady central fixation

OS: steady central fixation

Subjective responses: Mrs. Z was enthusiastic regarding the improvement in her vision in the left eye, which she now considered to be quite usable. The increase in depth perception was also much appreciated. She felt that the effort and inconvenience of the therapy program were worth the advantages of almost normal binocular vision.

Disposition:

The 20/40 acuity appeared stable. No further improvement was expected and Mrs. Z was placed on a maintenance program. She read with a polarized reading bar 30 minutes per day. She was rescheduled for a progress check in 1 month. At that progress check there was no change in her visual status and she continued to be pleased with the results. She was asked to continue to use the reading bar about twice a week for the next 3 months at which time another progress check was completed. As a regular maintenance and monitoring procedure, Mrs. Z agreed to use the reading bar once a week indefinitely. If she noticed suppression or reduced resolution of the left eye she was instructed to return for testing. She was seen again in 6 months and since there was no deterioration in acuity or visual skills, she was then placed on a yearly recall schedule.

Case no. 2: Anisometropic and Strabismic Amblyopia[70]

Abstract:

A 6-year-old female presented with anisometropia, esotropia, and amblyopia. This case report outlines the diagnostic and management principles that were employed to remediate the patient's visual deficiencies. (We thank Dr. Garth N. Christenson for permission to publish this case report.)

Case History:

KB, aged 6 years, was referred by an optometrist who diagnosed her condition as esotropia and amblyopia. She presented with no complaints and her parents reported that they had not "really noticed" the eye turn until the referring optometrist pointed it out. There was no history of birth or developmental problems. The child was reported to be in good health and was not taking any medication. Additionally, the

parents reported that KB had not received any previous treatment for her eye condition.

Diagnostic Findings:

Unaided Visual Acuity at 6 m:
OD 20/20, OS 20/200

Dry Retinoscopy:
OD +3.50 DS, OS +5.00 DS

Dry Subjective:
OD +1.25 DS 20/20, OS +4.50 20/200

Wet Retinoscopy:
OD +4.00 20/20, OS +6.00

20/60- (Snellen) 20/68
(Flom psychometric "S-chart" acuity)

Cover Test: Constant, comitant, unilateral, left esotropia of 20^Δ at 6 m and 40 cm. (without lenses)

Pursuits (4+ scale): OD 4+ OS 2+

Saccades (4+ scale): OD 4+ OS 2+

Visuoscopy: OD: central steady fixation

OS: central unsteady fixation

Correspondency Testing:

Bagolini: suggests HARC

Hering-Bielschowsky: unreliable results

Major Amblyoscope: suggests NRC; H = 20^ΔBO = S

Sensory Fusion:

Reindeer Test: 150 seconds of arc (Reindeer test)

Amblyoscope: Suppression with 2nd degree targets.

Worth-dot test: unreliable results.

Diagnosis:

Amblyopia left eye due to anisometropic hyperopia and accommodative esotropia.

Management and Results:

The initial spectacle prescription was OD +3.00 DS and OS +5.00 DS. The patient was instructed to wear the lenses full time and return to the clinic 2 weeks after dispensing. The parents were advised that a combination of prescription lenses, patching, and vision training would be necessary to attempt to correct the visual deficiencies. The prognosis was presented as fair-to-good providing compliance with patching and home therapy be maintained. Estimated treatment time was approximately 25 weekly office visits.

After 2 weeks of wearing spectacles, the visual acuity was: OD 20/20-1, OS 20/60-2 (S-chart: 20/68). The strabismus had substantially improved: constant, unilateral, left esotropia of 8^Δ at 6 m and an intermittent, left esotropia of 6^Δ at 40 cm. When the patient fused at near, stereopsis measured 45 seconds of arc. The Worth-dot test indicated central suppression of the left eye at far but normal sensory fusion at near.

After this first follow-up visit, a program of patching and home vision training was initiated. For patching, frosted tape was placed over the distance portion of the right lens. The patient's teacher was informed and arrangements were made for KB to sit in the front row. The tape was positioned so that binocular vision could be attained for nearpoint activities. In addition, complete patching of the right eye with an opaque occluder was prescribed for home therapy, 30 minutes per day. During this time the patient was provided with eye-hand coordination activities such as image tracing, directionality C's, line counting, puzzles, squirt gun and bubbles, toothpick and grapes, gross saccades with a flashlight, and flashlight chase pursuits.

During the first visit of office vision training (OVT), additional eye-hand coordination and gross pursuit and saccadic techniques were used, e.g., rotating pegboard, Groffman visual tracings, four-corner saccades, and the Wayne Saccadic Fixator. At the second week of OVT (and at approximately 2-week intervals thereafter) an S-chart testing was performed. The S-chart acuity at this time had improved to 20/45. As a result, techniques with higher visual discrimination demands were employed. Hart Chart saccades, dot-to-dot number drawings, smaller directionality C's, and other visual discrimination techniques were utilized during this phase of therapy.

Sensory and motor fusion training began with the third OVT session (2 weeks later). Gross fusion, antisuppression, and vergence therapy were initiated using the Brock string and beads, Quoits Vectogram, and a cheiroscope. By the end of the fifth visit of therapy (six weeks later), KB was found to have best corrected VA OS of 20/40 (Snellen 6 m) and 20/45 by S-chart. The cover test revealed a constant left esotropia of about 7^Δ at far and esophoria of 2^Δ at near. Central suppression at far was found by the Worth-dot test but "grade A" fusion at near. No significant change in refractive error was found on dry retinoscopy.

Patching instructions remained the same as before during the middle phase of training (Office visits 6 through 15). Monocular accommodative therapy using the Hart chart was initiated to emphasize awareness of the process of focusing and relaxing the eye. After 3 weeks, KB could demonstrate voluntary ability to clear and purposefully blur near targets with either the right or left eye. At that point ±1.50 D flipper lenses were introduced for accommodative facility training. Concurrently with accommodative rock, vergence training continued with Vectograms and Brock string and beads. With the Vectograms, awareness of SILO ("small in, large out") and convergence "strain" was taught. Home training involved the use of a cheiroscope and other techniques to work on monocular fixation in a binocular field. By the 15th office visit, the patient had best corrected acuity of 20/30 in the left eye. The cover test revealed a small left esotropia "flick" at far with low esophoria at 40 cm. Stereopsis (at near) had improved to 30" on the Reindeer test (lateral disparities) and 500" on Randot patterns. Again dry refraction suggested no change in the lens prescription.

During the final 10 office visits, the training goals were to break the remaining suppression at far and introduce high-level vergence techniques at the nearpoint. New techniques included presenting central targets in the amblyoscope and the AN and Dvorine cards on a Biopter (Brewster stereoscope) with double pointing. High-level vergence procedures included jump vergences, in the open environment, fusion training with Vectograms, Keystone "Lifesaver" cards (red-green fusion circles). Also during this phase, binocular accommodative therapy with a bar reader was done to check on nearpoint suppression. For home training, patching was discontinued, but eye-hand coordination activities were performed. Vergence training and antisuppression home techniques were the "Lifesaver" cards, the E series of Biopter cards, and cheiroscopic tracings.

Final Results

At the 25th office visit, the patient's visual status was as follows: Best corrected visual acuity at 6 m was OD 20/20 and OS 20/25-1 (Snellen), 20/30 (S-chart). The cover test revealed a small eso "flick" (eso microtropia) at 6 m and 2^Δ esophoria at 40 cm. Central suppression of the left eye was still found at far, consistent with the microtropia, but normal fusion was found at near with 30 sec. of arc of stereopsis and normal fusional vergence ranges. Accommodative facility was 14 c/m OD, 10 c/m OS, and 9 c/m binocularly. These findings were stable on 3 and 6 month progress evaluations.

Although there was a small amount of residual amblyopia (one line Snellen) and a left microtropia at far, vision therapy was considered successful. The improvement of visual acuity and development of normal binocular fusion reflexes and stereopsis at near are significant benefits in this case. The patient was given retainer exercises and regular follow-up visits were recommended to prevent regression.

REFERENCES

1. Wick B. Amblyopia: Case Report. *Am J Optom Arch Am Acad Optom*. 1973;50:727-730.
2. Pickwell LD. The management of amblyopia without occlusion. *Br J Physiol Opt*. 1976;31:115-118.
3. Revell MJ. *Strabismus: A History of Orthoptic Techniques*. London: Barrie & Jenkins; 1971:3-4.
4. Jastrzebski G. *Dynamics of Visual Acuity in Children*: A Model of Treatment and Prevention of Stimulus Deprivation Amblyopia. Berkeley Calif: University of California School of Optometry; 1982. Thesis.
5. Oliver M, Neumann R, Chaimovitch Y, Gotesman N, Shimshoni M. Compliance and results of treatment for amblyopia in children more than 8 years old. *Am J Ophthalmol*. 1986;102:340-345.
6. Garzia R. Efficacy of vision therapy in amblyopia: A literature review. *Am J Optom Physiol Optics*. 1987;64:393-404.
7. Saulles H. Treatment of refractive amblyopia in adults. *J Am Optom Assoc*. 1987;58:959-960.
8. Schoenleber DB, Crouch ER. Bilateral hypermetropic amblyopia. *J Ped Ophthalmal Strabismus*. 1987;24:75-77.
9. Kutschke PJ, Scott WE, Keech RV. Anisometropia amblyopia. *Ophthalmology*. 1991;98:258-263.
10. Birnbaum MH, Koslowe K, Sanet R. Success in amblyopia therapy as a function of age: a literature survey. *Amer J Optom Physiol Optics*. 1977;54:269-275.
11. Hiscox F, Strong N, Thompson JR, Minshull C, Woodruff G. Occlusion for amblyopia: A comprehensive survey of outcome. *Eye*. 1992;6:300-304.
12. Wick B, Wingard M, Cotter S, Scheiman M. Anisometropic amblyopia: is the patient ever too old to treat? *Optom Vis Sci*. 1992;69:866-878.
13. Wilson ME. Adult amblyopia reversed by contralateral cataract formation. *Brit J Ophthalmol*. 1992;29:100-102.
14. Lithander J, Sjostrand J. Anisometropic and strabismic amblyopia in the age group 2 years and above: a prospective study of the results of treatment. *Br J Ophthalmol*. 1991;75:111-116.
15. Kageyama CJ, Loomis SA. Central fixation amblyopia: a case report. *Optom Mon*. 1980;71:333-336.
16. Wesson MD. Use of light intensity reduction for amblyopia therapy. *Am J Optom Physiol Optics*. 1983;60:112-117.
17. Hokoda SC, Ciuffreda KJ. Different rates and amounts of vision function recovery during orthoptic therapy in an older strabismic amblyope. *Ophthal Physiol Opt*. 1986;6:213-220.
18. Ludlam WM. Orthoptic treatment of strabismus: A study of 149 non-operated, unselected, concomitant strabismus patients completing orthoptic training at the Optometric Center of New York. *Am J Optom Arch Am Acad Optom*. 1961;38:369-388.
19. Flom MC. The prognosis in strabismus. *Am J Optom Arch Am Acad Optom*. 1958;35:509-516.
20. Shippman S. Video games and amblyopia treatment. *Am Orthopt J*. 1985;35:2-5.
21. Leyman IR. A comparative study in the treatment of amblyopia. *Am Orthopt J*. 1978;28:95-99.
22. Von Noorden GK, Romano P, Parks M, Springer F. Home therapy for amblyopia. *Am Orthopt J*. 1970;20:46-50.
23. François J, James M. Comparative study of amblyopic treatment. *Am Orthopt J*. 1955;5:61-64.
24. Sen DK. Results of treatment of anisohypermetropic amblyopia without strabismus. *Br J Ophthalmol*. 1982;66:680-684.
25. Mitchell DE, Howell ER, Keith CG. The effect of minimal occlusion therapy on binocular visual functions in amblyopia. *Invest Ophthalmol Vis Sci*. 1983;24:778.
26. Leguire LE, Rogers GL, Bremer DL. Amblyopia: the normal eye is not normal. *J Ped Ophthalmol Strab*. 1990;27:32-38.
27. Goel BS, Maheshwari R, Saiduzaffar H. Penalization in amblyopia. *Indian J Ophthalmol*. 1982;31:307-311.

28. Gauthier CA, Holden BA, Grant T, Chong MS. Interest of presbyopes in contact lens correction and their success with monovision. *Optom Vis Sci.* 1992;69: 858-862.

29. Von Noorden GK, Attiah F. Alternating penalization in the prevention of amblyopia reoccurrence. *Am J Ophthalmol.* 1986;102:473-475.

30. Bartlett JD, Jaanus SD. *Clinical Ocular Pharmacology.* Stoneham, Mass: Butterworth; 1989:131.

31. Von Noorden GK. Amblyopia caused by unilateral atropinization. *Ophthalmology.* 1981;88:131-133.

32. Repka MX, Gallin PF, Scholz RT, Guyton DL. Determination of optical penalization by vectographic fixation reversal. *Ophthalmology.* 1985;92: 1584-1586.

33. Von Noorden GK, Milam JB. Penalization in the treatment of amblyopia. *Am J Ophthalmol.* 1979;88: 511-518.

34. Ron A, Nawratzki I. Penalization treatment of amblyopia: a follow-up study of two years in older children. *J Pediatr Ophthalmol Strabismus.* 1982;19:137-139.

35. Repka MX, Ray JM. The efficacy of optical and pharmacological penalization. *Ophthalmol.* 1993;100: 769-773.

36. Brinker WR, Katz SL. A new and practical treatment of eccentric fixation. *Am J Ophthalmol.* 1963;55: 1033-1035.

37. Binder HF, Engel D, Ede ML, Loon L. The red filter treatment of eccentric fixation. *Am Orthoptic J.* 1963:64-69.

38. Von Noorden GK. *Binocular Vision and Ocular Motility.* 4th ed. St. Louis: CV Mosby Co; 1990:470.

39. Pigassou R, Toulouse JG. Treatment of eccentric fixation. *J Pediatr Ophthalmol.* 1967;4:35-43.

40. Rubin W. Reverse prism and calibrated occlusion in the treatment of small angle deviations. *Am J Ophthalmol.* 1965;59:271.

41. Brack B. Penalization and prism: New results obtained with the method of treating squint amblyopia with eccentric fixation. In: Moore S, Meine J, Stockbridge L., eds. *Orthoptics: past, present and future.* New York: Stratton Intercontinental Medical Book Corp; 1975:99-103.

42. Banks RV. Campbell FW, Hess R, Watson PG. A new treatment for amblyopia. *Br Orthopt J.* 1978;35:1-12.

43. Schor C, Wick B. Rotating grating treatment of amblyopia with and without eccentric fixation. *J Am Optom Assoc.* 1983;54:545-548.

44. Griffin JR, Sherban RJ, Seibert P. Amblyopia therapy: a case report. *Optom. Monthly.* 1978;69:619-620.

45. Ciuffreda KJ, Levi DM, Selenow A. *Amblyopia: Basic and Clinical Aspects.* Stoneham, Mass: Butterworth-Heinemann; 1991:398-406.

46. Gould A, Fishkoff D, Galin MA. Active visual stimulation: a method of treatment of amblyopia in the older patient. *Am Orthopt J.* 1970;20:39-45.

47. Callahan WP, Berry D. The value of visual stimulation during constant and direct occlusion. *Am Orthoptic J.* 1968;18:73-74.

48. Bahill AT, Adler D, Stark L. Most naturally occurring human saccades have magnitudes of 15 degrees or less. *Invest Ophthalmol.* 1975;14:468-469.

49. Ciuffreda KJ, Kenyon RV. Accommodative vergence and accommodation in normal, amblyopes, and strabismics. In: Schor CM, Ciuffreda KJ, eds. *Vergence Eye Movements: Basic and Clinical Aspects.* Boston: Butterworth; 1983:101-73.

50. Kirschen DG, Kendall JH, Riesen KS. An evaluation of the accommodative response in amblyopic eyes. *Am J Optom Physiol Optics.* 1981;58:597-601.

51. Kirschen DA, Flom MC. Visual acuity at different retinal loci of eccentrically fixating functional amblyopes. *Am J Optom Physiol Optics.* 1978;55:144-150.

52. Bailey I. Night Vision: *Current research and future directions, NAS-NRC Committee on Vision monograph.* Washington, DC; Natl Academy Press; 1987.

53. Ciuffreda KJ, Levi DM, Selenow A. *Amblyopia: Basic and clinical aspects.* Newton, Mass: Butterworth-Heinemann; 1991:331-332.

54. Caloroso E. After-image transfer: a therapeutic procedure for amblyopia. *Am J Optom Arch Am Acad Optom.* 1972;49:65-69.

55. Farrall D. After-image transfer in the treatment of amblyopia. *Ophthalmic Optician.* 1978;18:352-354.

56. McCormick BJ. After-image transfer therapy in nonstrabismic amblyopia. *Ophthalmic Optician.* 1978;18: 641-643.

57. Wick B. Anomalous after-image transfer: An analysis and suggested method of elimination. *Am J Optom Physiol Optics.* 1974;51:862-871.

58. Ciuffreda KJ, Levi DM, Selenow A. *Amblyopia: Basic and Clinical Aspects.* Stonehem, Mass: Butterworth-Heinemann; 1991:389-391.

59. Baldwin WR. Pleoptics: historical developments and overview of the literature. *Am J Optom Arch Am Acad Optom.* 1963;39:149-162.

60. Bangerter A. Cited by Meyer A. Observations on squint therapy in Switzerland. *Br Orthopt J.* 1952;9:89-93.

61. Revell MJ. *Strabismus: A History of Orthoptic Techniques.* London: Barrie & Jenkins Ltd; 1971:187-198.

62. Revell MJ. *Strabismus: A History of Orthoptic Techniques.* London: Barrie & Jenkins Ltd; 1971:198-202.

63. Ciuffreda KJ, Levi DM, Selenow A. *Amblyopia: Basic and Clinical Aspects.* Newton, Mass: Butterworth-Heinemann; 1991:398-400.

64. Vodnoy BE. Personal communication. 1974.

65. Priestley BS, Hermann JS, Nutter AH. Home pleoptics. *Arch Ophth.* 196;70:616-624.

66. Wick B. A home pleoptic method. *Am J Optom Physiol Optics.* 1976;53:81-84.

67. Wick B. Modified strobe flash for home pleoptics. *Am J Optom Physiol Optics.* 1977;54:187-188.

68. Caloroso EE, Rouse MW. *Clinical Management of Strabismus.* Stoneham, Mass: Butterworth-Heinemann; 1993:196-197.

69. Grisham JD. *Case Report: Anisometropic amblyopia. Examination for Diplomate in Binocular Vision and Perception.* Nashville, Tenn: American Academy of Optometry; December 1991.

70. Christenson GN. *Case Report: Anisometropic and strabismic amblyope. Examination for Diplomate in Binocular Vision and Perception.* Nashville, Tenn: American Academy of Optometry, December 1989.

Chapter 11 / Anomalous Correspondence Therapy

Therapy Precautions   323
Sensory and Motor Therapy
  Approaches   324
Occlusion Procedures   325
  Constant, Total Occlusion   325
  Binasal Occlusion   326
  The Graded Occlusion Method of
   Revell   326
Optical Procedures   327
  Prism Overcorrection   327
  Ludlam's Method   328
Major Amblyoscope   328
  Classical Techniques with the
   Amblyoscope   329
   Flashing Targets at the Objective
    Angle (T11.1)   329
   Macular Massage (T11.2)   331
   Vertical Displacement of Targets
    (T11.3)   331
   Alternate Fixation (T11.4)   331
   Entoptic Tags (T11.5)   332
   Open Space Training on an Amblyoscope
    (T11.6)   334
   Divergence Technique for Esotropia
   (Flom Swing) (T11.7)   334

Training in the Open Environment   337
  Binocular Luster Training (T11.8)   337
  Afterimages at the Centration Point
   (T11.9)   338
  Prism-rack Afterimage Technique
   (T11.10)   339
  Haidinger Brush Technique (11.11)   339
  Bagolini Lens Technique (11.12)   341
Exotropia and ARC   341
  Theoretical Considerations   341
  Gross Convergence for Exotropia with
   ARC (T11.13)   341
Surgical Results in Cases of ARC.   343
Case Management   343
Case Examples   344
  Case Report no. 1 Prism
   Overcorrection   344
  Case Report no. 2 Stimulating
   Covariation in Constant
   Exotropia.   345
  Case Report no. 3 Flom Swing
   Technique   346

Before deciding how to treat anomalous "retinal" correspondence (ARC), one should seriously consider whether or not to treat the condition. The functional prognosis for constant strabismus associated with ARC is generally not good (as reviewed in Chapter 6). It ranges from poor to fair depending on the type of strabismus and associated conditions. In some cases, there is also a chance of causing intractable diplopia.

THERAPY PRECAUTIONS

ARC therapy is generally not regarded as a primary care responsibility and often requires referral to a binocular vision specialist. Many of the most effective techniques require the use of a major amblyoscope or other special instruments not ordinarily found in a primary care practice. Most procedures demand much concentration and effort by both doctor and patient, which also translates into time and money. In some cases, patients experience severe eyestrain during therapy and prolonged double vision may be the only outcome. The benefits of normal binocular vision to the patient must be weighed against all these and other negative factors. Patients or parents need to be aware of the costs and potential dangers before undertaking specific therapy for ARC. The doctor and patient (or parents) should discuss all relevant factors before attempting to change anomalous correspondence to normal.

Intractable diplopia is often associated with unharmonious ARC secondary to strabismus surgery. Fortunately, most strabismic patients with ARC, even post-surgical cases, have harmonious anomalous retinal correspondence (HARC); the subjective angle is zero. HARC is a rudimentary form of peripheral binocular vision for a strabismic patient resulting in single vision, some peripheral stereopsis, and often vergence eye movements that tend to keep the angle of deviation stable. After surgery, particularly late surgery for strabismus in cases of early onset, the patient may not properly readapt the anomalous correspondence completely to the new angle of deviation, i.e., angle A does not equal angle H. This meets the definition of unharmonious ARC. Sometimes the unharmonious correspondence is of a paradoxical type (Paradoxical ARC type I or II), which presents significant complications to treatment. (See Chapter 5 for descriptions of these types of ARC.) Diplopia after surgery may result. Fortunately, in may cases, suppression prevents diplopia, although the correspondence remains unharmonious. Most of the training techniques used in ARC therapy are effective in breaking suppression. However, if normal correspondence cannot be established, the patient may have diplopia.

The cautious clinician should only admit ARC patients into vision therapy who show HARC in the normal environment. The Bagolini test is particularly useful for making this clinical distinction. *Patients with unharmonious ARC in the open environment, particularly adults, present an unacceptable risk for treatment in our opinion.* Children, fortunately, usually can learn to suppress to prevent diplopia when ARC therapy is unsuccessful.

Horror fusionis is another contraindication for ARC therapy. Horror fusionis is the inability to obtain binocular superimposition even at the subjective angle with haploscopically presented targets. On an amblyoscope, as the targets approach superimposition, they seem to slide or jump past each other without apparent fusion or suppression.[1] In cases of strabismus with ARC, this central fusion deficit may be due to the notch in the horopter.[2] In these cases, horror fusionis is a common observation using foveal sized targets on an amblyoscope, but fusion can sometimes be achieved using large, second-degree targets. If horror fusionis is evident using both central and peripheral targets, ARC therapy is contraindicated. The chance of achieving a functional cure is remote. Vision training will probably result in failure after a major investment of the patient's time, energy, and money. Horror fusionis, however, needs to be distinguished from several other conditions that are easily confused. The differential diagnosis includes deep central suppression, aniseikonia, and lack of fusion due to head trauma.[3] Suppression can usually be treated (Chapter 10) and aniseikonia can often be managed with iseikonic lens corrections (Chapter 16).

SENSORY AND MOTOR THERAPY APPROACHES

Therapy approaches are usually based on either the sensory adaptation theory or the motor theory of ARC genesis. The *sensory adaptation theory*[4] maintains that ARC develops as a secondary adaptation to early onset strabismus when visual directionalization is plastic, as with many other visual functions. ARC localization is slowly superimposed on the innate, infantile NRC localization system and becomes embedded with reinforcement as the child lives with a constant strabismus. The rehabilitation approach consistent with this theory suggests that ARC needs to be inhibited and NRC localization stimulated and reinforced. Early intervention is desired for a successful outcome; the earlier the better. Full-time occlusion is often prescribed for strabismic patients, even cases in which amblyopia is not present. Patching prevents ARC from becoming embedded. Overcorrecting prisms or other optical intervention may be prescribed to disrupt ARC adaptation. Many specialized active training techniques have been designed specifically to bring out the latent NRC system in an instrument environment, and later on, in open space.

The *motor theory*[5,6,7] proposes that ARC occurs simultaneously with the strabismus due to a neural dysfunction of the vergence system. When the strabismic deviation occurs, the change in motor innervation is "registered" within a perceptual neural network controlling spatial localization. This theory regards ARC as an all-or-none phenomenon rather than having various depths as proposed by the sensory adaptation theory. The common finding of covariation in cases in intermittent exotropia and some intermittent esotropes provides evidence for the motor theory. Vision training is directed toward producing appropriate vergence eye movements to straighten the eyes, thus stimulating covariation whereby ARC changes to NRC. (See Chapter 5 for a more detailed discussion of these theories.)

We believe that both the sensory and motor theories are, in part, correct. The nature of ARC is not well understood at this time. In a particular patient, one or both mechanisms may be factors in the etiology of ARC and strabismus. We will, therefore, discuss rehabilitation procedures based on both these approaches and suggest when one may be more clinically appropriate than the other.

Before ARC therapy begins, amblyopia, if present, should be treated. (Refer to Chapter 10.) Even though treatment is hampered by the patient's not having 20/20 (6/6) in each eye, it may be necessary to begin binocular treatment despite reduced acuity of an eye. At least 20/60 (6/18) acuity should be achieved before proceeding with ARC therapy. As discussed in the preceding chapter, many patients show further improvement in visual acuity of the amblyopic eye as a result of appropriate binocular training.

Good monocular skills (saccades, pursuits, fixation, and accommodation) should be developed in each eye before administering binocular treatment of ARC. Once monocular acuity and motility approach normal levels of performance, ARC therapy procedures are introduced. ARC therapy techniques may involve occlusion, optical procedures, instrument training, training in open space, and extraocular muscle surgery.

OCCLUSION PROCEDURES

The purpose of occlusion in ARC therapy is to disrupt habitual ARC localization and prevent its reinforcement. Additional benefits of occlusion in cases of strabismus include breaking suppression and treatment of amblyopia. The method and schedule of occlusion selected for a patient depends on the age of the patient, the characteristics of the condition, and several practical considerations.

Constant Total Occlusion

ARC is associated with early-onset comitant strabismus. Whenever there is an onset of constant strabismus before age 7 years, the doctor should consider occlusion to prevent the occurrence or continuance of ARC. The most common form of occlusion is constant total patching. Patching is also effective in preventing suppression and amblyopia. If the patient has intermittent strabismus, the doctor should be cautious in prescribing occlusion because "occlusion strabismus" may result. This principle is particularly true in cases of heterophoria of high magnitude that may decompensate and become strabismic if dissociation (i.e., occlusion of an eye) continues over a long period. When there is constant strabismus, constant occlusion is appropriate provided there is alternation of occlusion appropriate for the age of the patient (to prevent "occlusion amblyopia"). Often, however, the chief problem is not the risk of undesirable sequelae but getting the patient to cooperate wearing the patch on a full-time basis.

Constant occlusion should be recommended during times between office treatments for ARC.[8] Once the patient has started on

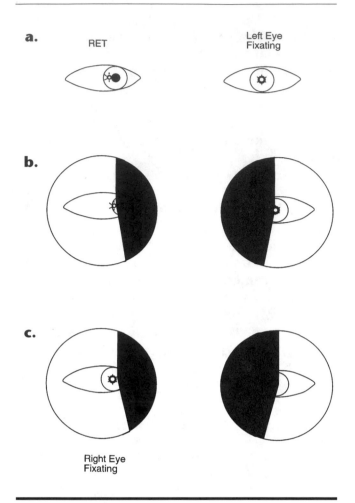

FIGURE 11-1—Binasal occlusion in the case of esotropia of the right eye. (a) Hirschberg illustrations. (b) Binasal occlusion with corneal light reflex seen in each eye. (c) Patching width increased for left eye to encourage fixation with the right eye.

an active therapy program, it is easier to motivate him to patch at home during the intervals between training. Since ARC does not exist under monocular conditions, occlusion facilitates office training for the successful elimination of ARC and the ultimate achievement of normal fusion.

Binasal Occlusion

Binasal occlusion is advocated by some clinicians for the prevention and treatment of ARC associated with esotropia. Opaque strips of tape are cut to conform to the nasal areas of the patient's spectacle lenses. The tape can be tapered slightly to allow for convergence at the nearpoint (Figure 11-1). Greenwald's[9] criterion

for placement of the tape on the spectacle lens is that "there be a visible pupillary reflex in both eyes, just beyond the edge of each tape while the patient fixates a near and far muscle light." Greenwald contended that if the objective angle of deviation is reduced as a result of wearing the binasals, the prognosis for functional cure is fair to good. However, if angle H increases, "either eye being 'thrust' behind the tape (to avoid simultaneous awareness)," the prognosis is poor.

We recommend binasal occlusion in some cases of esotropia and ARC, especially with children under 7 years old. The purpose of the method is to promote alternate monocular fixation while preventing bifoveal stimulation (Figures 11-1b and 11-1c). This approach promotes equal visual acuity, full abduction of each eye, and possibly breaks down ARC. The patient will tend to use the right eye to fixate targets in the right field of gaze and the left eye for targets in the left field. The temporal peripheral field of each eye is stimulated, so the patient experiences his full field of vision, that is to say "panoramic vision."[10] If there is strong ocular dominance and the patient resists alternating fixation, then the tapes should be moved to break the unilateral fixation habit. The tape on the dominant eye should be moved to obscure the central field and the tape on the nondominant eye moved a corresponding amount in the same direction until alternate fixation is achieved. The spectacles, of course, must rest in the proper position on the patient's face to be effective. This requirement is a major disadvantage of the method, especially with highly active children. Another problem is that some children resort to frequent and large head movements to achieve alternate fixation.[10] These head movements may be cosmetically distracting. As with all forms of occlusion, frequent office visits are recommended to ensure proper application and to evaluate effectiveness.

Graded Occlusion Method of Revell

An attenuating filter or fogging lens placed before the dominant eye may be used in some cases to eliminate ARC. Such penalization procedures are also referred to as graded occlusion.

In a few cases, when a dark filter (either neutral density or colored filter) is placed before the dominant eye, ARC localization spontaneously shifts to normal "retinal" correspondence (NRC). A case was reported by Revell[11] in which he used a frosted lens (a graded occluder) to force a unilateral esotropic patient to alternate fixation to her nondominant eye. Using Bagolini striated lenses to monitor the state of correspondence, he observed that an ARC response occurred with the dominant eye fixating but an NRC response was found when the nondominant eye fixated. If, in fact, there is a shift to NRC with the strabismic eye fixating, the patient is instructed to wear a full-time graded occluder on the dominant eye to reinforce NRC. The least amount of attenuation is prescribed that allows constant fixation with the nondominant eye. A Fresnel prism, with power equal to or exceeding the deviation, is also placed before the dominant eye thus providing bifoveal stimulation and, over time, normal fusional abilities. The patient wears this prescription for several months to reinforce NRC and central fusion. If long-term prismatic neutralization of the deviation is not cosmetically acceptable, the patient should be referred for surgical correction of the deviation. The mechanism for a shift in correspondence is unknown, but it is consistent with Bagolini's concept of ARC in natural environments and NRC in unnatural ones, a version of the sensory adaptation theory.[12] Since the patient is unaccustomed to fixating with the strabismic eye, latent NRC localization is stimulated. We recommend checking every unilateral esotropes and exotrope with ARC for a change in correspondence using forced alternation of fixation. If the change in correspondence is verified with Bielschowsky afterimages or Bagolini striate lenses, then this graded occlusion and prism compensation can be attempted with reasonable hope of success.

OPTICAL PROCEDURES

Prism overcorrection of the deviation and Ludlam's method are consistent with the sensory adaptation theory of ARC. These procedures work best with younger patients and attempt to disrupt ARC localization while stimulating a latent NRC localization system.

Prism Overcorrection

Several practitioners recommend using prism overcorrection in the treatment of ARC.[13-17] This approach is most effective with patients younger than 16 years. The idea is to disrupt ARC adaptation by inducing diplopia. In some cases when diplopia occurs, the latent NRC localization manifests itself. The great advantage of this method, if it is successful, is that little doctor time or patient effort is required. The major disadvantage is cosmetic acceptance. To an observer, the strabismus appears to be a larger deviation than before prism application. Also, some patients cannot tolerate diplopia during the initial stage of therapy.

Fleming et al.[14] recommended keeping the patient about 15^Δ overcorrected to disrupt the ARC and possibly elicit NRC. For example, a 15^Δ constant esotrope, far and near, would be given 30^Δ base-out Fresnel prisms. With the prisms in place, the patient may be thought of as having "sensory" exotropia. Since prism adaptation is expected, the patient's deviation should be checked each week. Additional Fresnel prisms can be added, if necessary, to maintain "sensory" exotropia or, hopefully, exophoria. Fresnel prisms can be easily removed and reapplied for this purpose. Some patients experience diplopia and asthenopic symptoms. Indeed, diplopia is desirable, for treatment purposes, since it may stimulate a normal fusion response. If symptoms are intolerable, however, constant occlusion can be prescribed, interspersed with short periods of prism wearing. Caloroso and Rouse[15] recommended wearing overcorrecting prism only 30 minutes to 1 hour per day. We suggest trying a more vigorous approach by prescribing constant wear of the prism, or for as much time as the patient will accept. In this way, NRC localization is more likely to develop quickly.

When ARC is disrupted and eliminated by this procedure after a few weeks or months of constant wear, a second stage of prismatic correction is applied. When NRC is repeatedly found on the Bielschowsky afterimage test, the ideal prism power is that to equal the objective angle of deviation (15^Δ base-out in our example). The patient should experience "sensory orthophoria" and fusional vergence training may proceed. The prism power can slowly be reduced over time as the patient develops fusional control of the deviation. Both home and in-office training procedures can be given to strengthen sensory and motor fusion skills. If the deviation is too large for the patient to develop comfortable fusional control, extraocular surgery is probably required.

Amigo[16] and Arruga[17] recommended very strong prism overcorrection. They suggested the prism amount should be 2.5 to 3 times the magnitude of the objective angle of deviation to keep the deviation from running ahead of the power of the prism through prism adaptation. Fresnel prisms would usually be placed before both eyes. The very large amount of prism overcorrection is necessary in cases with large magnitude of prism adaptation. (See case report no. 1.) After "sensory exophoria" has been established for 1 or 2 months, the prism power may be gradually reduced to equal the objective angle of deviation, assuming NRC is present. Again, if the strabismus is large, surgery is necessary.

Ludlam's Method

Ludlam[18] suggested a randomized approach for disruption of ARC by optical means, sometimes referred to as the "Rockum Sockum" method. He stated that a stable, full correction of hyperopia is not advisable in cases of esotropia with ARC as this may allow ARC to become more embedded. With undercorrection of hyperopia, the angle of deviation would necessarily be more variable because of the accommodative convergence. Whether the full refractive correction is worn, Ludlam contended that various combinations of lenses and/or prisms should be worn during the intervals between office training. For instance, one day the patient may wear 20^Δ base-out over the left eye, the next day 20^Δ base-in, then 20^Δ base-up, etc. Fresnel prisms are ideal for this purpose. Various lenses may be used, e.g., a minus lens-add over one eye, and then over the other eye on the following day.

The same sort of randomized wearing of plus lens-adds can be applied. Fresnel lenses and prisms are ideal since they can be re-applied many times. In this manner, the angle of deviation never stabilizes, which tends to break down the ARC localization. However, we have reservations how well patients, even young ones, accept this aggressive optical approach. Rather, we generally prefer simply to prescribe prism overcorrection prior to office visits for binocular training. In some cases, ARC may be eliminated completely by optical means, but in many cases, other vision therapy approaches, including training and/or surgery, are also necessary.

MAJOR AMBLYOSCOPE

According to the sensory adaptation theory, there is less chance of ARC responses when testing is done in a reduced environment (less natural) rather than in the open environment (more natural). This observation is one reason for beginning ARC training in closed-space instruments. Although many instruments and devices can be used, the major amblyoscope is the best single instrument for this purpose. Normal binocular localization is trained first in a controlled visual environment using a variety of techniques and then the learned visual skills are transferred into open space.

The amblyoscope was originally designed by Claude Worth, a century ago, primarily for the orthoptic treatment of strabismus.[19] Amblyoscopic techniques for attacking ARC and promoting NRC that have evolved over the years have become known as the "Classical method of ARC treatment." Classical techniques attempt to elicit bifoveal NRC localization by stimulating the latent NRC system. Amblyoscopic targets are directed to the fovea of each eye and are flashed to stimulate NRC. The length of time the patient has had strabismus of early onset is a key element in the depth of ARC adaptation. Likewise, a key element in rehabilitating NRC is the amount of time involved in bifoveal stimulation. Most of the amblyoscope techniques represent variations on the theme of intensive bifoveal stimulation. When the patient is not being treated with the amblyoscope, one eye is constantly patched or he wears prisms or lenses designed to disrupt ARC. Classical methods are also applicable for the constant exotrope with ARC.

There are numerous combinations of procedures involving real images, Haidinger's brushes, and afterimages. Synoptophores, as well as other modern major amblyoscopes, are equipped with attachments to make these auxiliary procedures possible. Table 11-1 lists amblyoscope procedures discussed later in this chapter. We have no rigid sequence of training when dealing with anomalous correspondence; however, it is best to begin with conditions in which an NRC response can be elicited. Some procedures are limited by the patient's immaturity, poor cooperation, or lack of perceptual awareness. The doctor may, therefore, be limited to using the more simple procedures and must necessarily begin training with these.

Classical Techniques with the Amblyoscope

Strabismic ARC patients who respond favorably to classical techniques on the major amblyoscope have certain clinical characteristics (Table 11-2). They tend to be young children; from a functional standpoint, the younger the better. However, most children under age 4 often are incapable of cooperating with amblyoscopic methods. Furthermore, the later the onset of the strabismus, the better. The adaptation theory implies that NRC localization may be stronger and easier to revive in late onset cases. A favorable age of strabismus onset is 1 year or, preferably, much later. Also, the adaptation theory suggests that the larger the angle of deviation, the less embedded is the ARC localization. In addition, patients should have good acuity in each eye, comitancy, and harmonious ARC. Patients can be accepted for treatment who vary from these recommendations, but the prognosis will be worse and the management more complex. Ideally, an intensive training program consists of at least three office visits per week of 1 hour and supplemented by home training and occlusion. Using classical techniques on an amblyoscope, it is common for ARC therapy to take between 3 to 6 months of concentrated effort by doctor and patient.

TABLE 11-1. *Procedures for the Major Amblyoscope*

- Flashing of targets at angle H (T11.1)
- Macular massage (T11.2)
- Vertical displacement (T11.3)
- Alternate fixation (T11.4)
- Use of entoptic tags (T11.5)
- Open space training with an amblyoscope (T11.6)
- Divergence technique (T11.7)

TABLE 11-2. *Clinical Characteristics Favorable for Classical Techniques to Treat ARC*

- Patient's age should be between 4 and 10 years. Younger children have difficulty cooperating and older patients tend to have deeply embedded ARC.
- The later the onset of the strabismus and ARC, the better. Infantile esotropic individuals did not have sufficient developmental time to establish normal binocularity.
- With full optical correction, the strabismus should be greater than 20^Δ because ARC seems to be less embedded in larger angles of deviation.
- Esotropia should be constant and comitant. Intermittent cases usually do not require classical techniques. Noncomitant deviations may have a poor prognosis regardless of ARC or NRC.
- Visual acuity should be 20/40 (6/12) or better. Good acuity is necessary for good binocularity.
- The patient should have harmonious ARC in the open environment, otherwise there is a chance of causing intractable diplopia if unHARC. (Check for HARC with Bagolini lenses.)
- The patient should demonstrate NRC on at least some testing procedures. This finding suggests the ARC adaptation may not be deeply embedded.

Flashing Targets at the Objective Angle T11.1

The first classical training technique usually attempted is superimposition of two dissimilar targets (first-degree targets) at the objective angle of deviation. Illumination of the amblyoscopic targets (for example, a circle and a star) is increased to the maximum while the room

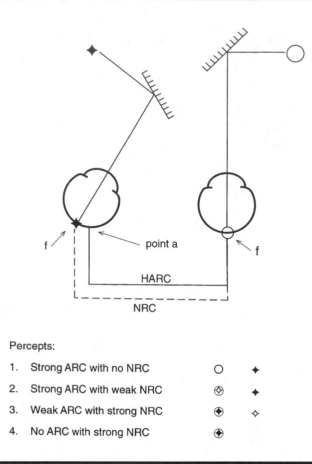

Percepts:

1. Strong ARC with no NRC
2. Strong ARC with weak NRC
3. Weak ARC with strong NRC
4. No ARC with strong NRC

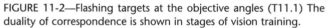

FIGURE 11-2—Flashing targets at the objective angles (T11.1) The duality of correspondence is shown in stages of vision training.

illumination is dimmed. The automatic flashing unit is set to a rapid alternate flash. Since the patient has ARC and the foveas are being stimulated, the two targets will not appear to be in the same visual direction. The images will be separated by an amount equal to the angle of anomaly (angle A) (Figure 11-2, percept #1). This percept is considered to be ARC projection. Over time, the bifoveal stimulation revives the latent NRC localization system. When this occurs the patient will notice a faint ghostlike image (star) from the nondominant eye appearing in the center of a dominant eye's image (circle) (see Figure 11-2, percept #2). This percept is called "binocular triplopia." The dominant eye sees one image and the nondominant eye sees two under binocular conditions. At this point there is a duality of localization systems, both ARC and NRC. This percept of "binocular triplopia" represents an intermediate stage in

the rehabilitation process. With reinforcement, the poorly defined ghost image (the NRC image of the star) grows in clarity and the peripheral image (ARC localization of the star) fades in vividness (see Figure 11-2, percept #3). The training process under these stimulus conditions is complete when the patient is aware of only the NRC projection. The star will only appear inside the circle when both foveas are simultaneously stimulated (see Figure 11-2, percept #4). Throughout this rehabilitation process, the patient should be encouraged to use "mental effort" in the attempt to see the ghost image for NRC, at least part of the time. Depending on how embedded ARC is, the treatment time to achieve consistent NRC responses on the amblyoscope can vary widely from a few weeks to several months with 3 to 5 hours of in-office training each week.

It is important to point out that some patients do not experience "binocular triplopia" when targets are flashed at the objective angle of deviation.[20] There can be an abrupt shift in correspondence from anomalous to normal, although the triplopia may be perceived fleetingly by some patients. The patient starts reporting that the two targets are seen in the same visual direction and they do not appear separated as before. On occasion, one target may appear to move suddenly to reach the position of the other even though the amblyoscope tubes remain locked at the objective angle of deviation. The above responses indicate that NRC localization is being revived.

Other types of flashing, besides rapid alternate flashing, can also be used to stimulate NRC localization. Unilateral flashing of the nondominant eye at the objective angle represents one variation. Stimulation may be varied from slow to rapid, and the light and dark phases can be modified to promote superimposition. The goal, in this case, is to have the patient superimpose the circle and the star (or similar first-degree targets) at the objective angle when flashing is stopped and the two targets are seen simultaneously. During simultaneous flashing, the patient can also look for NRC localization of both images and try to maintain NRC superimposition during the moments after flashing is discontinued.

This rehabilitation process requires the patient merely to keep looking in the instrument while the foveas are stimulated. The time required to reach binocular triplopia may be from only one session of training to many. Some patients never achieve this stage, but most take about 10 to 20 sessions. Since patients may become bored with the therapy, the therapist should have a large number of appropriate major amblyoscope slides for the sake of variety. Another good 1° slide pair for the early stage of training is the "soldier and the sentry box" (see Figure 5-6). Initially, peripheral first-degree targets are introduced, but later central first-degree and all sizes of second-degree targets (having suppression controls) are also utilized. Success with classical techniques requires a therapist skilled in communication with children, particularly story telling. Other classical techniques can be introduced for the sake of variety and interest, besides their therapeutic benefit.

Macular Massage T11.2

The method of "macular massage" is another classical amblyoscopic technique described in the following example. In a case of esotropia of 15^Δ of the left eye with harmonious ARC (subjective angle of zero), the circle seen by the right eye would be moved back and forth from approximately 10^Δ base-out to 20^Δ base-out, approximately 5^Δ to either side of the objective angle. The speed of movement may be varied from slow to fast. Care should be taken to avoid the subjective angle, which is a common mistake. The moving image is on the dominant eye, because NRC is more likely to occur when the nondominant eye is steadily fixating.

Initially, the two images are seen in different locations. At some point, more or less suddenly, the movements of the circle reach the star. When the patient is able to report the circle superimposed on the star as the targets pass the objective angle, NRC is being elicited. Some patients may report seeing the "binocular triplopia" response as ARC is broken down and NRC localization occurs. Since the patient's angle of deviation in the amblyoscope may be variable, the therapist should not rely completely on the prismatic scale. He/she should also observe the corneal light reflections to monitor the angle of deviation (as in Hirschberg testing) during this training. Better yet, the therapist should verify that the targets remain at the objective angle by the exclusion "douse" test described in Chapter 4.

When macular massage is effective in breaking ARC with the nondominant eye fixating, the dominant eye should then be given the opportunity to fixate the stationary target. The technique is then repeated with the oscillating target clued to the nondominant eye. NRC is less likely to occur when the habitually dominant eye is fixating; and consequently, superimposition of the targets at angle H may be more difficult to achieve than before.

Vertical Displacement of Targets T11.3

Vertical displacement of the targets is another amblyoscopic technique that may cause superimposition at the horizontal angle of deviation (angle H). For example, the left eye may fixate the star while the Synoptophore carriage arm for the right eye is elevated to cause a displacement of the circle above the star. The two images can then possibly be aligned subjectively at angle H provided enough base-out prismatic compensation is given; this is assuming peripheral retinal stimulation has triggered NRC localization. The therapist gradually reduces the vertical displacement in an attempt to have the patient superimpose the circle and star. Often, the targets quickly separate due to horror fusionis as the circle target invades the foveal area. This procedure is repeated until the targets jump apart less often. When superimposition is achieved with the left eye steadily fixating, the procedure is repeated with the right eye steadily fixating.

Alternate Fixation T11.4

Alternate fixation on the amblyoscope is a procedure that may help in breaking ARC. This technique demonstrates an incongruity between the patient's image perception and eye movements. The targets are set in a position of neither the objective angle nor the subjective angle, but at a point usually between the two. The patient is instructed to fixate alternately the star and the circle, for example. At first, the therapist may have to flash the targets alternately to get the patient started. With alternate fixation, the ARC patient usually sees the images jumping and has the feeling that his eyes are moving. The patient alternately fixates as rapidly as possible for several minutes. This procedure tends to disrupt stable localization of the two images. The targets are then slowly moved to the subjective angle where they appear superimposed. However, the patient soon becomes aware that eye movements are necessary to fixate each target. The targets are then placed at the objective angle and the patient realizes that eye movements are no longer necessary to fixate each target alternately. This mismatch in kinesthetic-perceptual feedback helps to break ARC localization. In theory, the patient will now be more likely to respond successfully to other classical amblyoscopic techniques such as flashing targets at the objective angle (T11.1).

Entoptic Tags T11.5

Consistent with the adaptation theory of ARC is the observation that NRC is present if there are no contours in the visual field, since NRC is innate. This phenomenon can provide a starting point in treatment of ARC in the open environment filled with complex contours. Most major amblyoscopes come supplied with slides and flash units that can generate afterimages. Slides S3, a horizontal streak, and S4, a vertical streak, are used in the Synoptophore. Each has a central red fixation mark. As with the Hering-Bielschowsky test (Chapter 5), it is customary to flash the dominant eye first with the horizontal streak, and then flash the nondominant eye with the vertical streak. With the older instruments, the opal diffusing screen should be removed from the optical pathway when each eye is flashed, providing a much stronger afterimage than would otherwise be generated. Most new instruments have an afterimage mode with intensified illumination and removal of the diffusing screen is unnecessary. The background illumination in the Synoptophore is kept low enough so that the afterimages are not washed out. The afterimages are

sustained by an automatic background flashing feature of the instrument. The timing of light and dark phases and the speed of flashing can be adjusted conveniently as desired.

Positive afterimages are considered less natural than negative; therefore, NRC is more likely elicited when positive afterimages are seen. In order to see them, long dark phases should be emphasized initially. If the patient can see a perfect cross with the positive afterimages, the dark phase can be shortened, and the negative afterimage can be made visible more of the time. It is not unusual for the patient to report seeing a cross (NRC) in the dark phase, but seeing a noncross (ARC) in the light phase. In such a case, various adjustments of the automatic flashing unit may help in developing a cross response with the negative afterimages. The goal is to have the patient achieve a perfect cross with both eyes being flashed simultaneously indicating NRC.

When NRC with afterimages can be achieved, real images may be incorporated into the training. The traditional slides used initially in this technique are a ring and a dot. The amblyoscope arms are adjusted to the angle of deviation, all targets are removed and the afterimages are properly applied. The patient must see a perfect cross of the afterimages. In the case of left esotropia, a dot is presented to the left eye as the patient tries to continue seeing a perfect cross indicating that NRC is maintained. Achieving this, a ring is introduced to the right eye. The patient now tries to superimpose the dot and ring while maintaining an AI cross that is centered on the superimposed targets. ARC localization is indicated when the afterimages separate forming an uneven cross. The targets should be removed, NRC reestablished with blank fields, and then contoured targets can be reintroduced. As NRC localization is achieved, more complex targets are introduced and the training process is repeated.

An ARC response is indicated if the AI cross comes apart (Figure 11-3a). The doctor should be aware that ARC also may be present even when there is a perfect cross (see Figure 11-3b). This percept may occur because the afterimage is unnatural enough to show NRC, but the real targets may induce ARC at the very same

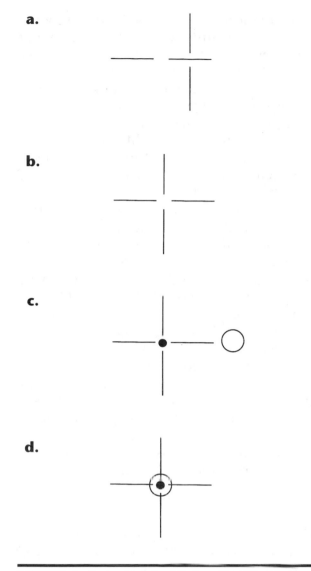

a.

b.

c.

d.

FIGURE 11-3—Esotropia of the left eye with ARC with the amblyoscope set at angle H. (a) Noncross with horizontal afterimage seen by the right eye and the vertical by the left eye. (b) An NRC response may occur because of the relative unnaturalness of the afterimages. (c) Real targets (dot and ring) are seen separated, indicating ARC for more natural targets but NRC for less natural targets (afterimages). (d) Goal in training is superimposition of real targets and afterimages. Caution in interpretation is required if the setting of the amblyoscope is at angle S rather than angle H.

moment (see Figure 11-3c). The goal is to achieve superimposition of the AIs and the real targets (see Figure 11-3d). The doctor must be cautious when interpreting the patient's subjective reports and not falsely assume there is an NRC response for the real targets. It is possible that the strabismic deviation has changed during the training session in the amblyoscope.

The patient may be superimposing the real targets at his subjective angle. The douse target test can verify whether the patient is superimposing at angles S.

Many of the Synoptophores come equipped with attachments to produce Haidinger brushes (clinically referred to as Haidinger brush, HB). An HB may be for the left eye, the right eye, or for each eye binocularly. Patients with ARC frequently are unable to superimpose two real images, but they may be able to superimpose less natural targets such as two HB images. The tubes of the Synoptophore should be locked at the objective angle. One HB should be rotating clockwise and the other counterclockwise, so superimposition can be monitored. Superimposition is indicated when the HBs appear together with a fluttering and flapping of the composite image.

Haidinger brushes are more easily seen if the Synoptophore targets are printed in black and white on transparent film. Colored slides tend to wash out the images of the HBs. (Clement Clarke offers several black and white slides: F 161 and 162, F 163 and 164, and F 165 and 166.) Similar slides also may be custom-made for use in the Synoptophore.

The following description suggests a training sequence using combinations of entopic tags and real targets. First, have the nondominant eye perceive an HB. Then, introduce a real target to the dominant eye. Have the patient superimpose them. A blue filter (small insertable lens that comes with the Synoptophore) before the dominant eye is used to equalize the light intensities so that the HB can be seen by the nondominant eye under binocular conditions. If the patient has trouble superimposing these, the real target is removed and a vertical afterimage is generated on the dominant eye. The patient then attempts to superimpose the HB and the AI. Flashing the instrument lights, either manually or by various settings of the automatic unit, may help the patient achieve superimposition. When this is done, a real target (dot, circle, square, or any suitable line drawing on a clear slide) is placed in the tube for the nondominant eye to fixate. If superimposition of this combination can be maintained, another real target is presented to the dominant eye. Ideally, the patient should have superimposition of the two real images, in conjunction with the superimposed HB and the vertical AI. (This technique requires central fixation in each eye.) These foveal tags are excellent monitors of the state of correspondence. The variations of different combinations are many. It is good to try a number of these on each patient, because some of them might be very effective in helping the patient break ARC whereas others may not be.

Open Space Training with an Amblyoscope T11.6

Although the major amblyoscope is good for training in a reduced environment, the fact remains that the conditions of seeing in such an instrument are very different from those of habitual everyday seeing. Some patients have difficulty transferring visual skills achieved in the amblyoscope to the open environment. Some modern amblyoscopes come equipped with Stanworth mirrors.[21] When these mirrors are flipped into position, the patient can superimpose ordinary amblyoscope targets as if the targets were in open space. The patient looks through the half-silvered mirrors at a distant blank wall while simultaneously seeing the targets in each tube of the amblyoscope. This modification allows for the treatment of ARC under more natural conditions than could otherwise be done using a standard amblyoscope. All the previously described classical methods can be applied now in a relatively natural environment.

Divergence Technique for Esotropia (Flom Swing) T11.7

Drs. Merton Flom and Gordon Heath devised a divergence technique on the amblyoscope (also known as the Flom Swing Technique) for treatment of small-angle esotropia with ARC.[22] The technique is based on Morgan's motor theory of ARC. Morgan held that fusional vergence eye movements can stimulate covariation between ARC and NRC in some strabismic patients. When the eyes are in the strabismic position, ARC exists, but when the patient makes a fusional vergence eye movement and straightens the

eyes, covariation results in NRC. The essence of the divergence technique with the amblyoscope for small angle esotropes is to establish "ARC fusion" at the subjective angle and then slowly diverge the eyes through the angle of deviation, using fusional divergence demands, until the eyes are physically straight. The patient is then taken out of the instrument while concentrating on holding the eyes straight in the ortho position. Hopefully, the patient will covary to NRC in open space since the eyes are straight. If he does covary, the patient temporarily becomes nonstrabismic, shows NRC localization, and experiences a dramatic awareness of stereopsis in the open environment. One of the virtues of the divergence technique is that if it is going to work with a patient, it works relatively quickly. The training program takes only a few weeks instead of months using classical methods.

Only certain esotropic patients qualify for the divergence technique. Table 11-3 lists qualification criteria we recommend. Besides having comitant deviations, good acuity, and HARC, patients should be older (teenagers or adults) because the technique requires much concentrated effort and usually is associated with visual discomfort. Patients should have an angle

---

TABLE 11-3. *Qualification Criteria for the Divergence Technique (Flom Swing Technique)*

- Patients should be teenagers or adults because the technique requires intense concentration and tolerance for discomfort.
- Esotropia with full optical correction should be 20^Δ or less because this amount approaches the limit of fusional divergence that can be trained at far.
- Esotropia should be comitant and the visual acuities 20/40 (6/12) or better.
- The patient should have harmonious ARC in the open environment, otherwise there is a chance of causing intractable diplopia. (Check for HARC with Bagolini lenses.)
- The patient should demonstrate the ability to fuse the targets placed at the subjective angle in the amblyoscope, maintain seeing the suppression controls, and perceive at least some peripheral stereopsis.

of deviation of 20$^\Delta$ or less. We have found this magnitude to be about the training limit for divergence. Patients who match this clinical profile have the best chance for functional cure of strabismus.

The divergence technique proceeds as follows (Figure 11-4). After the patient's angles H and S have been measured, a pair of peripheral, third-degree fusion slides are placed in the major amblyoscope at the patient's angle S. The swing slides are frequently used targets for this procedure (Figure 11-5). Background room illumination should be dim. The automatic flashing unit is set for alternate flashing at a rapid rate of 2 to 3 cycles per second. Under these stimulus conditions, the patient should have a vivid percept of the "fused" swing targets with perception of a stereoscopic effect and aware of suppression controls (i.e., both flowers) in view. At this point there is "ARC fusion," although not true fusion. Starting at angle S, the targets are diverged at a normal rate to test the patient's divergence limit, i.e., the break point. After recovery, the targets are again diverged, but this time very slowly (about 2$^\Delta$ per minute) while the patient maintains a percept of a single image with suppression clues and stereopsis. Patients usually experience eyestrain as they diverge their eyes. This sensation of eyestrain is important and can be utilized as part of the technique. The patient is encouraged to experience the stressful "feeling" of diverging his eyes, as unpleasant as this may be. When diplopia or suppression occurs, the divergence demand is decreased until fusion is *reestablished* that is, fusional vergence recovery. Alternate rapid flashing continues at the recovery point for several minutes to reinforce sensory and motor fusion; then divergence is again very slowly increased. This procedure continues until maximum divergence can be held. The eyes should be diverged maximally in a series of breaks and recoveries for approximately 20 minutes. The goal is to straighten the eyes physically. In other words, the magnitude of fusional divergence eye movement is equal to the magnitude of angle H. When alignment is accomplished in the amblyoscope, the patient attempts to hold alignment in the open environment. If, however, alignment of the eyes is

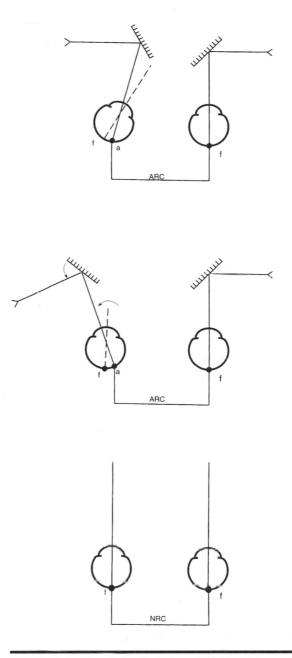

FIGURE 11-4—Flom Swing Technique (T11.7). (A) Esotropia of the left eye with ARC in the major amblyoscope. The instrument is set for Angle S. (B) Sufficient base-in demand is introduced until there is sufficient divergence so that Angle S is exo and angle H becomes zero. There is still ARC since superimposition is with points *a* and *f*. (C) The patient views objects in the open environment attempting to have NRC while the eyes are held in the ortho position.

not achieved after about 20 minutes of divergence training, the patient is taken out of the instrument for a much needed rest. If divergence is accomplished, the room illumination is slowly raised and the patient is instructed to

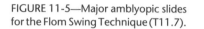

FIGURE 11-5—Major amblyopic slides for the Flom Swing Technique (T11.7).

concentrate on keeping the "feeling" of eyestrain. On many occasions when the patient meets the fusional divergence demand in the open environment, he experiences NRC fusion with vivid stereopsis. The patient looks at real objects across the room and appreciates "depth," perhaps for the first time in his life. The therapist should closely observe the patient's eyes as he looks above the instrument and should note if there is a rapid shift back to the esotropic position. If the eyes appear straight, patients who still experience eyestrain in the open environment should be allowed to reinforce alignment for a few minutes before doing a cover test to verify that the eyes are indeed aligned. The cover test is, of course, dissociative and the patient may not be able to regain fusion afterwards. If the patient lapses back into the esotropia, the above steps should be repeated until the patient can reflexly fuse in the open environment and hold the eyes in alignment for relatively long periods of time.

Successful treatment may take 10 or more intensive office visits along with home training. Ideally, office visits for amblyoscope training can be scheduled two or three times per week to achieve rapid progress in getting covariation. We recommend constant patching out of the office, except for a 30-minute daily home training session to practice divergence using a mirror stereoscope. Caloroso and Rouse[23] recommended using other home training instruments to build the patient's range of "anomalous divergence" in the open environment, e.g., Brewster stereoscopes and Vectograms®. Patients who achieve a functional cure of strabismus and become esophoric should be given retainer exercises to prevent regression. We recommend 15 minutes of divergence training once a week indefinitely using a Minivectrogram at near distances. Progress visits are scheduled for 3-month intervals during the first year to see if the retainer exercise schedule is sufficient to control the deviation.

Using the divergence technique, Grisham's success rate for a functional cure of small-angle esotropia with ARC is about 33%.[24] Wick reported a remarkable 56% cure rate (9 of 16) for these patients in a private practice setting.[25] These cured patients have straight eyes all or nearly all day, markedly increased stereopsis, but they may need to wear prisms for esophoria. If these patients do happen to lapse back into an esotropia (e.g., after a long workday), they do not usually see double since they also covary back to ARC. About one-third of our patients who complete 10 sessions end up with a microesotropia, smaller than the original deviation, and usually have some stereopsis. We believe that these cases are partial cures. The remaining third were not successful and showed no change in their condition. Fortunately, they did not invest much time or money in the attempt for a functional cure. An important point to remember is that the successful treatment of small-angle esotropia with ARC in adulthood is far from hopeless, as some authorities in the past have believed. Cure rates between one-third and one-half are acceptable for a therapeutic intervention that avoids surgery and does not involve a lot of training time. In geographical locations where binocular vision specialists offer this service, we strongly recommend that patients who qualify for the divergence procedure be informed that this option exists and be referred for treatment.

TRAINING IN THE OPEN ENVIRONMENT

Although ARC training in cases of esotropia can be done in the open environment, we believe it is generally a good rule to break ARC using the major amblyoscope before free-space techniques are introduced. Some practitioners prefer training almost exclusively in free space. In many respects training techniques in open space at the centration point are similar to those performed in the Synoptophore; both foveas are stimulated simultaneously. Many of the open space procedures, however, are difficult to administer in all but the most cooperative patients. Nevertheless, successful results are sometimes obtained, and various open-space procedures may enable the shortening of treatment sessions.

Techniques of open environment training can utilize binocular luster, afterimages, Haidinger Brushes, a prism bar (rack), Bagolini lenses, real objects, and combinations of these (Table 11-4). These techniques are usually applied at the centration point in cases of esotropia with the centration point add in place. They can also be used in cases of constant exotropia with ARC providing a centration point can be achieved with minus adds and the gross convergence technique (T11.13) described later in this chapter.

Binocular Luster Training T11.8

Ludlam[18] advocated a binocular luster technique to establish NRC. There are numerous ways to elicit luster, but the best in cases of ARC is to set up conditions to promote red-green color fusion (see Figure 5-38). For home training, the patient may view a brightly illuminated blank white wall while wearing red-green filters, but illumination should be evenly distributed without shadows. When the patient stands between the source of illumination and the viewing screen, this condition is difficult to meet. For this reason, a retro-illuminated gray screen is preferable for in-office training.

The esotropic patient with ARC may be better able to appreciate luster if plus lenses are used and a blank screen is placed at the patient's centration point. Under these conditions, it is hoped the patient will be able to see red-green fusion (luster) over the entire screen since there are no contours in the field. The perception of form with sharp contours is thought to trigger the ARC split-field response. If, however, the patient reports seeing a split red-green field, no attempt is usually made for further training because of the poor prognosis indicated by such a response. Seeing the Swann Split Field effect in a contourless field indicates a deeply embedded ARC response (see Figure 5-39).

The patient tries to maintain binocular luster (indicating NRC) while targets are introduced at the edge of the peripheral visual field. Placing targets initially in the superior quadrant seems to work best. If a split-field response results, the object is removed from the patient's view, and he is instructed to perceive luster in the formless field as before. The process of slowly introducing an object into the periphery is repeated until the patient is able to maintain luster as the object approaches the centration point. When objects are placed in the central visual field,

TABLE 11-4. Open Environment Techniques for ARC (Usually esotropia)

- Binocular luster training (Ludlam's method) (T11.8)
- Afterimages at the centration point (T11.9)
- Prism-rack afterimage technique (T11.10)
- Haidinger Brush technique (T11.11)
- Bagolini lens technique (T11.12)
- Gross convergence for exotropia with ARC (T11.13)

there is a strong tendency to elicit a split-field response. At first it may be necessary to "over-plus" the patient in relation to the fixation distance of the screen. A blurred image may promote luster better than clear distinct contours. This training process is repeated until the patient is able to maintain the perception of luster when a small target (such as a black dot) and, later, complex targets are centrally fixated.

With the appropriate addition lenses in place, fusion training can proceed at the centration point. Theoretically the patient has "sensory orthophoria" in relation to the fixated target; normal color fusion is indicated if the patient continually notices luster. There is no assurance, however, that central fusion is actually being developed. It may well be that only peripheral fusion exists at this stage of treatment. Consequently, the luster method can be refined by projecting small red and green targets on the screen to monitor for central suppression.

Motor fusion training can be started once normal central sensory fusion is demonstrated. Only small amounts vergence demand are introduced at first because the patient's ability to maintain NRC is very tenuous; an ARC response is likely to reoccur with any change in sensory or motor fusion stimulation. The best way to induce vergence eye movements is to have the patient move slowly back and forth (only a few centimeters at first) from the screen and attempt to maintain fusion of the target. Peripheral fusion targets (e.g., large Brock red and green rings) may be required initially, but eventually, the patient should be able to fuse small targets while he is moving back and forth. Sensory and motor fusion training continues until the patient has developed his maximal range of motor fusion under these conditions. In combination with the binocular luster technique, Ludlam[18] recommended using the "Rockum Sockum" optical method of disrupting ARC between daily home training sessions. (See previous section on optical methods.) Simple occlusion or binasal occlusion may also serve the same purpose. Training for NRC in this manner with children may take from 1 to 3 months for maximum results.

Afterimages at the Centration Point T11.9

This method with afterimages is similar to the open-space luster procedure. The Hering-Bielschowsky test is the recommended procedure for generating afterimages (see Figures 5-40 to 5-44). Positive afterimage training is given first in dim room illumination, followed by working with negative afterimages in normal lighting conditions. This is also similar to training in the Synoptophore, except the patient views the afterimages in open space. The first goal is to have the patient perceive a perfect cross for both the positive AI and the negative AI. With a centration-point add in place, the esotropic patient initially views a blank field at the centration point while trying to hold a perfect AI cross (NRC) in perception. If NRC occurs under blank field conditions, then targets and real objects are moved toward the centration point as the patient attempts to maintain NRC localization. The final goal with this technique is for the patient to hold a perfect AI cross while bifixating a variety of targets at the centration point.

Hugonnier et al.[26] recommended a free-space training procedure called "direct attack at the objective angle in space" (Figure 11-6). A target such as a pencil point is placed at the centration point, and the patient attempts to see a Hering-Bielschowsky cross superimposed on the tip of the pencil. This picture is an indication of NRC, but the unilateral cover test should be performed since the AI could be seen with NRC, whereas the pencil tip is seen with ARC. A movement of the uncovered eye on the unilateral cover test would indicate ARC. In this eventuality, a higher plus add and a closer training distance should be attempted. Bagolini lenses can be used for further training (See Figures 11-6b, 11-6c and 11-6d).

There are many combinations of procedures that can be used in cases of ARC. Real images may be provided by targets such as black dots,

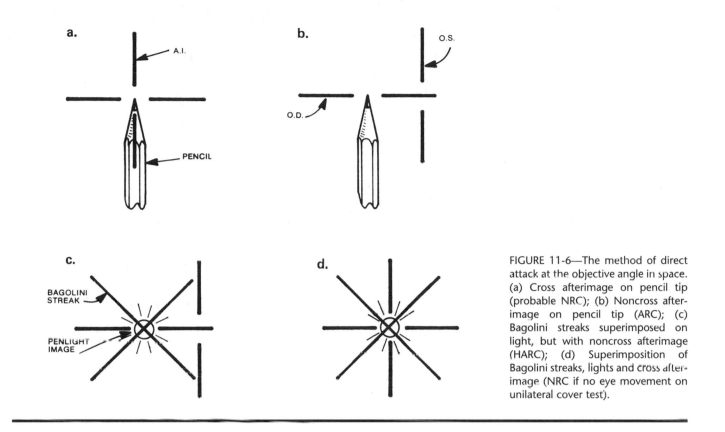

FIGURE 11-6—The method of direct attack at the objective angle in space. (a) Cross afterimage on pencil tip (probable NRC); (b) Noncross afterimage on pencil tip (ARC); (c) Bagolini streaks superimposed on light, but with noncross afterimage (HARC); (d) Superimposition of Bagolini streaks, lights and cross afterimage (NRC if no eye movement on unilateral cover test).

anaglyphs, vectographic targets, and a penlight. These may be used together with entoptic phenomena and/or afterimages. Only a few representative procedures can be discussed since the number of possible variations and combinations are legion.

Prism-Rack Afterimage Technique T11.10

Ronne and Rindziunski[27] reported a prism-rack afterimage technique. This simply involves the placement of a horitzontal prism bar before one eye, while the patient is perceiving afterimages. The prism bar should be slowly racked up and down as the patient reports any changes in AI localization. They found that on the Hering-Bielschowsky test, a noncross may become a cross, in some cases, as a result of the introduction of various prisms. Possibly covariation is stimulated with this procedure or overcorrection of the deviation with prisms may stimulate an NRC response. When an NRC response

occurs (a perfect cross), the patient attempts to hold it as other prism powers are introduced in small increments. This technique can be performed with a blank field, if necessary, or with real targets in open space utilizing a centration point add.

Haidinger Brush Technique T11.11

The combination of the Haidinger Brush (HB), a transferred afterimage (AI), and a black dot is sometimes useful in ARC therapy (see Figure 5-45). An AI is generated on the fovea of the right eye. The centration-point add is used to allow for bifixation in open space (the right eye is not occluded in this training techniques). A device to generate an HB (e.g., Bernell MITT) is placed at the centration point. Suppose a patient has a left esotropia and HARC. The patient should fixate with the left eye so that the HB is on the black dot (assuming central fixation); the transferred AI would be seen to

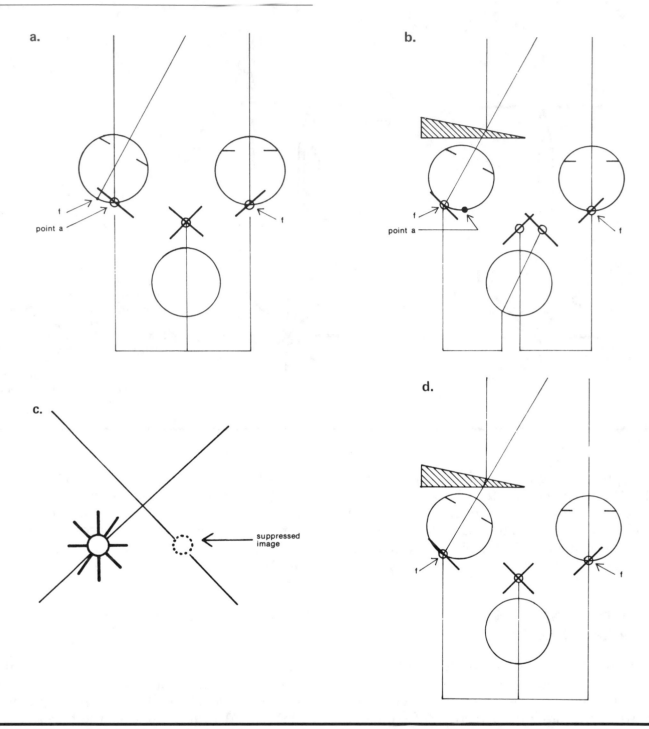

FIGURE 11-7—Bagolini striated lenses and prisms for treatment of anomalous correspondence. (a) Harmonious ARC response. (b) Harmonious response with compensating prism. (c) Only one light seen because of foveal suppression of the left eye. (d) NRC response after ARC has been eliminated and angle of strabismus fully compensated by prism.

the left of the HB (ARC localization to point "a" in the left eye). A flashing light near the right eye intensifies the perception of the transferred afterimage. The patient is instructed to try mentally to reduce the angle of anomaly so that all

the images (dot, HB and AI) are superimposed (NRC localization). The use of a pointer for tactile/kinesthetic stimulation and feedback often helps in this type of training. Hopefully, visual stimulation with an HB and AI will help to break ARC localization. When the patient achieves NRC localization using a dot, other real targets of various sizes and complexity are introduced.

Bagolini Lens Technique T11.12

Bagolini lenses with prisms can be used in a later stage in open space training for the elimination of ARC (Figure 11-7). Since most cases of strabismus with ARC show HARC on the Bagolini lenses, the patient sees the "ortho" response with the light centered in the X (angle S = 0) (see Figure 11-7a). If the full compensating base-out prism is worn, the image of the light is now on the fovea of the deviating eye and no longer on point "a." This causes the patient with HARC to report seeing lights below the intersection of the streaks (see Figure 11-7b). Since the fovea of the deviating eye is usually suppressed, only one light is seen in most of these cases (see Figure 11-7c). Rapidly introducing and removing the prism may be sufficient in disrupting ARC and an underlying NRC may emerge as a result of extensive training of this nature. The patient should then see the light centered in the cross, which indicates NRC (providing the strabismic angle is fully compensated by prism) (see Figure 11-7d).

Another variation of this technique is to stimulate diplopia in open space (without a compensating horizontal prism). Spontaneous diplopia is not easily seen in free space by a patient who is strabismic; therefore, the environment may have to be less than natural at times. For this purpose, graded occluders, lowered room illumination, and bright fixation targets may be helpful. For example, a bar of graded filters (either gray or red) is useful for eliciting an NRC response with the Bagolini lens procedure. The attenuators are placed over the dominant eye and progressively increased until the patient reports diplopia of the light that indicates NRC localization. Once NRC diplopia is appreciated, it should be extended to all distances and fields of gaze using anti-suppression techniques of flashing, blinking, increasing stimulus contrast, and focusing the

patient's attention (see Chapter 12). The patient is not left diplopic at this point in strabismus therapy; sensory and motor fusion should be expanded maximally using methods described in Chapters 13 and 14. Any residual angle of deviation may need to be compensated for with prisms, lenses, or surgery. On the other hand, if a patient does not show the ability to fuse the diplopic images produced with these techniques, training should be discontinued immediately. Intractable diplopia is an undesirable outcome.

EXOTROPIA AND ARC

ARC is a less significant factor influencing the prognosis for a functional cure in exotropia, compared with esotropia. Even though over 50% of exotropic patients have ARC, there are reasons why it is of less concern.

Theoretical Considerations

Exotropia is generally much easier to cure, regardless of the state of correspondence. The prognosis is better because the age of onset is usually later for exotropia than for esotropia, thus the re-education of fusion is easier. Normal fusion had the early opportunity to develop in many of these patients before the onset of strabismus. More importantly, most exotropes are intermittent (compared with esotropia that tends to be constant); ARC is also intermittent because of covariation. When the eyes are straight, the patient is fusing with NRC. Covariation is consistent with Morgan's motor theory of ARC and seems to be independent of the magnitude of exotropia. Training to eliminate ARC in exotropia is, therefore, a form of motor fusion training. Consequently, sensory training specifically for eliminating ARC can usually be bypassed except for some cases of constant exotropia.

Gross Convergence for Exotropia with ARC T11.13

Gross convergence training involves the use of pushup targets, minus adds, and afterimages.

This technique is helpful primarily in cases of constant exotropia, but can also be used in cases of intermittent exotropia with a remote nearpoint of convergence. The essence of the technique is to give the patient as much feedback as possible to help him make a gross convergence movement, ultimately to achieve bifoveal fixation and sensory fusion on a nearpoint target using fusional convergence. Gross convergence should be attempted with all exotropes as part of the initial treatment sequence.

The first step in gross convergence training, assuming the refractive error is corrected, is to build the patient's awareness of the eyes in motion. This training develops a tactile-kinesthetic sense of convergence. Initially, the patient can simply practice moving the eyes in all directions of gaze while increasing his awareness of sensation associated with these movements. The sensation probably arises from the lid margins, extraocular muscles, and orbital tissue. Monocular saccades can also be stimulated with various prism powers with the patient learning to sense subtle eye movements. Large accommodative shifts should be made, far to near to far, under binocular conditions. The patient should be sensitized to changes in convergence using accommodative convergence. This sensitization phase of training may take several sessions to develop the patient's awareness of convergence eye movements, an important source of feedback.

The next step is to apply Hering-Bielschowsky afterimages to provide visual feedback when covariation is occurring. The afterimages will appear uncrossed or displaced (ARC) when the eyes are in the exotropic position. When fusional convergence is stimulated during the next step in the technique, the patient will see the afterimages joining to become a perfect cross (NRC) as the eyes move toward bifoveal alignment on a nearpoint target. This visual feedback is a strong incentive for the patient to continue exerting fusional convergence.

The final phase in this technique is to stimulate accommodative convergence sufficiently in the attempt to trigger a fusional (disparity) convergence response. Merely stimulating accommodative convergence with minus adds cannot be expected to result in a shift of correspon-

dence,[6] but it may recruit a fusional vergence eye movement that is associated with covariation. For example, a 12-year-old boy has a comitant, constant, alternating exotropia of 40^Δ at far and near with HARC. With vision training the patient is aware of eye movements, particularly accommodative convergence, but he cannot yet fuse intermittently at near. Bielschowsky afterimages are applied and appear uncrossed (ARC). A -2.00 D add is placed before the patient's spectacle lenses (using Halberg clips for example) to reduce the angle of deviation and provide a stimulus to accommodation. With the minus add in place, the resultant deviation is 30^Δ XT. The patient is asked to look far away and close his eyes. A small, detailed, colorful target (e.g., a sticker on a stick) is held just beyond the patient's nearpoint of accommodation. The patient is asked for open his eyes, focus rapidly on the target, and to try to "pull the eyes together." This is done while sensing the crossing of the eyes (tactile-kinesthetic feedback) and joining the afterimages (visual feedback). Similar to a personal exercise trainer, the therapist gives strong verbal encouragement and feedback about performance, whether or not there is alignment of the eyes. On the first few attempts, convergence may be inadequate. The goal is for the patient to increase convergence until the afterimages join. As the training proceeds, different nearpoint targets are used for the sake of variety. The procedure is practiced at home and in-office until the patient can hold nearpoint alignment and perfectly crossed afterimages for about 5 minutes. The doctor can verify bifoveal alignment and covariation by testing with Bagolini lenses and the unilateral cover test. In this example, further management might include constant patching of an eye between therapy sessions. After gross convergence has been achieved, standard vergence training can proceed at near using loose prisms, Vectograms, Tranaglyphs, and binocular accommodative flippers. Extraocular muscle surgery may be recommended depending on the results of the sensory and motor fusion training. (See Chapter 13 for a discussion of vision therapy for exo deviations.)

Occasionally, an exotropic patient with ARC may require amblyoscopic sensory training similar to that given in esotropia with ARC. This happens in some cases of large-angle constant exotropia with deeply embedded ARC when the gross convergence technique is unsuccessful. Open space alignment by means of base-in prisms and training may be tried, but this is usually not as successful as when the eyes are actually in the ortho position (i.e., with the minus lens and gross convergence method). Training in a reduced environment of the major amblyoscope for exotropia follows the same principles applicable to esotropia.

SURGICAL RESULTS IN CASES OF ARC

Surgical correction of strabismus may possibly result in changes in correspondence, even in adults. If NRC existed prior to strabismus surgery, however, NRC will persist following the operation.[28] On the other hand, normalization of correspondence in esotropic or exotropic ARC cases may occur after an operation.[28-31] Rutstein et al.[28] reported a retrospective analysis of 20 strabismic patients who showed presurgical ARC. Seven of these patients (35%) were found to have NRC postsurgically. Most of these cases were surgically overcorrected for their strabismic deviation; esotropes became consecutive exotropes and exotropes became esotropes. Undercorrection of the strabismus, even slightly, is not likely to trigger the NRC response. These patients tend to redevelop HARC. Two separate studies, Hugonnier[29] and de Decker,[31] reported that about 70% of their surgically overcorrected esotropes (consecutive exotropes) developed NRC. Jampolsky[32] has also proposed surgical overcorrection as a way of jolting the fusion mechanism, creating diplopia, and awakening a dormant normal correspondence system. He called this effect "surgical orthoptics." These reports are very interesting especially considering the positive results with prism overcorrection;[14,16,17] the same or a similar mechanism of action may be responsible for the shift in correspondence. When de Decker[31] combined surgical overcorrection of esotropia with prism overcorrection, so that patients had about 12^Δ exo, his results

improved to 82% for developing NRC and 46% for a cure (or partial cure) of the strabismus. However, surgical overcorrection of esotropia sometimes necessitates a second operation due to a cosmetically unacceptable consecutive exotropia, an undesirable outcome. With these results in mind, one possible strategy in cases of esotropia associated with ARC might be to attempt a slight surgical overcorrection, 5^Δ or less, supplemented by prism overcorrection to insure that the patient remains with either "sensory" exotropia or binocular fusion. Fresnel prisms can be conveniently applied post-surgically with frequent changes as needed. We believe some pre- and post-surgical vision training usually improves the chance of either permanent functional cure or partial cure of strabismus.

The exact mechanism of the shift in correspondence with surgery remains unknown. Sensorial results are essentially unpredictable. Unfortunately, a few cases result in intractable diplopia.[33] Flom et al.[34] reported a detailed case study of a 37-year-old intermittent exotropic female with covering ARC. She showed an immediate change in the angle of anomaly with a surgical change in the ocular deviation. The investigators proposed that post-surgical diplopia served as a stimulus for the change in correspondence to normal or near normal. The result after two operations was a small exophoria with NRC when bifixating; however, HARC persisted when fusion was disrupted and an exotropia was manifest. Further research is needed to illuminate the nature of these changes in correspondence associated with surgical and prism overcorrection, as well as spontaneous changes in the angle of deviation.

CASE MANAGEMENT

When considering treatment of constant strabismus associated with ARC, the question must be raised: "What is the price and the chance of successfully training normal binocular vision?" Clinicians and patients value this goal differently and there is nothing approaching a consensus. In their extensive review of the literature, Wick and Cook[25] estimated that about

50% of esotropic patients having ARC can be expected to achieve normal binocular vision provided sufficient time (up to 12 months) is devoted to re-education. Based on our experience, we do not prescribe vision therapy when we do not think we can cure a strabismic patient with ARC (using all therapy approaches including surgery) within a year. We often accept patients, however, for ten training sessions to verify the prognosis and assess the patient's responses to active therapy. This is called "diagnostic therapy."

If possible, we prefer to treat ARC by stimulating covariation. The fusional vergence mechanism of shifting ARC to NRC is often applicable in exotropia up to 50^Δ and esotropia of 20^Δ or less. For exotropia, the gross convergence technique in open space (T11.13) and the Flom swing technique (T11.7) in an amblyoscope can both be used. In cases of exotropia, the Flom swing technique is applied to generate convergent eye movements rather than divergence. For small-angle esotropes who qualify for this method, Flom's divergence technique offers a fair chance for success within a reasonable period. Once the patient has learned to covary and utilize this mechanism when straightening the eyes, the diverging ability seems permanent. Surgery, however, is sometimes necessary to reduce the magnitude of the deviation. Regression is prevented by assigning retainer vergence exercises on a regular schedule. (Refer to Chapters 13 and 14.)

Besides having a major amblyoscope, applying classical techniques successfully requires considerable skill in managing children over a period of several months. The techniques are not inherently entertaining. Regular amblyoscopic training, 3 to 5 sessions per week, is time intensive and, therefore, expensive. Since we see similar or better rates of success in normalizing correspondence by simply prescribing prism overcorrection, this is our preferred initial approach with preschool and elementary school children. Often the prism spectacles are not acceptable for full time wear, particularly at school, so the patient is given constant occlusion during school hours and wears the prism spectacles at home, 3 to 4 hours per day. If and when NRC is established, the prism power is reduced to become neutralizing prisms. Home and in-office training activities help to consolidate normal sensory and motor fusion at this point. (See Chapters 12, 13, and 14.) Extraocular muscle surgery may be necessary to achieve comfortable binocular vision unless large amounts of prism are worn. Using effective therapy options, many patients with constant strabismus and ARC can develop good binocular vision and maintain straight eyes within 3 to 6 months.

Following these recommendations, the prognosis for a complete or partial cure of strabismus with ARC can conservatively be estimated at 50%. Frequently, the result of therapy in cases of ARC is microtropia. The patient may achieve fair stereopsis (e.g., 200 seconds) and almost normal fusional vergence ranges despite the presence of ARC with a small angle of anomaly. This outcome can be considered a partial cure and is, in our opinion, clinically acceptable. When a patient has successfully undergone vision therapy to establish NRC and there is no microtropia, the next therapy goals involve breaking any remaining central suppression and developing good visual skills. Chapters 12, 13, 14, and 16 discuss these vision therapy procedures.

CASE EXAMPLES

Case Report no. 1: Prism Overcorrection in Esotropia

Christenson[35] presented a case of a 6-year-old female with a history of an eye-turn since the age of 3. This case demonstrates the efficacy of prism overcorrection combined with vision training and extraocular muscle surgery. There was no previous treatment. The onset was gradual, but the strabismus later became constant. The diagnosis of the deviation was: comitant, constant, alternating (left eye dominant), esotropia of 30^Δ at 6 m and 40 cm. Cycloplegic refraction:

OD +1.00 − 1.00 x 150   20/20 (6/6)

OS +1.00 − 1.00 x 035   20/20 (6/6)

Associated conditions included HARC (Bagolini striated lens test), no motor fusion, and no stereopsis.

A prism adaptation test was performed. Fresnel prisms were placed on plano lenses in a frame fitted to the patient. A total of 40^Δ base-out (20^Δ each eye) was worn for 10 minutes but resulted in an eso movement on the alternate cover test. Prism adaptation had occurred. The procedure was repeated with a total of 50^Δ base-out with the same result as before. When a total of 60^Δ was worn for 30 minutes, there was no eso movement on the cover test. The patient was then instructed to wear the overcorrecting prism spectacles for 30 minutes per day while performing active visual tasks. At all other waking hours, the patient wore a patch on an alternating daily schedule.

After 2 weeks, the patient again showed an eso movement with the alternate cover test. A total of 80^Δ base-out was prescribed for daily wearing of 30 minutes each day along with patching. After 1 month, there was an exo movement on the cover test. The Fresnel base-out prism power was reduced to 70^Δ, and the same regimen as before was carried out. After 2 months, NRC was found with the major amblyoscope (angles H and S approximately 40^Δ).

At this juncture, the second phase of the therapy was initiated. Overcorrecting prism of 60^Δ was prescribed for 30 minutes per day with constant patching at all other times. In-office procedures began with peripheral first-degree and second-degree targets on an amblyoscope and sensory-motor fusion procedures at the centration point. Home training included monocular pencil saccades and accommodative facility training with Hart Charts. With training, the fusional vergence range increased to 30^Δ converging and 15^Δ diverging from the objective angle, but the patient was unable to appreciate stereopsis, although she did report SILO ("small-in" with base-out and "large-out" with base-in). Fusional vergence training around the objective angle continued in the open environment using Vectograms.

After a total of 36 office visits, the diagnosis was: comitant, constant, alternating esotropia of 30^Δ at 6 m and 40 cm; there was NRC and a large fusional divergence range. At this point,

the patient was referred to an ophthalmologist for extraocular muscle surgery. The operation consisted of a 5.5 mm bimedial rectus recession. Postsurgically, a monofixation pattern of the right eye was indicated by the unilateral cover test and the 4^Δ base-out test at far. A small right eso flick was seen with unilateral cover test with the paradoxical finding of 10^Δ base-in on the alternate cover test (i.e., patient having an exo deviation when dissociated). Suppression of the right eye was indicated with the 4^Δ base-out test. However, 2^Δ of esophoria was found at the 40 cm fixation distance. Amblyoscope testing indicated NRC, but stereopsis was not found with either the Reindeer or Randot tests.

Ten weekly office training visits followed the post-surgical evaluation. Vision training was done with Vectograms and stereoscopes to attempt to break central suppression and increase fusional vergence ranges. Although vergences were strengthened with training, there was still no stereopsis; the four base-out prism tests revealed a small central suppression zone of the right eye. Subsequently, the exo deviation at far on the alternate cover test decreased and the esophoria at near increased to 8^Δ. Plus-adds were prescribed in the form of bifocal lenses. Rx: OD +0.50 - 1.00 x 170; OS +0.50 -1.25 x 010 with +2.50 adds. With this prescription, the patient maintained an eso monofixation pattern at distance and 2^Δ esophoria at near. Follow-up evaluation 2 years later showed the deviation to be stable. This patient's binocular status satisfied most of Flom's criterion in the "almost cured" category.[36] There was clear, comfortable, single binocular vision present at all distances, normal ranges of motor fusion, but lack of stereopsis. The patient was happy with her improved binocular status.

Case Report no. 2: Stimulating Covariation in Constant Exotropia.

Wick[37] presented a detailed case report of a 13-year-old patient with constant, alternating exotropia of 45^Δ and HARC on all tests. Constant occlusion was prescribed between training sessions (both office and home). He used a variation of the gross convergence technique (T11.13) to stimulate fusion at near and covariation to NRC. Minus 2.00 D adds were worn to induce convergence at far. Afterimages were used so that correspondence could be monitored during forced convergence at near. The minus additions were not used at near. The Pola-Mirror (See Chapter 12) was included so that suppression could be monitored during convergence while the patient maintained a perfect AI cross. The patient was able to achieve this after 2 weeks of vision therapy. Red-green TV antisuppression training was then done in conjunction with afterimages at far, with the −2.00 D addition lenses being used. After 3 weeks the patient was able to achieve an AI cross without suppression on the red-green TV trainer. Extraocular muscle surgery reduced the deviation to 20^Δ and the patient became exophoric afterwards. Postsurgical vision therapy consisted of base-out training with the TV trainer, single Aperture Rule Trainer, and various chiastopic fusion procedures. (Refer to Chapters 12, 13, and 14). The patient had no symptoms and all visual functions became normal. The important point of this case is that ARC may be present when exotropia is manifest, but there is NRC when the eyes are in the ortho position.

Case Report no. 3: Flom Swing Technique for a Small Angle Esotropic Patient.

Ms. B, a 23-year-old female student, was referred by an optometrist, who fitted her with RGP contact lenses, because of her persistent asthenopic complaints that seemed related to deficient binocular vision. She complained of headaches initiated by reading, itching and burning eyes that increased in intensity throughout the day, and reduced reading time. College studies required her to read several hours per day. She reported good general health and no medications, but she had had surgery for esotropia at about 2 years of age.

Ms. B's visual acuity was slightly reduced with her contact lenses: OD: +2.00 DS 20/25 and OS: +1.50 DS 20/25-. The strabismus evaluation revealed a constant, comitant, alternating (left eye preferred for fixation) esotropia of 12^Δ at 6 m and 40 cm with the contact lenses. Cosmesis of the strabismus was good. Sensory fusion testing indicated HARC, deep central alternate suppression, and 400 sec. "reported" on the Stereo Fly test. Although her accommodative amplitude was normal for her age (10 diopters each eye), binocular accommodative facility was reduced. Ms. B took 2 minutes to clear 20 cycles using ±1.50 D flippers. A cycloplegic subjective refraction showed the following refractive error:

OD: +2.50 −1.75 axis 176 20/20

OS: +2.25 −3.00 axis 17 20/20

Keratometry readings confirmed the astigmatism:

OD: 42.50 @ 170; 44.75 @ 80

OS: 42.00 @ 5; 45.37 @ 95

Ordinarily, patients having a small angle constant esotropia, central suppression and ARC are free of binocular vision symptoms. However, in this case, we suspected that the combination of high vision requirements, only rudimentary binocular vision, accommodative infacility, and uncorrected astigmatism caused her visual complaints and reduced reading time. Rather than just treating her on a symptomatic basis, we suggested that she could attempt a functional cure of the strabismus and the accommodative disorder in addition to wearing a full correction for her refractive error. Ms. B was agreeable to this approach.

In-office training, 1-hour weekly sessions consisted primarily of the divergence technique (Flom Swing) on an amblyoscope (T11.7). The central suppression was overcome by the automatic, rapid, alternate flashing and increasing the illumination to the right (non-dominant) eye. During the initial training session on the amblyoscope, Ms. B appreciated stereopsis on the swing slide, held both suppression controls in perception, and demonstrated some divergence skill as base-in demand was gradually increased. She was unable, however, to diverge her eyes through the entire angle of deviation until the third training session. For 20 minutes per day of home training, a Mirror Stereoscope was assigned with large second- and third-degree fusion targets. She achieved sensory fusion with these targets at her subjective angle, then attempted to build fusional vergence ranges using sliding vergences with emphasis on divergence. She also spent 10 minutes per day training monocular accommodative facility using Hart Charts and accommodative flipper lenses.

Progress in building divergence and accommodation was rapid. After 4 weeks of in-office and home training, Ms. B could voluntarily straighten her eyes in the open environment and hold them aligned at distance and near for several minutes. She noticed an increase in perception of stereopsis when the eyes were straight, but there was also a sense of eyestrain. Monocular accommodative facility was within normal limits. By cover test, she showed an intermittent, comitant, 12^Δ esotropia of the right eye at far and near. Stereopsis had increased to 40 seconds of arc at 40 cm (Fly Stereo test) when she voluntarily aligned her eyes. Response time, however, was slow. After 8 weeks of training, normal sensory and motor fusion was maintained on a reflex level most of the day. In the evenings she would occasionally lose fusional control of her deviation and experience some intermittent diplopia.

In an attempt to increase fusional control and comfort, the following prism spectacle lenses were prescribed:

OD: +2.25 −1.25 axis 175 3^Δ BO 20/20

OS: +2.25 −2.75 axis 017 3^Δ BO 20/20

Also, +1.50 D Fresnel flat-top adds were also applied to reduce the deviation at near. Ms. B discontinued contact lens wear except for some social occasions.

The patient continued the fusional vergence training with the Mirror Stereoscope at home. Vectograms® (Mother Goose and Spirangle) were also introduced with a total training time of 30 minutes per day. Accommodative facility training was discontinued since the patient had achieved normal monocular and binocular facility. Vergence ranges continued to increase over a 1-month period and then stabilized. Since the patient was essentially symptom free at this point and vergence skills had been trained to a high stable level, Ms. B was given retainer exercises of 30 minutes, twice a week, using the Mirror Stereoscope and released from therapy. Vergence skills generally regress faster in strabismic cases compared with phoric cases due to the resultant stress on fusional vergence and recurrent suppression, so a vigorous retainer program was required.

Ms. B was released from active therapy completely symptom free and fusing normally with bifoveal fixation 99% of the time, a cured case by Flom's criteria.[36] A periodic schedule of progress checks was initiated with 6-month intervals. She occasionally lost fusion at intermediate distances, but not at far or at near (even without the bifocals). She experienced diplopia at these times; blinking initiated the required vergence eye movement to align the eyes properly. This finding suggests that NRC was present, even when fusion was lost. The Fresnel adds were removed without a noticeable reduction of visual skills. In summary, the patient gained normal stereopsis and visual functions within a reasonably short period of active vision training. In this case, partial prism compensation was also necessary to achieve maximum results.

REFERENCES

1. Bielschowsky A. Lectures on motor anomalies. *Dartmouth College Publications.* Hanover, NH: Dartmouth College; 1943:72.
2. Flom MC. *The empirical longitudinal horopter in anomalous correspondence.* Berkeley, Calif: University of California; 1953. Thesis.
3. Caloroso EE, Rouse MW. *Clinical Management of Strabismus.* Stoneham; Mass: Butterworth-Heinemann; 1993:162-163.
4. Von Noorden GK. *Binocular Vision and Ocular Motility: Theory and Management of Strabismus.* 4th ed. St. Louis: CV Mosby Co; 1990:255-256.
5. Morgan MW. Anomalous correspondence interpreted as a motor phenomenon. *Am J Optom.* 1961: 131-148.
6. Kerr KE. Instability of anomalous retinal correspondence. *J Am Optom Assoc.* 1968;39:1107-1108.

7. Cook D. Considering the ocular motor system in the treatment of anomalous retinal correspondence. *J Am Optom Assoc.* 1984;55:109-117.

8. Folk ER. *Treatment of Strabismus.* Springfield: Charles Thomas; 1965:72.

9. Greenwald I. Re-evaluation of binasal occlusion. *Optom Weekly.* 1974;65:21-22.

10. Caloroso EE, Rouse MW. *Clinical Management of Strabismus.* Newton, Mass: Butterworth-Heineman; 1993: 117-118.

11. Revell MJ. Anomalous retinal correspondence: A refractive treatment. *The Ophthalmic Optician.* 1971;2: 110-112

12. Bagolini B. Sensorial anomalies in strabismus (suppression, anomalous correspondence, amblyopia.) *Doc Ophthalmol.* 1976;41:1-22.

13. Berard PV. The use of prisms in the pre- and post-operative treatment of deviation in comitant squint. In: Fells P, ed. *First Congress of the International Strabismological Association. Acapulco, Mexico.* St. Louis: CV Mosby Co;1971:227-234.

14. Fleming A, Pigassou R, Garipuy J. Adaptation of a method of prismatic overcorrection for testing strabismus in children 1 and 2 years old. *J Ped Ophthalmol.* 1973;10:154-159.

15. Caloroso EE, Rouse MW. *Clinical Management of Strabismus.* Stoneham Mass: Butterworth-Heinemann; 1993:117-118.

16. Amigo G. Present trends in orthoptics and pleoptics in Giessen. *Am J Optom.* 1970;47:713.

17. Arruga A. *First International Congress of Orthoptists.* St. Louis: CV Mosby Co; 1968:69.

18. Ludlam WM. Lecture. San Jose, Calif: San Jose Vision Training Seminar; 1970.

19. Revell, MJ. *Strabismus: A History of Orthoptic Techniques.* London: Barrie & Jenkins; 1971:30-36

20. Caloroso EE, Rouse MW. *Clinical Management of Strabismus.* Newton, Mass: Butterworth-Heinemann; 1993:209.

21. Revell, MJ. *Strabismus: A History of Orthoptic Techniques.* London: Barrie & Jenkins; 1971:160-163.

22. Wick B. Visual therapy for small angle esotropia. *Am J Optom Physiol Optics.* 1974;51:490-496.

23. Caloroso EE, Rouse MW. *Clinical Management of Strabismus.* Newton, Mass: Butterworth-Heinemann; 1993:213.

24. Grisham JD. Treatment of binocular dysfunctions. In: Schor C, Ciuffreda KJ, eds. *Vergence Eye Movements: Basic and Clinical Aspects.* Boston: Butterworth; 1983:637-639.

25. Wick B, Cook D. Management of anomalous correspondence: efficacy of therapy. *Am J Optom Physiol Optics.* 1987;64:405-410.

26. Hugonnier R, Hugonnier S, Troutman S. *Strabismus, Heterophoria, Ocular Motor Paralysis.* CV Mosby Co; St. Louis 1969:573-580.

27. Ronne G, Rindziunski E. The diagnosis and clinical classification of anomalous correspondence. *Acta Ophthalmologica.*, 31, cited by Borish IM. *Clinical Refraction.* 3rd ed. Chicago: Professional Press; 1970:1235.

28. Rutstein RP, Marsh-Tootle W, Scheiman MM, Eskridge JB. Changes in retinal correspondence after changes in ocular alignment. *Optom Vision Sci.* 1991;68:325-330.

29. Hugonnier R. The influence of the operative overcorrection of an esotropia on abnormal retinal correspondence. In: Arruga A, ed. *International Strabismus Symposium.* New York: Basal. S Karger; 1968:307-310.

30. Katsumi O, Tanaka Y, Uemura Y. Anomalous retinal correspondence (ARC) in esotropia. *Jpn J Ophthalmol.* 1982;26:166-174.

31. DeDecker W. Result of surgery versus prism tolerated overcorrection therapy of anomalous correspondence. In: Fells P, ed. *Proceedings of the Second Congress of the International Strabismological Association.* Marseilles, France: Diffusion Generale de Librairie; 1976:279-282.

32. Jampolsky A. The postoperative use of prisms. In: Fells P, ed. *Proceedings of the Second Congress of the International Strabismological Association.* Marseilles, France; Diffusion Generale de Librairie; 1976: 291-294.

33. Gruzensky WD, Palmer EA. Intractable diplopia: a clinical perspective. *Graefe's Arch Clin Exp Ophthalmol.* 1988;226:187-192.

34. Flom MC, Kirschen DG, Williams AT. Changes in retinal correspondence following surgery for intermittent exotropia. *Am J Optom Physiol Opt.* 1978;55: 456-462.

35. Christenson GN. Treatment of esotropia with anomalous correspondence: a case report. *J Am Optom Assoc.* 1992;4:257-261.

36. Flom MC. Issues in the Clinical Management of Binocular Anomalies. In: Rosenbloom AA, Morgan MW, eds. *Pediatric Optometry.* Philadelphia: Lippincott Co; 1990:222-223.

37. Wick B. Visual therapy for constant exotropia with anomalous retinal correspondence: a case report. *Am J Optom Physiol Opt.* 1974;51:1005-1008.

Chapter 12 / Antisuppression Therapy

Occlusion Antisuppression Therapy 350
General Approach to Active
   Antisuppression Training 350
   Antisuppression Variables 351
     Attention 351
     Brightness 351
     Target Contrast 351
     Color 352
     Target Size 352
     Intermittent Stimuli 353
     Target Movement 353
     Tactile and Kinesthetic Senses 354
     Auditory Sense 354
     Combinations 354
   Four-step Approach to Antisuppression
     Training 354
     Step One 354
     Step Two 355
     Step Three 355
     Step Four 356
Specific Antisuppression
   Techniques 356

Translid Binocular Interaction Trainer
   T12.1 356
Major Amblyoscope T12.2 358
   Illumination Gradient and Flashing
     358
   Chasing 358
   End Point Suppression 358
Penlight and Filters T12.3 359
Hand-Mirror Superimposition
   T12.4 359
Cheiroscopic Games T12.5 360
   Counting 360
   Coloring and Drawing 360
   Point-to-Point Chasing 361
   Tracing 361
Modified Remy Separator T12.6 361
Brock String and Beads T12.7 362
Television Trainers T12.8 364
Pola-Mirror T12.9 365
Reading Bars T12.10 366
Management Considerations. 366
Case Example 367

Suppression is active cortical inhibition of all or part of one eye's binocular field under binocular viewing conditions. The perception of a suppressed image cannot always be rejuvenated by simply calling the patient's attention to that image. Suppression occurs when sensory or motor fusion is overly taxed. Uncorrected anisometropia, aniseikonia, amblyopia, and strabismus are conditions often associated with suppression. Suppression is an active process to prevent diplopia and relieve visual discomfort. Generally, the longer suppression is present, the deeper it is and the more difficult it is to treat. Many heterophoric patients with ver-

gence anomalies also have some degree of suppression. Suppression, therefore, is an important consideration in the treatment of most binocular vision disorders.

More than 100 years ago, Javal[1] pointed out the importance of antisuppression to effect a binocular cure in cases of strabismus. Antisuppression training was fundamental to his therapeutic approach and is still considered to be of primary importance in the management of all binocular vision anomalies. Javal believed that obstacles to sensory fusion should be removed before efforts are made to align the eyes with vergence training or surgery. One of his basic principles of effective vision therapy is providing targets that have suppression clues (controls) for monitoring and training purposes. Appropriate targets are presented either with an ortho demand or with forced vergence demands. When suppression of an eye is found, active antisuppression techniques are immediately used to enliven the suppressed image and establish sensory fusion. Once sensory fusion is established, sensory and motor fusion demands can be increased until a suppression response occurs again. This antisuppression process is continued until suppression is completely eliminated within a zone of clear, single, comfortable, binocular vision. Theoretical aspects of suppression and testing procedures are discussed in detail in Chapter 5. This therapy chapter describes: (1) General approaches (passive and active therapy) to breaking suppression; (2) Targets and stimulus variables for breaking suppression; and (3) Specific antisuppression techniques.

OCCLUSION ANTISUPPRESSION THERAPY

There are two antidiplopia mechanisms in strabismus, anomalous "retinal" correspondence (ARC) and suppression. Just as in ARC, patching an eye also prevents suppression since it does not occur under monocular viewing conditions. Occlusion can be thought of, therefore, as a passive form of vision therapy to prevent and break suppression. Suppression is an active process that tends to deepen with abnormal visual experience. Occlusion helps to break through suppression by preventing its reinforcement.

The typical occlusion regimen in cases of deep suppression associated with constant strabismus is constant patching during all times in which active vision training is not being done. Occlusion allows for maintaining the gains made in active antisuppression training during daily activity at school, work, or play. In cases of moderate suppression, the patching regimen can be relaxed somewhat with the patient wearing the patch part of the day but always under concentrated seeing conditions, such as reading, writing, and watching television. If the suppression is only shallow, the patch need only be worn while reading or watching television in the evening for 1 or 2 hours. Some cases of shallow suppression require only antisuppression training activities, without the necessity of occlusion.

Graded occlusion may be applied when suppression is shallow. (Refer to Chapter 5 for testing the intensity of suppression.) In most cases of deep suppression, however, an opaque occluder is required between active therapy sessions. Note that these active therapy sessions may be either in-office or out-of-office (home training). When suppression is moderate, a graded occluder may be prescribed to promote fusion, but only in cases of anisometropic amblyopia or in which the strabismus is only occasional. Graded occlusion can break suppression while reinforcing sensory and motor fusion. When suppression is only shallow, mild attenuating occluders may be effective in promoting sensory fusion. The concept of graded occlusion is consistent with the naturalness concept of testing the intensity of suppression (Chapter 5). In short, the deeper the suppression, the more unnatural the occluding procedure should be. For example, a dark red lens could be worn over the dominant eye when the suppression is moderately deep. If the suppression is only shallow, a light pink lens over the dominant eye may suffice to break the suppression of the nondominant suppressing eye. A neutral density filter of appropriate transmittance can also provide effective graded occlusion and can be attached to the spectacle lens with adhesive tape.

GENERAL APPROACH TO ACTIVE ANTISUPPRESSION TRAINING

There are hundreds of active antisuppression training instruments, targets, and techniques. Many training methods are variations of tests used to detect suppression, such as stereoscopes and colored filters. Although only a few antisuppression techniques are presented, the concepts we discuss can be applied to most innovative methods the therapist originates.

Antisuppression Variables

When active antisuppression training is assigned, a number of important variables must be considered when designing an appropriate training method. Factors that should be considered in procedures requiring active training are listed in Table 12-1.

Attention

The attention factor is a very important consideration in the treatment of suppression. When the therapist presents a new target or device, each eye should be occluded in turn and all suppression controls should be pointed out to the patient. The therapist should continually remind the patient to make a conscious effort to hold the suppression controls in perception. This mental concentration can momentarily stop the suppression. Antisuppression training is, therefore, an active process and the patient is expected to exert "mental effort" to hold the suppression controls in perception. Although attention is necessary, it alone is not always sufficient to break through a suppression response.

Since attention is such an important variable, the therapist should select targets that are of interest to the patient, particularly in the case of children. Polarized or anaglyphic TV trainers or reading bars are antisuppression instruments that are popular with most patients. Cheiroscopic training can also peak the interest of children who enjoy drawing and tracing. For older children and adults, we have found the Bernell 500 series of Tranaglyphs showing sports figures are well designed for antisuppression training to hold the patient's interest.

Brightness

The target before the suppressing eye should be brighter than the target before the nonsuppressing eye. This difference in the level of brightness must be large if suppression is very intense (deep). Even patients who have deep suppression are unlikely to suppress when the dominant eye has a dim image and the nondominant eye has a bright one. Differential brightness of the targets for each eye may be

TABLE 12-1. *Antisuppression Variables*

- Attention to target
- Brightness of target
- Contrast of target
- Color of target
- Size of target
- Flashing of target
- Movement of target
- Tactile and kinesthetic effects on suppression
- Auditory effects on suppression

created either by raising and lowering the luminance of the targets or by using graded (attenuating) filters before the eyes. Instruments such as the Synoptophore have rheostats for this purpose. Home training and simple office devices can accomplish this by direct illumination from a penlight or desk lamp to the target of the nondominant eye. Background room illumination can also be lowered so that the dominant eye has a dimly illuminated target. Figure 12-1 shows how this principle is applied to an instrument such as the Aperture Rule Trainer. The dominant eye can view the target in low illumination while the suppressed target can be illuminated with a penlight.

Target Contrast

Contrast between figure and ground is a factor in the treatment of suppression. If the contrast is high, there is less likelihood of suppression. The suppressing eye should be presented with a high-contrast target. This is one of the reasons why suppression is more likely under natural seeing conditions, since figure-ground contrast is relatively low. On the other hand, simplified targets in a major amblyoscope with high contrast are less likely to be suppressed. For practical purposes with home training devices, a neutral gray overlay can be placed over the target of the dominant eye to reduce its brightness. The contrast may also appear to be diminished, as when a dark gray target is on a light gray background. This penalization of the dominant eye, as to brightness and contrast, helps break suppression of the nondominant eye.

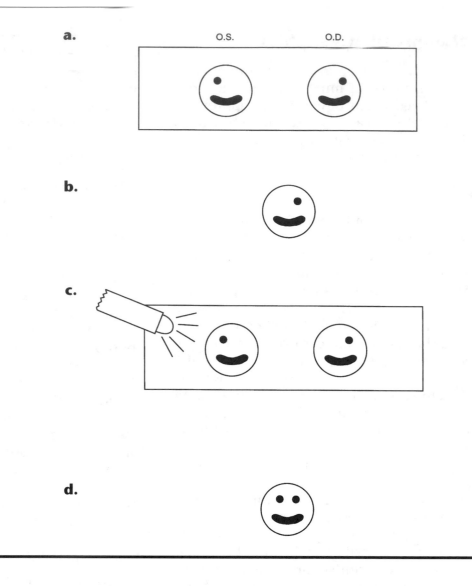

FIGURE 12-1—Example of the use of target brightness to break suppression of the left eye: (a) Actual target; (b) Patient's perception; (c) Target of the left eye is illuminated with a penlight; (d) Patient's perception when suppression is broken. Note that the room illumination is lower so that the dominant eye sees a target with low lluminance.

Color

Generally, colored targets hold the patient's attention better than black and white ones. Targets are usually colored for both eyes, but it may be helpful to use a black and white target for the nonsuppressing eye, and one that is colored for the suppressing eye. This is particularly applicable to first-degree targets such as shown in Figure 12-2. The circle can be brightly colored with the X being black.

Target Size

Target size and the size of suppression controls should be tailored to the size of the patient's suppression zone in a particular instrument. Refer to Table 5-1 for zone classification and dimensions. The choice of appropriate target size usually proceeds on a trial-and-error basis. Also, the distance of a target from the patient determines its size according to the inverse square relationship. A target size or distance is chosen so that the patient can hold the suppression controls in perception most of the time (about 80%) but not all the time. If the patient is successful all the time, the target has little training value. Similarly, if a control is suppressed most of the time, the task may be too demanding, thereby frustrating the patient.

In cases of strabismus with deep suppression, large superimposition targets (first-degree targets) are initially presented in an amblyoscope (see Figure 12-2). Smaller targets are gradually introduced as the suppression zone shrinks as the result of therapy. Rapid progress often occurs at first, since it is much easier to treat peripheral rather than central suppression. Progress becomes slower as the fovea is approached. Flat fusion (second-degree) and stereopsis targets are introduced later as suppression is broken to build both sensory and motor fusion skills.

In cases of heterophoria, foveal-sized suppression controls should be selected. As fusional vergence ranges are stressed as part of motor fusion training, end-point suppression needs to be detected and broken. The goal is to develop normal, or above normal, ranges of fusional convergence and divergence that are free of foveal suppression.

Intermittent Stimuli

Flashing a target or an eye is very effective in breaking down suppression. The visual system responds vigorously to any rapidly changing stimulus.[2,3] A flashing stimulus is difficult to suppress. Jampolsky[4] suggested there is a latency period needed for suppression and a flashing pattern interferes with this period. One of the most powerful methods is flashing one or both targets using the automatic flashing unit on a major amblyoscope. Some deeply suppressing strabismic patients require this level of intervention. Clinicians may prefer unilateral flashing of the suppressed target to elicit its perception. Others prefer alternate flashing to force the suppressing eye to see the controls when the dominant eye is occluded. Both types of flashing should be tried to discover which is more effective in a particular case. We often use rapid automatic flashing in the amblyoscope, which seems to work well in most cases. At home, in case of deep strabismic suppression, a circuit breaker can be put in the socket of a desk lamp, transforming it into an automatic flashing unit. The light from the flashing desk lamp can then be directed onto the suppressed field in a mirror stereoscope, set up with fusion targets at the patient's objective angle of deviation. The patient is asked to make a conscious effort to hold all the suppression controls in perception once they are seen.

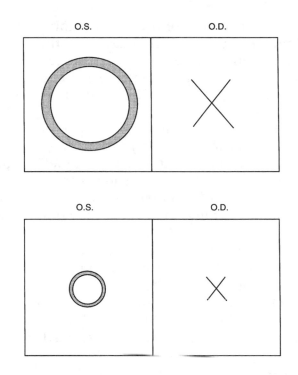

FIGURE 12-2—Example of size change of superimposition targets in antisuppression training.

Flashing can be easily done in free space (open environment) in several ways. The therapist or patient can quickly cover and uncover an eye with a paddle occluder. This popular technique for breaking suppression can be applied to many training instruments if there are suppression controls in the field. Another method is simply asking the patient to blink one or both eyes when suppression occurs. This also helps to enliven a suppressed image if it is not carried on for a long time, resulting in visual fatigue. A penlight flashing technique can be applied with free space instruments (Figure 12-1c). These three techniques are the most frequently used methods for breaking suppression and establishing sensory fusion both in the office and at home.

Target Movement

Movement of the suppressing eye's target is effective for several reasons. One is that noncorresponding points are being stimulated by the oscillation of the target. These points are less likely to be suppressed than corresponding points. Movement of the target before one eye stimulates new retinal areas and the visual system generally responds to change. Also, a moving target is apt to draw the patient's attention, tending to keep the target from being suppressed.

Movement of one target under binocular conditions can be done in various ways. In the office, the major amblyoscope is ideal. Some models have an oscillator switch; others require back and forth movement of the carriage arm. For home training, the patient may hold a mirror that is angled before one eye in such a way that he can superimpose two different objects in the room. Getz[5] suggested that a television can be used for one eye, while the other eye sees an object in the room through the mirror. Jiggling the mirror can create the desired target movement. (This technique will be discussed later.)

Tactile and Kinesthetic Senses

Tactile and kinesthetic stimulation can be used for antisuppression purposes. In many instruments, such as a Mirror Stereoscope, the therapist can ask the patient to touch each eye's suppression control simultaneously with pointer sticks. The physical act of touching can break through a suppression response at least temporarily. The pointers also become suppression controls when introduced into the field of view. Cheiroscopic drawing is another well-known procedure utilizing the tactile and kinesthetic senses (Figure 12-3).

Auditory Sense

Auditory stimulation can be helpful, and it is an effective way to hold the patient's attention. Therapy time may be reduced when auditory feedback devices are incorporated in the training program. Instruments such as the Perceptual-Motor Pen (discussed in Chapter 10) can be used in conjunction with anaglyphic red-green filters to monitor suppression while the sound of the buzzer alerts the patient when tracing is inaccurate. Home training using auditory clues can be done during cheiroscopic drawing by tapping the pencil tip to make a noise. The patient can tap the pencil to create attention to the tip. Attending to the pencil tip tends to prevent its being suppressed. Involvement of

the tactile/kinesthetic and auditory senses helps break suppression more quickly than if the patient merely looks at stereograms without pointing. The patient soon becomes aware of the relation between motor performance and suppression; this feedback enhances awareness of sensory fusion.

Combinations

More than one variable in antisuppression training is usually utilized in any particular therapeutic procedure. The effectiveness of a procedure generally increases when several antisuppression variables are included. With the cheiroscope, for instance, the therapist can design the procedure to include colored pencils, pencil movement, having the patient blink the suppressing eye (intermittent stimuli), and tapping the pencil tip for auditory stimulation. The therapist should keep in mind these antisuppression variables and apply the appropriate ones for a particular instrument or procedure. On the other hand, the therapist should not add so many variables to confuse the patient in a particular antisuppression activity.

Four-step Approach to Antisuppression Training

The following four-step method represents a general approach to antisuppression training that can be applied using any specific instrument (Table 12-2).

Step One

The first step is to design the appropriate training environment for the patient's level of suppression. The antisuppression variables listed in Table 12-1 are used for this purpose. If suppression is deep, the initial training environment should be relatively unnatural, e.g., use of an alpha rhythm flasher (TBI), major amblyoscope, and red-green television trainer. If the suppression is shallow, a relatively natural training environment is appropriate, e.g., using Vectograms, Brock string, and Pola-Mirror. Working with a specific instrument, stimulus and target parameters are chosen that allow the patient to succeed at the antisuppression task about 70% to 80% of the time. The appropriate variables are found

a.

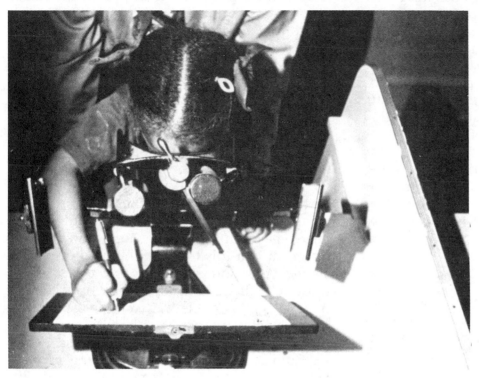

b.

FIGURE 12-3—(a) Cheiroscopic Tracing: an example of tracing while the tactile and kinesthetic senses aid antisuppression therapy; (b) A commercially available instrument suitable for home training is the Bernell Single Oblique Stereoscope. (Photo courtesy of Bernell Corp.)

TABLE 12-2. *Four-step Approach To Antisuppression Training*

1. Design an appropriate training environment. Select the instrument, targets, and stimulus conditions. The patient should not suppress more than 30% of the time in a particular environment.
2. Stimulate perception of the suppressed targets or controls. Common stimuli: flashing targets, blinking, target movement, pointing and touching.
3. Motivate the patient to exert "mental effort." Set time goals for suppression-free sensory fusion, e.g., 1 minute under specific stimulus and target conditions.
4. Increase the sensory and motor fusion demand. Progress to smaller suppression controls and higher vergence demands. Prisms and lenses can be used to extend the training range of a particular environment. The process is repeated with more challenging instruments or environmental conditions until normal fusional vergence ranges are developed and free of foveal suppression.

empirically by trial and error. The training task should neither be too easy to accomplish nor too difficult for the patient.

Step Two

This step is to stimulate perception of the suppressed image. When suppression does occur, an antisuppression stimulus is applied to break down the suppression response and enliven the suppressed image or control. Flashing a target (intermittent light stimulation) is the most commonly used stimulus. Other important antisuppression stimuli are blinking, movement of a target, and pointing or touching. The type and strength of the stimulus must be appropriate for the depth and extent of suppression; simultaneous perception of all targets or suppression controls in the binocular visual field is the goal.

Step Three

In this step, the patient is encouraged to make a "mental effort" to hold the targets or suppression controls in perception for a specified length of time. For example, the patient is asked to count aloud slowly as long as both images are seen at the same time. When suppression occurs, counting is stopped. Counting aloud provides convenient performance feedback to both therapist and patient. Each number is spoken at the rate of approximately 1 digit per second. The initial goal may be to reach the count of 10. When that is achieved consistently, a higher number is chosen. A practical goal is for the patient to avoid suppression for at least 1 minute under a particular set of training conditions. When accomplished, more challenging training conditions are given and the process is continued, e.g., flashing of the target is discontinued or brightness is diminished.

Step Four

The last step is to increase the sensory and motor fusion demand. Antisuppression therapy also involves building the quality and quantity of sensory and motor fusion. This is done by changing the target parameters listed in Table 12-1 and varying the stimulus to accommodation and vergence. For example, smaller targets or controls are introduced with the goal of using foveal-sized ones in the final stages of therapy. Loose prisms and accommodative flipper lenses can be included to increase the motor fusion demand of antisuppression tasks. The training goal is for the patient to achieve sufficient fusional vergence ranges without foveal suppression.

As the limits of sensory and motor fusion development are reached with a particular instrument or environmental condition, a more demanding instrument or environment is chosen for the patient. The progression is also toward more natural viewing conditions. With each new procedure, the training process is repeated (steps 1 through 4) until the patient has eliminated suppression under all environmental conditions and instruments, including the open environment.

SPECIFIC ANTISUPPRESSION TECHNIQUES

Most vision therapy instruments and targets contain suppression controls since suppression is an omnipresent consideration in binocular vision remediation. For purposes of this discussion, we have selected only those procedures we have found to be the most effective and practical in a direct assault on pathological suppression. A list of ten specific antisuppression techniques is presented in Table 12-3. These techniques are loosely sequenced from those appropriate for deep peripheral suppression to those for shallow foveal suppression. This sequence is based on our experience with patients.

Extreme unnatural visual conditions are necessary when attempting to break deep suppression. The suppressing eye is bombarded with relatively bright, large, flashing, and moving targets or controls to break the suppression response. As suppression is broken, the clinician must be vigilant to ensure that sensory fusion occurs, or is possible, rather than generating unresolvable diplopia. The clinician should ensure that normal retinal correspondence is present and that normal sensory fusion is possible before these techniques can be efficaciously applied. If, during the course of therapy, sensory fusion is discovered to be an unrealistic objective (e.g., in cases of horror fusionis, large aniseikonia, lack of fusion potential), antisuppression therapy should be stopped immediately before intractable diplopia is the result.

Translid Binocular Interaction Trainer T12.1

Allen introduced the Translid Binocular Interaction Trainer (TBI), that provides strong inter-

---

TABLE 12-3.	Antisuppression Techniques
T12.1	Translid Binocular Interaction Trainer
T12.2	Major Amblyoscope
T12.3	Penlight and Filters
T12.4	Hand Mirror Superimposition
T12.5	Cheiroscopic Games
T12.6	Modified Remy Separator
T12.7	Brock String and Beads
T12.8	Television Trainers
T12.9	Pola-Mirror
T12.10	Reading Bars

mittent photic stimulation.[6,7] The battery powered instrument consists of a pair of small transparent lightbulbs that are alternately flashed for each eye. This is done by a free-running multivibrator at a rate of approximately 7 to 10 hertz, which approximates the alpha rhythm. The bulbs are separated by a distance equal to the patient's IPD; they are gently placed against the closed upper eyelids so that they barely touch (Figure 12-4a). Ideally, a protective shield should be placed between the exposed bulb and the eyelid to prevent the possibility of the bulb breaking and causing eye injury. The lights flash alternately so that impulses arrive at the visual cortex asynchronously. Each pulse has a duration of approximately 1/40th second. This rate of alternate flashing is thought to make suppression impossible. Flashing continues for a 10 minute period as the patient experiences

pulsating light patterns seen through the lids. This procedure seems effective in preparing the patient to break through a suppression response on other instruments, with the eyes open (Figure 12-4b). Physiological diplopia training (Figure 12-4c) and chiastopic fusion training (Figure 12-4d) can also be done. We recommend such flashing lightbulbs that can attach to spectacle frames or to instrument fusion targets. Such flashing provides a strong anti-suppression stimulus that can be utilized for home training purposes. Using tape or clips, the therapist attaches a light over each fusion target, e.g., in a Brewster stereoscope, Mirror Stereoscope, or Aperture Rule Trainer.

The TBI and other rhythmic flashing units should not be used with patients having a history of epileptic seizures. Grand mal or petit mal seizures may occur in a small portion of the

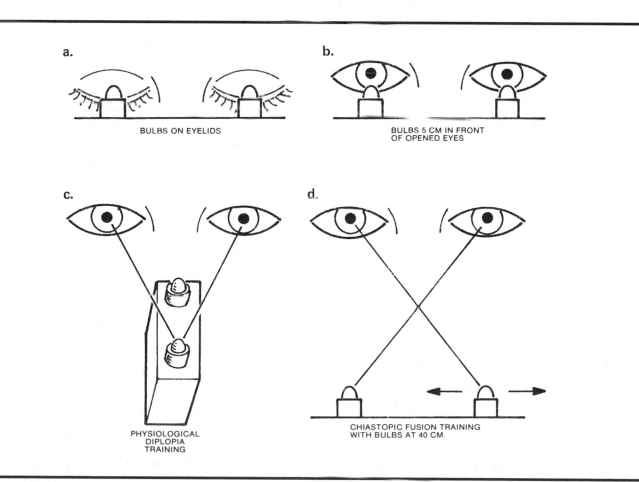

a.

BULBS ON EYELIDS

b.

BULBS 5 CM IN FRONT
OF OPENED EYES

c.

PHYSIOLOGICAL
DIPLOPIA
TRAINING

d.

CHIASTOPIC FUSION TRAINING
WITH BULBS AT 40 CM.

FIGURE 12-4—Translid Binocular Interaction Trainer for alternate flashing at the alpha rhythm: (a) Light source placed directly on eyelid; (b) Lights flashing in front of opened eyes; (c) Physiological diplopia training; (d) Chiastopic fusion training with variable vergence demands produced by changing target separation distance.

population when viewing a flashing light source. Closing the eyes and having the light go through the lids, however, supposedly reduces the likelihood of this type of reaction. Because of the possibility of seizures, treatment time should always be short, and made even shorter or discontinued if there is any sign of discomfort. The doctor should not prescribe TBI therapy for home use until there is certainty as to the patient's reactions to the TBI and complete understanding of its proper use.

Major Amblyoscope T12.2

In many ways, the modern major amblyoscope is an ideal instrument to break down pathological suppression associated with strabismus and amblyopia. The intensity of illumination can be varied over a large range. An automatic flashing unit provides many options in the rate, periodicity, and type of flashing. Some instruments come with Stanworth mirrors that allow targets to be projected into the open environment, thereby aiding the transfer of learned visual skills from instruments to natural seeing conditions. Also, hundreds of slides of various sizes and parameters are available that are appropriate for patients of all ages.

Illumination Gradient and Flashing

In cases of deep extensive suppression, large targets and suppression controls are selected. A bug target is a good example (see Figure 5-7). With these second-degree fusion targets aligned at the objective angle of deviation in the amblyoscope, illumination is increased for the suppressing eye and decreased in the dominant eye until the patient can see all four wings simultaneously most of the time (about 70% to 80%). Manual or automatic flashing or target movement is used to break the suppression response when it occurs. The patient makes a "mental effort" to hold the controls in perception with sensory fusion as long as possible or meet a specific goal, e.g., 1 minute. As the patient makes progress, the illumination gradient between the two eyes is reduced. Flashing is also used sparingly. The bug target also has foveal-sized suppression controls on its body. As peripheral

suppression is eliminated, a smooth transition can be made to central fusion training using the small dots to control for foveal suppression.

Chasing

Another variation of antisuppression training using the major amblyoscope is chasing, a break-and-join task. The procedure stimulates both sensory and motor fusion. A second-degree target is set at the objective angle and the illumination is adjusted to create the optimum training environment to minimize suppression. Rather than flashing when suppression occurs, the therapist moves a carriage arm of the amblyoscope to a new vergence setting, either BI or BO. This breaks sensory fusion and creates diplopia when one of the targets is moved out of the suppression zone. The patient then slowly moves the other arm of the amblyoscope to join the two images. "Mental effort" is encouraged to hold simultaneous perception of the two images when diplopic and again when they are joined into a single fused image with all suppression controls present. As soon as suppression is again reported, the therapist moves the arm to a new vergence setting. This process continues until the patient no longer experiences suppression when the images are fused. At this point, stimulus conditions are changed or new more demanding second-degree targets are selected. The therapist should note that the patient may report sensory fusion before he moves the amblyoscope arm an equal amount compared with the vergence stimulus introduced by the therapist. This discrepancy is desired since it suggests that the patient is making fusional vergence eye movements to gain sensory fusion. As before, central fusion targets and suppression controls are used as peripheral suppression decreases.

End-point Suppression

After suppression at the objective angle has been eliminated, suppression-free fusional ranges, both BI and BO, should be increased maximally. End-point suppression can be broken by very rapid flashing of the suppressing eye so as not to break sensory fusion. Also, slight movements of the target can be introduced by oscillation or by simply jiggling the amblyoscope arm. When the suppression control reappears, the vergence demand is further increased as the patient tries to keep the controls in view.

Penlight and Filters T12.3

A powerful and convenient in-office technique for establishing simultaneous perception (pathological diplopia) with a strabismic patient involves the use of a penlight and anaglyphic filters. The patient, wearing red-green filters, views a bright penlight held by the therapist in a dark room. Working at a close distance from the patient, the therapist moves and flashes the light in an attempt to elicit a diplopic response. The patient can blink or rapidly cover and uncover an eye. If necessary, a vertical prism can be held by the patient in front of the suppressing eye to move the image outside the suppression zone. The prism itself can also be rotated to add another dimension of movement. When diplopic images are seen, the patient exerts "mental effort" to maintain both images as the therapist backs away across the room. In this way, both brightness and image size are reduced. Background illumination can be raised to reduce contrast as training proceeds. Other variations of this technique are listed in Table 12-4. The end-point is to establish diplopia for lights and objects in a normal environment simply by the patient's visual attention.

An effective variation of this technique is to add a prism equal in amount to the patient's objective angle of deviation. Initially the prism is held vertically before the suppressing eye to stimulate diplopia. When the double images are seen, the prism is slowly rotated so the images are joined, i.e., base-out for esotropes and base-in for exotropes. The nondominant image should appear to move diagonally toward the dominant one, assuming NRC. As the moving image approaches the suppression zone, suppression may occur. When this happens, the patient blinks and the prism is jiggled to reestablish diplopia. The process continues until the two images are joined into one and color fusion occurs. The prism should be horizontal (if there is no vertical deviation) when this happens and the patient

TABLE 12-4. *Variations on Antisuppression Training with a Penlight and Filters (T 12.3)*
1. Penlight fixation with patient wearing red and green filters, in darkened room, and intermittent, rapid occlusion of deviating eye
2. Same, but with red lens over fixating eye (no green lens)
3. Same, but with red lens over deviating eye
4. Same, but without intermittent occlusion
5. Same, but with pink lens over fixating eye
6. Same, but with pink lens over deviating eye
7. Same, but with no lens over either eye
8. Repeat procedures 1 through 7, but with normal room illumination
9. Fixation of ordinary object in room while deviating eye is intermittently and rapidly occluded or blinked
10. Same, but without intermittent occlusion or blinking of the deviating eye

has second-degree sensory fusion. This procedure might be described as "macular massage" to break suppression. Background illumination can be slowly raised as the patient practices this technique working toward a natural visual environment. At some point, the filters are removed and the process repeated. The prism amount can also be reduced in small increments, 1 or 2 prism diopter steps. This modification requires the patient to supply the necessary fusional vergence to join the diplopic images when they reach the horizontal meridian. With this technique, diplopia training can be transformed into a sensory and motor fusion training method.

Hand-Mirror Superimposition T12.4

This excellent open-environment mirror training technique, described by Getz,[5] is particularly appropriate for deep extensive suppression. All the antisuppression variables listed in Table 12-1 can be applied and it is practical for use as a home training procedure. Assume a patient has deep suppression of a strabismic left eye. A handheld mirror can be aligned before the left eye at the bridge of the nose to view a bright desk lamp. The right eye observes an-

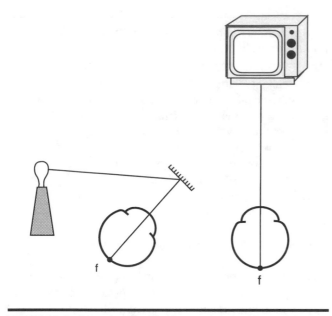

FIGURE 12-5—Example of hand-mirror superimposition training.

other stimulating target, e.g., a television (Figure 12-5). The patient can consciously attend to the television program during this procedure, which makes it a popular technique. The training task is to hold the lamp and television in simultaneous perception and superimposition as long as possible. The mirror can be angled so the image of the lamp is seen in the same direction as the television to promote bifoveal stimulation. Retinal rivalry may be seen if the different contours of the targets overlap, which is expected when differing images are superimposed. The images can be made brighter by moving closer and reducing the background illumination. When suppression occurs, the patient blinks and moves the mirror slightly to stimulate its perception. Conditions can be altered to make the task more difficult as progress is made by increasing background illumination and target distances and selecting less stimulating targets (e.g., vases and door knobs). This technique effectively stimulates superimposition (first-degree fusion), but once that is achieved, it is important move on quickly to other techniques that build higher degrees of sensory fusion.

Cheiroscopic Games T12.5

The cheiroscope is a binocular vision training instrument, a closed nearpoint space, in which the two fields are separated by a diagonal mirror (see Figure 12-3). The Mirror Stereoscope/Cheiroscope from Bernell Corporation is available for this purpose, as is the single oblique mirror stereoscope (SOMS) Trainer. In most training situations, the dominant eye fixates a target field through the mirror while the suppressing eye directly views the other field. Lenses in some instruments place the target fields at optical infinity, but this is usually unnecessary unless there is a large esotropia. To help break suppression in one field, a desk lamp light can be directed onto that field. Many other targets and stimulus variables are also available in the cheiroscopic training environment to make cheiroscopic games interesting and effective. Children usually enjoy this vision training technique.

Counting

This simultaneous perception technique requires the patient to hold the perception of various objects in the two fields at the same time. The type of objects, real and drawn, is limited only by the therapist's imagination and the patient's interests. Targets can be glued to paper, drawn, or held in place. At first the objects are counted: such as pennies, small seashells, or grains of sand. If successful, the therapist asks the patient to retain the images as long as possible as the patient counts out loud in a consistent manner. Suppression is represented by silence. Blinking, flashing, increased light, and movement activate the suppressed image, and counting can continue. An agreed on goal of the number of objects and time is set, achieved, and a new goal chosen. Counting can certainly be challenging and fun.

Coloring and Drawing

This variation is a fill-in task. A suitable line drawing at the patient's level of suppression serves to capture interest. The patient uses colored pencils or crayons clued to the suppressing eye to color the drawings. This first-degree fusion task requires that the patient only fill-in within the perceived lines and not draw the contours of the target. Coloring will be done at the subjective angle of directionalization; therefore, it should appear in the same direction as the target of regard. The therapist needs to emphasize clarity of the target to control accommodation. Otherwise, the coloring seems to be moving because of the effect of variable accommodative convergence. The crayon tip and the colored portion will tend to be suppressed since they are clued to the nondominant eye. When suppression occurs, the crayon is jiggled to activate perception of that image. The patient is instructed not to color the target unless the contours and the crayon tip are seen at precisely the same time. As the patient exhibits less suppression, the target contours are made smaller and the selected crayon color should be less vivid, e.g., yellow or gray instead of red or green. When a drawing is completed the patient should attempt to maintain the target and colored area in continuous perception for at least 1 minute. Slight displacements of the two images are acceptable since there is no true sensory fusion of the dissimilar images.

A cheiroscopic drawing variation is the circle and X technique. The therapist quickly draws circles on a paper in the dominant eye's field as the patient attempts to place an X in each in his suppressing field. The therapist's speed is governed by experience with the patient. The circle sizes are varied for the sake of challenge. At the end of this speed task, the patient attempts to hold both targets and drawings in perception for 1 minute before suppression occurs. Blinking, flashing, and intensity are variables readily available for antisuppression purposes.

Point-to-Point Chasing

Vodnoy[8] reported a chasing technique that can be easily done on the cheiroscope. A pointer or pencil held by the therapist is slowly moved in the dominant eye's field. The patient holds a pointer or pencil on the baseboard and positions the tip to superimpose it with the tip of the therapist's target. The patient attempts to keep the tips superimposed as the therapist's target is moved at increasingly faster rates. The therapist gauges the rate based on performance. The patient reports when suppression occurs. Antisuppression variables are used as necessary, e.g., blinking, flashing, and illumination differential. Point-to-point chasing requires active

participation and usually captures a patient's interest (including adults).

Tracing

Cheiroscopic tracings can be an excellent antisuppression exercise, both in and out of the office. Simple cartoons or drawings are initially used as targets for the dominant eye. More complex designs can be included as the patient masters this procedure. The nondominant eye views a blank white sheet of paper and a pencil that is held by the patient. The patient attempts to trace the design seen in the mirror with the instructions to draw only when the lines and the pencil tip are seen at exactly the same time. The pencil tip and the line need to be viewed simultaneously without alternate suppression or memory of the position. When the pencil tip disappears, the patient shakes it to break the suppression and then continues the tracing. If the line disappears, illumination is increased for that eye. Blinking is usually helpful. As the patient succeeds in breaking suppression, the therapist selects targets with more detail and finer lines. Parents can find cartoons or comic strips of interest to their child and mount these as targets for cheiroscopic tracing at home.

Cheiroscopic games can be done with either Brewster or Wheatstone stereoscopes. The factors of attention, brightness, target size, intermittent stimuli, target movement, contrast, and color can all be applied to break suppression. Many stereoscopes have the additional benefit of allowing binocular pointing (tactile-kinesthetic sense) as an antisuppression method. The fused target is seen with the two pointers converging to the fixated portion (Figure 12-6).

Modified Remy Separator T12.6

The Remy separator can be used for antisuppression therapy.[9] This simple device consists of a handheld septum dividing two targets set at a nearpoint distance. The septum can be made for home training by using a rigid material such as a file folder placed in the midsagittal plane in front of the patient's nose (see Figures 13-15 and 13-16 illustrating the Remy Separator). In cases of strabismus, two dissimilar objects or

a.

b.

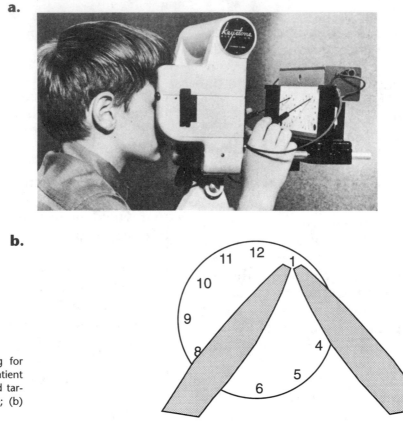

FIGURE 12-6—Double pointing for antisuppression training: (a) Patient pointing to homologously fused targets in a Brewster stereoscope; (b) Patient's perception.

drawings can be initially placed on either side of the septum. The patient attempts to fixate the two targets alternately at a regular rhythm without suppression. The use of prism neutralization is usually necessary in cases of strabismus so that superimposition can be achieved. The training goal is stable superimposition of the two images for at least 1 minute duration. Antisuppression stimuli applicable to this training environment are target size, color, differential illumination, blinking, flashing, and pointing. When the patient can binocularly perceive foveal targets the size of small dots, the technique has reached its limits of first-degree fusion. Second- and third-degree targets can then be attempted. (Refer to Chapter 13 for further discussion.)

Brock String and Beads T12.7

A popular physiological diplopia training technique is Brock string and beads. This anti-suppression technique works well with patients having intermittent strabismus, anisometropic amblyopia, or heterophoria. The patient holds one end of a 3-meter string to the tip of his nose with the other end tied to a distant object such as a doorknob (Figure 12-7). Directing visual attention, the patient should be able to see two strings apparently intersecting wherever the horizontal components of the visual axes meet (Figure 12-8a). Seeing only one string or a portion of one missing, indicates pathological suppression (Figure 12-8b). Three brightly colored beads on the string usually serve as fixation targets. When one bead is fixated and seen as single, the other two beads should appear to be diplopic. A double image of the string should also appear to intersect at the fixated bead. This represents the proper physiological diplopic percept. Patients with binocular anomalies, of course, may not see this correct image. Suppression is indicated when only one image of the nonfixated beads or only one string is totally

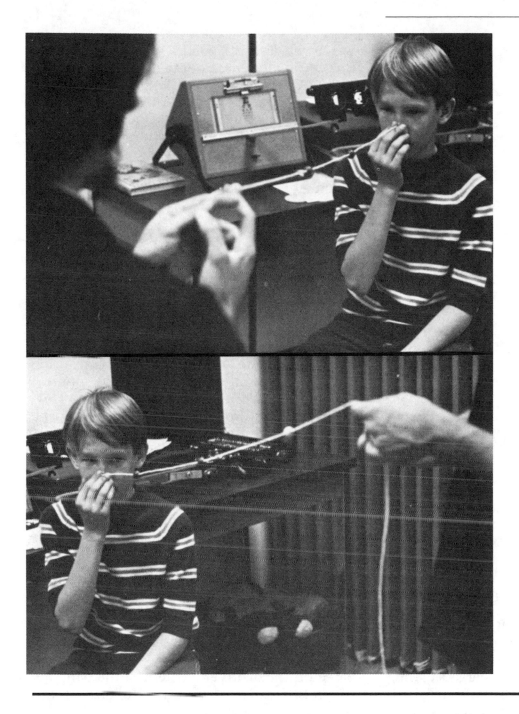

FIGURE 12-7—Brock string and beads: (a) Training in the primary position of gaze; (b) training in a secondary position of gaze.

seen. An inadequate vergence response is indicated when a double image of the fixated bead appears or the string intersects either in front of or behind that bead. Antisuppression stimuli for the string and beads include blinking, flashing, movement of the string (jiggling), and increasing illumination. A particularly strong stimulus is to place a penlight by the suppressed bead and flash it as the patient makes a "mental effort" to see physiological diplopia under these conditions. The patient can also wear red-green filters to introduce color contrast to break suppression. One image of the string should appear red and the other green. Inadequate vergence responses can be neutralized with loose prisms or a prism bar. Sufficient prism is used to join the double image of the fixated bead into one as the technique requires.

String and beads are a simple and versatile antisuppression technique suitable for home

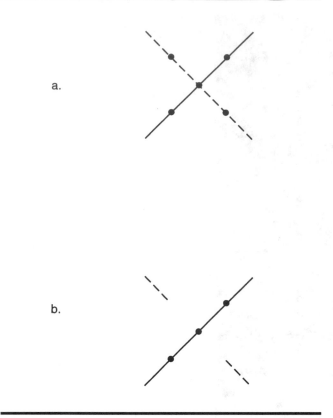

a.

b.

FIGURE 12-8—Patient's perception of Brock string: (a) Middle bead is bifixated with images of string intersection it. Nearest bead is seen with heteronymous diplopia (bead on dashed line seen only by the left eye). Farthest bead is seen with homonymous diplopia (bead on dashed line seen only by the left eye and on the left side). (b) Central suppression of the left eye (portion of dashed line missing).

training. Several vergence and oculomotor techniques can be done using the string and beads as a free-space control for suppression. The patient can make near-far jump vergence movements from one bead to the next. Prisms can be introduced for step vergences. The patient can also build up gross convergence using the tromboning method while holding physiologic diplopia of the nonfixated targets as the fixated bead is moved closer. Rotations can also be conveniently done. A major drawback of Brock string and beads, however, is that some patients quickly become bored. Children often have difficulty training with string and beads for more than 1 or 2 weeks. The therapist should remember that physiological diplopia training does not need to be confined to the string and beads. A physiological diplopia control for suppression can be introduced with many other methods. For example, a child can

watch television or read a comic book while holding a pointer stick or pencil in front of the target. A double image of the pointer or pencil would indicate physiological diplopia. When suppression occurs during the activity, the patient should blink or shake the pointer to activate the diplopic image. As one might expect, this variation of physiologic diplopia training is much more popular than string and beads with some patients.

Television Trainers T12.8

Most patients can find at least 30 minutes in their day when they can watch television. Since training compliance is usually not a problem, the TV trainer can be an effective antisuppression method of home use. The technique may be inappropriate, however, for patients with constant strabismus or deep extensive suppression, unless the strabismic patient wears a Fresnel prism equal to the deviation. The patient should be able to have fusion of a television screen at some distance before this technique can be used. Suppressing patients who have intermittent strabismus, anisometropic amblyopia, and heterophoria are generally good candidates for this technique.

Television trainers are available in red-green and polarized materials (Figure 12-9). The red-green models work better with young children who tend to tilt their head and in patients with deep suppression. In contrast, polarized models are more appropriate for adults and patients with shallow suppression. TV trainers usually come in large and small sizes. Selection can be based on the depth and extent of the patient's suppression and, necessarily, the size of the patient's TV screen.

The TV trainer is attached to the television screen vertically with suction cups. The appropriate filters are worn by the patient over spectacle or contact lenses, if recommended. The therapist or patient should alternately occlude each eye to make sure each filter mutually excludes part of the television screen. The patient moves as close to the screen as necessary to a position where the images can be seen without suppression. The patient should then slowly step back from the screen until a viewing dis-

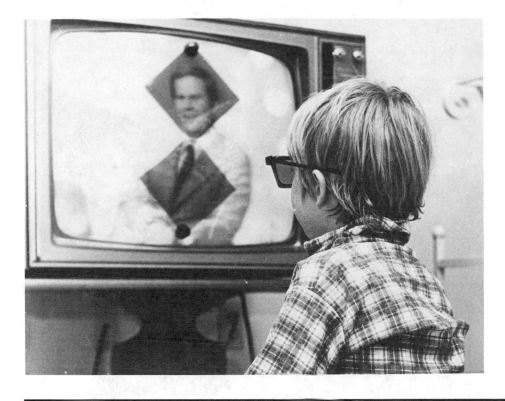

FIGURE 12-9 Television trainer to treat suppression.

tance is found at which there is either unilateral or alternate suppression about 20% to 30% of the time. That position is the correct training distance for the patient. If the patient suppresses more than 30% of the time, the viewing distance may be too far or the trainer unit too small.

Once the proper training distance is established, the task is for the patient to watch a 30-minute program while breaking suppression every time it occurs. Suppression is indicated when one portion of the trainer darkens to obscure that part of the TV screen. Antisuppression variables that are readily applicable are blinking, rapidly flashing an eye (cover-uncover), moving toward the screen, and increasing contrast by dimming the background room lights. As suppression is overcome at a near distance, the patient should take a step back from the TV until suppression is seen again, and then continue the training process. The patient should always exert visual attention to avoid suppression while watching a TV program. This procedure can be mentally exhausting and frequent rest periods are advised.

When the procedure is mastered, prisms can be used to introduce vergence demands. The TV trainer in this case serves as a suppression control for end-point suppression.

Pola-Mirror T12.9

The Pola-Mirror[10,11] can be used for vision training in heterophoric patients with central suppression. Wearing polarized filters, the patient fixates an image of his face in a mirror. Each eye can see only an image of its eye. Both eyes are visible under binocular viewing conditions if there is no foveal suppression. The filter before a suppressing eye appears darkened, obscuring the image of that eye. The technique is for the patient to get close enough to the mirror so that both eyes can be seen (Figure 12-10). The patient then moves the mirror away and tries to keep seeing with both eyes. Blinking, moving the head, and increasing illumination are effective ways to break suppression when it occurs. The procedure is repeated with the patient trying to increase the fixation distance each time. A realistic goal is for the patient to see both eyes

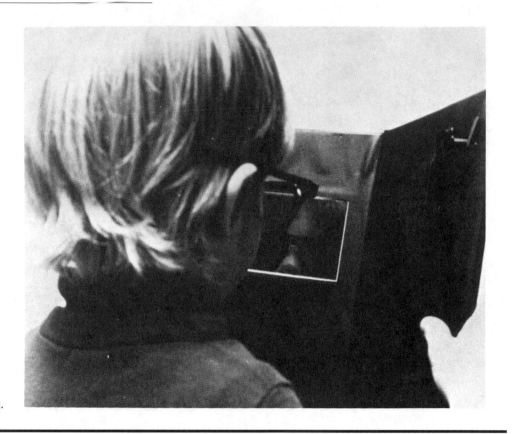

FIGURE 12-10—Pola-Mirror training.

at a distance of about 75 cm from the mirror, a total of 1.5 meters when looking in the mirror.

Reading Bars T12.10

Reading bars have been a popular antisuppression method even in the time of Javal.[12] The patient can concentrate on any reading material he chooses while working to break central suppression. This home training technique does require sufficient motor fusion at the reading distance before it can be used effectively. Reading bars, placed directly on the printed page, are available in polarized and red-green filter materials. Strips of filter material are interspaced on transparent plastic and alternately clued to the eyes (see Figure 10-21). The patient wears the appropriate filters over any needed refractive correction. Suppression will be recognized by the patient when a filter strip appears dark, decreasing the visibility of print beneath it. The patient's task is to read across lines of print or look at pictures (for young children) free of suppression for a certain length of time. Often 10 minutes is required as a training inter-

val. Suppression can be broken by blinking, flashing an eye by occlusion, moving toward the book, or increasing illumination. As suppression is overcome, the book and reading bar can be held farther away from the patient to work on foveal suppression. When suppression is broken at the ortho position, flipper lenses and prisms are often assigned to expand accommodative and vergence skills while monitoring for end-point suppression. Also see T10.23 in Chapter 10 on amblyopia therapy for further discussion on training with a reading bars.

MANAGEMENT CONSIDERATIONS

Antisuppression training also has the effect of building sensory and motor fusion. As suppression diminishes, stereopsis and motor fusional ranges usually increase. Antisuppression training naturally evolves into sensory and motor fusion training. When the emphasis changes to the training of fusional vergence ranges, motor training is temporarily stopped if end-point suppression is found; the suppression should be broken before continuing. Therefore, antisuppression, sensory fusion, and motor fusion training consists of a reciprocally interwoven process. Antisuppression training builds sensory and motor fusion, conversely, establishing good sensory and motor fusion prevents the reoccurrence of suppression.

Suppression is deepest in cases of strabismus with normal retinal correspondence since it is the only antidiplopic mechanism available. Because the strength of the antisuppression stimulus must match or exceed the depth and extent of the suppression zone, in-office procedures that are unnatural such as the TBI (T12.1) and amblyoscope training (T12.2) are appropriate and necessary during the first phase of vision training. Effective home training techniques include red filters (T12.3) and hand mirror superimposition (T12.4). Progression of targets is from peripheral to macular to foveal sizes with each technique. At some point in the training, many patients begin to alternate suppression, particularly with foveal-sized targets. Central suppression controls in each eye's field of view are, therefore, necessary.

Some intermittent strabismic patients show good sensory fusion when the eyes are aligned but deep suppression when an eye deviates. It is important for the patient to get visual feedback of pathological diplopia when the eye turns. The break-and-join technique using the red lens and filters (T12.3) is particularly effective in such cases. However, if the intermittent strabismus is associated with covaring ARC, the training objective should be different. In these cases, there is usually little of no suppression; diplopia may not occur even if suppression is broken because of the ARC. A better strategy is to increase the patient's fusional vergence reserves maximally to prevent loss of bifixation.

Antisuppression training is an important step in the management of amblyopia, particularly anisometropic amblyopia. Holopigian et al.[13] reported that amblyopia and suppression are often inversely related. The deeper the amblyopia, the less the suppression. Our clinical experience is not in accord with this concept. Consequently, most cases of amblyopia require antisuppression therapy. Elimination of suppression is essential to prevent

regression of amblyopia after vision therapy has been completed. In cases of anisometropic amblyopia when there is a potential for normal fusion, several antisuppression techniques are particularly effective to improve visual acuity. [Three techniques were discussed in Chapter 10 on amblyopia therapy: red filter and red print (T10.21); visual tracking with a stereoscope (T10.22); and bar reading and tracking (T10.23).] Several techniques described in this chapter are also appropriate when acuity in the amblyopic eye has been improved to 20/80 (6/24) or better. These include: cheiroscope games (T12.5); Brock string and beads (T12.7); TV trainers (T12.8); and the Pola-Mirror (T12.9).

Suppression is also a consideration in minimal binocular dysfunction cases of heterophoria, fusional vergence deficiency, and accommodative deficiency. Very small foveal suppression controls are usually necessary to identify suppression if it exists. When training is given for improved vergence ranges, foveal suppression clues should be present for each eye so that alternate suppression can be detected and broken if it occurs. Double pointing techniques are useful in these cases since they do not break motor fusion. Using red pointer sticks, the patient simultaneously touches the suppression control for each eye. This usually breaks the suppression response and vergence training can proceed (see Figure 12-6).

CASE EXAMPLE

The Problem: Trish, a 15-year-old female straight-A student, presented for an eye examination with neither symptoms nor a chief complaint.[14] She had worn the following spectacle prescription for the previous 4 years: OD: +2.50 −0.50 axis 10 (20/25−), OS: +0.50 DS (20/20). The examination revealed that she had 3 diopters of additional uncorrected axial anisometropia, intermittent central suppression, and reduced stereopsis.

Clinical Data: Pertinent clinical findings are summarized as follows: Keratometry: OD: 42.75 at 180, 44.00 at 90; OD 42.50 at 180, 43.25 at 90. Retinoscopy: OD: +6.50 −0.50 axis 180; OS

TABLE 12-5. *Trish: Results of Treatment: Full Anisometropia Spectacles and Antisuppression Training*

		Initial Exam	1 Month	2 Months	8 Months
Visual Acuity	OD:	20/25	20/25+	20/20	20/15–
	OS:	20/20	20/15–	20/15	20/15
Stereopsis Test (Fly)		200"	140"	40"	50"
Suppression		Interm. central	Interm. foveal	None	None

(Note: All data were collected with the patient wearing the full anisometropic spectacle lenses.)

+1.25 –0.25 axis 180. Turville infinity balance subjective: OD: +6.25 –0.50 axis 157 (20/25); OS +1.00 DS (20/20). These refractive data were confirmed by cycloplegic examination using 1% Cyclogyl. Cover test with subjective Rx: Orthophoria at 6 m and 5^Δ exophoria at 40 cm. Worth dot test with full spectacle correction: intermittent central suppression of the right eye at all distances. Stereo Fly Test with full correction in place: 200 seconds of arc. Internal and external ocular health was within normal limits.

Management: Although Trish was symptom free, we explained to her that her visual performance may increase if she could adapt to the full anisometropic prescription and break the central suppression. Although we thoroughly discussed the expected adaptive symptoms when correcting 5 diopters of anisometropia with spectacle lenses, the patient expressed her willingness to wear the full optical correction. Spectacle lenses were selected because the anisometropia was axial rather then refractive, judging from the K readings, and theoretically should result in relatively little aniseikonia. She was also instructed in the use of a polarized reading bar (T12.10) to break suppression and was assigned home training for 1 hour a day during her study periods for a duration of two months. No other training techniques were given.

Results: (See Table 12-5.) During the initial 3 days of wear, Trish experienced minor headaches, occasional double vision, some spatial disorientation and misjudgment of distances. Within a week all adaptation symptoms disappeared and the patient reported clearer vision and an increased sense of depth when viewing near objects. No suppression was found at the 2 month progress check. Stereopsis had improved to 40 seconds of arc, and good results persisted in later examinations. It was noted that the stereopsis improved as the suppression was eliminated. Eikonometer measurements indicated no aniseikonia. She rarely noticed diplopia in spite of the induced prismatic difference between the lenses when viewing is off the optical centers. Trish was very pleased with her increased depth perception and visual skills. We believe that the antisuppression training was an important addition to the optical correction in eliminating the obstacles to normal sensory fusion in this case. Two years later, she was fit with rigid gas permeable contract lenses and adapted well to them without aniseikonic or other symptoms.

REFERENCES

1. Revell MJ. *Strabismus: A History of Orthoptic Techniques.* London: Barrie & Jenkins; 1971:15
2. Bagolini B. Sensorial anomalies in strabismus. *Doc Ophthalmol.* 1976;41:1-22.
3. Schor CM. Visual stimuli for strabismic suppression. *Perception.* 1977;6:583-593.
4. Jampolsky A. Characteristics of suppression in strabismus. *Arch Ophthalmol.* 1955;54:683-696.
5. Getz DJ. *Strabismus and amblyopia.* Duncan, Oklahoma: Optometric Extention Program; 1974;46:series 1, number 12.

6. Allen MJ. The Bartley phenomenon and visual rehabilitation: a home training technique. *Optom Weekly*. 1966;57:21-22.

7. Allen MJ. Shock treatment for visual rehabilitation. *Opt J Rev Optom*. 1969;106:616-624.

8. Vodnoy BE. Orthoptics with the PSC Variable Prismatic Mirror Stereoscope-Cheiroscope kit with correlary techniques. *Am J Optom*. 1963;40:84.

9. Kramer ME. *Clinical Orthoptics*. 2nd ed. St. Louis: CV Mosby Co; 1953:161-163.

10. Griffin JR, Lee JM. The Poloroid-Mirror method. *Optom Weekly*. 1971;61:29.

11. Griffin JR. Screening for anomalies of binocular vision by means of the Polaroid-Mirror method. *Am J Optom*. 1971;48:689-692.

12. Revell MJ. *Strabismus: A History of Orthoptic Techniques*. London: Barrie & Jenkins; 1971:16-20.

13. Holopigian K, Blake R, Greenwald MJ. Clinical suppression and amblyopia. *Invest Ophthalmol Vis Sci*. 1988;29:444-451.

14. Thal LS, Grisham JD. Correcting high anisometropia: two case reports. *J Optom Physiol Optics*. 1976;53: 85-87.

Chapter 13 / Vision Therapy for Eso Deviations

Diagnostic Variables   372
Vision Therapy Sequence for Comitant
    Esotropia   372
    Correction of Refractive Error   372
    Elimination of Major Sensory
        Anomalies   373
    Compensating Prisms and Lens
        Additions   373
    Centration Point Training   374
    Sensory and Motor Fusion Training   374
    Changing Viewing Distance   376
    Surgical Management   376
    Follow-up Care   377
Vision Therapy Sequence for
    Esophoria   377
Specific Training Techniques   378
    Amblyoscopic Divergence Technique
        T13.1   378
    Bernell Mirror Stereoscope T13.2   379
    Brewster Stereoscope BI Training   380
        Isometric and Step Vergences
            T13.3   382
        Stereoscope Tromboning T13.4   383
    Anaglyphic Fusion Games T13.5   384
    Brock String and Beads T13.6   385
    Peripheral Fusion Rings-BI Training at Far
        T13.7   386
    Vectograms® and Tranaglyphs   386

Divergence Training at Near
    T13.8   388
    Divergence Walk-aways T13.9   390
    Projected BI Slides T13.10   390
Binocular Accommodative Rock
    T13.11   390
Vergence Rock Techniques (Flipper
    Prisms) T13.12   391
Aperture-Rule Trainer (Double Aperture)
    T13.13   391
Remy Separator T13.14   393
Orthopic Fusion T13.15   394
Computerized Divergence Procedures
    T13.16   395
Case Management and Examples   396
Convergence Excess Esotropia   396
    Management Principles   396
    Case Example   398
Basic Esotropia   398
    Management Principles   398
    Case Example   400
Divergence Insufficiency Esotropia   401
Microesotropia   402
    Management Principles   402
    Case Example   402
Esophoria   403
    Management Principles   403
    Case Example   404

Many doctors prefer to manage esotropia either optically or surgically. These are often important and necessary approaches in vision therapy, although sometimes the results are only cosmetic improvement. Optical and surgical approaches do not exhaust the options available to the clinician who is dedicated to achieving a functional cure of esotropia. Other than treating amblyopia, vision training in cases of esotropia may not be a serious consideration by some clinicians. This may be due to their impression that fusional divergence ranges cannot be significantly increased. This impression is incorrect; divergence ranges and facility can be

TABLE 13-1. *Vision Therapy Sequence for Comitant Esotropia.*

1. Full correction of any significant ametropia, particularly latent hyperopia
2. Amblyopia therapy, if needed, improving visual acuity to at least 20/60 (6/18).
3. Training of basic ocular motility in each eye: fixation, saccades, pursuits, and accommodation.
4. ARC therapy, if prognosis for its elimination is favorable.
5. Sensorial alignment of the eyes at some or all distances using any combination of prisms and added lenses (assuming NRC).
6. Antisuppression therapy, if NRC, to establish diplopia awareness and basic sensory fusion.
7. Central sensory and motor fusion training, if NRC, to achieve good stereopsis and maximum fusional vergence ranges, free of suppression, at all viewing distances.
8. Strabismus surgery, if necessary, to reduce the angle of deviation to within the range of reflex fusional vergence.
9. Prescription of compensatory prisms and added lenses as needed.
10. Development of good monocular and binocular efficiency skills.
11. Maintenance home exercises and periodic progress checkups.

increased.[1-3] Similarly, some clinicians prescribe prisms or lenses for symptomatic esophoric patients without thought of including vision training. When patients are properly selected, we have found vision training an effective and practical solution to treating both esophoric and esotropic deviations. When optics and/or surgery are applied without vision training, we have frequently observed that the patient's level of binocular functioning remains deficient. We hope all options for binocular treatment are given serious consideration in the patient's best interests.

DIAGNOSTIC CONSIDERATIONS

Eso deviations, whether tropic or phoric, are generally classified into three categories: (1) divergence insufficiency (DI), having a low AC/A; (2) basic eso (BE), having a normal AC/A; and (3) convergence excess (CE) having a high AC/A. (See Chapters 3 and 7 for discussions on these classifications.) In this scheme, however, not all nine diagnostic variables of a deviation are taken into account. Only the near and far magnitudes are considered. (The AC/A can be calculated from the far and near deviations.) The use of a limited number of variables is convenient to avoid the hundreds of possible diagnostic permutations arising when nine variables are considered. For this reason, the discussions of therapy strategies in this chapter follow this simplified classification. It should be remembered, however, that a complete strabismus diagnosis and prognosis should include a description of all nine variables: constancy, comitancy, laterality, direction, magnitude, AC/A, variability, dominancy, and cosmesis (Chapter 4). Diagnosis of heterophoria would exclude constancy, laterality, and possibly variability and cosmesis.

VISION THERAPY SEQUENCE FOR COMITANT ESOTROPIA

Our recommended sequence of steps in the management of comitant esotropia with vision therapy is outlined in Table 13-1. Prospective vision therapy patients should have a reasonably good prognosis for functional cure (Chapter 6).

Correction of Refractive Error

Optical management of eso deviations, particularly esotropia, requires full plus correction of any significant refractive error, based usually on a cycloplegic refraction. Many cases of accommodative esotropia can be completely resolved by correction of the full amount of hyperopia. (Refer to discussions in Chapter 7.) The patient is encouraged to wear these lenses, full time, even if visual acuity at far is initially blurred. Children usually relax the spasm of accommodation in a matter of days while young adults often take longer, a few weeks, depending on the amount of latent hyperopia present. In cases of esotropia in infants and toddlers, some doctors even overcorrect the full hyperopia by as much as 1.00 D in an effort to improve alignment at near distances. Any residual esotropia or esophoria may require compensation, at least in part, with base-out prism and/or plus addition lenses. This optical treatment is beneficial if there are no major sensory anomalies of deep amblyopia, suppression, or ARC.

Elimination of Major Sensory Anomalies

This discussion of vision therapy approaches in esotropia assumes that major sensory anomalies have been partially or totally eliminated. Before sensory and motor fusion techniques are applied, the patient should be generally free of amblyopia, ARC, and deep suppression. (See Chapters 10, 11, and 12, respectively.) In some esotropic cases, the clinician may have to continue therapy procedures for these sensorial anomalies along with developing bifoveal fusion and improving motor fusional ranges. Also, before fusional divergence training begins, the doctor should ensure that basic monocular skills (i.e., fixation, saccades, pursuits, and accommodation) are adequate for each eye. (See Chapter 2 for normative values.) The strabismic and/or amblyopic eye frequently has deficient ocular motility.[4] If ocular motility is deficient, vision training is usually necessary to develop these oculomotor skills before a concerted effort is made to increase fusional divergence. (See Chapter 16 on therapy for vision efficiency skills.)

Compensating Prisms and Lens Additions

If a residual eso deviation is present after full correction of the refractive error, the effect of compensating prisms and/or added plus at near needs to be evaluated. If sensory fusion with optics can be achieved at some distance, open-environment training can be used; this provides the best chance for successful treatment. Normal retinal correspondence must be present for prisms and adds to be effective. When compensating prisms and adds are prescribed, the patient should be checked frequently for the possibility of prism adaptation (See Chapter 6).

Although it is important to correct the full hyperopic refractive error in all cases of eso deviation, plus–lens additions at near are not very effective in cases of DI. This is because the AC/A is low. However, in some cases of basic esotropia, bifocals may be recommended. This distance portion of the spectacle lenses should not be overcorrected with plus lenses since blurred vision at far is unacceptable. An exception may be made in esotropic infants since most of their visual requirements and interests are at near distances. In BE cases, base-out prism compensation may be necessary to keep the patient fusing and, therefore, prevent the recurrence of amblyopia, ARC, and/or suppression. In cases of DI, prisms are usually needed only for far vision. This can be accomplished by applying the Fresnel prism segment only over the "distance" portion of the lenses. Note that an overall base-out compensating prism, while good at far, is contraindicated at near, because it would make the DI patient have to converge, as though having convergence insufficiency. Fusional convergence training is not advised in the initial stages of therapy; rather, fusional divergence ranges must be developed. As the magnitude and quality of sensory and motor fusion increase with vision training, the amount of compensating prism can be reduced considerably or totally removed in some cases.

A problem often arises with base-out prism compensation for esotropia if normal sensory fusion has not been established; otherwise, the deviation will usually increase due to ARC or, possibly, suppression.[5] When prism adaptation is not a problem, base-out compensation is an ideal way to maintain fusion. This, along with fusional divergence training, often allows for a gradual reduction of the compensating prism power. In DI or BE cases with prism adaptation, one alternative during a vision therapy program is to increase the prism amount until adaptation ceases. Using Fresnel prisms, it is possible to apply as much as 60^{Δ} base-out to compensate for an eso deviation. A greater amount of base-out power can be obtained by also having prism ground into the spectacle lenses. The sum of that with the Fresnel prisms allows for prismatic compensation exceeding 60^{Δ}. An alternative is patching of an eye between vision training sessions to prevent ARC and suppression. If sensory alignment of the eyes is not possible with prisms and plus lens additions at any viewing distance, the patient must wear a patch for distances while involved in vision therapy.

The CE esotropic patient benefits greatly from plus lens additions, usually in the form of bifocal spectacles. We have also found that bifocal contact lenses are effective particularly with children. Also, prism compensation may be needed for the far deviation if it is significantly large. (The use of plus-addition lenses is discussed extensively in Chapter 7.) The minimal amount of plus power to achieve a sensory and motor fusion response at near should be prescribed so the patient can read and work at a comfortable viewing distance.

Centration Point Training

As part of esotropia management, Vodnoy[6] pointed out the importance of finding a fixation distance at which fusion can be established. He recommended beginning training at the nearpoint where the visual axes cross in esotropia for the best chance to achieve good binocularity. The proper amount of plus power at the centration point (where visual axes cross) can easily be calculated using the following formula: Diopter= H^Δ/IPDcm. For example, suppose the esotropia is 15^Δ at far and the interpupillary distance (IPD) is 60 mm. Fifteen divided by 6 is 2.50 D, making the centration point 40 cm from the patient's eyes. (Refer to Chapter 6.)

The centration point concept can be applied to any esotropic patient who has a constant deviation at far. This is a theoretical calculation, and the visual system does not always respond in a mechanical and predictable manner. In some cases of esotropia, even with NRC, plus lenses seem to have little or no immediate effect. If there is ARC, the add for the centration point is often ineffective, probably due to the influence of vergence adaptation to the habitual anomalous corresponding point in the deviating eye. In any case, an attempt to align the eyes at the centration point should be made in all cases of esotropia when vision therapy is being considered.

There are several advantages to training an esotropic patient in open space as opposed to using closed space instruments such as the major amblyoscope, not the least of which is the transfer of learned sensory and motor fusion skills to the natural visual environment. If the calculated amount of the centration point add does not completely neutralized the deviation, the clinician should try an add with higher power while placing the fixation target at the appropriate closer fixation distance. Hopefully, a nearpoint distance can be found at which the patient has the opportunity for bifoveal fixation under these conditions. The next step would be to establish sensory fusion at the centration point by breaking suppression, e.g., using Brock string and beads (T13.6). Vision training for fusional divergence can also start at this position. Several instruments and procedures can be used effectively with centration point adds as high as +5.00 D, e.g., Vectograms® and Tranaglyphs (T13.8) in conjunction with prism flippers for step vergence demands (T13.12).

Sensory and Motor Fusion Training

The patient with an eso deviation must be sensorily ready (i.e., having at least flat fusion and hopefully stereopsis) before motor fusion demands can be introduced in vision training procedures. This is not problem in esophoria, but often so in esotropia; intensive therapy for elimination of ARC and suppression may be required to develop flat fusion. (Refer to therapy techniques in Chapters 11 and 12.) Sensory fusion is usually established after ARC and suppression are broken. When motor fusion training is begun, the monitoring of suppression is, in effect, a training procedure that enhances both flat fusion and stereopsis when appropriate targets are used to emphasize these sensory fusion skills.

In addition to sensory fusion development, ocular motility must be good. (Evaluation of saccadic and pursuit eye movements and fixation is discussed in Chapter 2.) It is usually important to include duction (monocular) and version (binocular) motility training prior to and during the early part of the motor fusion training program for eso deviations. This is particularly applicable when there is a noncomitant deviation. Even in cases of comitant eso deviations, one or both eyes may have limited abduction, particularly in unilateral esotropia of long standing.

Assuming the patient demonstrates some stereopsis, targets with stereopsis clues are introduced as soon as possible. Various combinations of antisuppression stimuli for breaking suppression and enhancing the fusion percept may be required for the patient with constant esotropia. These procedures may include flashing, large target size, brightness, movement, etc. (See Chapter 12.) Foveal suppression should be monitored frequently and, if found, should be immediately broken. Eliminating foveal suppression promotes development of motor fusion ranges. When sensory fusion is steady and consistent for a particular pair of targets, a vergence demand for the patient should be introduced. If, for example, angle H is 15^Δ eso on the major amblyoscope, the tubes are slowly moved from the 15^Δ base-out setting to a 20^Δ base-out setting. Training fusional convergence initially, builds the patient's confidence. If the patient is able to converge 5^Δ, the tubes are reset at 15^Δ base-out and then a relative 5^Δ base-in demand is introduced. (This means that the setting on the instrument scale actually reads 10^Δ base-out.) Other instruments, such as the Dual Polachrome Illuminated Trainer, may also be used in this manner. Divergence training is repeated until the patient's fusion range, with clear vision, increases beyond the ortho demand setting on the instrument scale. This goal, however, is not always achievable at this point in vision therapy.

Accommodative changes will blur the fused image; blur indicates that pure fusional vergences are not in play. When the target becomes blurred, the patient is relying on accommodative vergence changes (decreasing accommodative response in an eso case) to maintain single vision. The goal at this point is to achieve clear vision with maximum fusional ranges, free of foveal suppression, around the angle of deviation.

Most patients with esotropia are ready to leave instrument training and begin open-environment training when the motor fusion range at the angle of deviation is 10^Δ in either direction. However, the patient should not be allowed to lapse into strabismus, if possible. The patient should be kept fusing most of the time by means of compensating prisms and/or plus addition lenses. During active vision training, either in or out-of office, vergence demands are introduced in the open environment (free-space). There are numerous methods for changing vergence demand (Table 13-2).

Sliding vergences can be introduced with convenient and available mirror stereoscopes, split Vectograms, Tranaglyphs, etc. Such proce-

---

TABLE 13-2. *Methods for Changing Vergence Demand*

A. Prisms
  1. Risley
  2. Loose prisms
  3. Prism bar
     a. Conventional glass or plastic
     b. Wick's Fresnel bar
B. Use of Septums
  1. Brewster stereoscope (homologous point separation increased for BI and decreased for BO demands)
  2. Wheatstone stereoscope (mirror angle changed for BI or BO demands)
  3. Remy Separator (BI demand increased with target separation increase)
C. Vectographic and colored filters (separation varied for prismatic demands)
D. Plus and minus spherical lenses
  1. BO demand with plus
  2. BI demand with minus
E. Chiastopic and orthopic fusion
  1. BO demand with chiastopic
  2. BI demand with orthopic
F. Changing fixation distance
  1. Inside instruments (e.g., Brewster stereoscope, BI demand far to near and BO demand from near to far)
  2. In open environment (e.g., Bagolini lenses used with penlight push-ups and push-aways)

dures simulate the smoothness of movement afforded by a major amblyoscope. Sliding vergence ranges are initially trained because they are generally easier to achieve than step vergence responses. Step vergences are introduced later on, beginning with small prismatic demands and allowing ample time for the patient's responses. Rapid step changes in vergence demand are conveniently done with the use of a prism bar. Wick[7] described a bar made with Fresnel Press-On™ prisms that has the advantage of less weight and bulkiness than conventional prism bars made of glass or plastic. Prism flippers are also good for step vergence training. Base-out prism may have to be used exclusively at first until the patient can learn to fuse when base-in prism is flipped into place. The important rule is that the demand must be within the patient's ability. As the motor fusion range expands, the difference between base-in and base-out demands can be increased. The range is eventually expanded to include an adequate base-in range. An ideal goal is to have a base-in range that is twice the magnitude of the eso deviation, while maintaining clear vision (Sheard's criterion).

Changing Viewing Distance

One principle of vision therapy for strabismus is that open-environment training is started at a distance where the patient can fuse (or when fusion can be established with prisms and lenses). Eventually, the patient works toward those distances where fusion is deficient. The DI and BE esotropic patient is encouraged to maintain fusion at the centration point, and then slowly walk backward while keeping fusion. The power of the training add (e.g., trial case lenses) should be reduced accordingly so that the patient's vision is not blurred as viewing distance is increased. In cases of DI, it is easy to visualize how a receding target requires an increasingly greater demand on fusional divergence. This is because the eso deviation becomes greater when viewing is changed from near to far. (Refer to discussion in Chapter 3.) Even in BE cases, the receding target is more difficult to fuse at far than at near fixation

distances; stereopsis diminishes with increasing distance and stereopsis is a strong stimulus to maintain fusional divergence. There are other factors at near that help an individual maintain alignment of the eyes. The relatively larger retinal images at near also provide more "glue" for sensory-motor fusion. Also, tactile-kinesthetic clues at near help the patient attend to the act of fusing the target with both eyes. These aids to fusion are lacking at far. Increasing the fixation distance from near to far, therefore, is useful in several training procedures for both divergence insufficiency and basic eso deviations.

In cases of CE with a high AC/A, the eso deviation becomes greater with decreasing viewing distance. Pushups with a bifixated target are effective in training of fusional divergence. This is because the patient must use fusional divergence to maintain bifixation while absolute convergence is increasing at near (Figure 3-19 illustrates graphically the relation between the ortho demand line and the AC/A line). This counterintuitive concept of pushup training in these cases of eso deviation becomes rational when the relation between the demand line and the AC/A are visualized.

Surgical Management

Extraocular muscle surgery is necessary in cases of esotropia when the magnitude of the deviation is too large for compensating prisms to be worn with acceptance by the patient. As to prognosis for functional cure, an esotropia is considered large if the magnitude exceeds 20^Δ. (See Chapter 4.) A common surgical procedure is bimedial rectus recession. This not only reduces the magnitude of the angle of esotropia but also tends to lower the AC/A. A lowered AC/A is particularly helpful in cases of convergence excess (CE) (Table 13-3). The symmetrical operation (medial rectus on each eye) helps in maintaining comitancy, as opposed to recession and resection on one eye only. In cases of DI, surgeons often prefer a bilateral lateral rectus resection; this symmetrical operation tends to preserve comitancy and increase the AC/A. Another operation popular with strabismus surgeons for basic esotropia is the recession–resection operation. (Strengthening and weakening approaches in surgery are discussed in Chapter 6 along with other aspects of surgical management.)

At the beginning of a vision therapy program for esotropia, the doctor should introduce the concept of possibly needing extraocular muscle surgery. If the deviation remains cosmetically obvious after full correction of the refractive error, discussing this possibility is essential for good management. If the residual eso deviation at near, but particularly at far, measures 20^Δ or more, an operation is often necessary for the sake of long-term comfortable and efficient binocular vision. In our experience, fusional divergence can be effectively trained, but there are realistic limits.

Follow-up Care

If a postsurgical patient had compensating prisms or plus–added lenses to establish fusion prior to the operation, it is important that new prescription lenses be given to the patient immediately following surgery. Hopefully the prisms and lens additions will no longer be necessary. Fresnel Press-on™ prisms can be applied to new spectacle lenses as needed to resolve any significant diplopia in the primary position or at the reading distance, but patching is usually not recommended.

Vision therapy can be started again about 2 weeks after an operation. Immediately following surgery, the eye(s) are sensitive to irritation and bright lights, so a little time-off from training is appropriate. If presurgical vision training and the operation have been successful, the patient quickly establishes fusion in the open environment and the angle of deviation rapidly stabilizes during the healing process. Vision training is directed toward identifying and breaking any suppression that may occur. Motor fusion ranges and vergence facility are again maximally increased. If there is any restriction of ocular motility in some fields of gaze, training may help to reduce the restriction. In all cases, whether post-surgical or not, when vergence skills are maximally increased, retainer

TABLE 13-3. *Common Surgical Procedures for Esotropia*

Divergence Insufficiency Esotropia:
Strengthen both lateral rectus muscles with a bilateral resection procedure that decreases deviation at far primarily.

Convergence Excess Esotropia:
Weaken both medial rectus muscles with a bilateral recession that decreases deviation at near primarily. Can be combined with Faden procedure, e.g., suturing a medial rectus muscle to the sclera 11–15 mm posterior to its insertion.

Basic Esotropia:
1. A unilateral or bilateral recession and resection operation depending on the size of the deviation.
2. A bimedial rectus recession operation: weakening both medial rectus muscles.

Immediate Post-Surgical Goal:
10^Δ undercorrection to ortho.

exercises are then given to the patient and a regular recall schedule is established based on quality of results.

VISION THERAPY SEQUENCE FOR ESOPHORIA

Most cases of esophoria and intermittent esotropia can be successfully managed with some combination of prisms, added lenses, and vision training. Surgery is not frequently required. In our experience, a home vision training program of 30 minutes per day for 8 to 12 weeks (with weekly office visits) is usually sufficient to eliminate symptoms and meet release criteria. If the patient is not making adequate progress in a home based program, an in-office training program with 2 or 3 visits per week may be necessary for successful treatment.

Therapy for esophoria is a continuation of that for esotropia, as though a finishing process of the strabismus. A general sequence of vision therapy for esophoria is outlined in Table 13-4. This sequence parallels that for esotropia, but excludes management of major sensory condi-

---

TABLE 13-4. *Vision Therapy Sequence for Esophoria*

1. Fully correct any significant ametropia, particularly latent hyperopia.
2. Prescribe compensatory prism and added lens combinations as needed.
3. Train good monocular and binocular fixation, saccades, pursuits, and accommodation.
4. Central sensory-motor fusion training to achieve good stereopsis and maximum fusional vergence ranges free of suppression.
5. Development of good vergence facility and stamina.
6. Maintenance home exercises and periodic progress checkups.

---

tions and surgery is not frequently required. The emphasis is on breaking foveal suppression and building the quantity and quality of fusional vergence.

In DI esophoric cases in which the deviation is greater at far, push-away and walk-away training are given. Examples include: Brock string and beads (T13.6), Vectograms and Tranaglyphs (T13.9), penlight and anaglyphic filters (T12.3), Pola-mirror (T12.9), and Television Trainer (T12.8). Vision training from near-to-far also applies to BE cases, even though the eso at near and far are approximately of the same magnitude. As discussed previously, the fusion "glue" is stronger at near than at far; this allows the patient to achieve the more easy tasks initially before attempting the more difficult ones at far. Failure at far is likely without prior training at near. Failure should be avoided and success should always be emphasized in vision therapy. In CE cases where the deviation is greater at near, a push-up procedure can be given using the same instruments mentioned above.

SPECIFIC TRAINING TECHNIQUES

Sixteen exemplary vision training procedures particularly appropriate for cases of eso deviations are presented. There are numerous other effective techniques clinicians can utilize;

many doctors and therapists improvise techniques based on their experiences treating patients. The techniques we present here generally follow a sequence from treating the most difficult cases, as in esotropia with poor sensory and motor fusion, to treating the least difficult cases, as in esophoria with relatively minor deficiencies of sensory and motor fusion. Another way to look at this sequence is to consider the first techniques in the series of procedures as relatively easy for the patient to master. The clinician should always be flexible, however, and choose those techniques that are most appropriate for the particular skill and interest level of each patient.

Amblyoscopic Divergence Technique T13.1

The amblyoscopic divergence technique discussed in this section is similar to that presented in Chapter 11 for esotropia with ARC (T11.7), but the emphasis here is on improvement of the fusional divergence range in the instrument with the assumption that NRC is present. This procedure is usually applied in cases of esotropia, but can also be used for esophoria when little or no progress has been made using other techniques. Large stereoscopic targets with suppression controls are utilized, e.g., the swing slides (see Figure 11-5). Rapid alternate flashing intensifies the perception of stereopsis and breaks suppression that may be present. With the targets initially set at the subjective angle, the amblyoscope arms are slowly diverged until the images become diplopic or suppression occurs. The divergence demand is then reduced just enough for the patient to re-establish fusion. This vergence demand is held stationary for 1 or 2 minutes as an isometric procedure. The arms are then slowly diverged again and the technique is repeated until maximum divergence has been achieved within a 20-minute period. The emphasis in this training technique is to expand the divergence range within the instrument, then have the patient view distant objects in the open environment while trying to maintain the achieved divergence. In cases of esotropia, partial prism compensation is usually necessary to help the patient maintain binocular alignment in the open environment. Besides seeing diplopically for feedback when motor fusion is lost, the patient also utilizes the sensation of eyestrain to provide subjective feedback that free-space motor fusion is occurring. At some point, the doctor must use the unilateral cover test to monitor bifoveal alignment; this breaks fusion if it has been achieved. The patient should be encouraged to rejoin the images after the cover test as a break-and-join training procedure. Other techniques [e.g., mirror stereoscope (T13.2), Vectograms and Tranaglyphs (T13.8)] can similarly be used for isometric exercises to transfer the learned skill of fusional divergence in the major amblyoscope to the open environment.

Bernell Mirror Stereoscope - BI Training T13.2

The Mirror Stereoscope from Bernell Corporation is a Wheatstone stereoscope (Figures 13-1 and 13-2). The instrument has two mirrors mounted on arms that are in the shape of the letter W, hence its colloquial clinical name, "Flying W." Prismatic changes are made by varying the angle between the mirrors. A range of 40^Δ BI to 50^Δ BO can be measured by simply adjusting the angle of the instrument. This large range makes it particularly useful in cases of strabismus. For measurement purposes, a scale calibrated in prism diopters is placed at the bottom of the instrument. Base-out is induced by narrowing the angle of the instrument (narrow W) and base-in demand is created by widening the instrument's angle (wide W). The fixation distance from each eye via the mirror to the target is approximately 1/3 meter; therefore, optical infinity can be created by using plus lenses of approximately 3.00 D. This plus addition can be in the form of trial lenses worn over the CAMP lenses. Training at optical infinity is an important goal in cases of DI and BE esotropia. Plus-addition lenses are usually not needed in cases of CE esotropia unless the nearpoint deviation is beyond the base-out scale of the instrument.

The initial phase of T13.2 is to help the patient achieve fusion at some vergence de-

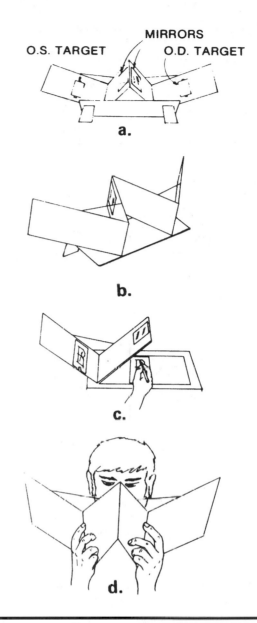

FIGURE 13-1—Bernell Mirror Stereoscope, four views: (a) Front view; (b) back view; (c) adaptation as a cheiroscope for antisuppression therapy; (d) wheatstone type of stereoscope for prismatic variation for first-, second-, and third-degree fusion demands.

mand, possibly base-out prism if necessary. Targets with the appropriate level of difficulty are placed in the target holders and can be aligned at the patient's subjective angle of deviation. Some of the fusion targets have large suppression controls, important in cases of deep suppression. An auxiliary light source (e.g., a desk lamp) can be shined directly onto the target of the suppressed eye. When the patient achieves

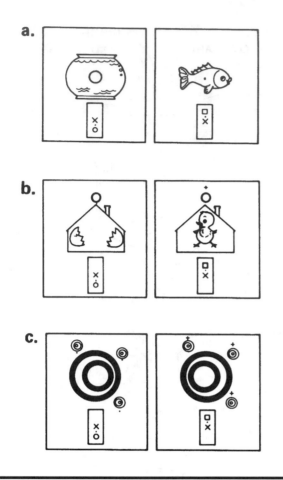

FIGURE 13-2—Examples of targets used in the Bernell Mirror Stereoscope: (a) Fish and bowl, first-degree fusion; (b) chick and egg, second-degree fusion; (c) doubled circles, third-degree fusion. (Courtesy of Bernell Corp.)

sensory fusion, base-in demands are gradually increased (or base-out decreased) as the patient attempts to maintain fusion. This sliding (tonic) vergence procedure helps to increase fusional divergence. The instrument can also be conveniently changed into a cheiroscope if an intensive attack on suppression is needed; this is applicable if there is NRC, but not if there is ARC.

An intermediate goal is for the patient to achieve sliding vergence ranges from a 10^Δ BO to 10^Δ BI range around the angle of deviation, not necessarily clearing the ortho setting of the instrument. Vergence training is done in both horizontal directions with an emphasis toward the BI direction. An ideal goal would be to increase vergence ranges (e.g., blur/break/recovery) to conform to the normative nearpoint

values listed in Chapter 2. Training can be done either in the office or at home. The typical training period for this technique is 10 minutes of continuous activity of moving the targets between the limits of convergence and divergence. The patient's goal at this point is to increase vergence ranges, not speed, while maintaining clear, single, suppression-free, binocular vision.

Brewster Stereoscope BI Training

The refracting type of stereoscope was invented by Brewster a decade after the first Wheatstone (mirror) stereoscope was devised. Unlike the Wheatstone stereoscope, a septum without mirrors is used for dissociation. Base-out prisms are incorporated for purposes of increasing the lateral field of view in this instrument and allowing for more range in lateral vergences. The compactness of this stereoscope compared with the Wheatstone instrument led to its popularity for clinical usage (and also for entertainment purposes as a parlor stereoscope). There are several commercial varieties of the Brewster stereoscope, but all have a similar optical design.

The schematic top view of such an instrument (Keystone Telebinocular in this example) is shown in Figure 13-3. The Telebinocular is illustrated in Figure 13-4. The eyepieces are +5.00 D spherical lenses (which can be made from a single spherical lens that is cut in half, with each center placed on opposite sides). Base-out prismatic effect is created by the optical centers being far apart relative to the patient's interpupillary distance (IPD). The standard separation between optical centers is 95 mm and designated by the letter S. Fixation distance is designated by the lower case letter u and is 0.2 m (20 cm) for farpoint testing, which is optical infinity for the +5.00 D lenses. The target separation distance representing an ortho demand for vergence is designated by the lower case letter h. In Figure 13-3 the homologous points are the star seen by the left eye and the circle seen by the right eye. The formula to calculate h (target separation) in millimeters is as follows:

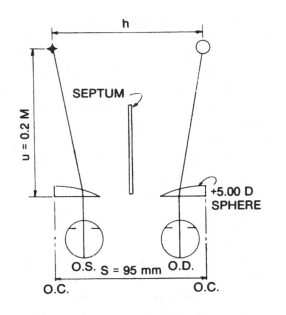

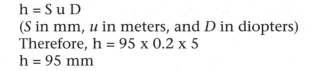

FIGURE 13-3—Schematic top view illustrating the optics of the Brewster stereoscope.

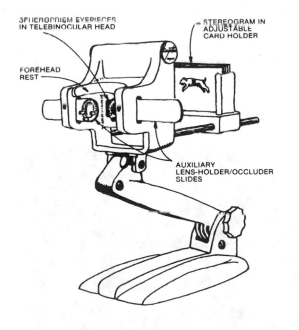

FIGURE 13-4—Keystone Telebinocular.

h = S u D
(S in mm, *u* in meters, and *D* in diopters)
Therefore, h = 95 x 0.2 x 5
h = 95 mm

This means that when the homologous points at optical infinity are 95 mm apart, the demand on vergence is zero. In other words, the points are in the ortho position. For any target separation (*h*) other than 95 mm, a vergence demand is created. A rule to remember is that at 0.2 m fixation distance (optical infinity), it takes 2 mm to equal 1^Δ. For example, suppose the star and circle were separated by only 87 mm instead of 95 mm. There is now a difference of 8 mm, which represents 4^Δ base-out demand. Conversely, if the *h* value is 103 mm, divergence of 4^Δ is required to superimpose the star and circle.

While it is true that 95 mm is the theoretical separation for homologous points on a stereogram that represents an ortho demand at optical infinity, the practical clinical *h* value most often used is 87 mm. This is because most people, on average, converge approximately 4^Δ when viewing in a closed environment such as the Brewster stereoscope. This, in effect, compensates for the average amount of proximal (psychic) convergence. The separation of 87 mm represents 4^Δ base-out and is the practical distance that compensates an eso postural shift caused by the proximal convergence. This is the reason stereograms designed for an ortho demand have homologous point separations of approximately 87 mm. Note that standard Brewster stereoscopes have an optical-center separation distance of 95 mm and the 87 mm homologous point separation applies. (Some small stereoscopes vary in this standard and the doctor should measure the optical-center separation when in doubt.)

When nearpoint training (closer than optical infinity) is performed in a Brewster stereoscope, new target separation values (*h*) represent the ortho demand setting of this instrument. A nearpoint accommodative stimulus of 2.50 D is represented by a distance of 0.133 m (13.3 cm) within the collapsed optical space of the stereoscope. The 0.133 m distance has a dioptric value of 7.50; and since the 0.2

m distance has a dioptric value of 5.00 D, the total demand on accommodation is 7.50 – 5.00 = 2.50 D. The *h* value is calculated for nearpoint as follows:

$$h = 95 \times 0.133 \times 5$$
$$h = 63 \text{ mm}$$

This means that if the homologous points are separated by a distance of 63 mm, the vergence demand at this nearpoint distance of 0.133 m is ortho. At this particular distance of 0.133 m (1.33 decimeters), it takes 1.33 mm lateral displacement on a stereogram to equal 1^Δ. For example, if the circle and star are 59 mm apart, the base-out demand is 3^Δ (4 divided by 1.33). At the farpoint (2 decimeters), every 2 mm on the stereogram equals 1^Δ, and every 1.33 mm equals 1^Δ at the nearpoint (traditionally at 2.50 D demand with fixation distance of 1.33 decimeters). Any prismatic demand can be determined using this "decimeter rule" when stereograms are used in a Brewster stereoscope.

Isometric and Step Vergences T13.3

One of the most widely used Brewster stereoscopes is the Keystone Telebinocular (see Figure 13-4). The Biopter and the Bernell-O-Scope are two of the many examples of small Brewster stereoscopes used for home training purposes. Many training procedures can be performed with such instruments as these. The first phase of training is to have the patient fuse a stereogram and appreciate stereopsis while monitoring suppression. Initially, the homologous points may need to be relatively close together to create a base-out compensation for the esotropic or esophoric patient. For example, the separation of the targets could be 77 mm to help the patient fuse, by providing a 5^Δ base-out compensation (87-77/2 = 5) for the eso deviation. The patient can maintain fusion on the target for a period of time, e.g., 1 to 2 minutes, as an isometric exercise. When there is good fusion, the target separation can be increased to, say, 87 mm for an ortho demand. With time, the patient should attempt to fuse the targets when the separation becomes wider, thus creating base-in demands to stimulate fusional divergence.

The next phase of training with the stereoscope is to introduce vergence steps. Figure 13-5 shows a typical stereogram providing step vergence demands. The top pair of targets has a relatively more base-in demand than does the

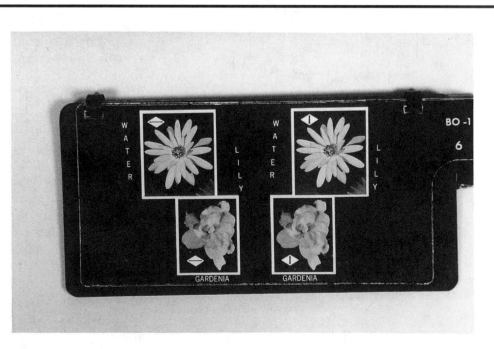

FIGURE 13-5—Example of a stereogram of step vergence training, a Bioptogram. (Reprinted with permission from Stereo Optical Co.)

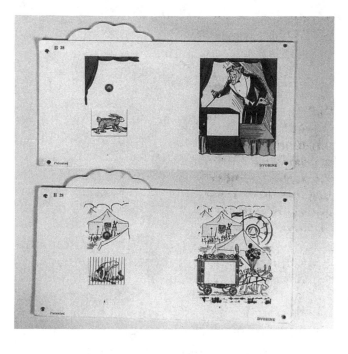

Figure 13-6—Example of Dvorine stereograms. (Reprinted with permission from Keystone View, Division of Mast/Keystone.)

bottom pair. Later in training as the patient improves his fusional divergence ability, BO demands are placed on the bottom and relatively large BI demands are on the top of the stereogram. This is training vergence facility,

also referred to as "vergence rock." This is phasic (fast) vergence training, as opposed to the initially easier procedure for steady isometric vergence training. (Refer to Chapter 2 for goals for fusional vergence ranges and facility.)

If there is suppression, an external light source can be directed toward the suppressed image; also bimanual pointing can be added to break the suppression response (see Figure 12-6). Corporations, such as Keystone View, Bernell, and other suppliers, provide a large variety of stereograms designed for most levels of sensory and motor skill and different patient's interests. Examples of stereograms designed specifically for young children are the Dvorine cards (Figure 13-6). Stereograms appropriate for older children and adults include the Biopter BI and BO cards (Figure 13-7). Fortunately, the base-in range of the Brewster stereoscope can exceed its base-out range-making it an ideal instrument for building divergence abilities. This point is made explicit in the following discussion of the tromboning technique.

Stereoscope Tromboning T13.4

Although some stereograms are split to allow for sliding vergence training with Brewster

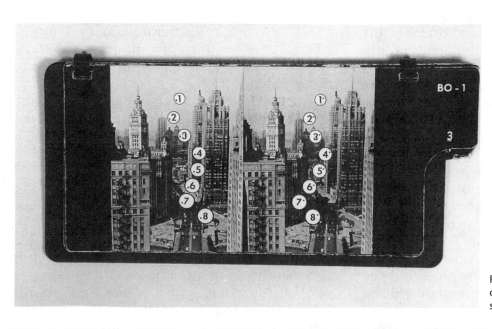

FIGURE 13-7—Example of a stereogram of the Biopter. (Reprinted with permission from Stereo Optical Co.)

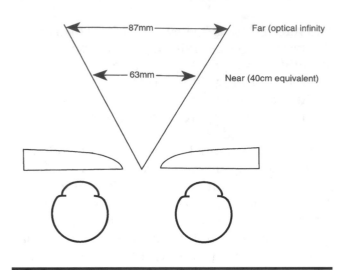

FIGURE 13-8—Ortho demand resulting from decreasing target separation on stereograms in a Brewster stereoscope as fixation distance is decreased. Theoretically, there is no target separation for an ortho demand at the plane of the lenses. Since the ortho distance goes from 87 mm at far to 63 mm at near, base-in fusional divergence is required (e.g., target separation of 87 mm on the stereogram) as the tromboning goes from far to near.

stereoscopes, this procedure is more easily done with a Mirror Stereoscope that provides gradual changes in BO and BI prismatic demands. However, the Brewster stereoscope is uniquely designed for the application of tromboning vergence training (T13.4) Donder's line of vergence demand in the Brewster stereoscope is represented at near accommodative demands by decreasing target separation distances. At far (optical infinity) the target separation for ortho demand (distance between homologous points for no vergence demand) is 87 mm; at the equivalent of 40 cm, it is 63 mm: and at closer distances, the target separation of ortho demand is progressively smaller (Figure 13-8). This optical fact has implications for training given for eso deviations. Most stereogram targets have a fixed target separation; so when they are slowly tromboned on the instrument, the vergence demand becomes progressively more divergent. Even if the stereogram vergence demand at optical infinity is convergent, as the target is tromboned to nearpoint distances, the convergent demand decreases; at some point along the accommodative scale there is a base-in demand. Tromboning on this instrument, therefore, increases the stimulus to

accommodation and divergence simultaneously. The beneficial effect of this "shaking up" technique is that the patient learns to dissociate accommodation from convergence in this paradoxical process of diverging while focusing at near.

Because of this optical relationship, almost any stereogram can be used to expand the range of fusional divergence with tromboning. In the case of esotropia, base-out cards (e.g., the Dvorine cards) with appropriate target separation can be selected so the patient can easily fuse them. As the target is slowly moved closer, the patient consciously attempts to maintain fusion and stops the procedure momentarily when suppression or diplopia occurs. The position of the stereogram on the accommodative scale is noted; on subsequent trials, the patient attempts to increase the range of fusion. The therapy goal during a 10-minute training period is to increase the range of response with this technique, but not necessarily the speed of responses. Speed of tromboning can be introduced as a goal after the patient's fusional range has been maximally expanded.

In esophoric cases, base-in stereograms (e.g., BI Biopter cards) may be fusible for the patient and can be introduced from the start. As these cards are tromboned along the accommodative scale, the BI demand to the patient increases rapidly making the technique quite challenging.

The isometric technique can be repeated when progress with tromboning slows or stops. Here the patient simply holds sensory and motor fusion for several minutes at a challenging divergence and accommodative demand setting without changing stimulus conditions.

Anaglyphic Fusion Games T13.5

This sensory and motor fusion technique, designed by Grisham, is particularly appropriate for young esotropic children, ages 2 to 6. The technique (or game) is intended to establish a child's gross sensory and motor fusion while playing with a parent at home. The child's success in the game provides feedback to the trainer about the development of fusion skills. This procedure can be applied in cases of amblyopia if the acuity is at least 20/80 in the affected eye.

The first step, as usual, is full correction of any significant refractive error. Next, the strabismic deviation is neutralized with Fresnel prisms and/or a centration-point add at the child's nearpoint working distance for this game. Prism power is increased as needed if there is prism adaptation (discussed in Chapter 6). The parent is given or acquires the following items: (1) one square yard of black felt material; (2) red-green plastic filter "glasses" with an elastic band; and (3) at least 30 small plastic toys of various sizes in three colors: red, green, and yellow. We have used small cars, animals, Lego blocks, pegs, and beads that can usually be found in abundance at most toy stores. The red and green toys must appear as black when viewed through the opposite filter (i.e., mutual exclusion). Also, the yellow toys should appear red through the red filter and green when viewed with only the green filter.

The anaglyphic game proceeds as follows: Wearing the prism glasses and red-green filters, the child sits on the piece of black felt placed on the floor. The toys are strewn randomly on the felt in front of the child. The task is to have the child find and separate the toys into three piles based on their color (red, green, or yellow). The yellow toys will only be seen as yellow (or some color different from the others) if there is sensory and motor fusion at the moment of selection. If the child suppresses or sees double, the yellow toys will appear to the child as either red or green and will, therefore, be place in the wrong pile. At the end of the game, the child and trainer look at the piles without the red-green glasses to check successes and errors. The parent may like to develop a reward system (e.g., verbal praise, stickers, or stars) to reinforce participation or success in the game depending on the child's wishes.

The difficulty level of the game and the sensory and motor fusion stimuli can be changed to meet the needs in each case. When deep suppression occurs, large colored toys and high background illumination is provided. With shallow suppression, a lot of small colored pegs or beads can be used. Motor fusion demands can be increased by reducing the

amount of Fresnel prism compensation or by introducing flipper lenses or prisms that demand fusional vergence. The child's success rate in the game provides a check on the level of fusion skill the child is developing. For optimum training results based on our experience, the child should correctly select the yellow toys at least 70% of the time, but not consistently 100% of the time. If less than 70%, a child often becomes frustrated and 100% success usually means the game is too easy to have training value.

Brock String and Beads - BI Training T13.6

Breaking suppression and establishing physiological diplopia with the Brock string and beads (see Figure 12-7) has been previously discussed (T12.7); however, this procedure can also be used for fusional divergence training. Base-in training to build fusional divergence ranges and reflexes in the open environment can be done effectively at home or in the office in selected cases of esotropia and esophoria. In esotropia, the first step is to provide the patient the opportunity for sensory fusion by using prisms and/or a centration-point add. One bead is placed at the ortho demand setting along the string and a second bead is positioned to create a small fusional divergence demand, e.g., second bead behind the first bead in cases of divergence insufficiency. The patient attempts jump vergences between the two beads and tries to perceive physiological diplopia with each fixation. Any suppression that occurs may be broken by blinking an eye, or by movement of the string; this should be done before the technique is continued. The procedure is timed for a selected number of cycles for each set. With training, the speed and amplitude of the jumps are increased maximally.

In cases of basic esotropia or esophoria, a step vergence variation of T13.6 is more effective than jump vergences. Step vergences, particularly emphasizing base-in demands, are introduced with either flipper prisms or loose prisms. It is important to begin with reasonably small vergence stimuli so the patient does not struggle excessively during this procedure. The patient sequentially fixates each of three beads placed along the string at prescribed training distances. Physiological diplopia is established and maintained by antisuppression procedures during the entire exercise (See T12.7). Working for speed, the patient completes 60 cycles of step vergence on each bead while noticing physiological diplopia. The time is recorded for the entire sequence. The distances between the beads are increased as training proceeds.

Peripheral Fusion Rings - BI Training at Far T13.7

There are several good peripheral stereopsis devices for enhancement of fusional divergence at far. A popular example is the Root Rings target (Figure 13-9). In this farpoint procedure, the red filtered eye sees only the red rings and the green filtered eye sees only the green rings. (The colored rings are printed on a black background.) The patient is instructed to fixate the center configuration while wearing red-green spectacles (red on right eye and green on left eye). The outer complementary colored rings are laterally disparate creating a stereoscopic effect. The outer rings should appear to float forward in relation to the central fixation area. Even in cases of strabismus, if the farpoint angle is smaller than 10^Δ, many patients can appreciate the floating of the rings. Some patients, esophoric and esotropic, take several minutes of intense target viewing before the full stereopsis effect is perceived. Even many orthophoric individuals with good binocular vision may require a minute or more to perceive the maximum stereoscopic effect. The latency period of

perception, however, tends to decrease with repeated training sessions.

A DI or BE eso deviation should be neutralized with base-out prism. The patient stands about 2 m from the target and is instructed to maintain the floating effect while slowly walking as far away as possible, while fusing the target. As fixation distance is increased, the rings should appear to float closer. They may appear 1 to 3 meters closer than the wall on which the target is attached. This is so for the outer rings that have the largest lateral disparity. The smaller rings also have a dramatic floating effect but not to the extent as the larger ones. Fusional divergence ranges are built up by gradually reducing the BO compensation and eventually by introducing BI prism of progressively greater power. Later, flipper prisms are used to increase vergence facility at far.

Other similar anaglyphic target for T13.7 are the Bernell 500 and 900 series, e.g., ring target shown mounted in lower portion of the Dual Polachrome Illuminated Trainer in Figure 13-11. Stereo Targets with suppression controls are transparent and can be attached to a television screen. An isometric technique would be to increase the BI prism demand to maximum acceptance while the patient watches television for an extended period, e.g., 30 minutes. A BI Fresnel or loose prism can be attached to the spectacles to create the appropriate divergence demand for the patient.

Vectograms and Tranaglyphs

Vodnoy popularized a set of polarized training targets, printed on rigid photographic sheets, called Vectograms that helped revolutionize orthoptic management of strabismus and heterophoria. These vectographic slides probably set the standard for open-environment sensory and motor fusion training (Figure 13-10). These targets are of interest to children and adults and have suppression controls of various sizes; they provide both crossed and uncrossed disparity for stereopsis. Crossed-polarizing filters, oriented at 45 and 135 degrees, are worn to dissociate the images. Relatively natural seeing conditions are simulated when the targets are fused. Three of the Vectograms are nonvariable

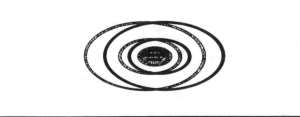

FIGURE 13-9—The Root Rings target.

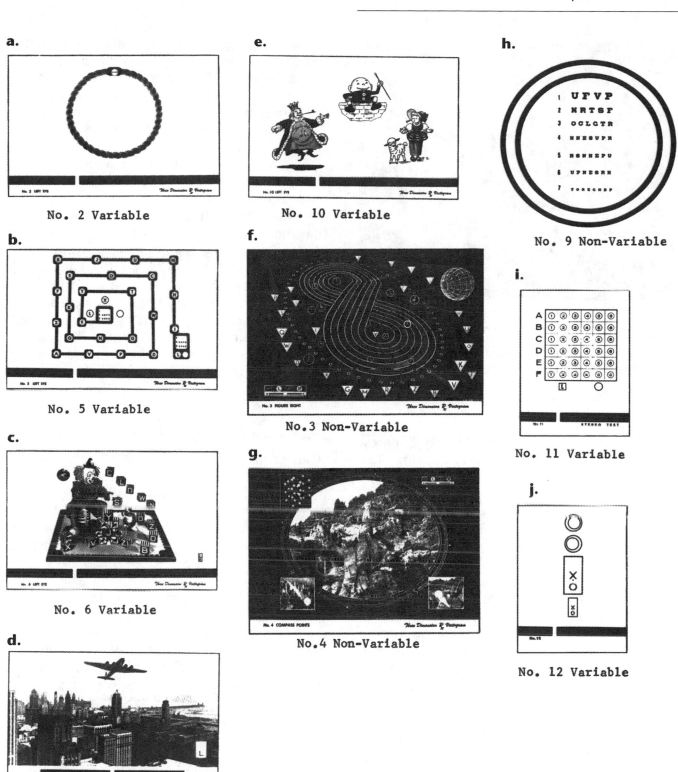

a.

No. 2 Variable

b.

No. 5 Variable

c.

No. 6 Variable

d.

No. 7 Variable

e.

No. 10 Variable

f.

No.3 Non-Variable

g.

No.4 Non-Variable

h.

No. 9 Non-Variable

i.

No. 11 Variable

j.

No. 12 Variable

FIGURE 13-10—Ten Vectograms for the Bernell Dual Polachrome Illuminated Trainer (previously named the Polachrome Orthopter): (a) Quoits, no. 2; (b) Spirangle, no. 5; (c) Clown, no. 6; (d) Chicago Skyline, no. 7; (e) Mother Goose, no. 10; (f) Figure 8, no. 3; (g) Compass Points, no. 4; (h) Acuity Suppression, no. 9; (i) Stereo Test, no. 11; (j) Basic Fusion, no. 12. Note that there is no no. 1 or no. 8 target. Vectograms numbers 3, 4, and 9 are not split but the others are, so that varying base-in and base-out demands can be induced with these. (Courtesy of Bernell Corp.)

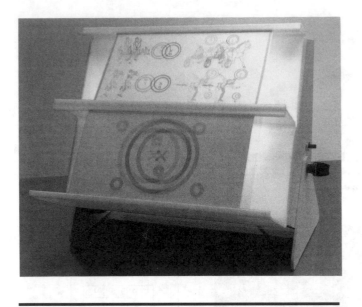

FIGURE 13-11—Nonvariable Tranaglyph mounted in the top portion of a Bernell Dual Polachrome Illuminated Trainer; example of a 500 series variable Tranaglyph is shown in the bottom portion. (Courtesy of Bernell Corp.)

eye sees only the green target and the green-filtered eye can see only the red target. There are several available Tranaglyph slide sets, either of the variable (500 and 600 series) or nonvariable (50 series) type (Figure 13-11). There is even a set devoted to training vertical vergence, the 70 series.

Tranaglyphs are used in the same manner in free space as Vectograms, but the stereopsis content of the slides tends to be less vivid. The advantage of Tranaglyphs over Vectograms is that they are relatively inexpensive, more durable, and the subject matter seems more motivating for teenagers and adults, e.g., sports action pictures. Also, head or target tilting is no problem as it can be for polarizing devices (i.e., polarization effect lost with significant tilting). They can be placed in a handheld slide holder or in a Dual Polachrome Illuminated Trainer. Most slides have adequate suppression controls for each eye.

Divergence Training at Near T13.8

If an esotropic patient has NRC, split Vectograms and Tranaglyphs are placed at the angle of deviation (the objective and subjective angles being the same) in an attempt to establish sensory fusion at 40 cm. At this distance the vergence scale on the slides reads directly in prism diopters. On a Vectogram, the numbers represent base-out demands and the letters, base-in, e.g., "D" represents 4^Δ BI. An add or prisms can be worn if the size of the nearpoint deviation is large. The Mother Goose Vectogram (Figure 13-10e) is particularly helpful for children at this basic level of training, because it has large suppression controls for all three figures. As each figure is fused in turn (they have slightly different step vergence demands), suppression may be broken with blinking, reduction of the overall vergence demand, or by pointing with a stick. As the patient continues making the small step vergence movements from one figure to the next, the slides are slowly separated in the base-in direction. The patient uses "mental effort" to keep the images fused and free of suppression. Sliding vergence ranges are trained in both BI and BO directions, alternating from one limit to the other, but emphasizing the divergence range two-thirds of the

(unsplit); these slides are the "Acuity Suppression," "Stereo Test," and "Basic Fusion." The remaining seven are variable (split); these can be set to compensate for the patient's horizontal angle of deviation to establish sensory and motor fusion. Fusional vergence skills can then be increased with sliding, step, jump, tromboning, and isometric vergence training techniques. In cases of esotropia and esophoria, the emphasis is on developing and expanding suppression-free, fusional divergence ranges, and step divergence reflexes that are fast and accurate. Some valuable attributes of the Vectograms are their variety and flexibility. They can be used with many types of patients (strabismic and phoric, either eso and exo) in many ways and at various viewing distances. Because of their expense and vulnerability to damage, most vision therapists utilize them for in-office training. Split Minivectograms (horizontal and vertical) are also available and appropriate for home training purposes.

Tranaglyphs are sets of translucent vergence training slides, printed in red and green, which were introduced and popularized by Vodnoy. The patient wears red-green filters to give mutual exclusion of the images. Because of the white illuminated background, the red-filtered time. Training in both horizontal directions ensures that the zone of clear, single, binocular vision is expanded and not merely shifted in the base-in direction. When diplopia occurs, the demand is reduced sufficiently to allow recovery of fusion; the patient continues making small step vergence movements for a minute or more before the divergence demand is again increased. Smoothness of disparation with lack of suppression is an important goal as is expanding the vergence ranges. The patient notes each blur (if any is perceived), break, and recovery point in each direction and records the highest values during the training interval of about 10 minutes. Split Tranaglyphs are used is a similar manner. When progress has been made with the Mother Goose slide, increased sensory fusion demands can be introduced with the Spirangle Vectogram (Figure 13-10b). This split Vectogram contains subtle stereopsis and suppression clues that challenge most patients. The goal is to achieve a normal range of fusional convergence and divergence that is free of suppression.

Later in the training program, other split Vectograms can be added (e.g., using the Dual Polachrome Illuminated Trainer). The top target is set at the patient's maximum divergence limit and the bottom target is set at the convergence limit. The patient is then instructed to fixate rapidly from one Vectogram to the other, fusing each in turn to train the speed of step vergences, i.e., vergence facility.

Step vergences can also be trained using the 50 series of nonvariable Tranaglyphs. This series of sports action figures has a different vergence demand for each figure. The first card in the series consists of four figures having the following demands: 1^Δ BI, 1^Δ BO, 2^Δ BO, and 4^Δ BO. The other figures in the series increase in vergence demand by 2^Δ steps to a maximum of 30^Δ (Figure 13-11). Convergence demands can be switched to divergence demands by simply turning the rigid vinyl card over or by reversing the left-right placement of the red and green filters worn by the patient. Also, flipper prisms can be used for step vergence training (Figure 13-12).

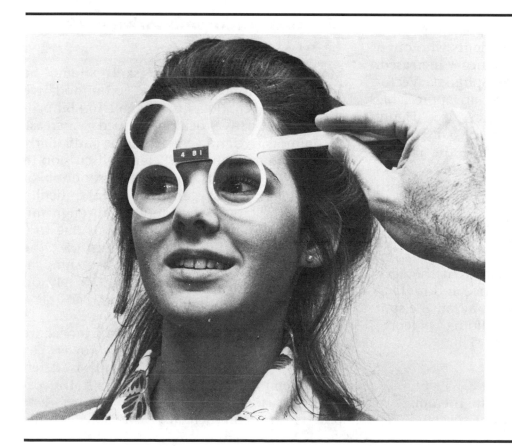

FIGURE 13-12—Flipper prisms for expanding the range of motor fusion.

For esotropic or esophoric patients, the therapist selects a BO demand target that can be easily fused. A second target with less BO demand is set in the holder above the first target. The patient alternates fixation between the two targets as quickly as possible, fusing each in turn, while monitoring for suppression. If suppression occurs, the patient should break it by blinking and/or moving closer to the targets. The patient is instructed to count the number of fixation cycles. Twenty cycles are often prescribed and the patient attempts to better his time with each set. The therapist prescribes as many sets as the patient can complete within a 10-minute training session. The size of the vergence steps can be increased as the patient's proficiency improves. The last stage of training with vectographic or tranaglyphic targets is when the patient can make steps from a large BO demand to his maximum BI demand with good facility and without suppression. This phasic vergence training technique is particularly effective since the targets have stereopsis content and good suppression controls.

Divergence Walk-Aways T13.9

Split Vectograms and Tranaglyphs are particularly helpful for DI and BE patients who often lose fusion as the fixation distance is increased. A good pair of targets is the Spirangle Vectogram, which is large and has an appreciable stereopsis effect at far distances (see Figure 13-11b). The base-in demand should be increased maximally at near while the patient maintains fusion. As the patient slowly walks away, the spiral figure appears more in depth and the base-in demand decreases theoretically and should make fusion easier for the patient. For example, 12^Δ BI at 40 cm translates to only 6^Δ BI at 80 cm and only 3^Δ at 160 cm, and so on. Patients are delighted to realize that they can fuse at far; this builds confidence and motivation. Once the patient is fusing at far, the split targets are further separated (sliding vergence) to increase fusional divergence skill.

Projected BI Slides T13.10

Using an overhead projector, the therapist can project split Vectograms onto a special screen for fusional vergence training. The images must fall on a metallic surface (or special vinyl material) so that the polarization qualities are not lost. The patient wears crossed-polarizing filters as the target separation is increased in the base-in direction. In esotropia, particularly the DI and BE types, the targets are initially aligned to the patient's subjective angle of deviation, a base-out setting. This procedure is ideal for training sliding vergence at far due to the fusional lock of stereopsis. Besides sliding vergence, step (using two pairs of targets at the same distance) and jump (alternate near-far viewing) vergence procedures can be used to build the range and facility of fusional divergence.

Tranaglyphic projection may be a more practical choice for some vision therapists since they are printed in red and green and do not require any special surface for projection other than a blank wall. The Bernell 500 or 600 Tranaglyph Kits are good choices for this procedure. These split tranaglyphic procedures are carried out in the same manner as with split Vectograms.

Binocular Accommodative Rock T13.11

Monocular accommodative skills should be adequate before binocular accommodative training is given. (Refer to Chapter 16.) Binocular accommodative rock can be used to increase accommodative and vergence skills particularly with esophoric patients. (Refer to discussion in Chapter 2.) Patients with basic esophoria or convergence excess generally have difficulty clearing the target when looking through minus lenses. Binocular facility is poor due to a limited range of fusional divergence (i.e., the eso deviation increases with the accommodative stimulus and the patient has to rely on fusional divergence to maintain single and clear binocular vision).

The therapist should start this procedure with small amounts of minus lens power, i.e., −0.50 D to −1.00 D. The amount is determined empirically by working with the patient. Equal plus and minus flipper lens powers are commercially available or the therapist can prepare unequal powers as needed using a clip demonstrator lens holder and trial case lenses. The nearpoint target should have suppression controls appropriate for the patient's level of sensory fusion. Various targets can be used for this purpose, e.g., strip reading bars, Minivectograms, and Mini-Tranaglyphs (see Figure 16-6). The technique requires the patient to flip the lenses (keeping them horizontally aligned with the eyes), fuse and clear the target, note the suppression controls, and build the speed of alternation. The lenses are not flipped until the target is perfectly clear and the suppression controls are present. The patient, or therapist, records the number of cycles within a prescribed time interval (1 to 2 minutes) or the amount of time the patient takes to complete an assigned number of cycles. These numbers are logged to chart progress. With short rest periods of about 30 seconds between sets, the patient continues this exercise for 10 minutes each day until proficiency is achieved. For nonpresbyopic adults, the binocular flipper rate should eventually be 20 cycles per minute using ±1.50 D flippers. Using ±2.00 D flippers, children aged 8 years and older should achieve at least 10 cycles per minute. We have found these training goals to be realistic and effective in preventing regression of vergence skills. Binocular accommodative rock is a procedure easily combined with other vergence training procedures, e.g., with Vectograms (T13.8), Brock string (T13.6), or Aperture-Rule Trainer (T13.13).

Vergence Rock Techniques (Flipper prisms) T13.12

Flipper prisms or loose prisms are effective for training step vergences at far or near either in the office or at home (see Figure 13-12). If the eso patient is initially unable to fuse when a base-in demand is introduced, base-out prism compensation may be necessary until divergence ranges are developed to meet step (phasic) demands. The important rule to remember in vision training is that the demand must be within the patient's capability; the demand is increased only as the patient's ability increases.

Likewise, as the step vergence range increases, the power difference in BO and BI prism flips can be made greater. Speed and range of vergence facility are then trained. The goal is to have vergence facility and stamina that at least meet the criteria presented in Chapter 2 (5 cycles per minute with 8^ΔBI-8^ΔBO at near and 4^ΔBI-8^ΔBO at far). Vergence rock can often be combined with other training techniques, e.g., Brock string (T13.6), peripheral fusion rings (T13.7), and Vectograms or Tranaglyphs (T13.8-13.10).

Bar reading (T12.10) with prism rock is a demanding exercise that is often given in the final stages of training and as a retainer exercise. A loose prism of low power is held by the patient using the thumb and index finger to grasp the bottom of it. With the bar strips placed vertically over the reading material and the prism held before one eye, the patient reads across the line noting any suppression and trying to break it by blinking. After reading each line, the patient shifts the prism to the other eye with one quick movement of the hand. The prism, therefore, changes direction from BI to BO. Reading in this manner is continued for a 10-minute period. With practice, patients can learn to read passages for meaning without thinking about sensory or motor fusion. The prism amount can be increased each week as needed.

Aperture-Rule Trainer (Double Aperture) T13.13

The Vodnoy Aperture-Rule Trainer (ART) is a good instrument for both office and home training. A double aperture is used to create base in demands (Figures 13-13 and 13-14). This procedure is very difficult for most CE and BE patients, because of a significant eso deviation at near and because the aperture acts as a septum, which is dissociative. For this reason, this instrument is usually not introduced at the beginning of a vision therapy program. The patient is instructed to look at the pair of targets through the double aperture. The pair of targets is placed at the "O" position and remains there throughout the training procedure; the distance is 40 cm. This is actually orthopic fusion

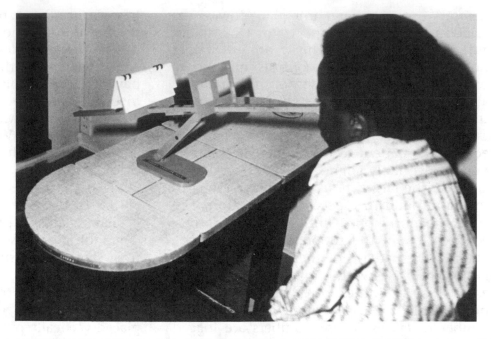

FIGURE 13-13—Double aperture septum used on the Aperture-Rule Trainer for base-in demands.

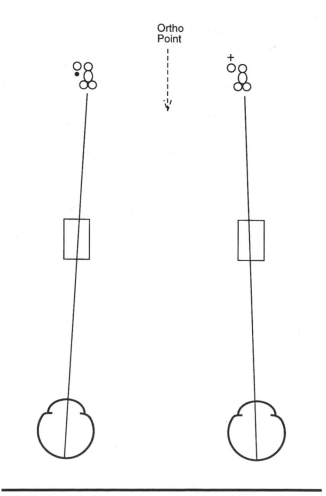

FIGURE 13-14—Fusional divergence demand with two apertures.

(discussed in the next section); however, the ART has the dissociative factor of a septum. If there is difficulty fusing the first few cards, the patient is instructed to look above the apertures to a pointer stick placed at the end of the rule, or farther away if necessary. Fixation on the pointer helps to diverge the eyes so the patient can initially fuse the pair of targets even though they may appear blurred. Plus-addition lenses can be used so the patient can see the fused target clearly.

There are 12 pairs of targets increasing in separation, ranging in demand from 2.5^Δ BI (card AP1) to 30^Δ BI (card AP12). The prismatic demand is calculated simply by multiplying the target number by a factor of 2.5. For example, card AP2 would create a 5^Δ demand. The goal is for the patient to progress to cards with higher step prism demands while perceiving all suppression clues. Vodnoy[8] suggested that for building divergence, card AP7 represents a reasonable goal for most esophoric patients, but many patients can go higher. The therapist or patient must remember to move the septum slider (with the apertures) appropriately with each change of target so that the septum does not block the view of either eye. For example, card #6 requires that the septum be on the

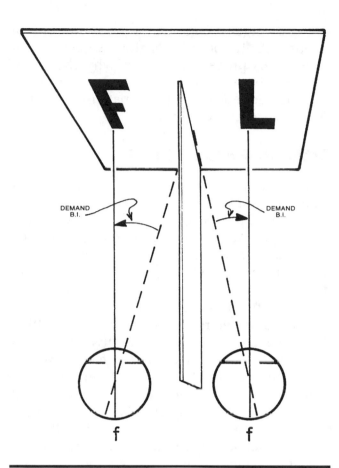

FIGURE 13-15—Top view of a Remy Separator illustrating base-in vergence demand.

for antisuppression training, it is also useful for eso therapy since this technique presents base-in vergence demands (Figure 13-15). Because there is no optical system involved, the vergence demand can be figured quite simply. Suppose the fixation distance is 30 cm. If the separation between the F and L is 6 cm, the fusional divergence demand is 20^Δ.

This is calculated as follows:

1. At a 30 cm (or 3 decimeters) fixation distance, every 3 mm equals 1 pd (i.e., the decimeter rule)
2. Convert 6 cm to 60 mm
3. To find prism diopters, divide 60 by 3.
4. Therefore, the BI demand is 20^Δ.

marker designated as position 6 on the scale of the rule.

An effective jump vergence technique using the Aperture-Rule Trainer is to have the patient converge and focus on a target placed centrally on the septum and then diverge to the targets seen through the apertures. These back and forth fixations should be as rapid as possible. A divergence target almost at the patient's limit is chosen. The patient records the time for the number of cycles achieved within 2 minutes and is given instructions to repeat this procedure at least five times each day. Suppression should be monitored and broken, if it occurs, before continuing with this jump technique.

Remy Separator T13.14

The Remy Separator is an excellent training instrument that utilizes a septum. As in T12.6

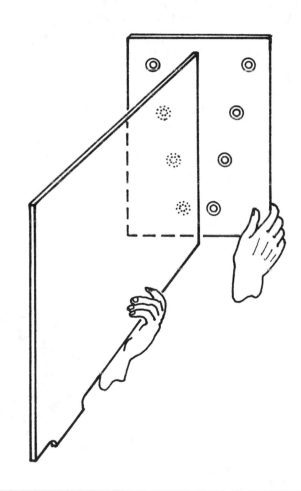

FIGURE 13-16—Custom-made training instrument based on the principle of the Remy Separator. An ordinary file folder is used as a septum as the patient views a Keystone Colored Circles Card. The card should be transparent initially; later an opaque card can be used as fusional divergence improves with training.

The BI demand can be increased by making the target separation greater and decreased by making the separation less. It should be noted that the eso deviation must be overcome by the patient, in addition to the base-in demand of the target from the ortho position. If the patient has an esophoria of 10^Δ at 30 cm fixation distance, he would have to diverge a total of 30^Δ to fuse the F and L into an E in this example. At first, most esotropic and many esophoric patients cannot perform this procedure without the aid of either plus-add lenses (to reduce accommodative convergence) or base-out prism compensation. These optical aids are useful in the beginning, but the patient should be gradually weaned from them as soon as possible. Any set of fusion targets, either flat fusion or stereopsis demands, can be used with the Remy Separator.

A convenient and inexpensive Remy Separator for home training is the use of a septum and a "Lifesaver" card (Figure 13-16). The patient views the card as though performing orthopic fusion in free space while the septum is in the midline and perpendicular to the card, a difficult challenge to fusion. Once fusion is established on the least demanding set of red-green circles, the patient attempts to make step vergence responses to the other targets. Fu-

sional divergence requires a great amount of "mental effort" because of the dissociative nature of this procedure. This is why the Remy Separator is introduced toward the end of the training sequence, after the patient has mastered the easier techniques.

Orthopic Fusion T13.15

A difficult training procedure for most esotropic and esophoric patients is orthopic fusion. This is done in free space using targets printed on transparent material, for example, Keystone Eccentric Circles (Figure 13-17). Before this technique is introduced, the patient should have developed fairly normal divergence ranges with other training procedures. Orthopic fusion refers to fusing targets on which the visual axes of the two eyes diverge beyond the plane of the fixated targets, yet the images are maintained in clear focus. When using Eccentric Circles, the right eye fixates the right target and the left eye fixates the left target. One way to help the patient with this difficult vergence demand is to have him hold the targets at arm's length with the A's together. The patient looks through the *transparent* cards at a blank wall. If the eyes are properly aligned

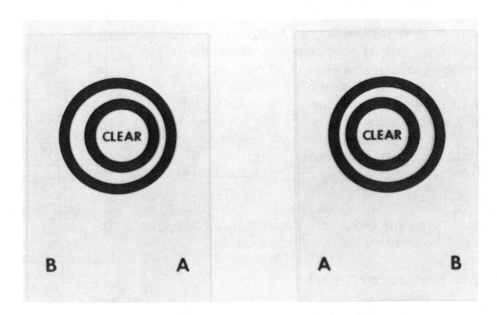

FIGURE 13-17—Keystone Eccentric Circles.

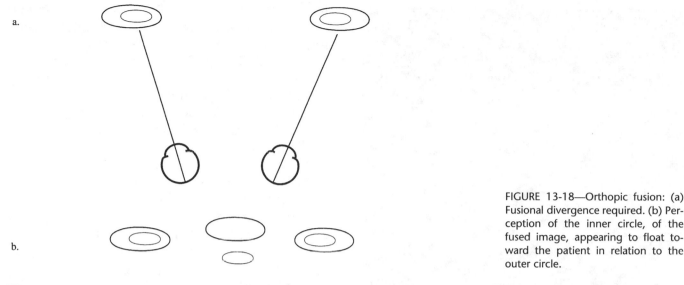

FIGURE 13-18—Orthopic fusion: (a) Fusional divergence required. (b) Perception of the inner circle, of the fused image, appearing to float toward the patient in relation to the outer circle.

with the Eccentric Circles, the patient will notice a fused image centered between two unfused images. Stereopsis should be perceived if the fused target is seen clearly. The smaller inner circle should appear to float in front of the larger outer circle (Figure 13-18). (Refer to Chapter 1 for discussion of principles of stereopsis and the effects of crossed and uncrossed disparity.) Patients often need the help of a plus add to see the fused image clearly. Sometimes base-out prism also helps the patient get started so that orthopic fusion can be learned. A training goal is to wean the patient from these optical compensations.

When orthopic fusion is established, the targets can be slowly separated to induce a sliding divergence demand. The patient uses "mental effort" to relax convergence and maintain fusion as the cards are separated. The patient smoothly diverges the eyes to the limit of his range and, then, decreases the demand appropriately. We recommend patients be instructed to build vergences with such cards by using 2-minute training intervals. Since eyestrain may be induced, rest periods between the intervals can be at the patient's discretion. Five sets of 2-minute training intervals would complete the daily requirement for this procedure. The patient and clinician should not expect large increases in the base-in range with this technique; however, improved ease, smoothness, and speed indicate progress. Other targets are also convenient for home training, e.g., two thumbs or two coins. The drawback, however, is that there is no stereopsis clue to indicate that the targets have been fused correctly. For example, if chiastopic fusion (discussed in Chapter 14) is mistakenly done rather that orthopic fusion, the patient would perceive the inner ring floating farther away in relation to the outer ring. This perception indicates the targets have been fused incorrectly and the sliding technique is increasing convergence rather than divergence. The correct perception of stereopsis during orthopic fusion training should be closely monitored by both the doctor and the patient.

Computerized Divergence Procedures T13.16

Computerized vision therapy programs have become widely used for a variety of vision problems, including fusional vergence training. Many programs employ complementary colors for mutual exclusion of each target. An anaglyphic program may have red and blue targets that are displayed on a video screen while the patient wears red-blue spectacles of matching colors. A special feature of such programs for

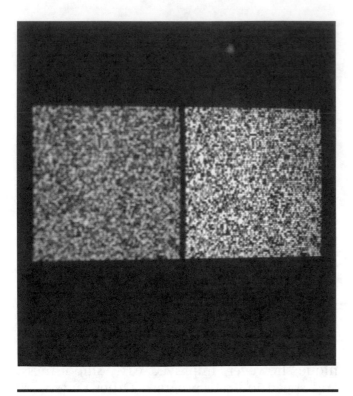

FIGURE 13-19—Example of random dot targets for vergence training with stereopsis on the Opti-Mum Computer Vision Therapy program.

fusional divergence training is the use of random dot stereograms.[9] (See Figure 13-19.) They have no monocular clues to stereopsis and the forms can be seen only if there is binocular fusion. The stereopsis image randomly appears in one of four locations, up, down, left, or right. The patient must fuse the target to indicate the correct position of the stereoscopic image using a joy stick. The targets can be disparated smoothly at various speeds or in steps of various magnitudes to build vergence ranges. Children and adults appreciate the game features of such programs. We recommend these programs because of the patient interest and motivation they stimulate. An excellent program (using red and green colors) designed by Ludlam is the Opti-Mum Computer Vision Therapy produced by Learning Frontiers, Inc. Bernell corporation also offers vision therapy software.

Computer Orthoptics by Dr. Cooper introduced a powerful computer combined with high-speed liquid crystal filters for mutual cancellation of targets for the right and left eye. The patient wears these instead of red and blue filters. The liquid crystal filters alternately darken at 60 Hz, allowing for stabilized binocular viewing. High resolution and color stimuli can be presented. Our patients report being aware, however, of a flickering background but usually not of significant annoyance.

Major et al.[2] found that base-in ranges could be significantly improved by using computerized tonic and isometric divergence demands. The computer is a welcomed development as it can ease the labor intensive in-office practice of vision therapy and make it more affordable to patients than in the past. Many of the procedures discussed earlier in this chapter can be applied with computerized programs for improving fusional divergence ranges, facility, and stamina.

CASE MANAGEMENT AND EXAMPLES

Convergence Excess Esotropia

Management Principles

Convergence excess (CE) esotropia and esophoria are characterized by a nearpoint deviation that is substantially larger than at farpoint. If the patient is phoric or intermittently strabismic at near, visual symptoms may be reported (e.g., intermittent blur, diplopia, asthenopia, and inefficient reading). Many CE cases have considerable suppression at near; therefore, symptoms of discomfort do not always result.[10] Convergence excess is usually caused by an abnormally high AC/A with inadequate fusional divergence. However, a "nonaccommodative" type of CE was reported by von Noorden and Avilla[11] In their series, there was a larger esotropia at near compared with far, but plus addition lenses did not reduce the nearpoint deviation as would be expected in the case of high AC/A. They proposed that increased tonic vergence somehow resulted in the larger deviation at near. The gradient AC/A was low or normal. Although this "nonaccommodative" type of CE esotropia does not benefit from wearing bifocals, it can be successfully managed in many cases with vision training and strabismus surgery.

Most patients having a high AC/A type of convergence excess, on the other hand, show esotropia at near that can usually be treated successfully. Our vision therapy approach involves fully correcting the refractive error, prescribing appropriate bifocals to control the near deviation, and initiating a vigorous vision training program. Amblyopia and ARC usually do not develop in CE cases that maintain fusion at far. This is one reason why these patients generally have a better prognosis than BE esotropes who tend to have a constant deviation, particularly at far.

The effect of plus–addition lenses can be remarkable in cases of CE since the AC/A is high. For example, a patient with a 60 mm IPD with 6^Δ of esotropia at 6m and 16^Δ at 40 cm has a calculated AC/A of 10/1 and probably a gradient AC/A of 7/1 or 8/1. (Refer to Chapter 3.) This high AC/A implies that for every diopter of plus lens addition that is worn, the eso deviation is reduced by at least 7^Δ. Therefore, a +1.00 D addition would cause the deviation at near to be reduced to about 9^Δ eso, and +2.00 D addition to about 2^Δ eso. These are theoretical values, since the esotropic patient does not always respond to the plus additions mechanistically. The clinician must directly observe and measure how the patient responds to plus-addition lenses at near before a lens prescription is written. We recommend wide flat-top segments, 28 to 35 mm, which give good optics for near work. Caloroso and Rouse[12] recommend the top of the bifocal segment be placed at midpupil for children under 5 years old, because children tend to look over the top of the segments. For children, aged 5 to 8 years, the top should be at the lower margin of the pupil; for older patients, the segment height would be at the lower lid margin. They also advocate progressive addition lenses (PAL) for the sake of cosmesis and promoting fusion at intermediate distances.[12] The top of the PAL segment should be placed 4 mm above the center of the pupil for children under 8 years of age and 2 mm above for older patients. We concur with their advice.

In cases of accommodative esotropia, especially CE cases, there is usually the need for active vision training to break suppression and build vergence ranges and facility. Bifocals only correct the nearpoint deviation in CE at one particular viewing distance, whereas patients habitually use many nearpoint distances in real life situations. The deviation, therefore, can easily decompensate if sensory and motor fusion are weak. Von Noorden et al.[13] reported the best long-term results were achieved by those patients who underwent fusional vergence training in addition to bifocal management. We believe the most effective management of accommodative esotropia includes a relative short program of vision training to maximize sensory and motor fusion, then the prescription of retainer exercises, and regular progress visits, once or twice a year, to ensure successful long-term results.

The emphasis of the vision training is to break the deep suppression often found at near, even with a bifocal add, and to extend the motor fusion ranges to compensate for an eso deviation at all nearpoint viewing distances. Specific training techniques, used in combination with a bifocal, which we have found particularly effective with CE cases, include Brock string and beads (13.6), Vectograms and Tranaglyphs (T13.8), binocular accommodative rock with minus lenses (T13.11), and vergence rock techniques (T13.12). Push-up training should be emphasized with all these techniques to extend the range of sensory and motor fusion to very near distances, within 10 cm.

Convergence excess patients with a very high AC/A are usually difficult to manage successfully with adds, even when vision training is included. This is because such CE patients tend to redevelop suppression at near and regress quickly.[10] In those cases where the AC/A is over $12^\Delta/1D$, the potential for needed strabismus surgery (a bimedial recession) as part of a vision therapy program significantly increases. (Refer to Chapter 7.)

In most cases of CE when fusion can be established with bifocals at some near distance, vision training usually takes from 2 to 4 months to complete. These cases can often be managed on a home training basis with weekly office testing and training visits. A good retainer exercise is bar reading with prism (T13.12) since it monitors for suppression and trains the reflex aspects of fusional vergence. Fifteen to 20 minutes of bar reading with prism, once a week, is usually sufficient to prevent regression of trained binocular skills.

Case Example

A 4-year-old female arrived with her parents for her first complete eye and vision examination. The parents reported they saw her left eye cross several times a day when she looked carefully at nearpoint toys and other objects. They had noticed this for about 6 months, but it was becoming more frequent. There was no family history of strabismus or other major eye problems, nor was there any birth complication. Questions regarding general health, trauma, medications, allergies, and development, were answered all in the negative.

The relevant clinical findings follow:

A cycloplegic refraction (1% Cyclogyl gtt) revealed a moderate amount of hyperopic astigmatism:

OD: +3.25 −1.25 x 090   10/10
OS: +4.25 −1.75 x 090   10/20

With the prescription lenses in place, visual acuity testing using Lighthouse cards indicated slightly reduced far vision of the left eye, equivalent to 20/40 (6/12). Near acuity testing using the AO picture card indicated about the same difference between the eyes. Wearing lenses to correct the ametropia, the patient had 2^Δ esophoria at far and a comitant, constant, unilateral, left esotropia of 25^Δ at 25 cm (her working distance) when she focused on a nearpoint target. No oculomotor restrictions or overactions were found. The patient showed central suppression of the left eye at far and uncrossed diplopia at near by Worth Dot testing that suggested NRC. The eye health examination proved negative. The diagnosis was uncorrected hyperopic astigmatism, convergence excess esotropia, and shallow amblyopia of the left eye.

The parents agreed to follow the recommended vision therapy plan:

1. Full correction of the refractive error with spectacles for constant wear.

2. A +2.00 D add for near was given in bifocal form to help control the nearpoint deviation due to her high AC/A.
3. Direct occlusion (right eye) for 3 hours a day for 1 month to stimulate the development of acuity in the amblyopic eye. An Elastoplast occluder was worn.
4. Anaglyphic fusion games (T13.5) were encouraged during the child's play time with her mother.

At a 1-month progress evaluation, the patient's condition had improved considerably. The little girl had complied well with the wearing of the spectacles and the patch, but had only occasionally played the anaglyphic games, although she liked them. The parents had not noticed a crossed eye except on rare occasions when she looked over the bifocal segments at near and when she removed the spectacles. No change in the refractive error was found. The corrected visual acuities were almost equal: OD 10/10; OS 10/12. With the bifocal spectacles, the deviation measured 1^Δ esophoria at far and 5^Δ esophoria in downgaze through the add. She demonstrated normal reflex fusion responses to a 4^Δ BI prism at near. Only occasional central suppression of the left eye was found at far. The parents were pleased with the vision therapy results. They were instructed to continue to patch the right eye 3 hours a day, on weekends only, to reinforce the improved acuity. The child and mother were instructed in the use of an anaglyphic reading bar (T12.10) for antisuppression training with picture books. Another progress evaluation was scheduled in 3 months.

Basic Esotropia

Management Principles

Most cases of basic esotropia (normal AC/A), have an associated accommodative component that requires full optical correction. Sometimes esotropia is caused solely by uncorrected hyperopia. Once the patient adapts to wearing the cycloplegic spectacle or contact lens correction, a strabismus may not be found. Esotropic patients should be encouraged to wear their glasses full-time and to put up with the minor inconvenience of farpoint blur during the spectacle adaptation period. Latent hyperopia may take several weeks to relax in some cases. Even if the strabismus is not completely corrected, the deviation may be significantly reduced, thus improving the prospects for success with other therapy approaches.[14]

Since most cases of BE of moderate to large magnitude are constant from an early age, the doctor must frequently treat amblyopia and ARC to effect a functional cure of strabismus. Chapters 10 and 11 are dedicated to these discussions. Once these sensory adaptations are basically resolved, the clinician establishes normal sensory fusion at some position in space, usually at near, with optics. Spectacle prisms, Fresnel prisms, centration-point add, plus-add bifocals (based on the AC/A), or some combination of these are the optical tools available for this purpose. If sensory fusion cannot be achieved at some distance by these means, then the patient wears a patch on one eye for all distances. When optical alignment can be achieved at near in BE cases with a combination of prisms and add, but not at far, the top portion of one lens is occluded with tape or plastic. While in a vision therapy program, the patient is not allowed to "practice his strabismus." The next step toward a functional cure requires vigorous, usually in-office, vision training.

There are innumerable ways that vision training can be programmed. We present here an example of one training program for basic esotropia that we think is effective in many cases. Only a brief discussion of each technique can be given; the reader should refer to other sections for details. When possible, we start vision training at near distances in the open environment, as recommended by Brock,[15] expanding sensory and motor fusion as much as possible, then work to extend the learned skills to the farpoint. Wearing an add and/or prisms for training at the centration point, the patient attempts to break suppression using a strong stimulus if necessary, e.g., Brock string and beads (T13.6), except that two penlights are used rather than two beads. The patient attempts to make small vergence jumps between lights recognizing physiological diplopia at all

times. With progress, the therapist replaces the lights with beads, but initially they are directly illuminated with penlights while the room illumination is dim. The Mother Goose Vectogram with its large suppression controls is introduced at the centration point and vergence ranges are expanded in both horizontal directions (T13.8). With good suppression controls and stereopsis clues in the visual field, vergence rock techniques (T13.12) are introduced to build reflexive step vergences. As binocular skills increase, the amount of plus-addition lenses and prism compensation is reduced and the training distance is increased. The walk-away technique (13.9) can be used to extend the training environment to farther distances from the patient. Projected Vectograms and Tranaglyphs (T13.10) and peripheral fusion rings (T13.7) help consolidate sensory and motor fusion at the farpoint. The Mirror Stereoscope (T13.2) and the Brewster stereoscope (T13.3 and 13.4) are excellent initially for home training. Other techniques should also be introduced for the sake of variety, patient interest, and generalization of learned skills. If the patient does not progress as expected using the above techniques, amblyoscopic divergence training (T13.1) can be intensively applied in an attempt to establish basic fusion.

Suppression is broken within the maximum vergence ranges that can be trained at all viewing distances. Vergence facility and stamina, besides the perception of stereopsis, are all increased. These are the initial therapeutic goals even if the esotropia is not totally resolved with training.

Alignment of the strabismus comes with the training of fusional divergence in some cases, prism and add compensation in many, and others require strabismus surgery. After full correction of the refractive error, the magnitude of the resultant deviation usually determines whether or not an operation is required. When that angle measures 20^Δ or greater, even in cases having NRC, an operation is often necessary if the goal is clear, comfortable, single, binocular vision. We have seen patients with 20^Δ of esophoria with no symptoms and good stereopsis, but they are indeed rare. Occasionally with vision training, there is an apparrent spontaneous reduction in the angle of deviation. Trained fusional vergence can become like a conditioned reflex and will not dissipate quickly with occlusion, as on a conventional cover test. Reductions in the angle of deviation following vergence training, as revealed by cover test, can be transitory following training and may not represent the permanent dissociated tonic vergence position of the eyes. In many cases, the doctor will easily determine which patients require surgery and which do not, after 1 to 2 months of vision training. The rate of skills improvement, the motivation and compliance of the patient in vision training, and the size of the resultant deviation are prime indicators. There are also cases, however, in which this issue is not easily resolved. The patient or parents may be extraordinarily determined to avoid an operation. Progress may be slow, but steady. The patient has fusion most of the time following training, but comfort and visual efficiency may not be acceptable, as in a case of esophoria of 20^Δ or greater. Should training be continued or the surgeon consulted? We have an arbitrary guideline to deal with this difficult question. If the strabismic patient has not achieved a satisfactory binocular vision result within a 6-month period of active vision training with full compliance, we suggest a surgical evaluation and support the surgeon's recommendation in most cases. (See Chapter 6 for a discussion of surgical considerations.) Postsurgical care would proceed as previously described (in the previous section on vision therapy sequence) in this chapter. Six-month progress evaluations are advisable in cases of BE managed with vision therapy, especially if amblyopia has been part of the condition. We usually recommend bar reading with prism rock (T13.12) as a retainer exercise, once a week, to prevent regression; the retainer training schedule, however, depends on the findings of each progress evaluation.

Case Example

The following case is of a 9-year-old boy with basic esotropia of approximately 11^Δ at near and far. The patient had been given the following lens prescription:

O.D. +3.25 –0.25 x 95 with
3^Δ base-out 20/25+2
O.S. +3.75 –0.25 x 90 with 3^Δ
base-out 20/25-1
+2.25 add (25 mm straight-top bifocal)

Through the distance portion of the lenses the diagnosis of the deviation was as follows: comitant, constant, alternating (right eye preferred), esotropia with central suppression, NRC, only some peripheral sensory fusion with central suppression, and poor motor fusion ranges.

A series of 12 vision therapy visits was prescribed along with home vision training. Procedures included: cheiroscopic tracing, loose BI prism training, vectographic training to improve stereopsis, various antisuppression techniques, Mirror Stereoscope BI training, centration-point training, major amblyoscope for suppression and motor fusion training, monocular and binocular accommodative rock, and Root Rings for peripheral stereopsis with fusion walk-aways. Progress evaluation showed improvement in stereopsis from 550 to 300 seconds of arc; increased motor fusion range, improved from 3^Δ to 7^Δ (being able to fuse from 6^ΔBO to 1^ΔBI). Central suppression was less deep and only foveal (previously macular in extent).

Additional vision therapy was recommended. Another series of 12 office visits and home training included: Pola-Mirror and Vis-A-Vis (no mirror but patient and therapist wearing crossed-polarizing filters), pencil pushups, fusion walk-aways, 3-dot card, Keystone Eccentric Circles, Brock string, major amblyoscope, and Polachrome Illuminated Trainer with Vectograms. In the major amblyoscope the BI break was 12^Δ with recovery of 10^Δ BI; BO break was 12^Δ with 9^Δ recovery. In the open environment with vectographic slides the BI break was 11^Δ with 9^Δ recovery; BO break was 31^Δ with 24^Δ recovery. Another series of 12 visits was prescribed, and many of the vision training techniques mentioned above were repeated. Based on cycloplegic and manifest refractive findings, a new prescription for spectacle lenses, including Fresnel prisms, was given:

O.D. +3.75 –1.00 x 90 with 3^Δ base-out
O.S. +3.75 –1.00 x 80 with 3^Δ base-out
+2.00 add (Executive bifocal)

Visual acuity was 20/20 (6/6) in each eye. Stereoacuity had improved to 60 seconds of arc (contoured targets). There was no strabismus on the cover test with the above spectacles but a residual esophoria of 2^Δ prism diopters was found when testing through these lenses (thus a total of 8^Δ eso deviation). At near the patient was orthophoric through the bifocal additions. The patient was able to maintain fusion for several minutes without the aid of the base-out prisms, but could not do so when the hyperopic lens correction was removed. The patient was advised to continue wearing the bifocal spectacles with prism. Subsequent progress checks indicated that the patient passed all 15 cards of the Keystone Visual Skills Test and had suppression-free ranges from 8^ΔBI to 42^ΔBO on the major amblyoscope. On phorometry testing the NRC was 17^Δ, PRC 31^Δ, and NRA and PRA were normal. The spectacle frame needed to be replaced and a prescription for 6^Δ BO was continued and the prescription remained the same in all other respects.

While there had been no significant cosmetic problem in this case, there was a functional cure of the esotropia according to the criteria of Flom (Chapter 6). The patient was happy and expressed the feeling that his successful results of vision therapy were worth the time and effort.

Divergence Insufficiency Esotropia

Divergence insufficiency (DI) is a relatively infrequent vergence anomaly in which the eso deviation at far is greater than the eso deviation at near, a low AC/A case. The characteristics of DI esophoria were discussed in Chapter 3. The same principles apply to DI esotropia except that more intensive and extensive vision therapy is required for the strabismic condition, particularly if the magnitude of deviation at far is large. Differential diagnosis is important in cases of DI as discussed in Chapter 7. A divergence paralysis originating from a midbrain lesion can sometimes imitate DI esotropia.

Many patients with DI usually have NRC, therefore BO prisms can possibly be of benefit. A major problem with prism compensation for the farpoint eso deviation, however, is that the nearpoint deviation is consequently increased in an exo direction. Some patients, therefore, should wear the prism spectacles only for dedicated far viewing and switch to another pair without prism for reading. Others may find it disturbing and difficult to adapt to constantly changing glasses. A temporary solution might be to attach an appropriate power Fresnel BO prism to only the top half of the lenses. Base-out prism may be prescribed, with caution, for some patients not needing more then 10^Δ of compensation at far. Convergence training is sometiimes necessary because of the induced nearpoint exo deviation, but more importantly, fusional divergence training to help control any remaining eso deviation at the farpoint is most definitely required in such cases.

Increasing the fusional divergence range at far with vision training is not easy. Progress is often slow; asthenopic symptoms frequently intensify. If the far eso deviation exceeds 20^Δ, strabismus surgery (most likely a bilateral resection) often is necessary for a satisfactory outcome. Our approach to vision training in DI cases is similar to that for BE patients. Sensory and motor fusion is enhanced initially at near where the patient has best control of the deviation. As the patient's fusion skills increase, the training distance is also increased toward the farpoint (e.g., Tranaglyph walk-aways T13.9). Finally, large stereo targets (e.g., peripheral fusion rings T13.7 and projected Vectograms T13.10) are introduced at the farpoint to help the patient make the required divergence movements without suppression. In-office and home training may take 3 to 4 months. We have found that rigorous retainer exercises are usually needed to maintain the results of divergence training. We suggest using either a loose prism or flippers for vergence rock (T13.12) combined with a television trainer. The goals are to build divergence facility while monitoring suppression for 30 minutes, at least once a week.

Microesotropia

Management Principles

Microtropic patients generally have a stable binocular condition and do not complain of visual symptoms. ARC and reduced stereopsis are expected and many have amblyopia. If the amblyopia in these cases is worse than 20/30, we often recommend a short term patching program to improve it. The goal is to ensure that the patient has good visual acuity in each eye even though there is no central fusion. Other than treating amblyopia (Chapter 10), we rarely try to cure the microtropia unless the patient has asthenopic symptoms. We have found that in cases of symptomatic microtropia, symptoms often abate with standard sensory and motor fusion training. Prisms usually do not help because of prism adaptation, but a plus-add may if accommodative dysfunctions exist. Suppression can be broken with a TV trainer (T12.8) and Brock string and beads (T13.6). Vergence ranges are increased with sliding Vectograms (T13.8), the Mirror Stereoscope (T13.2), and the major amblyoscope (T13.1) if necessary. But in most cases, after symptoms are resolved, the microtropia as detected by unilateral cover test persists. Patients, nevertheless, usually consider this a satisfactory result and we accept their judgment. These patients have enhanced peripheral sensory and motor fusion and have resolved their visual symptoms.

There are some cases, however, in which the microesotropia is not associated with ARC. In these cases, patients often experience intermittent diplopia and asthenopia. This type of microtropia represents an intermediate condition between esophoria with fixation disparity and a manifest esotropia. These patients with microesotropia often respond well to prism compensation, plus adds, and antisuppression and divergence training as the following case example demonstrates.

Case Example

A 16-year-old male presented with the complaint of blurred vision at far with his myopic spectacles and wanted to have contact lenses. He was more comfortable reading without his glasses and occasionally noticed double vision when he was tired. Only pertinent data regarding binocular status are included in this case example.

Habitual lenses and acuities were:
O.D. −3.00 DS 20/40 (6/12) J1 at 40 cm
O.S. −3.00 DS 20/40 (6/12) J1 at 40 cm

With the patient wearing his habitual lens correction, the unilateral cover test showed a constant, unilateral, right, esotropia of 3^Δ at 6 m and a constant, unilateral, right esotropia of 22^Δ at 40 cm. There was a latent deviation at 6 m on the alternate cover test of 20^Δ. When the cover was removed, there was a fusional recovery movement to within 3^Δ of ortho at far, but no recovery was evident at near. Hirschberg testing in all fields of gaze indicated comitancy with good pursuit and saccadic eye movements. The Worth dot test showed moderate suppression O.D. at far and homonymous diplopia of five dots at near. Hering-Bielschowsky afterimage testing indicated NRC and Bagolini striated lens testing showed that angles S and H were equal. The microtropia at far was neutralized with 3^Δ BO; there was no movement on the unilateral cover test, but a large esophoric movement was observed. Subjective refraction (dry) was:

OD −4.00 −0.25 x 120 20/15 (6/4.5)
OS −4.00 −0.25 x 180 20/15 (6/4.5)

With these CAMP lenses, a +3.00 D add and 3^Δ BO neutralized the esotropia at near. With this optical combination the patient had 60 seconds of arc on the Stereo Fly test. Motor fusion ranges, however, could not be measured because of suppression.

These binocular findings are unusual because the microesotropia was not associated with eccentric fixation or ARC at far as well as there being a manifest deviation of 22^Δ at near. The patient demonstrated peripheral fusion at far, but not at near. (Refer to the discussion of microtropia in Chapter 7.) It is likely that the potential for sensory fusion was always good because the patient would habitually read without his spectacles, as though having an add for fusing at his centration point.

The vision training plan included prescribing CAMP spectacle lenses to solve his problem of blurred vision at far, his only complaint. The plan also included prescribing base-out prism and an add at near in the form of bifocals to promote fusion at far and near. The patient was reluctant, however, and wanted contact lenses for cosmetic reasons. The patient made a compromise and agreed to accept the following: Soft contact lenses for social occasions and, for study and critical viewing occasions, plano spectacles having 4^Δ base-out overall (for fusion at far) and a bifocal add of +3.00 (for fusion at near) worn with the contact lenses.

Vision training with weekly office visits and daily home training was done for 3 months. The procedures and sequence generally followed the program for basic esotropia discussed previously. Emphasis, however, was on the use of physiological diplopia with the Brock string and beads, TV trainer and prism rock, and the Spirangle Vectogram. At the conclusion of vision therapy there was no movement on the unilateral cover test at far or near, although there was a latent eso deviation of 20^Δ at far and 2^Δ at near (testing done with contact lens-spectacle combination). Motor fusion ranges with the Spirangle Vectogram were 15^Δ BI and 20^Δ BO and free of suppression. Stereopsis was 40 seconds of arc (Stereo Fly test).

The patient had not shown any regression in binocular skills after 2 months. His vergence ranges had not diminished but had actually increased. The patient had no symptoms and was happy with the contact lens-bifocal combination. He was instructed to continue home vision training for 10 minutes once a month to monitor fusion skills, but to return for evaluation if fusional control started to diminish. The patient's binocular status appeared stable and he was advised to have another progress check in 6 months.

Esophoria

Management Principles

Our preference in treating symptomatic esophoria, all three types, is to correct fully any significant refractive error, then prescribe fusional divergence training to determine if symptomatic and performance problems can be abated. If not we may prescribe prisms, plus adds, or some combination. In regard to prism prescribing, we usually apply one of three clinical criteria: (1) Clinical wisdom recommends completely compensating for the eso deviation if the deviation measures 10^Δ or smaller. Larger deviations are given partially compensating prisms; (2) Sheard's criterion should be met; and (3) Associated phoria as measured by the Mallett or Bernell unit with a central fusion target should be neutralized.

Sensory and motor fusion training proceeds much in the same pattern as recommended for the corresponding types of esotropia. (Refer to the section of vision therapy sequence for esophoria and Table 13-4.) Initially, we suggest an emphasis on training ocular motility including accommodation if a dysfunction exists. When vergence skills are introduced, it is prudent to include convergence ranges as well as divergence ranges. This is because convergence ranges expand quickly, which is an encouraging result for the patient. Divergence ranges expand slowly, but divergence facility may increase rapidly with training. We, therefore, emphasize phasic exercises (i.e., step and jump) more than tonic (i.e. sliding and tromboning) when training divergence. Isometric exercises also are an efficient approach in the treatment of esophoria. The patient can be instructed to read while wearing a base-in prism or a minus-lens add for a period of time. This procedure may cause some eyestrain; frequent breaks may be needed.

In our experience, vision training can often be effective in cases of esophoria using a home-based program augmented with in-office therapy. The length of training usually takes 8 to 12 weeks to complete. Without retainer exercises, divergence skills tend to regress more so than convergence skills in exophoric cases. Good retainer exercises are Aperture-Rule Trainer (T13.13) and orthopic fusion (T13.15). Either or both of these can be assigned for a 20-minute period once a week. If the patient notices a decrease in divergence skills or a reoccurrence of suppression, he should return for a progress evaluation and, probably, a more rigorous retainer program.

Case Example

The following example is a patient with basic esophoria. Surgical management is infrequently necessary in cases of esophoria. We have, however, seen patients with large esophoric deviations who benefited from an operation. One example is a college student who coped with a basic esophoria of approximately 20^Δ at far and near for many years. She wore 8^Δ base-out in her spectacle lenses and had completed a vision training program. Sheard's criterion was partially met but not completely, even with the compensating prisms in her spectacles. She had occasional symptoms of asthenopia, for many years, especially when fatigued; but because of lack of time and finances while in college, she deferred extraocular muscle surgery until graduation. The deviation was reduced to about 5^Δ eso with a unilateral recession of the medial rectus of the nondominant eye. The patient was able to discontinue wearing the base-out relieving prisms. Although her symptoms were mostly abated, she continued regular home vision training to maintain good vergence ranges, facility, and stamina. This case was treated successfully with a combination of several modes of vision therapy, i.e., lenses, prisms, vision training, and surgery. Surgery for esophoric patients is the exception, rather than the rule.

REFERENCES

1. Griffin JR. Efficacy of vision therapy for nonstrabismus vergence anomalies. *Optom Vision Sci.* 1987;64:411-414.

2. Major D, Pirotte P, Griffin JR. *Orthoptic therapy with microcomputer: a comparative study.* Fullerton, Calif: Southern California College of Optometry; 1985. Research project, on file, in the M.B. Ketchum Library.

3. Vaegan. Convergence and divergence show large and sustained improvement after short isometric exercise. *Am J Optom Physiol Opt.* 1979;56:23-33.

4. Ciuffreda KJ, Levi DM, Selenow A. *Amblyopia: Basic and Clinical Aspects.* Newton, Mass: Butterworth-Heinemann; 1991:196-220.

5. Postar SH. *Ophthalmic prism and extraocular muscle deviations: the effect of wearing compensatory prisms on the angle of deviation in cases of esotropia.* Fullerton, Calif: Southern California College of Optometry; 1972. Research project, on file in the M.B. Ketchum Libary.

6. Vodnoy BE. The basis and practice of orthoptics. *Optom Weekly.* 1972;63:16.

7. Wick B. A Fresnel prism bar for home visual therapy. *Am J Optom.* 1974;51:576-578.

8. Vodnoy BE. Aperture orthoptics for the non-strabismic. *Am J Optom Arch Am Acad Optom.* 1956;33:537-44.

9. Cooper J, Cirton M. Micro computer produced anaglyphs for evaluation and therapy of binocular anomalies. *JAOA.* 1983;54:785-788.

10. Pratt-Johnson JA, Tillson G. The management of esotropia with high AC/A ratio (convergence excess). *J Ped Ophthalmol Strabismus.* 1985;22:238-242.

11. Von Noorden GK, Avilla CW. Nonaccommodative convergence excess. *Am J Ophthalmol.* 1986;101:70-73.

12. Caloroso EE, Rouse MW. *Clinical Management of Strabismus.* Newton, Mass: Butterworth-Heinemann; 1993:80-81.

13. Von Noorden GK, Morris J, Edelman P. Efficacy of bifocals in the treatment of accommodative esotropia. *Am J Ophthalmol.* 1978;85:829.

14. Flom MC. Issues in the clinical management of binocular anomalies. In: Rosenbloom AA, Morgan MW, eds. *Principles and Practice of Pediatric Optometry.* Philadelphia: JB Lippincott; 1990:238-239.

15. Brock FW. A simple and direct clinical method of controlling the squinter to normal visual habits. *J Am Optom Assoc.* 1941;13(4)132-145.

Chapter 14 / Vision Therapy for Exo Deviations

Diagnostic Considerations   406
Vision Therapy Sequence for Comitant
  Exotropia   406
  Correction of Refractive Error   406
  Elimination of Major Sensory
    Anomalies   407
  Gross Convergence Training   408
  Compensating Prisms and Lens
    Additions   408
  Sensory and Motor Fusion
    Training   409
    General Considerations   409
    Changing Viewing Distance   410
    Efficacy of Treatment   410
  Surgical Management   410
    General Considerations   410
    Efficacy of Treatment   411
  Follow-up Care   412
Vision Therapy Sequence for
  Exophoria   412
Specific Training Techniques   413
  Voluntary Convergence T14.1   413
  Amblyoscopic Convergence Technique
    T14.2   414
  Peripheral Fusion Rings T14.3   415
  Bernell Mirror Stereoscope T14.4   415
  Physiological Diplopia   416
    Brock String and Beads T14.5   416
    3-Dot Card T14.6   416
  Brewster Stereoscope   417
    Isometric and Step Vergences
      T14.7   417
    Stereoscope Tromboning T14.8   418

Vectograms® and Tranaglyphs   418
  Convergence Training at Near
    T14.9   418
  Convergence Walk-aways
    T14.10   419
Projected BO Slides T14.11   419
Aperture-Rule Trainer (Single Aperture)
  T14.12   419
Pencil Pushups and Push-aways
  T14.13   420
Chiastopic Fusion T14.14   422
Binocular Accommodative Rock
  T14.15   425
Vergence Rock Techniques   425
  Television Trainer and Prisms
    T14.16   426
  Bar Reader with Prisms T14.17   426
  Framing and Prisms T14.18   426
Pola-Mirror Vergence Techniques
  T14.19   427
Computerized Convergence Procedures
  T14.20   427
Case Management and Examples   427
  Divergence Excess Exotropia   427
    Management Principles   427
    Case Example   428
  Basic Exotropia   429
    Management Principles   429
    Case Example   430
  Convergence Insufficiency
    Exophoria   431
    Management Principles   431
    Case Example   435

Exo deviations are more prevalent than eso deviations. The ratio regarding strabismus is about 3 to 2 which translates into approximately 5 million people having some form of exotropia in the United States.[1] Approximately 80% of exotropes have fusion at some distance at least part time[2] and are, therefore, considered intermittent. Many of these individuals experience visual symptoms of eyestrain, fatigue, diplopia, blur, and photophobia. Exophoria has been associated with visual symptoms with reading and also with poor reading skills.[3,4] Since so many patients with exo deviations have some fusional ability and fusional convergence is relatively easy to increase with training,[5,6] vision training is often the preferred therapeutic option applied in these cases. Using vision training and surgery, Flom[7] reported the functional cure rate for most cases of constant exotropia to be about 40% to 50% and for intermittent exotropia, 70% to 80%. In an extensive review paper on vision training results in convergence insufficiency exophoria, Grisham[8] found a 72% cure rate that included relief from ocular symptoms as one of the criteria. Our clinical experience is consistent with these observations; exo deviations are generally easier to treat successfully than eso deviations and vision training is usually part of our treatment plan, often the most important part.

DIAGNOSTIC CONSIDERATIONS

Cases of exo deviations, either exotropia (XT) or exophoria (XP), may be categorized into three types: divergence excess (DE) with a high AC/A, basic exo (BX) with a normal AC/A, and convergence insufficiency (CI) with a low AC/A. (Refer to Chapter 3 for definitions and discussions.) Both DE and BX are considered to be primarily farpoint problems, since poor cosmesis, deficient sensory and motor fusion, and problems are relatively more likely with far rather than with near viewing. Although in BX cases the exo deviation is approximately the same at all distances, the fusional "glue" is weaker at far than at near, e.g., less stereopsis, smaller retinal images, and lack of tactile-kinesthetic feedback. On the other hand, convergence insufficiency exophoria and exotropia almost exclusively cause nearpoint problems. Compared with DE and BX,

patients with CI are usually easy to treat with good success.

It is worthwhile remembering that exotropia may present some diagnostic challenges and that accuracy in diagnosis affects the type and sequence of vision therapy. (See discussion in Chapter 7.) These challenges include: (1) Sometimes the true far and near angles of exotropia are larger in the open environment than found in the examination room, for as yet inexplicable reasons.[9] (2) There exists a high prevalence of "simulated" divergence excess exotropic cases, usually BX cases, that require a prolonged cover test to reveal the full magnitude of the near deviation.[10] A differential diagnosis must be made between a case of true DE and BX. (3) In cases of intermittent exotropia, abbreviated X(T), the clinician needs to be aware that fusional control of the deviation can vary considerably depending on the patient's general state of health and degree of fatigue. With these considerations in mind, the clinician may be helped in avoiding diagnostic errors that would result in case mismanagement.

VISION THERAPY SEQUENCE FOR COMITANT EXOTROPIA

Our recommended vision therapy sequence of steps in the management of comitant exotropia is outlined in Table 14-1. The clinician should administer only the steps that are appropriate for a particular case based on the diagnosis.

Correction of Refractive Error

Exotropes tend to have a higher prevalence of myopia and myopic anisometropia than people in the general population.[11,12] Even small degrees of myopia, astigmatism, and anisometropia (e.g., 0.75 D) can be an obstacle to the control of the deviation in some patients. Certainly in cases of exotropia when fusion is the goal, we believe that the clinician should correct small amounts of refractive error. Exotropic and exophoric patients can have any type of refractive error, even large amounts of hyperopia. Moderate to high degrees of hyperopia should be corrected; one report indicated

TABLE 14-1. *Vision Therapy Sequence for Comitant Exotropia.*

1. Correction of any significant ametropia, even moderate to high hyperopia.
2. Treatment of amblyopia, if present, improving visual acuity to at least 20/60 (6/18).
3. Training basic ocular motility of each eye: fixation, saccades, pursuits, and especially accommodation.
4. Gross convergence training if there is no fusion at near, even in cases of ARC.
5. Classical ARC therapy, if gross convergence training is unsuccessful and prognosis for its elimination is favorable.
6. Sensorial alignment of the eyes at some or all distances using any combination of prisms and added lenses (assuming NRC).
7. Antisuppression therapy, if NRC, to establish diplopia awareness and basic sensory fusion.
8. Central sensory and motor fusion training, if NRC, to achieve good stereopsis and maximum fusional vergence ranges, free of suppression, at all viewing distances.
9. Strabismus surgery, if necessary, to reduce the angle of deviation to within the range of reflex fusional vergence.
10. Prescription of compensatory prisms and added lenses as needed.
11. Development of good monocular and binocular efficiency skills.
12. Maintenance home exercises and periodic progress checkups.

that some hyperopic exotropic children (ranging from 3 to 7 D) were cured with spectacle correction, whereas all others in this series of seven had improved their binocular sensory status.[13] Many moderate to high hyperopes do respond to plus with an increase in the exo deviation, as expected, based on the AC/A. Even so, it is advisable to relieve the stress on accommodation; sometimes the fusional status is remarkably improved as the previous report indicated.

Most authorities agree that large exophoria and intermittent exotropia in childhood tend to decompensate over time and may become constant strabismus if left untreated.[14-16] Hiles et al.,[17] however, reported a clinical series of 48 intermittent exotropes whose sole treat-

ment was correction of their refractive error. These patients were followed for several years; 65% became phoric and 73% reduced the magnitude of their exo deviation. We believe that correction of the refractive error remains the primary step in treating most binocular anomalies.

Elimination of Major Sensory Anomalies

Amblyopia is not usually associated with XT because most of these deviations are not constant. In patients with amblyopia, however, it is important to improve visual acuity to about 20/60 (6/18) before proceeding with binocular therapy. It is also necessary for the patient to have good fixation, pursuits, saccades, and accommodation. If these skills are deficient, they should be the immediate concern in vision training. (See Chapters 10 and 16.)

Anomalous "retinal" correspondence (ARC) is usually not a significantly unfavorable factor in cases of exotropia, and no problem at all in exophoria. (See discussion in Chapter 11.) Since most exotropes fuse at some distance, usually at near, they covary from ARC to NRC when fusional vergence movements align the eyes. When the exo deviation is manifest, however, they covary back to ARC. Even in cases of constant exotropia, ARC is often not an overriding consideration if the patient can learn gross convergence (T11.1). On the other hand, ARC does become a serious obstacle to progress in constant XT when gross convergence techniques fail to align the eyes at near, with covariation to NRC. If classical amblyoscope techniques for eliminating ARC are necessary in cases of constant exotropia, the same problems and restrictions limit success as in cases of constant esotropia (Chapter 11). Wick[18] demonstrated that success is possible, even in the case of an adult with XT (a 22-year-old female). We believe success is possible in many such cases; however, there are considerations that can make treatment impractical for the patient. For example, vision training may be time consuming, difficult, and expensive.

Deep suppression, if present, can also be a significant obstacle to establishing sensory and motor fusion. As with ARC, it is best to stimulate gross convergence (T11.13); hopefully, the patient can attain peripheral fusion at some near distance. Antisuppression training can begin at this position in the open environment.

Gross Convergence Training

As indicated in the previous discussion, we believe it is very important in cases of constant exotropia to attempt gross convergence training (T11.13) early in the therapy sequence. This procedure is usually unnecessary, however, in cases of DE because these patients frequently have fusion at near. The need arises more often in cases of BX of large magnitude and in cases of CI exotropia. Any exotrope not having near-point sensory and motor fusion should attempt this technique, even on the initial diagnostic visit. If successful, the prognosis for a functional cure increases. Training time usually decreases and the patient can avoid a lot of closed instrument training. Even when the procedure results in fusion at near for only 1 minute, the patient can be considered, for practical purposes, an intermittent exotrope. The prognosis dramatically increases by 30% according to Flom's chart[7] (see Table 6-4). We consider gross convergence important enough to spend two or three in-office training sessions trying to develop it before resorting to amblyoscope training (T14.2). Even then, it should be periodically attempted as vision training continues in closed space instruments. (Refer to the discussions on gross convergence in T11.13 and T14.1.)

Compensating Prisms and Lens Additions

Base-in prism compensation should be tried in cases of constant exotropia if NRC exists. The goal is to obtain sensorial orthophoria by optical means so that fusional reflexes are encouraged. Typically in cases of exophoria and exotropia, it is not necessary to prescribe the total amount of compensatory prism as measured by the cover test to elicit a fusional convergence response, 1/3 to 1/2 the angle may be sufficient. Many exotropes do not show prism adaptation in response to BI prism and their fusion remains stable for many years.[19] Patients in which ARC and suppression are present

when the eyes are in an exotropic position, may require BI prism compensation to be initially successful. A trial period of wear (a few days) using Fresnel prisms may help to determine efficacy of relieving prisms.

If the exo deviation has an associated vertical component, as is frequently the case,[20] the effect of vertical prism on the patient's control of the horizontal deviation should also be carefully evaluated. Vertical prism is usually necessary only when the vertical deviation is primary and not simply secondary to the exotropic posture of the eyes. If the patient can fuse, vertical fixation disparity measurement indicates the necessary prism priscription. If the patient cannot fuse, prisms adds can be used to get the eyes close to the ortho alignment, where the vertical deviation is measured (e.g., Maddox rod).

An efficient means to elicit fusional vergence is by aligning the eyes with minus-lens overcorrection. Calrider and Jampolsky[21] reported that 72% of their young (ages 2 to 13 years) intermittent exotropic subjects (N35) changed to well-controlled exophorias using minus-lens overcorrection as the sole intervention. The effect of minus adds should be evaluated with all nonpresbyopic exotropic patients, even convergence insufficiency cases, but particularly with those having a normal or high AC/A, i.e., BX and DE cases. Sometimes even a small amount of accommodative stimulus is sufficient to initiate a fusional convergence response. In other cases, 2 or 3 D of over-minus power may be required to reduce the angle of deviation substantially to within the range of reflex fusional vergence. When the patient has a large-angle basic exotropia, 40^{Δ} or more, minus adds usually have no significant effect. Nevertheless, we encourage the clinician to evaluate the effect of minus adds in many cases of exotropia. As part of their evaluation, some doctors have a stock of −3.00 D loaner spectacles they give to patients for a 1-week trial period. We have found this aggressive approach effective in many cases. In addition, it is often appropriate to assign some accommodative techniques for home training so the patient can get maximum benefit from the minus-add loaners. Some older children and adults may experience accommodative asthenopia due to the over-minus lenses; vision training may help to relieve this discomfort. Another possible adverse consequence to minus-lens overcorrection is that of causing or increasing myopia. However, a study by Rutstein et al.[22] found that the rate of myopia progression with minus-lens overcorrection was no greater than expected during the usual course of myopia development. Nevertheless, the clinician should remain alert for unexpected changes in the patient's refractive status during this treatment.

The amount of minus-add addition most effective for a particular patient must be determined by directly observing the effect of various lens powers on the angle of deviation and the patient's fusional control. The calculated AC/A can give the clinician an idea of which amount to try first. Typically, this amount yields less effect than would be expected by calculation, because patients usually do not fully accommodate in response to the lenses. It is usually unnecessary, however, to compensate the angle of deviation completely. One practical criterion is to prescribe the lowest amount of over-minus power that gives the fastest reflex fusion response. A trial and error method can be used to determine this amount. Trial lenses are placed before the patient's eyes. Using a cover paddle to break fusion, the clinician observes the speed of the fusional vergence recovery when the occluded eye is uncovered. Alignment should occur by reflex; the patient is instructed to avoid voluntary convergence. The shorter is the vergence response latency and the faster the velocity, the better. Additional increases in power do not always result in a more vigorous fusion reflex; therefore, the lowest power that produces the maximum response is selected.

An interesting and seemingly paradoxical use of added lenses to build fusional control of intermittent exotropia involves the prescription of a plus-lens bifocal. If the patient shows an exotropia at far and an exophoria at near (which is often the case), an isometric fusional vergence technique may be effective. The idea is to increase the habitual exophoria at near with a plus add. This increased exophoria requires the constant exertion of greater fusional convergence at near. Over time, this helps the patient control the farpoint deviation. The patient should be warned of nearpoint asthenopic symptoms and must be willing to endure them. This optical isometric method of training fusional convergence may be appropriate for those patients who cannot actively participate in a vision training program. Careful periodic monitoring of the effect of the lenses is needed to ensure control of the near deviation without suppression.

In an extensive review of the literature, Coffey et al.[23] found that the functional success rate in intermittent exotropia using base-in prism as the sole intervention was 28%. Minus–add as a sole intervention was also 28%. This review surveyed over 200 patients in each therapy category. We rarely use these as isolated treatment modalities. They are usually combined with sensory and motor fusion training.

Sensory and Motor Fusion Training

General Considerations

It bears repeating that during a vision training program for strabismus, the patient should never be allowed to reinforce the strabismus. If the strabismus is constant, so is occlusion to treat or prevent suppression or other sensory adaptations. For example, if after a good effort with gross convergence training in a CI exotropic case, fusion at near has not been achieved, except during active training, the patient must still wear a spectacle half-patch (lower portion of the lens) for nearpoint viewing. However, if this patient fuses 60% of the time and loses fusion in the afternoon and evening, the patch need only be worn during the latter part of the day. Patching alone may result in a cure of intermittent exotropia. In a clinical series reported by Cooper and Leyman,[10] 4 of 11 cases (36%) reverted to an exophoric condition using occlusion as the sole treatment.

Suppression must be worked on first. (Refer to Chapter 12 for antisuppression therapy.) Eliminating suppression at far is not always easy. The best approach is to have the patient achieve alignment, even if temporary, with minus-lens overcorrections and by mental effort (voluntary convergence). When the eyes are aligned, the ARC is eliminated with covariation; suppression can be more easily broken in the ortho posture with NRC than when the eyes are in the exo position with ARC.

As in training in cases of eso deviations (Chapter 13), the doctor should be sure that the monocular visual skills of saccades, pursuits, fixation, and accommodation are adequate before vergence training begins. The principal difference in vision training between cases of eso and exo deviations is the emphasis on base-in training for eso and base-out for exo deviations. Many of the techniques for both conditions can be used interchangeably with but minor differences in techniques. Only a few of many possible training procedures are included in this text, for the sake of brevity.

Changing Viewing Distance

The approach to sensory and motor fusion training in cases of farpoint exo deviation involves increasing the viewing distance of a fixated target. When a DE patient bifixates a receding object, there is an increasing demand on fusional convergence. This is because the exo deviation is larger at far than at near. (Refer to discussion in Chapter 3.) It seems counterintuitive at first to do push-aways and walkaways to cure exotropia, but the efficacy of this approach is understood when the relation between the AC/A and the ortho demand line is taken into account.

Changing the viewing distance in the open environment is an effective approach to building sensory and motor fusion skills in cases of intermittent exotropia and exophoria. Sensory and motor fusion training should ideally be introduced and enhanced at the distance the patient can successfully fuse in the open environment. If fusion is absent and gross convergence is unsuccessful, then training can start on the major amblyoscope in the office and with a mirror stereoscope at home. Usually the patient can fuse, at least part-time, at some distance. In this case, fusional skills are increased initially at that distance, then training is directed toward the distance or field in which control of the deviation is weak or lacking. Pencil pushups and push-aways techniques (T14.13), whichever is appropriate (based on the patient's AC/A) are introduced at a position in the open

environment where the patient can best maintain sensory and motor fusion. To extend the range of training distances, the patient can slowly walk away or walk toward the stimulus target (e.g., a Vectogram or Tranaglyph) while attempting to hold fusion. The goal is to extend sensory and motor fusion to all distances and fields of gaze in the open environment.

Efficacy of Treatment

Vision training, as a sole intervention, has been used extensively in the treatment of intermittent exotropia with good results. In one clinical series of 31 exotropes, mostly constant deviations, Sanfilippo and Clahane[24] reported a success rate of 64% and a failure rate of only 3% with little regression after 4 1/2 years. Success was defined as no strabismus at far or near and good fusional vergence ranges. These authors concluded that the size of the deviation and age of the patient were not important factors in achieving successful results, but patient motivation was. Goldrich[25] presented a series of 29 intermittent exotropes of the DE type, which are the most difficult types to treat solely with vision training. He reported a success rate of 82% having a phoric condition after treatment, no symptoms, and normal fusional ranges. Only one patient made no progress. The average number of in-office training sessions was 29 with a standard deviation of 14. There are other equally impressive clinical series reported in the literature.[26,27] In their literature review involving 740 cases of intermittent exotropia, Coffey et al.[23] reported a functional cure, by their strict criterion, of 59% with vision training as the sole therapeutic option.

Surgical Management

General Considerations

Generally speaking, if a patient has an intermittent exotropia greater than 25^Δ at far or near or a constant exotropia greater than 20^Δ, the possibility of strabismus surgery needs to be discussed with the patient, parents, or whomever appropriate. The larger the angle, the more likely that an operation will be required for successful long-term management. It is important to remember that intermittent exotropic patients should have a prolonged cover test; this is to determine the full angle of deviation and unmask any latent deviation. The degree of fusional control and the severity of the patient's symptoms, if any, are also important factors in assessing the appropriateness of surgery.

The general guidelines for surgical procedures vary according to the type of exotropia and are summarized in Table 14-2. In cases of true DE, the preferred operation is bilateral lateral rectus recession. This type of operation has the effect of reducing the AC/A while decreasing the magnitude of the exotropia. The generally preferred operation in CI cases is bilateral medial rectus resection, which has the effect of increasing the AC/A. In cases of BX, the surgeon may elect to perform a recession of the lateral rectus and a resection of the medial rectus of the same eye, usually the strabismic eye. This "R and R" procedure tends to have little affect on the magnitude of the AC/A. According to Helveston,[28] when the angle of deviation is larger than 50^Δ, the surgeon often operates on three muscles, e.g., an R and R on the strabismic eye combined with a lateral rectus recession of the dominant eye. Deviations larger than 75^Δ often require a four-muscle operation, a bilateral R and R. Although there are differences of opinion, most surgeons try to achieve an immediate post-surgical result of 10^Δ eso or less, a slight overcorrection.[29] The healing process often results in a shift back in the exo direction. Leaving a post-surgical residual exo deviation increases the risk that the patient will revert to an exotropia at a later time.[29] For this reason, some surgeons use adjustable sutures on one muscle so that post-surgical refinement of the deviation is possible.[30]

Efficacy of Treatment

The literature on surgical management of intermittent exotropia leaves much to be desired. Patients frequently regress to their previous deviation, often needing multiple operations for a successful outcome. Frequently, surgery is unsuccessful or only partially resolved. Intermittent exotropia is probably one of the toughest problems strabismus surgeons have to face.

TABLE 14-2. *Common Surgical Procedures for Exotropia*

Divergence Excess Exotropia

Weaken both lateral rectus muscles with a bilateral recession procedure that decreases the deviation at far primarily.

Convergence Insufficiency Exotropia

Strengthen both medial rectus muscles with a bilateral resection procedure that decreases the deviation at near primarily.

Basic Exotropia

If angle $<50^\Delta$, unilateral recession and resection.
If angle $>50^\Delta$ and $<75^\Delta$, a three muscle operation.
If angle $>75^\Delta$, bilateral recession and resection.

Immediate Post-Surgical Goal

10^Δ overcorrection to ortho.

Flax and Selenow[31] reviewed 22 journal articles dealing with surgical success in exotropia. They reported only a 34% success rate using the definition of functional cure as a phoric condition at all distances, sensory fusion, and demonstrable vergence ranges. The failure rate, as defined by the authors, was 22%, all other cases falling in between. In a later review by Coffey et al.,[23] surgical success for intermittent exotropia had apparently improved and was reported as 46% based on an accumulated total of 2530 cases.

A particularly revealing study that compared results of different treatment modalities was that of Cooper and Leyman.[10] In this retrospective study of 673 cases, "orthoptics only" had the highest success rate (59%) and lowest failure rate (5%) compared with the three other therapy approaches: (1) occlusion only; (2) surgery only; and (3) orthoptics and surgery (Table 14-3). The authors pointed out, however, that the smaller deviations tended to be found in the "orthoptics only" group, and the larger angles of strabismus in the two surgery groups. For this reason these data are not exactly com-

TABLE 14-3. Results of Surgical and Nonsurgical Treatment of Intermittent Exotropia[10]

A retrospective study of 673 cases.

	Number	Good	Fair	Poor
Occlusion only	11	36%	28%	36%
Surgery only	264	42%	41%	17%
Surgery and training	216	52%	38%	10%
Training only	182	59%	36%	5%

TABLE 14-4. Vision Therapy Sequence for Exophoria

1. Correction of any significant ametropia, even moderate to high hyperopia.
2. Training basic ocular motility of each eye: fixation, saccades, pursuits, and especially accommodation.
3. Antisuppression therapy to establish awareness of physiological diplopia.
4. Development of normal gross convergence amplitude including voluntary convergence ability.
5. Central sensory and motor fusion training to achieve good stereopsis and maximum fusional vergence ranges, free of foveal suppression, at all viewing distances.
6. Development of good binocular efficiency skills, e.g., facility and stamina of accommodation and vergence; normalize fixation disparity curve.
7. Prescription of compensatory prisms and added lenses as needed.
8. Maintenance home exercises and periodic progress checkups.

parable; however, when there is surgery and training, this combination tends to increase the success and diminish the failure rates.

Based on the many studies of therapy efficacy for exotropia, despite their scientific inadequacies, we think the following treatment recommendations can be made with assurance. (1) In cases of intermittent exotropia, 25^{Δ} or less (far or near or both), vision training is the preferred treatment option and may be combined with occlusion, prism compensation, and minus adds as each case demands.[23,32] (2) In cases of exotropia greater that 25^{Δ} at far or near or both, surgery becomes increasingly necessary to effect a cure as the angle of deviation increases. The amount of fusional control of the deviation is an important factor. Constant exotropia is far more likely to require an operation than intermittent exotropia. (3) In cases requiring surgery, either constant or intermittent, vision training and optical compensation used in conjunction increase the likelihood of a successful outcome.[10,33]

Follow-up Care

Compensating prisms (Fresnel) and minus-add lenses should be given to the post-surgical patient as soon as possible to aid the development and maintenance of sensory and motor fusion. Patching an eye is not recommended unless there are surgical complications such as an infection. Vision training can usually be started about 2 weeks after the operation without too much discomfort. If fusional skills exist at near, we usually recommend home training exercises, e.g., Minivectogram (T14.9), chiastopic fusion (T14.14), binocular accommodative rock (T14.15), and vergence rock techniques (T14.16 and T14.17). Any of these techniques can also be utilized as a retainer exercise for the patient to monitor regressions and to give periodic "booster" training as needed, perhaps once a month. Regular progress evaluations are scheduled consistent with fusional results of therapy.

VISION THERAPY SEQUENCE FOR EXOPHORIA

Management of exophoria is similar to exotropia, although there are slight differences and therapy is less intensive (see Table 14-4 and compare with Table 14-1). The clinician is usually not concerned with amblyopia, anomalous correspondence, or deep suppression. Correcting the refractive error, providing prism prescription, and initiating a short course of vision training are the principal modes of therapy in cases of exophoria. Patients are often highly motivated and cooperative patients in vision therapy; they want relief from their asthenopic symptoms and, in many cases, wish to improve vocational or avocational performance due to inefficient visual skills. Fortunately, progress in vision training is usually rapid.

We initially suggest vision training in most symptomatic exophoria cases rather than prism compensation. The rational is that developing good visual function is preferable to relying on a "crutch." Furthermore, most patients do not require prisms for visual comfort and efficiency after a successful training program. Some doctors, however, prefer to prescribe prism compensation to see if symptoms diminish or disappear, thus avoiding the inconvenience and effort necessary to maintain a training program. Whichever approach the doctor chooses, it should be done with informed consent of the patient after the options have been thoroughly explained.

Exophoria is often associated with accommodative deficiencies, particularly accommodative insufficiency.[34] We recommend training the accommodative dysfunction initially, if present, before effort is expended on convergence training. (Accommodative anomalies tend to have greater adverse effect on vergence than vice versa.) Also, training of accommodative skills progresses rapidly, thus increasing patient motivation. (See Chapter 16 for a discussion on training accommodative skills.)

Symptomatic exophoric patients frequently have shallow suppression that can be identified by: (1) the patient not seeing double at the endpoint of the nearpoint of convergence; (2) lack of perception of physiological diplopia; and (3) evidence of foveal suppression while testing vergence ranges. Conveniently, physiological diplopia awareness training can be combined with building of gross convergence and with training for voluntary convergence.

Motor fusion ranges, free of suppression, should be increased maximally in the horizontal, vertical, and torsional directions and for all distances, but emphasizing fusional convergence ranges. Most vision therapists also introduce training techniques for vergence facility (step and jump) at this stage in the sequence. Isometric training techniques should also be given since they help increase vergence amplitude and stamina.[35] Therefore, these two steps (vergence range training and building binocu-

lar efficiency skills) are often applied simultaneously, until release criteria have all been achieved. (See the section on exophoria management.)

Those cases of exophoria in which training has not resolved all the signs and symptoms of a dysfunction, prism compensation serves as a convenient option. Fortunately, patients with symptoms associated with heterophoria usually do not have prism adaptation; the prism effectively compensates for the condition.[19] We have seen a few symptomatic exophores who did not respond successfully to compensating prisms, due to abnormal vergence (prism) adaptation. Principal examples are patients with a type IV fixation disparity curve. Even vision training was not always effective in eliminating symptoms in such cases. A possible alternative to resolve the patient's symptoms is a monovision prescription for spectacles or contact lenses. (See Chapter 16.)

Most cases of exophoria, at least 70%,[8] are managed successfully with vision training within a 6 to 8 week period. It is wise to give patients retainer exercises to prevent regression, although this is seldom significant if the patient has met all release criteria.[36]

SPECIFIC TRAINING TECHNIQUES

Twenty vision training techniques are presented that are particularly appropriate of exo deviations. There are, however, many other techniques therapists can use. The techniques we present here generally follow a sequence from treating the most difficult cases, as in exotropia with poor sensory and motor fusion, to treating the least difficult cases, as in exophoria with relatively minor deficiencies of sensory and motor fusion. The clinician should choose those techniques that are most appropriate for the particular skill and interest level of each patient.

Voluntary Convergence T14.1

Voluntary convergence is the willful crossing of the eyes. The definition implies the lack of visual stimuli. Most exotropic patients can be taught voluntary convergence. The mechanism each person uses is not always known, but it is important to note that it can be learned, regardless of how it is achieved. If visual stimuli help in the learning process, that is fine. Some patients imagine seeing visual objects, such as a bug flying near the nose, to trigger the convergence response. After sufficient repetitive exercises, the patient begins to be aware of the proprioceptive feeling of his eyes converging, as opposed to remaining in the fusion-free exo deviated posture. The doctor and therapist can monitor the extent of convergence by using the Hirschberg test, and giving the patient feedback when the eyes are in the ortho posture. The "feeling" the patient has at that moment should be remembered and recaptured every time the eyes assume the ortho posture. Once the patient knows this feeling and can bring it about at will, he can practice voluntary convergence at home.

Voluntary convergence can also be aided by awareness of diplopia. The exotropic patient may have trouble noticing pathological diplopia, because point zero is on the temporal retina. If the patient is unable to perceive pathological diplopia, procedures designed to promote the awareness of physiological diplopia should be given. (Refer to Chapter 1 for discussions on pathological and physiological diplopia.) An example of physiological diplopia awareness training in conjunction with anti-suppression training is the Brock String technique (T12.13) discussed in Chapter 12.

The voluntary convergence technique can supplement the gross convergence technique (T11.13) that has been previously described as a treatment for ARC associated with XT. This procedure also applies in cases of constant XT at near with NRC; however, afterimages are unnecessary to monitor covariation since the correspondence is normal.

Once the patient with exotropia learns gross convergence or voluntary convergence, he should attempt isometric exercises to hold the eyes in a fully convergence posture for a reasonable time period, at least 1 minute. This exercise requires great effort and a high level of convergence control and stamina; consequently this often causes significant eyestrain. The patient should be given frequent rest breaks between training intervals.

Amblyoscopic Convergence Technique T14.2

In cases of constant exotropia when suppression is deep and fusion cannot be established with voluntary convergence, amblyoscope convergence training can be used to achieve sensory fusion. Patients are, ideally, scheduled for hourly sessions, two or three times per week. Constant occlusion is required when the patient is not actively training; this is to help break any existing suppression. The first slides introduced in the amblyoscope are usually first- or second-degree peripheral targets in an attempt to establish rudimentary fusion at the objective angle of strabismus. Suppression is broken with automatic, rapid, alternate flashing and by dimming the image of the non-suppressing eye. Initially, the patient's task is to use "mental effort" to hold in view the suppression controls for each eye simultaneously for a required time interval, e.g.,1 minute. When this goal is achieved, the stimulus characteristics of the targets are changed to challenge the patient further, and the process is repeated. Once suppression is consistently broken on a second-degree target set at the patient's angle of deviation, motor fusion demands can be introduced. The amblyoscope is designed to build sliding vergence ranges in horizontal, vertical, and cyclotorsional directions. In cases of exotropia, expanding convergence ranges are, of course, the primary concern, but building motor fusion skills in the other directions is ideal for the sake of generalization and reinforcement of learned skills. A reasonable goal for fusional convergence in the major amblyoscope is at least 20^Δ from the angle of deviation without suppression. When this level of skill is achieved, and perhaps less when the exotropia is of small or moderate magnitude, the patient can then learn to apply voluntary vergence movements to achieve and maintain fusion in the open environment. For sake of efficiency and effectiveness of training, every effort should be made to get the patient out of the instrument and into the open environment as soon as possible.

Peripheral Fusion Rings T14.3

The Root Rings target is a peripheral fusion target that can be used to build fusional convergence at far (see Figure 13-10). It is, therefore, particularly appropriate in cases of divergence excess (DE) and basic exotropia (BX). (This technique was described in the previous chapter for building divergence at far in cases of eso deviations, T13.7). The patient is instructed to fixate the center stereo configuration while wearing red-green spectacles (red on right eye and green on left eye). If sensory and motor fusion are present at some intermediate distance, the patient moves to that distance from the Root Rings to establish fusion initially. If the exotropia is constant at all distances, the deviation may require neutralization with base-in prisms, or possibly with minus-lens adds. The patient stands at the intermediate distance from the target and is instructed to maintain the floating effect while slowly walking away, as far as possible, while fusing the target. As fixation distance is increased, the rings should appear to be floating closer. (This is assuming the target is oriented upright to create crossed disparity for stereopsis.) This is a fascinating effect and motivates many patients to continue vision training. Fusional convergence ranges are gradually built up by reducing the BI compensation and eventually by introducing BO prism of progressively greater power.

Another similar anaglyphic target for peripheral fusion training is the Bernell 900 Stereo Trainer (Figure 13-11 shows the design of such a ring target). An advantage of this target is that it can be used on a television screen. This is ideal for isometric training at far and watching of television often improves training compliance with many patients. Base-out prism, either Fresnel or a regular loose plastic one, can be attached to the spectacles to create a challenging convergence demand. Later, flipper prisms are used to develop step vergence facility. Jump vergence facility can be introduced by using a pencil for nearpoint fixation and instructing the patient to alternate fixation from the fused rings at far to the pencil tip, continually repeating this procedure for several minutes.

Bernell Mirror Stereoscope T14.4

The Bernell Mirror Stereoscope can be set for an angle of deviation of 40^Δ base-in (see Figure 13-2). This instrument is ideal home training for exotropes who cannot achieve fusion at any distance either by gross convergence (T11.13) or by voluntary convergence (T14.1). Even larger angles can be considered by using base-in prism or a minus add. Sliding vergence training with a Mirror Stereoscope is similar to that described for T13.2 in the previous chapter in cases of esotropia. The emphasis in exo deviations, however, is to increase fusional convergence ranges rather than the divergence ranges, although training should ultimately include both horizontal directions. Second-degree targets with large suppression controls are initially aligned at, or close to, the subjective angle of deviation at which sensory fusion is most likely attainable. If suppression occurs, light from a desk lamp can be directed onto that field while the patient blinks the suppressing eye. A pointer can also be moved around and about in the suppressed field to break the suppression. When the patient achieves sensory fusion, base-out demands are slowly increased (or base-in decreased) as the patient attempts to maintain fusion. An initial goal is for the patient to achieve a sliding vergence range from 10^Δ converging to 10^Δ diverging around the angle of deviation. As training progresses, the patient attempt to reach the ortho position and go beyond it. Speed of vergence is not an initial objective, but this definitely is later in therapy. An ideal goal would be to increase vergence ranges (e.g., blur/break/recovery) to conform to the normative nearpoint values listed in Chapter 2, but this may be impractical depending on the size of exotropia. The usual training period for this technique is 10 minutes of continuous activity of moving the targets between the limits of convergence and divergence.

When the patient can fuse a great deal of the time, as in exophoria or intermittent exotropia, a break and join jump technique can be done with the Mirror Stereoscope. With central second-degree fusion targets in position, the wings of the instrument are adjusted to an appropriate convergence demand on the vergence scale for the patient's skill level. The patient looks over the top of the instrument at a distant target (e.g., television trainer with peripheral fusion rings), and fuses that target. Fixation is then quickly alternated to the targets in the Mirror Stereoscope and fusion attempted. This training variation allows for suppression monitoring at both distances. The patient's goal is to increase the speed of jump vergences maximally, without suppression. The rate of fusional recoveries is recorded at each training session to chart progress and to enhance motivation.

Physiological Diplopia

Brock String and Beads T14.5

The Brock string provides a convenient control for suppression (physiological diplopia) while motor fusion training proceeds (see Figures 12-7 and 12-8). This is especially appropriate for intermittent exotropic patients who have a tendency to suppress. The Brock string and beads technique has many variations, some being described for use with suppressing patients (T12.7) and esotropes (T13.6). With thorough instructions, most patients can effectively use this simple device for effective for home training.

Since most exotropes fuse at some distance, one bead can be set at that particular distance, and the others at more challenging positions on the string. The patient can make jump vergence movements from one bead to the others to build accuracy, range, speed, and stamina. The patient is instructed to perceive accurate bifixation (string images crossing at the fixated bead) and physiological diplopia of the other beads before changing fixation to a nearer or farther bead.

Gross convergence can be trained with a pushup variation of T14.5. The patient slowly moves a bead from arm's length toward his nose while maintaining bifixation on that bead and perceiving physiological diplopia of the other beads. The goal is to achieve vergence smoothness over a large range, i.e., tromboning. Flipper prisms combined with the Brock string and beads provide step vergence training. Vergence training in various fields of gaze is also conveniently accomplished by asking the patient to posture his head in various positions while holding the string to his nose and maintaining bifixation on a particular bead. This open environment technique, with its many variations, is appropriate in most cases intermittent exotropia and exophoria.

3-Dot Card T14.6

A 3-dot convergence card, such as the one printed by Allbee (Figure 14-1), is an excellent convergence stimulus at near. It can also be used effectively as a home training technique in most cases of exophoria and exotropia. Based on the same principle as the Brock string, the dots represent the beads; the patient should appreciate physiological diplopia of the non-fixated dots when one pair is fused. Since one side of the card has red dots and the other has blue, the fused dot should appear as a blend of purple. The dots are printed in three sizes and the card is held with the largest dot farthest away.

Because the septum is dissociative, the patient may have trouble converging. There are two things that may help. First, let the patient practice on the Brock string and beads. This would be relatively easy since the beads can be moved farther away and there is no septum involved. Another helpful means is to move the card a few centimeters away from her face to achieve fusion initially, even for the most remote dot. Once this is done, the card is brought closer to touch the nose, and fusion of the middle and nearest dots is then attempted. Another way to get the patient started on the 3-dot card is to remove the dissociating septum. This is done by cutting off the top portion of the card, down to the top of the dots (Figure 14-2). The patient can then look directly at the dots without dissociation. When the patient can quickly change fixation from one dot (fused pair) to another while appreciating physiological diplopia, the regular card (uncut) is substituted. The patient works on this technique until quick jump vergence responses without suppression are achieved. When suppression is noticed, the patient blinks her eyes and wiggles the card slightly to re-establish perception of physiological diplopia. Near-far jump vergence can also be trained by having the patient alternate fixation between a distant object and the 3-dot card. The goal of these jump procedures is to improve vergence facility as well as the nearpoint of convergence. The therapist can make these exercises easier for the patient by using minus adds or base-in prism and more difficult with plus-adds or base-out prism. This jump vergence training is effective, but very demanding; patients need to rest after each 2-minute training interval.

Brewster Stereoscope

The optics of the Brewster stereoscope were discussed in Chapter 13 along with its application to vision training in cases of esotropia and esophoria. The same principles apply for exo deviations except the emphasis is on fusional convergence training with base-out demands. The Brewster stereoscope is an important training instrument for farpoint exo deviations since the stereograms can be placed at optical infinity. For this reason it is used in cases of DE and BX but infrequently in CI cases.

Isometric and Step Vergences T14.7

Isometric vergence training is done when the maximum base-out demand can be met with the patient fusing and seeing the target clearly. The patient is shown a series of stereograms with varying separations and the one selected is that with maximum BO demand in which the patient can reasonably maintain clear, single binocular vision, but not necessarily with comfort. The patient monitors the suppression clues as fusion is held for a specific time, e.g., 2 minutes. Flashing, blinking, and increased illumination can be used to break suppression if it occurs. The patient completes at least 4 sets, of 2 minutes each, separated with short rest intervals. With continued training, comfort should be gradually achieved.

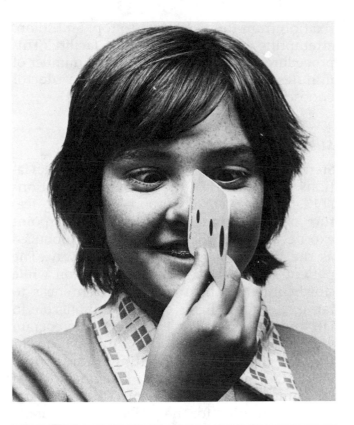

FIGURE 14-1—Nearpoint convergence training with a 3-dot card.

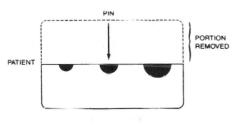

FIGURE 14-2—The 3-dot convergence card with the top portion cut off to facilitate bifixation. A pen is shown that can be stuck on the card to promote fusion of the middle-sized pair of dots (actually half-dots) in this example.

When progress reaches a plateau, the patient is introduced to step vergences. A stereogram with two pairs of targets on one stereogram, such as the example shown in Figure 13-5, is presented to the patient. The bottom pair of targets should have a base-out demand approximating that of the isometric maximum and the top pair with less BO demand. The patient is instructed to alternate fixation from top to bottom to top, and so on, attempting to increase vergence facility. This procedure is repeated for a specified number of minutes or cycles, whichever the doctor chooses.

Stereoscope Tromboning T14.8

Stereoscopic tromboning in cases of exo deviations is similar to that for eso deviations (T13.4). However, an important training feature of the Brewster stereoscope for farpoint exo deviations is that BO demand is produced as the target is tromboned farther away. The patient is instructed to maintain fusion while slowly moving the stereogram from near to far, and so on. This is especially applicable in DE and BX cases. For example, a stereogram with a target separation of 63 mm has an ortho demand at the near setting (simulated 40 cm distance) but has a BO demand of 12^Δ at far (simulated 6 m distance). This is a paradoxical sensation for the patient who naturally associates divergence with a receding target, rather than having to converge his eyes at greater distances. This dissociative maneuver on accommodation and vergence "shakes up" the patient's sensory and motor fusion pattern, thus creating a novel, motivating, and effective training technique.

Vectograms® and Tranaglyphs

These open-environment training materials, described in Chapter 13 (T13.8-T13.10), can be used in the office or at home and are distinguished by the variety of well designed and interesting targets with stereopsis and suppression clues. In exotropia and exophoria the emphasis is on developing and expanding suppression-free, fusional convergence ranges, and step convergence reflexes that are fast and accurate. Fusional convergence can be increased with sliding, step, jump, tromboning, and isometric training using Vectograms and Tranaglyphs. There are countless variations and embellishments on these familiar themes that result in more training procedures than can be described here. Innovation in vision training is limited only by the creativity of the therapist.

Convergence Training at Near T14.9

The majority of patients with exotropia have the ability to fuse at near, at least some of the time. In such cases, the target demand of a Vectogram or Tranaglyph is set at the ortho position and fusional convergence training can begin with the gradual introduction of base-out prism demand. The Mother Goose Vectogram is a good initial target because if has large suppression controls for all three figures (Figure 13-10e). As the patient makes small step vergences when fixating from one figure to the next, the slides are slowly separated in the base-out direction (numbers showing through the mask). The patient uses voluntary convergence and tries to maintain fusion with clearness and without any suppression, e.g., Little Bo Peep losing her sheep. The initial emphasis is on the base-out range, but eventually base-in demands are intermittently introduced so that fusional vergence can be strengthened in both directions.

When diplopia (break) occurs, the BO demand is reduced enough to allow for recovery of fusion. The patient continues to bifixate each target on the Vectogram for at least 1 minute before an increased BO demand is given. Smoothness of disparation requires the therapist to move each slide laterally and simultaneously at an appropriately slow speed for the patient. Later in training, the patient can learn to move the slides properly and at a faster rate commensurate with his ability to maintain fusion during the disparation. The patient should learn to perceive blur (if possible) and record this value along with break and recovery points. Each training interval should last about 10 minutes. Various split Vectograms and Tranaglyphs can be used for interest and for the special features on some of them, e.g., the Spirangle with its subtle stereopsis and suppression clues (see Figure 13-10b).

As progress is made, two pairs of split Vectograms or Tranaglyphs can be used on a Dual Polachrome Illuminated Trainer for vergence facility training. The top target can be a divergence demand and the bottom for convergence. The goal for the patient is to reach the maximum limit of vergence in either direction and recover fusion in each pair as quickly and accurately as possible. The clinician prescribes as many sets as the patient can complete within a 10-minute training session; this is also training for stamina.

In relatively rare cases of exotropia in which the patient cannot achieve any fusion at near, split Vectograms or Tranaglyphs can be placed at the patient's objective angle of deviation in an attempt to obtain sensory fusion. Fusional convergence training proceeds in a similar fashion as discussed above, except that the starting point may be with base-in compensation rather than at the ortho demand point. As progress is made, the BI demand is gradually reduced and, eventually, a normal base-out range is achieved. This procedure works well if there is NRC, but not if there is ARC when the exo deviation is manifest. (Refer to Chapter 11 for discussion of treatment of Exotropia with ARC.)

Convergence Walk-Aways T14.10

Split Vectograms and Tranaglyphs are particularly helpful for DE and BX patients who often lose fusion as the fixation distance is increased. A good pair of targets is the Spirangle Vectogram, which is large and has an appreciable stereopsis effect at far distances (see Figure 13-10b). The base-out demand should be increased maximally at near while the patient maintains fusion. When a good BO range is established, the patient is instructed to walk away from the target, slowly while maintaining fusion with clearness. The spiral figure should appear more in depth as fixation distance increases. Furthermore, the base-in demand decreases theoretically and should make fusion easier for the patient. For example, 12^Δ at 40 cm translates to only 6^Δ at 80 cm and only 3^Δ at 160 cm. Exotropic patients who previously could not bifixate at far are delighted to realize that they can fuse at far. The visual feedback of stereopsis and monitoring of suppression tells them so. This newly discovered skill builds confidence and motivation to continue to achieve in vision therapy. Once the patient can master fusing at

far with a small BO demand, the split targets are more widely separated (sliding vergence) to train for an increased fusional convergence range.

Projected BO Slides T14.11

As in T13.10 for eso deviations using an overhead projector, the therapist can project split Vectograms or Tranaglyphs with a base-out demand for fusional convergence training at far. In exotropia of the DE and BX types, the targets are initially aligned to the patient's subjective angle of deviation, a base-in setting. This procedure is ideal for training sliding vergence at far due to the fusional lock of stereopsis. Besides sliding vergence, step (using two pairs of targets at the same distance) and jump (alternate near-far viewing) vergence procedures can be used to build the range and facility of fusional convergence.

Aperture-Rule Trainer (Single Aperture) T14.12

The Aperture-Rule Trainer (ART) can be used as an in-office and home training instrument in cases of convergence insufficiency and basic exophoria. The design of the instrument was discussed in Chapter 13, specifically T13.13. A single aperture is used to create base-out demands (Figure 14-3). The patient looks at and fuses the pair of targets at the distance of 40 cm through the single aperture, i.e., chiastopic fusion. If there is difficulty fusing the first few cards, the patient is instructed to look at a pointer stick placed in the center of the aperture. Fixation on the pointer helps to converge the eyes so the patient can initially fuse the pair of targets even though they may appear blurred. With fusion, the pointer is quickly withdrawn and the patient is encouraged to maintain fusion. Blinking sometimes help to relax focus to the plane of the fusion targets.

The goal is for the patient to progress to cards with higher step prism demands, up to card 12, while perceiving all suppression clues. Initially, the patient may need minus-add lenses to achieve clear vision. The therapist or patient must remember to move the aperture

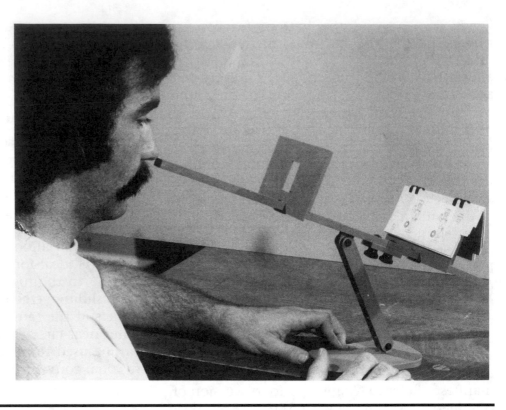

FIGURE 14-3—Patient doing convergence training with the Aperture-Rule Trainer with a single aperture.

slider appropriately with each change of target so the aperture slider does not block the view of either eye. Using loose base-out prisms, a prism bar, or prism or lens flippers can extend the range of the vergence demand if desired.

An effective jump vergence technique is to have the patient diverge the eyes and focus on a far target over the top if the ART and then converge to the targets seen through the aperture (Figure 14-4). The back and forth fixations should be as rapid as possible. The patient records the time for the number of cycles achieved within 2 minutes and is given instructions to repeat this procedure at least five times each day. Suppression should be monitored and broken, if it occurs, before continuing with this jump technique.

Pencil Pushups and Push-aways T14.13

The pencil pushup procedure is probably the most frequently assigned home training technique in clinical practice today. It is a simple convenient technique and is quite effective in cases of convergence insufficiency, if done properly. Patients of all ages can use it. Besides advancing the nearpoint of convergence (NPC), it can be used to established physiological diplopia, build vergence facility and stamina, and train accommodative skills. The downside, however, is that patients often find the technique boring. Therefore, compliance suffers, particularly when this technique is assigned as the sole training procedure; unfortunately, this happens too often in clinical practice. Vision training patients need variety in their exercise program for both psychological and physiological reasons, just as athletes do in theirs.

To utilize this technique, the patient must have a nearpoint of convergence within arm's length. A pencil, with its point up, is held at arm's length and is fixated bifoveally. The patient positions herself such that when fusing the pencil, a distant object across the room (e.g., a door knob or better yet, a small television screen) appears double as a normal physiological diplopic image. While maintaining a single image of the pencil and monitoring physiological diplopia of the distant target,

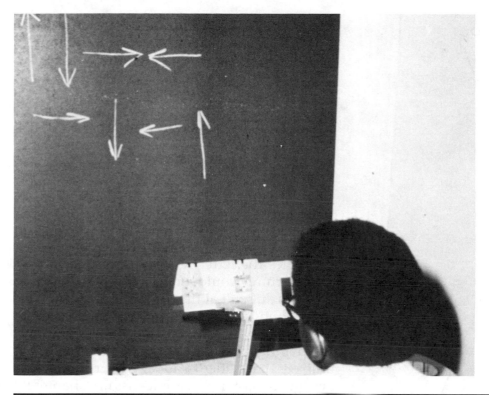

FIGURE 14-4—The single aperture is used for nearpoint fusion training. Fixation targets at far can be included for jump vergence training. A metronome can be incorporated to pace the vergence demands. The arrows challenge the patients directionality skills to promote automaticity of vergences.

the patient slowly moves the pencil toward her nose until the pencil tip doubles. Pushing the pencil away to regain fusion, the patient tracks the pencil back to arm's length again. If suppression occurs and one of the physiological diplopic images disappears, the patient should blink and shake the pencil a little bit to enliven the suppressed image before continuing. The technique is continued for a 10-minute period or for some other time interval the doctor judges feasible. Smoothness and amplitude of vergence tracking are trained, not necessarily speed. The goal is to train smooth vergence tracking with no "break and join" response along the way and to achieve an NPC of 5 cm or closer. The closest NPC achieved during the training session should be noted and recorded each day.

An emphasis on pencil push-aways is recommended in cases of divergence excess exotropia or exophoria since the far exo deviation is larger than the near. As progress is made and fusion occurs beyond arm's length, a walk-away technique is appropriate. The pencil becomes the physiological suppression control as the patient walks-away while maintaining fusion of the far target (e.g., the doorknob).

Convergence stamina can be improved through an isometric exercise. The patient steadily fixates a pencil placed just beyond the NPC for an assigned time period; we suggest 1 to 2 minutes at a time. Again, physiological diplopia should be monitored in the background. This technique builds gross convergence quickly,[35] but is often associated with considerable eyestrain. Sufficient rest periods, perhaps 5 to 10 minutes, are recommended between training intervals.

Vergence facility is trained using a jump vergence technique. The pencil is placed just beyond the nearpoint of convergence. The patient fixates a far target. For motivational purposes, we suggest a small television tuned to a commercial channel, but any distinct object will suffice, particularly a clock. At each commercial break, the patient completes as many cycles of jump vergence eye movements as possible between the television and the pencil, always noting or establishing physiological diplopia before the next jump is initiated. The

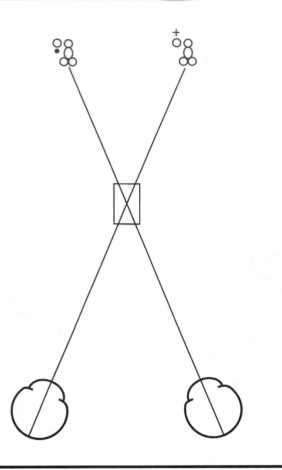

FIGURE 14-5—Illustration of chiastopic principle with a single aperture. The visual axes cross at the plane of the septum, intersection of an "X" resembling the Greek letter *chi*.

goal here, of course, is to increase speed of jump vergence eye movements without suppression.

Accommodative facility can be trained in much the same way as vergence facility, except using an alphabet pencil (letters printed on the pencil) or a detailed sticker attached to the pencil that serves as an effective accommodative stimulus. This modification is important to know because accommodative infacility is often associated with convergence insufficiency exophoria and gross convergence insufficiency[8,34] (Refer to Chapter 16 for discussions on accomodative training.)

Pencil pushups have become a traditional technique in vision training, but we would encourage clinicians to use their imagination, or better still, the patient's particular interests for selecting a pushup target. We have had success using toy cars, stamps, stickers, coins, can-

dies and other small objects that are of unique interest to the patient. And remember, in vision training, *variety* "spells" success.

Chiastopic Fusion T14.14

Chiastopic fusion and the Aperture-Rule Trainer are based on the same principle (Figure 14-5). Both techniques provide base-out demands for improving fusional convergence. The difference is that there is no aperture involved in chiastopic fusion, thus it is truly a free-space technique. Chiastopic fusion is the crossing of the visual axes (as in the Greek letter chi that resembles the letter X) at the plane on which the aperture would ordinarily be. Chiastopic fusion is difficult at first for most patients, especially younger ones. This is because there is no aperture to help direct the patient to the crossing point. In accord with Piaget's theory, it is unlikely that patients under 7 years of age will be able to master chiastopic fusion (Chapter 9).

A good procedure initially is the use of the Keystone Colored Circles ("Lifesavers") Card (Figure 14-6). The patient is instructed to follow a pencil tip placed between him and the card, approximately 40 cm away. The pencil should be moved back and forth slowly while being bifixated; this is done until the patient can perceive four circles from a single pair, i.e., two seen diplopically (because of physiological diplopia) equals four. When the pencil is at exactly the correct distance (as with the aperture of the Aperture-Rule Trainer), three circles should be perceived. The middle circle is the fused image and the outside two are merely diplopic images. These unfused circles (diplopic images) act as peripheral suppression clues. Central suppression clues are the missing letters for each eye, or the clinician's modification of added symbols such as arrows (Figure 14-7). The patient is instructed to continue this technique until chiastopic fusion can be achieved voluntarily and quickly. If the fused target appears blurred, the card may be moved slightly and slowly back and forth to achieve clearness. If that fails, the patient may try wearing minus-adds to help convergence and to extend the focus out to the plane of regard. (Note that exophoric or exotropic patients usually over

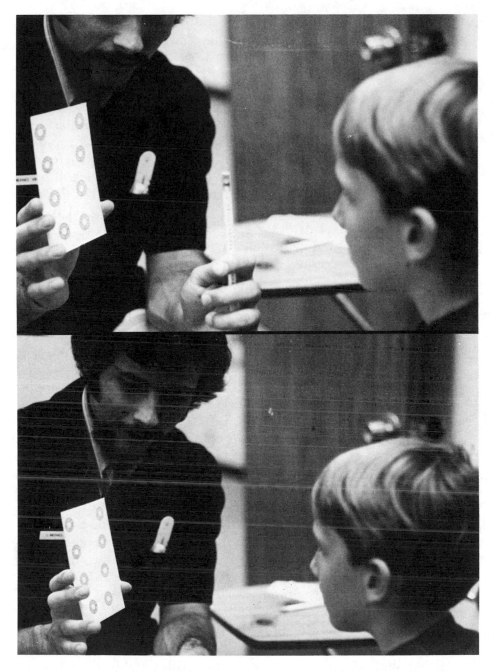

FIGURE 14-6—Chiastopic fusion training with the use of Keystone Colored Circles ("Lifesaver" card). (a) Use of pencil to aid convergence and teach patient to cross-fuse; (b) Chiastopic fusion without the use of pencil as aid to convergence.

accommodate to enlist accommodative convergence as an aid in the chiastopic fusion task.) The goal for the patient is to achieve chiastopic fusion quickly with clarity and with comfort, without any suppression. If suppression occurs, have the patient blink his eyes as an antisuppression method. All four pairs of circles, top being the most difficult, should be easily fused. The patient should strive to increase the speed

of step vergence responses by going from one pair to the next, up and down the card. The prism demand on fusional convergence for any particular pair can be calculated using the decimeter rule (Chapter 13).

The "Lifesaver" card is particularly applicable for patients with convergence insufficiency, either exotropia or exophoria. Once chiastopic fusion is achieved and the patient can make

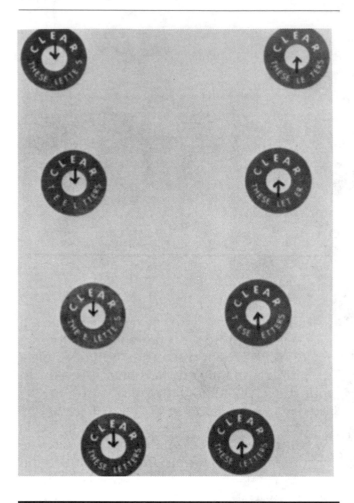

FIGURE 14-7—Modification of the Keystone Colored Circles for monitoring suppression. The missing letters and the added drawings of arrows monitor central suppression; Peripheral suppression is monitored by whether there is perception of three circles when the middle being chiastopically fused. Vertical marks such as arrows serve also to monitor fixation disparity during forced convergence.

step vergence movements on the card, tromboning can be introduced to build gross convergence much like the pencil pushup technique. This advanced variation is to have the patient make step vergence eye movements as he brings the card closer to his nose.

Another good nearpoint target for chiastopic fusion is the Keystone Eccentric Circles. These were discussed in Chapter 13 for orthopic (base-in) fusion (T13.15) for training in cases of eso deviations; the difference in training in cases of exo deviations is that chiastopic (base-out) fusion training should be given. A validity check by the therapist is to see if the patient is actually performing chiastopic fusion, rather than orthopic. The patient's perception of the

floating circle is the key. In Figure 13-17, the small circle in the chiastopically fused image should appear to float farther away than the larger circle when the cards are placed with the A's next to each other. If the patient reports that the smaller circle is floating toward him, the therapist knows that the patient is performing orthopic fusion, rather than chiastopic fusion as he should be doing. The goal for the patient is to achieve a base-out range comparable to the "very strong" values listed in Chapter 2 for blur, break, and recovery (23/28/18).

Another goal is for the patient to perceive SILO ("small, in; large, out"). As the patient converges to meet greater base-out demands (sliding vergence) with the targets being more widely separated, the middle fused target typically appears to be getting smaller ("small") and sometimes closer ("in"). This is a size constancy perceptual phenomenon and not a stereopsis response based on lateral disparity differences. Conversely with the SILO effect, as the base-out demand is reduced by decreasing the separation distance of the cards, the fused image appears to be getting larger ("large") and sometimes can be perceived as receding ("out"). The SILO effect is motivational and fascinating to patients and is a good check for the therapist that the patient is doing the prescribed technique properly. (Note that some patients may report a SOLI preception, i.e., "small, out; large in.")

Jump vergence training can be done with either the "Lifesaver" card or Eccentric Circles. The patient makes jump vergence eye movements from a chiastopically fused image at near to a distant object, such as a doorknob. A specific number of cycles or a specific time should be assigned for home training, and the patient records his results daily. Increasing both the amplitude of the jump and speed are training goals.

For DE and BX cases the chiastopic technique is done at far and can be done with two similar pictures for flat fusion, as in the Figure 14-8. The technique can be done with stereopsis targets by using enlarged Eccentric Circles, either home-made or purchased, e.g., Bernell Eccentric Circles (EC1). It is difficult for most DE or BX patients to begin chiastopic fusion at far. Nearpoint training on this technique is

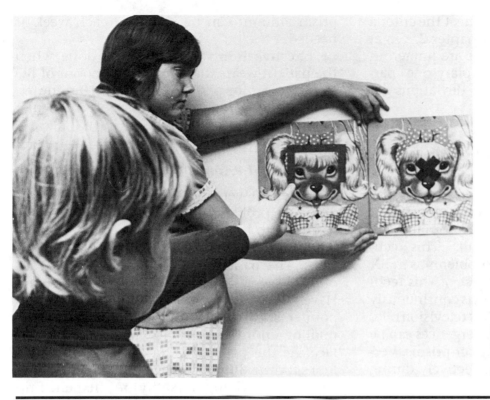

FIGURE 14-8—Chiastopic fusion training at far. Two similar pictures are cross-fused. The special markings act as suppression clues.

almost always essential before the fixation distance can be extended to far. This process takes considerable time to achieve, perhaps several weeks in some cases. The patient's goal is to achieve chiastopic fusion at a distance of 3 m or farther and be able to do this quickly (phasic training) with clear vision, perceive stereopsis, and have no suppression. The patient should be able to hold fusion (isometric training) comfortably for periods of 2 minutes.

Binocular Accommodative Rock T14.15

As in eso deviations (T13.11), binocular accommodative rock can be used to increase accommodative and convergence skills of exotropic and exophoric patients. The clinician should ensure good monocular accommodative skills before proceeding to binocular accommodative rock. (See Chapter 16.) Patients with CI usually have little or no difficulty with T14.15 by the time this phase of therapy is introduced. The reason is that the AC/A is low and lenses have relatively little effect on the demand for

fusional vergence. In BX cases the AC/A is normal and patients with large exo deviations may have trouble fusing the target clearly when plus lenses are introduced. This difficulty is usually exaggerated in DE cases because of the higher than normal AC/A. In summary, T14.15 is more necessary in DE cases, next in BX, and least of all in CI cases. The therapy procedure parallels that in T13.11 except that fusional convergence is emphasized rather than divergence. (Refer to Chapter 13 for details of this technique and goals.) Because convergence is potentially stronger than divergence and it is more easy to train and develop, most patients with exo deviations quickly pass through this phase of therapy.

Vergence Rock Techniques

Vergence rock training with flipper prisms can be done in cases of exo deviation in a similar way as for eso deviations (T13.12) (see Figure 13-12). Step convergence should be emphasized more than step divergence for patients with exotropia or exophoria, but both should be done. The training goal is to meet the criteria for vergence facility given in Chapter 2, i.e., at least 15 cycles per minute. There are numerous rock techniques but three exemplary ones particularly useful for treating exo deviations are presented here.

Television Trainer and Prisms T14.16

The use of television trainers was discussed in Chapter 12 for antisuppression training (T12.8). This procedure applies here but the emphasis is on motor fusion training to develop and improve fusional convergence skills. This technique applies to farpoint exo problems as in BX and DE cases. A beneficial aspect of this technique is that central suppression is continuously monitored as the patient watches television over extensive periods of time. Step vergences can be trained with either loose or flipper prisms. Vergence facility can be trained effectively during commercial breaks.

Isometric training is especially appropriate by having the patient wear the maximum base-out prism demand that allows clear, single, binocular vision. Greater BO prism power can be worn in subsequent training sessions if the patient can maintain fusion and be reasonably comfortable. The goal is to reach the maximum amount of prism that can be worn for 15 minutes without suppression.

Bar Reader with Prisms T14.17

Bar reading (T12.10) with base-out prism rock is especially helpful in CI cases, since training is done at near (see Figure 10-21). However, the technique can be used effectively for any type of exo deviation as long as there is nearpoint fusion. It is a demanding exercise that is often given in the final stages of training and as a retainer exercise. Step vergence training is done by having the patient alternately change the prism from BI to BO at the end of each line. If suppression occurs, the patient can blink her eyes, increase illumination, and move closer to the page. Reading in this manner is continued for a 10-minute period. With practice, patients can learn to read passages for meaning without thinking about sensory or motor fusion. The

prism amount can be increased each week as needed.

Effective isometric training is done when the patient wears the maximum amount of BO prism power for periods of at least 10 minutes. The goal is clear, single, comfortable, binocular vision without suppression.

Framing and Prisms T14.18

An excellent vergence rock technique for farpoint exo problems is framing with prisms. This is similar to bar reading for nearpoint training and it is especially applicable to BX and DE cases. The patient is instructed to look at an object, e.g., a penlight from across the room. Have the patient hold a pencil (or a bright red pointer stick) in the upright position in the midline approximately 40 cm away from his face. As the patient bifixates the penlight he looks for the diplopic images of the pencil. The patient then changes fixation to the pencil tip and tries to be aware of the diplopic images of the penlight. When this process of awareness of physiological diplopia is completed, the patient looks at the distant penlight and frames it symmetrically with the diplopic images of pencil. (Refer to a discussion of physiological diplopia in Chapter 1.) The two images of the pencil serve as peripheral suppression clues. If central suppression clues are desired, targets such as Vectograms, Tranaglyphs, TV trainers, and Root Rings can be bifixated at far while being framed by the pencil images.

Step vergence training with framing is done by having the patient place a loose prism before an eye, achieve fusion of the fixation target with framing, remove the prism, recover fusion, reinsert the prism, and so on. Base-out prism demands are emphasized, although base-in prism demands are eventually incorporated into the training routine. The training goal in step vergence is at least 15 cycles per minute using 4^Δ BI and 8^Δ BO (see criteria for "very strong" in Chapter 2).

For jump vergence training have the patient alternately fixate from the penlight to the pencil; the goal is to maximize the number of near-far fixations in 1 minute with recoveries of clear, single, binocular vision without suppression.

Pola-Mirror Vergence Techniques T14.19

Training with the Pola-Mirror was discussed in Chapter 12 as an antisuppression technique (T12.9) and shown in Figure 12-10. Because this monitors foveal suppression, vergence training can be done while bifixation is being ensured. In CI cases, the procedure is to do pushups with the Pola-Mirror to train fusional convergence. The patient is instructed to hold the mirror at arm's length and move it slowly toward him to about 5 cm. The patient is to see both eyes simultaneously. If one eye darkens, indicating suppression, the patient is to blink that eye and pay attention to it (mental effort) to break the suppression. The intermediate goal is to be able to see both eyes at all times from a range of about 1 m (note doubling of image distance by mirror) to about 10 cm. A final goal in CI cases can be to master this technique while wearing 20^Δ base-out over the polarizing filters during tromboning of the mirror.

In cases of BX and DE, the patient performs the above procedure but emphasis is on push-aways since the fusional convergence demand is greater at far. The procedure can begin at a near distance and the mirror is slowly moved farther away (or the patient walks away), to at least 75 cm (i.e., 1.5 m image distance). By adding base-out prism, the fusional convergence demand is increased even more so. The patient should practice this technique for 5-minute periods at least twice a day. The goal for the BX or DE patient is to achieve fusion continuously without suppression during push-aways.

Computerized Convergence Procedures T14.20

Computerized vision therapy programs for exo deviations have the same principles as for eso deviations (T13.16) Such programs provide excellent training procedures for step and sliding vergences. Vergence ranges are often improved quickly in children as well as adults because they appreciate the game features of computerized programs. We recommend these programs because of the patient interest and motivation they stimulate. Particularly fasci-

nating is Computer Orthoptics by Dr. Cooper with high speed liquid crystal filters for mutual cancellation of targets for the right and left eye. Most of the training techniques for patients with exotropia and exophoria can be done with computerized programs for improving fusional convergence ranges, facility, and stamina.

CASE MANAGEMENT AND EXAMPLES

Divergence Excess Exotropia

Management Principles

True divergence excess (DE) exotropia and exophoria are characterized by a farpoint deviation that is substantially larger than at near. These patients present with farpoint problems (e.g., asthenopia, diplopia, a cosmetic deviation) and often show normal fusional skills at near. Divergence excess is usually caused by an abnormally high AC/A with inadequate fusional convergence at far. It is the least prevalent type of exotropia although many exotropic patients initially appear to have it.[34] A prolonged cover test often reveals an increased nearpoint exo deviation indicating a "simulated" DE rather than a "true" DE.[10]

Our vision therapy approach in DE cases involves fully correcting any significant refractive error, possibly prescribing an appropriate minus add to help control the far deviation, and initiating a vigorous vision training program. The effect of minus addition lenses can be remarkable since the AC/A is high. For example, a patient with a 60 mm IPD with 20^Δ of intermittent exotropia at 6m and 10^Δ exophoria at 40 cm has a calculated AC/A is 10/1; the gradient is usually lower, e.g., 7/10. (Refer to Chapter 3.) This high AC/A implies that for every diopter of minus lens addition that is worn, the exo deviation is reduced by approximately 7^Δ. Therefore, a −1.00 D addition would reduce the deviation at far to about 13^Δ exo at far and 3^Δ exo at near, −2.00 D addition to about 6^Δ exo at far and result in 4^Δ *eso* at near. Of course these are only theoretical values since patients do not always respond to the addition lenses in a mechanistic way. The clinician must always observe and measure how the patient responds to minus addition lenses at far and near before a lens prescription is written. In this case example, the prescription of a −1.50 D add, in single vision form, might be the best choice; it may provide adequate control of the far deviation reducing it to about 10^Δ exo. The near deviation with the −1.50 D add should be close to ortho. This approach possibly avoids the need for a plus-add bifocal perscription for near viewing that would otherwise be needed if a minus add of higher power were prescribed.

The emphasis of the vision training is to break suppression, often found at far, and to extend the fusional vergence ranges at all viewing distances. If fusion cannot be quickly established at the farpoint with a minus add, a half-patch occluder to allow only nearpoint viewing must be worn until this is achieved. Magic Tape (by 3-M) or similar material over the top half of one spectacle lens is a convenient and effective method. Specific training techniques that we have found particularly effective in DE cases include voluntary convergence (T14.1), Brock string and beads at 3 meters (T14.5), Vectograms and Tranaglyphs (T14.9) using wide-field stimulation at distance,[25,37] and vergence rock techniques (T14.16). Push-aways (T14.13) and walk-aways (T14.10) techniques should be emphasized to increase the ranges of sensory and motor fusion at far distances.

Divergence excess patients with a very high AC/A or a large deviation at far are difficult to manage successfull, particularly with minus adds, even when vision training is included. When the patient looks up to the ceiling or sky, which is lacking in strong fusional stimuli, the deviation tends to become manifest. Suppression at far can quickly recur, and a patient can relapse into exotropia. Dissociation can also occur when the patient moves from a dimly lit space to a bright area. Many exotropic individuals tend to be dazzled and often close one eye, breaking fusion. (Refer to discussion in Chapter 7.) In these cases that do not respond to the combination of minus adds and vision training or those who show frequent relapses, strabismus surgery (usually a bilateral lateral rectus

recession) may be required for successful management.

In most cases of intermittent exotropia of the DE type, vision therapy usually takes from 2 to 4 months to complete. These cases can often be managed on a home training basis with weekly office testing and training visits. Biofocals (plus-adds) are often beneficial and may be prescribed at some time during therapy. The efficacy of biofocals in cases of DE is that isometric fusional convergence is trained at near. Also, the near and far magnitudes of exo deviation can be equalized. After dismissal criteria are met, a good retainer exercise is the TV trainer with prism (T14.16) since it monitors for suppression and trains the reflex aspects of fusional vergence at far. Thirty minutes per week of TV watching with prism rock during commercial intervals is usually sufficient to prevent regression of trained binocular skills.

Case Example

This case report is courtesy of Dr. Janice Scharre of the Illinois College of Optometry. Only a brief summary is presented here to exemplify vision training in a case of DE exotropia.

A 10-year-old female patient was referred because of an occasional outward eye turn, occurring more often at far. The time of onset was unknown, but she had had it "for a while." Her only symptom was occasional diplopia. She had been prescribed a patch by the referring doctor 6 weeks previously and was wearing spectacles with constant patching of her right eye. The patient's and family's eye and health histories were unremarkable. There was no history of eye surgery and she was doing well in school.

Pertinent clinical findings were as follows:

Habitual lenses: OD +0.25 −2.75 x 180 20/30+

(2 years old)   OS +1.00 −2.50 x 140 20/30

Refraction: OD +0.25 −2.25 x 015 20/30+3

    OS +1.00 −2.50 x 155 20/30+2

(Cycloplegic and manifest refractions were not significantly different.)

The binocular vision evaluation indicated a comitant, intermittent, alternating, exotropia of 20^Δ at far and 10^Δ exophoria at near. The Worth 4-dot test showed good fusion at near but intermittent suppression OS at far. Fusional vergences measured: at far BI X/8/2; BO X/10/4; and at near BI 10/12/10; BO X/10/4. The monocular accommodative amplitudes were reduced for her age, OD 9.00; OS 9.00, as was the relative accommodation, NRA +1.00; PRA −1.00. The NPC was normal, 8 cm, but stereopsis slightly reduced, 70 seconds of arc on Randot. Eye health examination proved unremarkable.

The diagnosis was moderate astigmatism with possible slight meridional amblyopia OU, divergence excess exotropia, NRC, suppression at far, slightly reduced stereopsis, and accommodative insufficiency.

Vision therapy in the office and home during the first 4 weekly visits emphasized accommodative training with minus lenses and Hart Chart, vergence training with pencil pushups and push-aways, Brock string with beads, and the Allbee 3-dot card. By the fifth visit after Vectograms, Aperture-Rule Trainer, Lifesaver card, and Tranaglyphs had been introduced, the patient was able to appreciate SILO and converge 18^Δ BO and recover 9^Δ BO at nearpoint. (Accommodative skills had improved.) By the seventh visit, she was able to do chiastopic fusion walk-aways with large Eccentric Circles and projected Vectograms.

The training results after week 7 indicated significant improvement in most binocular findings. No strabismus was found at near or far. Fusional vergences had increased to: BI X/14/12, BO 8/10/8 at far; BI 14/16/8, BO 18/30/18 at near. The relative accommodation was normal (NRA: +2.25; PRA −2.50) and amplitudes increased to 15 D each eye. Good fusion was found at far and near without suppression by Worth dots. Stereopsis improved to 50 seconds of arc. A trial frame refraction yielded more cylinder correction than previously and new lenses were prescribed.

OD +0.50 −3.00 x 010   20/25

OS +1.00 −3.25 x 160   20/25

Another seven office visits with home training were prescribed and completed with the follow-ing improvements: The patient was exophoric: 14^Δ at far, 6^Δ at near. There were normal fusional vergence ranges: BI X/18/10, BO 14/26/8 at far; BI 14/16/10, BO 30/40/14 at near. The NPC measured to the nose and stereopsis increased to 30 seconds of arc. The refractive findings were stable.

Disposition: Based on the results of therapy, the patient was dismissed as cured. Retainer exercises were prescribed using Eccentric Circles and lens flippers, every other day for approximately 10 minutes. A 6-month progress evaluation was scheduled.

At the progress evaluation 6 months later, the patient reported no symptoms and all clinical findings remained normal. The visual acuity of the right eye had increased to 20/20, but remained 20/25 in the left. The conclusion was that this patient's divergence excess exotropia had been successfully treated using vision training and meridional amblyopia was significantly reduced by using vision training and corrective lenses.

Basic Exotropia

Management Principles

Patients with basic exotropia (the normal AC/A type) tend to have the largest angles of deviation and the highest prevalence of constant deviations, although the majority are intermittent. Most BX patients have an intermittent strabismus at near and a constant one at far, as in DE cases. Exotropes in general have a better prognosis for a functional cure than esotropes, but as in esotropia, constancy of the deviation is a major consideration (a 30% factor) in predicting successful outcome.[7]

Our approach to therapy, in accord with Wick,[38] in cases of constant XT, whether associated with NRC or ARC, is to attempt to convert the constant deviation into an intermittent deviation at near distances as soon as possible. This step assumes that amblyopia is not present or has been successfully treated. As discussed previously, we train for fusion at near using gross convergence (T11.13) and voluntary convergence techniques (T14.1). If this training continues for 3 or 4 in-office sessions without success, we resort to more traditional techniques of building convergence on the major amblyoscope (T14.2). If, however, the patient is successful in getting fusion at near, even with great effort for short periods of time, we continue with open-environment training methods at near such as Brock string and beads (T14.5), Mirror Stereoscope (T14.4), and Vectograms (T14.9).

An attempt is made to find some satisfactory combination of BI prism and minus-add power to establish fusion at some distance, often at near. If the patient has adequate accommodative skills (or if they can be trained quickly), the effects of minus-add lenses are evaluated for a trial period of wear for 1 or 2 weeks. The minus-add is often a good stimulus to initiate fusional vergence eye movements even if the angle of deviation is not significantly reduced. With children under the age of 10, up to -3.00 D add should be tried; they can usually learn to tolerate the accommodative demand within 1 or 2 weeks. Older children and young adults also often benefit with minus adds, but lesser powers are more tolerable. It bears repeating that if sensory fusion cannot be achieved at a particular distance by any means, the patient must wear a patch on one eye for that fixation distance. While in a vision therapy program, the patient should not be allowed to view the world in his strabismic condition.

Auditory biofeedback is a promising alternative technique for achieving bifoveal alignment of the eyes in exotropia. Goldrich[39] reported his experience with twelve exotropic subjects and a training protocol he developed. The intermittent strabismics quickly achieved alignment at all distances and built adequate fusional convergence using this technique; the constant exotropes had mixed results. The suggested advantages of biofeedback therapy were shorter treatment time, elimination of lengthy home training exercises, and enhanced patient motivation. Auditory biofeedback instrumentation, unfortunately, is not readily available.

If the patient presents with fusion at near or it can be established quickly by optical methods and gross convergence techniques, the prognosis for functional cure with vision therapy is good, at least 70%.[7] Training proceeds as described in the sections on vision therapy sequence and management principles for DE. At this time the BX patient can be treated in the same way, for training purposes, as a DE patient who has fusion at near but strabismus at far.

Basic exo*phoria* is much more prevalent than basic exo*tropia*. These heterophoric patients are usually symptomatic and present with a moderate to large exo duration at far and near, deficient fusional convergence, and often, an associated accommodative deficiency. Base-in prism can be prescribed for symptomatic relief in these cases using one or several standard clinical criteria: Sheard's criterion, clinical wisdom (1/3 the angle of deviation), or associated phoria as measured on a Mallett unit. (Refer to Chapter 3 on heterophoria case analysis.) We often recommend a 6-to-8-week course in vision training for symptomatic exophoria, mostly home based. Within this time frame, functional deficiencies of fusional vergence and accommodation usually respond sufficiently to a consistent, well designed training program of approximately 30 minutes of home training per day. The specifics of the vision training program for basic exophoria is similar to that described previously for DE exophoric and for CI exophoria described in the next section.

Case Example

This example of vision therapy for basic exotropia was contributed by Garth N. Christenson, O.D., M.S.Ed., of Hudson, Wisconsin. A 7-year-old male was evaluated for binocular anomalies because his parents had noticed an occasional outward turning of an eye. The eye turn began 2 years previously but it had been getting worse. Case history was otherwise unremarkable and the patient had no complaints of blurred vision, diplopia, or asthenopia. Subjective refraction and acuities were:

OD +0.50 DS   20/20   (6/6)

OS +0.50 DS   20/20   (6/6)

Hirschberg testing was 0 mm OD and +1 mm OS, suggesting 22^Δ exotropia of the left eye. Cover testing at far indicated constant, alternating (right eye preferred for fixation) exotropia of 15^Δ, and at near, intermittent (strabismus approximately 10% of time), alternating exotropia of 15^Δ. The deviation was the same in all 9 diagnostic fields of gaze, indicating comitancy. The patient had poor pursuit and saccadic eye movements. Correspondence was tested with Bagolini striated lenses, major amblyoscope, and Hering-Bielschowsky afterimages; NRC was found on all tests. The patient had suppression at far on the Worth 4-dot test but good fusion at near. Stereopsis at near on a contoured test was 140 seconds of arc. Fusional vergence ranges were limited, being only 4^Δ diverging and 5^Δ converging around angle S in the major amblyoscope. The nearpoint of convergence was 15 cm to break and 20 cm to recover. Monocular accommodation was normal but binocular accommodative facility could not be tested because of suppression when plus lenses were introduced.

The above findings were discussed with the child's parents and recommendations for vision therapy were made. The possibility of surgery was discussed but not recommended due to the good prognosis for cure with vision training. The estimated treatment time was 20 to 25 office visits along with home training.

The first 8 weeks of vision therapy consisted of gross convergence training (pencil pushups, Brock string, and Allbee 3-dot Card), accommodative training (various procedures using a Hart Chart), and a variety of saccadic and pursuit training techniques. The next 7 weeks involved the following training techniques: (1) Sliding vergence techniques included Vectograms emphasizing BO demands and perception of SILO, Mirror Stereoscope, and major amblyoscope; (2) Step vergences included Vectogram, Mirror Stereoscope, major amblyoscope, and TV trainers (with −2.00 D over-correction to facilitate fusion at far); (3) chiastopic fusion with Lifesaver cards and Keystone Eccentric Circles (near and far) with −2.00 D over-correction at far when needed; (4) accommodative rock, monocular and binocular; (5) fusional "high level" vergence techniques, e.g., Delta Series Biopter Cards for far BO recoveries, projected vectographic slides, and accommodative rock combined with vectographic BI and BO demands.

After 15 weekly office visits and home training the exotropia was cured. There were normal vergence ranges, oculomotor deficiencies were abated as were accommodative infacility, suppression, and poor stereopsis. At the time of dismissal the patient was prescribed a home maintenance therapy program including Eccentric Circles at far and near, Lifesaver card, and lens rock with flippers. The patient was instructed to do home training twice a week and return for a progress evaluation in 3 months.

Convergence Insufficiency Exophoria

Management Principles

Convergence insufficiency exo deviation refers to a prevalent condition characterized by a low AC/A, a larger exo deviation at near than at far, deficient fusional convergence and, often, a reduced nearpoint of convergence, beyond 10 cm. Frequently, there exists an associated accommodative deficiency. Exophoric CI is far more prevalent than exotropic CI, but the management principles are essentially the same. Between 3% and 5% of the young adult population have CI.[40] Patients usually present with a slight exophoria at distance and a larger exophoria and, possibly intermittent exotropia at 40 cm. Visual symptoms include headaches, occasional diplopia, intermittent blurring, eyestrain, tired eyes, loss of concentration, and sleepiness, among other complaints. Convergence insufficiency has also been associated with reading problems.[8] Differential diagnosis requires distinguishing other etiologies than a low AC/A and deficient fusional convergence accounting for the "gross" convergence insufficiency as indicated by a reduced nearpoint of convergence. These other neuromuscular conditions include accommodative insufficiency resulting in "pseudo CI" and convergence "weakness" due to neurologic paresis or paralysis. (Another possible cause of a remote NPC is convergence excess esotropia; at near distance the esophoria increases beyond the limits of fusional divergence, resulting in a "break.")

Vision training has been the traditional therapy for CI. In most cases, it is an effective and practical approach; the training time does not take long. Grisham[8] evaluated the results of training in CI cases reported between 1940 and 1984. With a data base of 1931 cases, the a cure rate was 72%, an improvement rate was 19%, and a failure rate was 9%. Daum[41] analyzed the results in 110 CI patients and presented the clinical factors that correlated with success. Most of the training in this patient series was completed at home. The average training time was 4.2 weeks. The average age of the patients was 20 years, ranging from 2 to 46 years. Older ages were mildly associated with shorter lengths of treatment. This finding was presumably due to maturity of the patients and increased compliance with the training program. Over the course of training, there were statistically and clinically significant changes in the nearpoint of convergence, all the positive fusional convergence values (blur/break/recovery) far and near, the negative fusional divergence blur point at near, and the amplitude of accommodation. It has also been demonstrated that asthenopic symptoms reduce in response to the training of fusional vergence in CI cases.[42]

Another condition similar to CI is presbyopic exophoria. It is well known that presbyopic patients tend to show an increase in the nearpoint exophoria as the power of the reading add is increased over the years. (The increase is less than would be predicted simply by the decrease of accommodative convergence with accommodative response.) Frequently, presbyopic patients manifest an increased exophoria at near, a receding nearpoint of convergence, deficient fusional vergence responses, and increased fatigue and ocular discomfort if they continue with reading or other demanding nearpoint activities for extended periods of time. Some clinicians have recommended base-in prism in the form of single vision reading glasses or through the bifocal add in an attempt to increase patient comfort and efficiency. This is a valid and useful approach; however, relieving prisms do not always give satisfactory results. Vision training is a good alternative treatment option. There has been a clinical bias against applying vision training to elderly patients. The presumption was that the training would not be successful or acceptable to the patient. One study suggesting that this bias is

unjustified came from Wick.[43] He attempted a vision training program with 191 presbyopes, ages 45 to 89, having asthenopic symptoms associated with convergence insufficiency and presbyopic exophoria. The home-based program was 30 minutes per day; the average duration of therapy was less than 10 weeks. Home vision training was augmented with periodic office visits. The longest therapy program lasted 15 weeks. Using well defined and rigorous criteria for success, a 93% cure rate was reported immediately after the training program. A 3-month follow-up examination indicated that 48% of the previously cured patients needed some additional training, particularly those patients over 75 years old. This study indicates that age is only a factor in successful training for patients in their late presbyopic years. This factor is of minor clinical consequence because maintaining a successful result merely requires periodic reinforcement of learned skills. Wick's results have been confirmed by others.[44] A patient's age should not be the determining factor regarding the application of vision training presbyopes with convergence insufficiency exophoria.

A vision training program for convergence insufficiency can proceed as follows: As always, therapy starts with the correction of any significant refractive error. Even correction of low amounts of hyperopia can be beneficial since many CI patients have an associated accommodative deficiency. Many cases can be improved by prescribing spectacles for reading (+1.00 D add) and base-in prism for the convergence deficiency, but we usually reserve this approach for those patients who cannot, or will not, participate in a short vision training program.

If the patient does have accommodative deficiency, training accommodative skills becomes the initial goal of the program. Monocular and binocular exercises that are appropriate for accommodative training include accommodative tromboning (T16.21), jump focus (T16.22), and lens rock (T16.23). These techniques are described in Chapter 16. Accommodative facility for each eye can often be maximized within the first 3 weeks of a training program. Binocular accommodative rock (T14.15) is introduced after the monocular phase of training to help increase both accommodative and vergence facilities.

The next recommended goal in training is to establish physiological diplopia while building voluntary and gross convergence. This goal can be accomplished by using, primarily, three techniques: the Brock string and beads (T14.5), pencil pushups (T14.13), and the 3-dot card (T14.6). The specific training goal can be to build an NPC of 5 cm with smooth and accurate vergence and accommodation at all distances with full awareness of physiological diplopia.

The goal of enhancing central sensory and motor fusion can be achieved utilizing many techniques. Appropriate instruments and targets are designed to train vergence ranges, monitor for suppression, and enhance stereopsis. Clinicians and vision therapists are encouraged to explore their own creativity in designing and combining various methods. Some of the standard techniques that we recommend for this purpose can also improve binocular efficiency, i.e., speed, accuracy, integration, and stamina of accommodation and vergence. We find it efficacious to integrate vergence range training with techniques for binocular efficiency. Training techniques should include sliding, tromboning, step, jump, and isometric vergences. We tend to emphasize phasic (i.e., step and jump) techniques; they are reportedly slightly more effective.[45] Isometric techniques also have the advantage of being efficient, that is, they produce results in a relatively short period of time.[35] Some of our favorite techniques in CI cases are Vectograms and Tranaglyphs (T14.9), Aperture-Rule Trainer (T14.12), chiastopic fusion (T14.14), binocular accommodative rock (T14.15), and bar reading with prisms (T14.17). Even though in CI cases the initial training emphasis is placed on convergence skills, divergence should not be ignored. We suggest the ratio of 2/3 convergence training to 1/3 divergence to ensure that the entire zone of clear, single, comfortable, binocular vision is being expanded.

The specific training goals and release criteria are "very strong" convergence and divergence ranges free of suppression, far and near (listed in Chapter 2). An easy-to-remember ideal clinical guideline for release criteria is 20/30/20 (blur/break/recovery) for convergence and divergence at near but only for convergence at far. There should also be normal stereopsis (at least 40 seconds of arc), good nearpoint of convergence (5 cm or closer), and a normal fixation disparity curve with no measurable associated phoria on a nearpoint Mallett or Bernell Unit. Before being released, the patient should be free of symptoms and visual avoidance behaviors. We recommend training for at least 1 week after symptoms have disappeared to reinforce the newly learned skills. Most CI exophoric patients can achieve these goals within 6 to 8 weeks in a home-training program with periodic office visits; CI exotropes typically require a longer training period, perhaps 8 to 10 weeks or more, but are managed in essentially the same way. We suggest office visits once per week to monitor the patient's progress, prescribe and teach new training procedures and, importantly, continue motivating the patient. Most individuals undergoing any type of a training program need encouragement and reinforcement; vision training is no exception.

After a successful training program for CI is completed, in which all the release criteria have been met, little regression of skills is expected. This expectation is based on our clinical experience with these patients and two studies that have addressed the issue. Pantano[36] compared the long-term results of 207 CI patients on the basis of their success category immediately after training. Those who had been released as cured maintained the same result after 6 months and 2 years. Of those patients in the partially cured group, 79% remained asymptomatic after 6 months, but only 11% were asymptomatic after 2 years. There was also a slow decompensation of clinical findings. The failure group received no symptomatic relief and even the improved convergence skills were not maintained 6 months after therapy. This report illustrated the need to achieve a complete functional cure if regression of skills and reappearance of symptoms are to be avoided.

Grisham et al.[6] investigated the persistence of the vergence training effect in cases of exophoria at near and deficient fusional conver-

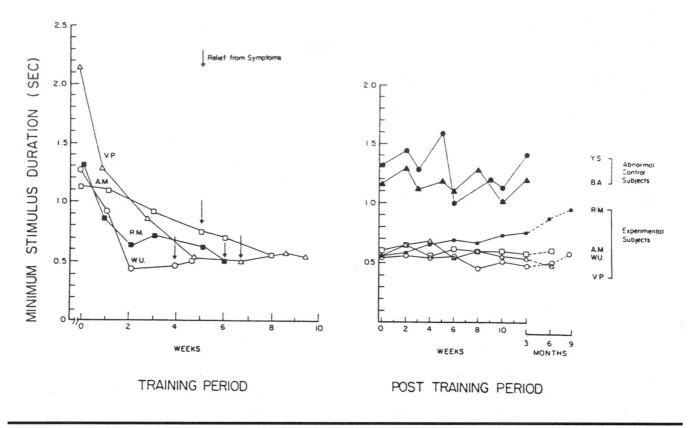

FIGURE 14-9—Vergence tracking rate of vergence-deficient exophoric subjects during and after vision training. All experimental subjects were successfully treated and the training effect was durable except that one subject, RM, had some regression that slowly occurred 9 months after cessation of training.

gence. They used vergence tracking rate, objectively determined from eye movement recordings, as an index of vergence performance (Figure 14-9). Four CI subjects received standard vision training for vergence deficiencies, two served as no-intervention controls, and all had their tracking rates monitored. The vergence tracking rate of each trained subject improved to normal levels within a period of 5 to 8 weeks; the controls showed no significant improvement. During the 6 to 9 month post-training period, three of the four trained subjects showed no significant regression in vergence tracking rate. These were the subjects who met all the release criteria for dismissal from the training program. However, one subject (RM) showed a slow linear regression of vergence tracking rate over the 9 months, almost to the pretraining level. That subject had discontinued the training prematurely before all release criteria were met. He also reported a gradual reoccurrence of visual

symptoms in association with reading activities and later was referred for further vision training. This study provides objective evidence supporting the validity of vergence training and demonstrates good short-term retention of trained skills, if all release criteria are achieved.

Even though regression in most cases is not expected, a maintenance home-training technique should be assigned after dismissal from vision therapy. At least, the patient can do self-monitoring for regression and return for "booster" training if needed. In cases of CI, we often recommend pencil pushups with physiological diplopia awareness (T14.13) for 20 minutes every 2 weeks as a retainer exercise. Bar reading with prisms (T14.17) is another good option. We have not seen regression of skills or reoccurrence of symptoms over several years in CI patients when they maintain this training schedule, even presbyopic exophores. Many patients accept this simple periodic exercise as a standard part of their general health maintenance.

Case Example

The following case of exophoria with convergence insufficiency was also contributed by Garth N. Christenson, O.D., M.S.Ed. of Hudson, Wisconsin. A 16-year-old female presented with complaints of frontal headaches after reading for about an hour, blurring of words, great difficulty concentrating during reading, and problems focusing from far to near. Health history was unremarkable. The refraction indicated only a slight amount of hyperopic astigmatism, which was considered clinically insignificant. The uncorrected visual acuities were 20/15 OD, OS, and OU. Pursuits and saccades were full and normal. Cover testing indicated a comitant orthophoria at 6 m and 7^Δ exophoria at 40 cm. Nearpoint of convergence was 5 cm to break and recovery was 7 cm; however, the break was 8 cm and recovery 10 cm after 5 attempts (indicating a possible problem with convergence stamina). There was good fusion on the Worth 4-dot test. The Randot Stereo test at near and The Vectographic Slide at far indicated normal stereoacuity. Fusional vergence ranges were: BI 6/4 at 6 m, 10/16/14 at 40 cm; BO X/10/4 at 6 m, and X/8/4 at 40 cm. The NRA was +1.25 and PRA −4.00. Monocular accommodative facility was normal but the patient had difficulty with binocular facility when plus lenses were introduced. A steep slope of the forced vergence curve was found on fixation disparity testing with the Disparometer.

The above clinical data indicated the diagnosis of convergence insufficiency (principally based on the exo deviation at near, low AC/A, decreased fusional convergence, low NRA, and poor binocular accommodative facility with plus lenses). The diagnosis was discussed with the patient and she became aware of the nature of her vision problems. She was informed that vision training provided the best choice for relieving her symptoms, but that she would have to decide if she would be willing to devote the time and effort necessary for successful results. The patient said she was willing to do so and planned on approximately 15 weekly office visits in conjunction with daily home training.

Vision training was done for 10 weeks and included the following approaches: (1) Gross convergence training to develop voluntary convergence and awareness of physiological diplopia; (2) increase sliding vergence blur, break, and recovery ranges; (3) improve step vergence skills; (4) integrate accommodative and vergence demands (BOP-BIM, i.e., base-out and plus add produce demand on fusional convergence; base-in and minus-add produce demand on fusional divergence); and (5) combine step (BI-BO) and jump (near-far) vergences with versions to simulate "real life" visual environment. Instrumentation was used such as the Mirror Stereoscope, Vectograms, lens flippers, Brock string, and Allbee 3-dot Card.

At the time of dismissal there was resolution of all visual symptoms. The patient was reading comfortably at all times and was enthusiastic about relief of symptoms. Clinical data were as follows: NPC to nose; BI at 6 m, 12/4; BO at 6 m, 20/44/40; BI at 40 cm X/16/15; BO at 40 cm, 28/32/30; binocular accommodative facility, 20 c/m; NRA, +2.25; fixation disparity curve, flat slope. A maintenance program for home vision training was prescribed and the patient was scheduled for a progress evaluation in 3 months. The maintenance program included procedures using the Allbee 3-Dot Card, Lifesaver card for orthopic and chiastopic fusion rock, and Keystone Eccentric Circles to ensure good vergence ranges. She was instructed to perform these techniques approximately 15 minutes, two times a week.

REFERENCES

1. Refractive Status and Motility Defects. *National Health Survey no. 206 1971-1972.* United States Vital and Health Statistics, Series 11; 1978.
2. Schlossman A, Boruchoff SA. Correlation between physiologic and clinical aspects of exotropia. *Am J Ophthalmol.* 1955;40:53-64.
3. Simons HD, Grisham JD. Binocular anomalies and reading problems. *J Am Optom Assoc.* 1987;58:578-587.
4. Simons HD, Grasser PA. Vision anomalies and reading skills: A meta-analysis of the literature *Am J Optom Physiol Optics.* 1988;65:893-904.

5. Cooper J, Feldman J. Operant conditioning of fusional convergence ranges using random dot stereograms. *Am J Optom Phyisol Optics.* 1980;57:205-213.

6. Grisham JD, Bowman MC, Owyang LA, Chan CL. Vergence orthoptics; validity and persistence of the training effect. *Optom Vis Sci.* 1991;68:441-451.

7. Flom MC. Issues in the clinical management of binocular anomalies. In: Rosenbloom AA, Morgan MW, eds. *Principles and Practice of Pediatric Optometry.* Philadelphia: Lippincott; 1990:222.

8. Grisham JD. Visual therapy results for convergence insufficiency: A literature review. *Am J Optom Physiol Optics.* 1988;65:448-454.

9. Burian HM, Smith DR. Comparative measurement of exodeviations at twenty and one hundred feet. *Trans Am Ophthalmol.* 1971; 69:188.

10. Cooper EL, Leyman IA. The management of intermittent exotropia: A comparison of the results of surgical and nonsurgical treatment. *Am Orthopt J.* 1977;27:61-67.

11. Jampolsky A, Flom MC, Weymouth FS, Moses LE. Unequal corrected visual acuity as related to anisometropia. *Arch Ophthalmol.* 1955;54:893.

12. Flom MC, Wick B. A model for treating binocular anomalies. In: Rosenbloom AA, Morgan MW, eds. *Pediatric Optometry.* Philadelphia: Lippincott; 1990:246.

13. Iacobucci IL, Archer SM, Giles CL. Children with exotropia responsive to spectacle correction of hyperopia. *Am J Ophthalmol.* 1993;116:79-83.

14. Jampolsky A. Ocular deviations. *Int Ophthalmol Clin.* 1964;4:567.

15. Von Noorden GK. *Binocular Vision and Ocular Motility.* 4th ed. St. Louis: CV Mosby; 1990:326.

16. Hardesty HH. Management of intermittent exotropia. *Binoc Vision.* 1990;5:145-152.

17. Hiles DA, Davies GT, Costenbader FD. Long-term observation on unoperated intermittent exotropia. *Arch Ophthalmol.* 1968;80:436-442.

18. Wick B. "Forced elimination" of anomalous retinal correspondence in constant exotropia: a case report. *Am J Optom Physiol Optics.* 1975;52:58-62.

19. Lie I, Opheim A. Long-term stability of prism correction of heterophorics and heterotropics: a 5 year follow-up. *J Am Optom Assoc.* 1990;61:491-498.

20. Davies GT. Vertical deviations associated with exo-deviations. In : Manley DR, ed. *Symposium on Horizontal Ocular Deviations.* St. Louis: CV Mosby; 1971:149.

21. Calrider N, Jampolsky A. Overcorrecting minus lens therapy for treatment of intermittent exotropia. *Am Acad Ophthalmol.* 1983;90:1160-1165.

22. Rutstein RP, Marsh-Tootle W, London R. Changes in refractive error for exotropias treated with overminus lenses. *Optom Vis Sci.* 1989;66:487-491.

23. Coffey B, Wick B, Cotter S, Scharre J , Horner D. Treatment options in intermittent exotropia: a critical appraisal. *Optom Vis Sci.* 1992;59:386-404.

24. Sanfilippo S, Clahane A. The immediate and long term results of orthoptics in exodeviations. In: *The First Congress of Orthoptics.* St. Louis: CV Mosby Co; 1968:299-312.

25. Goldrich SG. Optometric therapy of divergence excess strabismus. *Am J Optom Physiol Optics.* 1980;57:7-14.

26. Ludlam W, Kleinman B. The long term range results of orthoptic treatment of strabismus. *Am J Optom Arch Am Acad Optom.* 1965;42:647-684.

27. Cooper J. Intermittent exotropia of the divergence excess type. *J Am Optom Assoc.* 1977;48:1268-1273.

28. Helveston EM. Surgical Management of Strabismus: *An atlas of strabismus surgery.* 4th ed. St. Louis: CV Mosby; 1993:435-442.

29. Souze-Dias C, Uesugue CF. Postoperative evolution of the planned initial overcorrection in intermittent exotropia: 61 cases. *Binocular Vis Eye Mus Surg Qrly.* 1993;8:141-148.

30. Jampolsky A. Adjustable strabismus surgical procedures. In: *Symposium on Strabismus: Transactions of the New Orleans Academy of Ophthalmology.* St. Louis: CV Mosby Co; 1978;320-328.

31. Flax N, Selenow A. Results of surgical treatment of intermittent divergent strabismus. *Am J Optom Physiol Optics.* 1985;62:100-104.

32. Singh V, Roy S, Sinha S. Role of orthoptic treatment in the management of intermittent exotropia. *Indian J Ophthalmol.* 1992;10:83-85.

33. Carta A, Pinna A, Aini MA, Carta A Jr, Carta F. Intermittent exotropia: evaluation of results on the basis of different treatments. *J Français De Ophthalmologie.* 1994;17:161-166.

34. Daum K. Characteristics of exodeviations: 1. A comparison of three classes. *Am J Optom Physiol Optics.* 1986;63:237-243.

35. Veagan. Convergence and divergence show longer and sustained improvement after short isometric exercise. *Am J Optom Physiol Optics.* 1979;56:23-33.

36. Pantano F. Orthoptic treatment of convergence insufficiency: a two year follow-up report. *Am Orthopt J.* 1982;32:73-80.

37. Kertesz AE, Kertesz J. Wide-field fusional stimulation in strabismus. *Am J Optom Physiol Optics.* 1986;63:217-222.

38. Wick B. Visual therapy for contant exotropia with anomalous retinal correspondence: a case report. *Am J Optom Physiol Optics.* 1974;51:1005-1008.

39. Goldrich SG. Oculomotor biofeedback therapy for exotropia. *Am J Optom Physiol Optics.* 1982;59:306-317.

40. Kent PR, Steeve JH. Convergence insufficiency; incidence among military personnel and relief by orthoptic methods. *Milit Surgeon.* 1953;112:202-205.

41. Daum KM. Convergence insufficiency. *Am J Optom Physiol Opt.* 1984;61:16-22.

42. Cooper J, Selenow A. Ciuffreda KJ, Feldman J, Faverty J. Hokoda S, Silver J. Reduction of asthenopia in patients with convergence insufficiency after fusional vergence training. *Am J Optom Physiol Optics.* 1983;60:982-989.

43. Wick B. Vision training for presbyopic nonstrabismic patients *Am J Optom Physiol Optics.* 1977;54:244-247.

44. Cohen AH, Soden R. Effectiveness of visual therapy for convergence insufficiencies for an adult population. *J Am Optom Assoc.* 1984;55:491-494.

45. Daum K. A comparison of the results of tonic and phasic vergence training. *Am J Optom Physiol Optics.* 1983;60:769-775.

Chapter 15 / Management of Noncomitant Deviations, Intractable Diplopia, and Nystagmus

Infantile Noncomitant Deviations   437
    Diagnosis   437
    Management   438
Acquired Noncomitant Deviations   438
    Diagnosis   438
    Occlusion   438
    Prism Compensation   440
    Ocular Calisthenics   441
    Sensory and Motor Fusion
        Training   441
        Fusion Field Expansion T15.1   442
        Double Maddox Torsion Training
            T15.2   443
    Surgery and Follow-up
        Management   443
Intractable Diplopia   443
    Diagnosis   443
    Occlusion Strategies   445
    Prism Displacement   446
    Hypnotherapy   447

Congenital Nystagmus   447
    Diagnosis   447
    Optical Management   447
    Vision Training   448
        Afterimage Tag Techniques
            T15.3   449
        Intermittent Photopic Stimulation
            T15.4   449
        Auditory Biofeedback T15.5   450
    Surgical Management   452
Acquired Nystagmus   453
    Diagnosis   453
    Management   453
Case Examples   454
    Duane Retraction Syndrome   454
    Noncomitant Intermittent
        Hypertropia   456
    Acquired Third Nerve Palsy   457
    Intractable Diplopia   458
    Congenital Nystagmus   458

Patients who present with noncomitant deviations, diplopia, or nystagmus require a high level of professional attention. These conditions can be harbingers of neurologic disease; careful differential diagnosis and therapeutic management is needed. Although this chapter reviews some important diagnostic points of these conditions, the emphasis is on management approaches and specific treatments. The reader is referred to Chapter 4, which discusses testing procedures for noncomitant deviations, and to Chapter 8, which elaborates on the differential diagnosis and management of noncomitant deviations and nystagmus.

INFANTILE NONCOMITANT DEVIATIONS

Diagnosis

When an infant has a noncomitant deviation from birth or within the first year of life, the clinician must go through the same differential diagnostic process as would be the case with a deviation acquired later in life. There always exists the possibility that a disease process or injury has caused an extraocular muscle palsy and the etiology must be established and treated, if possible. However, many restrictive conditions affecting ocular motility, such as Duane and Brown syndromes, can and should be recognized early. Although rare, noncomitant deviations do occur during the traumatic process of childbirth, but often the cause of infantile noncomitant strabismus remains unknown. It should also be remembered that infantile comitant esotropia is frequently associated with overacting inferior oblique muscles occurring later for unknown reasons; this introduces a noncomitant vertical component to the strabismus as the child matures.

Management

Management of each type of noncomitant strabismus depends on the specific condition, age of treatment, associated conditions, along with other factors; therefore, general statements pertaining to all types are difficult to make. The clinician starts with correction of any significant refractive error. Occlusion and vision training may be indicated for amblyopia and eccentric fixation, if they exist, even if the prognosis of normal binocular vision is remote. If ARC exists (although rare in acquired noncomitancy), we usually recommend that no attempt be made to establish NRC since diplopia is a likely consequence. Surgical alignment of the eyes stands as the principal treatment, especially if the noncomitant strabismus is of neurogenic origin. (Discussion of surgical methods for these varied cases is beyond the scope of this text.) Patients needing an operation, which can be complex, should be referred to a strabismologist (ophthalmological specialist) rather than a general ophthalmologist for evaluation and treatment after the above mentioned management steps have been completed.

ACQUIRED NONCOMITANT DEVIATIONS

Diagnosis

When a patient of any age presents with an acquired noncomitant strabismus, often accompanied by complaints of diplopia, an active neurological condition must seriously be considered and ruled out. Often a referral to a neurologist or neuro-ophthalmologist is indicated in such cases to confirm or establish the diagnosis. The most common noncomitant deviations are due to sixth- and fourth-nerve palsies, in that order. (See Chapters 4 and 8 for strabismus diagnosis.) The specific etiology of the condition should be established, if possible, and professionally managed.

Our management approach for acquired noncomitant strabismus is not based on a wait-and-see attitude. Our efforts are directed toward preventing diplopia and contractures, re-establishing fusion at some fixation distance(s), and actively expanding ocular motility and binocular vision during the initial recovery period. Vision training, in these cases, is viewed as a form of physical therapy for eye movements (Table 15-1).

Occlusion

Diplopia is the most pressing problem facing patients with recent onset of extraocular muscle paresis. This annoyance can easily be eliminated by prescribing an occluder to be worn over the affected eye. Although this has been the traditional method in paretic cases, generally it is better to recommend alternate occlusion rather than confining the patch to the

---

TABLE 15-1. *Management of Acquired Noncomitant Deviations*

1. Referral for medical management of the primary etiologic factor(s).
2. Correction of any significant refractive error.
3. Prescription of Fresnel prism to promote fusion in a particular field of gaze and viewing distance.
4. Alternate patching to prevent diplopia, prevent contractures, and exercise the paretic muscle(s).
5. Vision training: Ocular calisthenics in the affected field of gaze to prevent contractures and remediate eye movements.
6. Vision training: Sensory and motor fusion training to build fusional control of deviation.
7. Consideration of need for strabismus surgery after 6 to 8 months of healing and vision therapy.

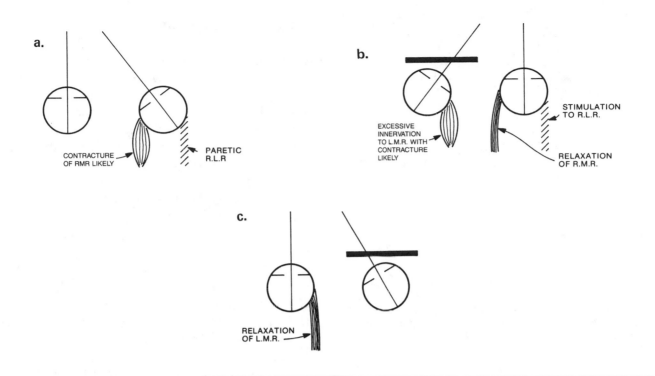

FIGURE 15-1—Alternate occlusion for prevention of contractures: (a) Paresis of the right lateral rectus with contracture of right medial rectus; (b) occlusion of the nonparetic eye to prevent contracture of the right medial rectus, and (c) occlusion of the paretic eye to prevent contracture of the left medial rectus.

paretic eye. Occluding the sound eye may provide beneficial stimulation to the paretic eye and can lead to eye movements into the field of action of the paretic muscle. Patching the unaffected eye may reduce the risk of secondary contracture of the homolateral antagonist. For example, if the right lateral rectus (RLR) is paretic, patching the left eye might encourage the patient occasionally to abduct the right eye in order to view objects in right gaze. This should occur unless the patient has become a head turner. When the patient abducts the right eye, the right medial rectus (RMR) relaxes (the homolateral antagonist) and, consequently, may help to prevent contracture of that muscle.

Continuous patching of the nonparetic eye can lead to trouble, because contracture may develop in the contralateral synergist. In this example of a paretic right lateral rectus, the yoke muscle is the left medial rectus (LMR), which will overact (risking contracture because of Hering's law) when abduction is attempted with the right eye. Therefore, alternate occlusion is preferable because of the possibility of contracture of either the homolateral antagonist (e.g., RMR), when the affected eye is occluded, or the contralateral synergist (e.g., LMR), when the sound eye is patched (Figure 15-1).

Although alternate occlusion seems the best approach to prevent diplopia and contractures, there is another important consideration. When the unaffected eye is patched and the patient looks into the field of gaze of the affected muscle (e.g., RLR), past pointing may occur. Since excessive innervation must be sent to the paretic muscle, the patient misjudges the spatial position of the target. As the patient practices eye-hand coordination with the nonparetic eye occluded, however, the disturbing sensation and misperception of direction either reduces or disappears. During all critical viewing tasks, such as driving or eye-hand coordination required on the job, the patient should simply occlude the paretic eye to avoid this problem.

Binasal occlusion can also be applied to prevent diplopia and contractures in cases of 6th nerve palsy. Binasal strips of opaque tape are positioned on spectacle lenses to promote

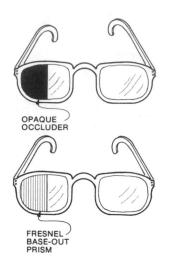

OPAQUE
OCCLUDER

FRESNEL
BASE-OUT
PRISM

FIGURE 15-2—Partial occlusion for relief of diplopia in cases of noncomitancy: (a) Occluder on temporal portion of spectacle lens in case of right lateral rectus paresis; (b) Base-out Fresnel prism so fusion can be obtained on dextroversion in case of mild paresis.

Prism Compensation

If possible in cases of recent diplopia, fusion should be maintained with Fresnel prisms without resorting to occlusion. This ideal seems achievable only when the extraocular muscle paresis is mild. We recommend trying Fresnel prism compensation even for cases of moderate paresis in which a deviation exists in the primary field of gaze at far and/or near. Fresnel prisms can easily be changed to keep up with changes in the angle of deviation during the healing period. In cases of moderate paresis, prisms can be prescribed for a specific distance and specific tasks, much like an optical aid is prescribed for a low-vision patient. The prisms usually do not result in fusion in all fields of gaze, but are utilized by the patient for a specific task for the sake of maintaining fusion and promoting recovery of the paretic condition. The prism spectacles can be worn for 1 to 4 hours per day for specific activities and the Fresnel prism can be removed when the patient does other tasks. The power should be on the conservative side, with the patient wearing just enough prism to maintain fusion, yet be comfortable at the same time. Weaning the patient from prism is gradual, reducing the powers commensurately with remission of the paresis and improvements in fusional control of the deviation.

alternation of fixation. (Refer to Chapter 11.) The right eye is used for fixation in the right field of gaze and the left eye for left gaze. In this way, abduction of each eye is continuously encouraged and thereby prevents contracture of the medial recti muscles. The procedure works well with cooperative adults who understand the importance of alternately abducting each eye as much as possible. The young child, however, is less apt to cooperate fully and tends to become a head turner, using only one eye for fixation. Total unilateral occlusion, alternated on a daily basis, is recommended in such instances.

Partial occlusion can be used to prevent diplopia in some cases of mild paresis. If the patient has a mild RLR paresis, for example, with diplopia only in right gaze, the temporal portion of the right spectacle lens can be occluded (Figure 15-2a). This type of occlusion allows the patient to maintain fusion in the primary position and in left gaze, possibly with a slight right face turn, which is therapeutically desirable. Diplopia is prevented with a version eye movement to the right field. Fresnel prism may also be tried (Figure 15-2b). Partial patching does not prevent contracture; fortunately, contracture is usually not of serious consequence in cases of mild paresis.

In some cases, the Fresnel prism might best be placed before the nonaffected eye, thereby lessening potential contracture of the homolateral antagonist.[1] For example, in the case of a right esotropia (paretic RLR), an appropriate power base-out Fresnel prism that gives fusion could be applied to the left spectacle lens. It should be remembered that the amount of prism needed to neutralize the secondary deviation is usually larger than that for the primary deviation. The left eye would then move in because of the prism and the right eye out, thus preventing contraction of the RMR.

When the angle of deviation has a vertical and horizontal component, each component is usually measured separately, and prisms are prescribed accordingly. However, when working with Fresnel prisms, this method has its limitations because two separate prisms cannot be applied to one lens. An alternative procedure for measuring both components at the same time can be done with the Maddox rod *vector method* (Figure 15-3). It is quick and quite accurate. This procedure, however, requires the patient to have NRC and minimal suppression. The patient fixates a small bright light with the dominant eye at the distance needing prism compensation. A Maddox rod, placed before the strabismic eye, is rotated so that the streak appears to pass through the center of the white light (Figure 15-3b). This axis is recorded. The Maddox rod is then rotated 90° (Figure 15-3c). Either Risley or loose prisms are used with the base oriented to the recorded axis to neutralize the separation between the light and streak (Figure 15-3d). The prism power at the particular axis is recorded for strabismic eye. For example, for a deviation of 8^Δ base-up and 18^Δ base-out of the left eye, the measurement and prescription would be approximately 20^Δ at 23° OS (Figure 15-4). This information is given to the optical laboratory for fabrication of either a ground-in prism or a single Fresnel prism.

Ocular Calisthenics

Physical therapy is recommended for paretic extraocular muscles. Exercises designed to force the paretic eye to move, particularly toward the field of action of the affected muscle, may help in restoring function and preventing contracture. Many pursuit techniques discussed in Chapters 10 (Therapy for Amblyopia) and 16 (Therapy for Vision Efficiency Skills) are appropriate here. Initially, the unaffected eye is occluded for monocular pursuit training of the affected eye. (Refer to Tables 16-5 and 16-6 for specific techniques.)

For training at home, we have found the Marsden ball technique (T16.14) effective. An afterimage (AI) placed on the fovea of the paretic eye can provide visual feedback to the patient as to the accuracy of the pursuit eye movement as the patient attempts to keep the AI on the swinging ball (T10.17). There are also several appropriate saccadic training techniques (T16.1 through T16.12) for therapy in the affected field of gaze described in the next chapter. Playing various eye-hand coordination games, such as ping-pong or computer

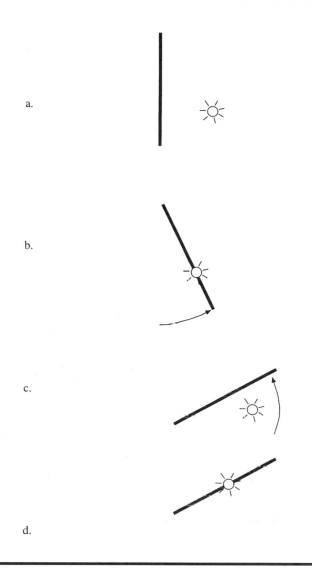

FIGURE 15-3—Maddox rod method for simultaneous measurement of vertical and horizontal deviations: (a) Image of Maddox rod of left eye and penlight of right eye; (b) Maddox rod rotated for superimposition; (c) Maddox rod rotated 90 degrees resulting in diplopia; and (d) neutralization of the left hypo and eso deviations.

games (T16.12), are effective and popular with patients.

Sensory and Motor Fusion Training

The patient should be fusing as much of the time as possible following an acquired extraocular muscle paresis. The majority of patients have a history of good binocular vision prior to the onset of noncomitancy. Sensory fusion training is usually unnecessary. The expansion

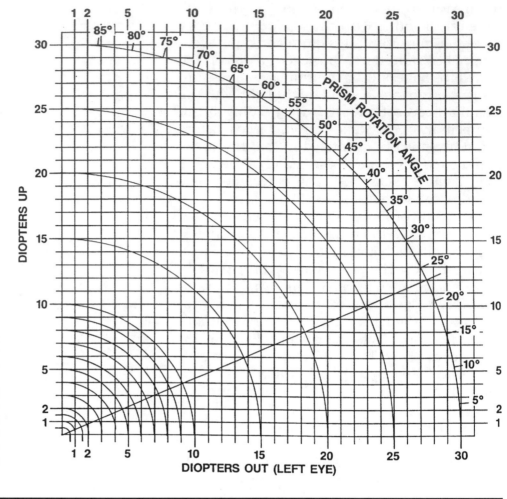

FIGURE 15-4—Nomogram for vertical and horizontal prism power when using one prism at various orientations of its base. In this example, the base is oriented 23 degrees out and up for the left eye. In this instance, 8 prism diopters base-up and 18 prism diopters base-out results in a vector oriented 23 degrees with a power of approximately 20 prism diopters.

of the motor fusion range, however, is recommended in practically all cases of recent origin. Sliding, isometric, and small step vergence training techniques seem easier and more effective than jump and tromboning techniques, at least initially. In cases of sixth nerve paresis, we have found the Mirror Stereoscope (T13.2), the Brewster stereoscope (T13.3), and Vectograms (T13.8-10), to yield good training results. The targets should have as much stereopsis content as possible to help expand the divergence ranges at near and far. In cases of fourth nerve paresis, vertical prism compensation is often required in combination with the above techniques and the two described subsequently, i.e., fusion field expansion (T15.1) and double Maddox torsion training (T15.2).

Erickson and Caloroso[2] described an example case of a 39-year-old female that illustrates the use of prisms and vision training. The patient presented with the complaint of constant diplopia following her first bifocal correction and was found have an esotropia and a noncomitant hyper deviation associated with a paresis of the superior oblique of long duration. A combination of compensating vertical prism and horizontal vergence training was utilized to re-establish fusion and resolve the patient's complaint. Many of the specific training techniques described in chapters 13, 14, and 16 are applicable in cases of noncomitant cyclovertical deviations when there is good potential for fusion.

Fusion Field Expansion T15.1

One effective technique for expanding the field of fusion is simply to establish a strong sensory fusion lock in an unaffected field of gaze and ask the patient to rotate her head slowly, thereby emphasizing sensory and motor fusion in affected fields of gaze. A vivid stereo target, such as the Spirangle Vectogram, can be used to stimulate sensory fusion. The patient slowly rotates her head so that the eyes move into the affected field of gaze while she makes a "mental effort" to maintain the stereo-percept. As soon as diplopia is noted, the head is moved to regain sensory and motor fusion; this break and join procedure can continue for a specified time. An isometric variation of this technique can be effectively used. The patient moves the eyes into a field of gaze where fusion is difficult, but can be maintained in this position for several minutes. The patient should try to continue this training process for a 10-minute period and then rest the eyes. Limitations of the fusion field in all affected directions can often be eliminated or diminished in this manner with repeated practice for 2 or 3 months.

Double Maddox Torsion Training T15.2

In cases of noncomitant vertical deviations, such as a superior oblique paresis, there is often an associated cyclotorsional component. Relatively few techniques, other than working on a major amblyoscope, are available to training cyclovergence. Wick[3] described a home training technique to expand the range of cyclovergence using two Maddox rods. The patient views a bright small light through a handheld Maddox rod placed before each eye. The axes of the streaks are rotated until their images are aligned and fused. Initially, fusion should be established in the least affected field a gaze. The axes of the Maddox rods are then slowly rotated as the patient attempts to maintain sensory and motor fusion. When fusion breaks and diplopia of the streaks occurs, the Maddox rods are rotated back so that fusion can be regained. For a 10-minute period the patient strived to increase the cyclofusional ranges, particularly of the compensating vergence, e.g., incyclovergence in cases of superior oblique paresis. As training progresses the fixation light is moved into the most affected field of gaze to increase the challenge to the patient. Isometric vergence training is also useful in these cases.

Surgery and Follow-up Management

The rate of partial or complete remission in cases of acute acquired noncomitant strabismus is high, about 70%.[4] Unless the affected muscle is completely paralyzed, surgery should not be contemplated for at least 6 to 8 month after the onset of the condition. There are few changes in the angle of deviation after this time unless there exists an active disease process, e.g., multiple sclerosis, diabetes. On the other hand, stroke or trauma patients usually have a stable condition after 6 months. During this time interval, the conservative approach is to manage the strabismus with lenses, prisms, occlusion, calisthenics, and motor fusion training. These procedures are done in conjunction with medical management of the primary condition responsible for the noncomitant deviation.

After the waiting period, if the residual deviation in the primary position exceeds 15^Δ esotropia, 20^Δ exotropia, or 12^Δ vertical strabismus and remains significantly noncomitant, extra-ocular muscle surgery should be considered as a treatment option.[5] Lesser degrees of deviation can often be successfully managed with a combination of compensating prisms and vision training.

These patients often need close follow-up care whether or not an operation is required. Usually some residual deviation may present a fusion problem to the patient. Six-month progress checks are realistic for many patients, but each case must be judged by the residual clinical features of the deviation.

INTRACTABLE DIPLOPIA

Diagnosis

When a patient presents with the complaint of double vision, the clinician must discover the cause because some etiologies are life threatening, e.g., a brain tumor. Several history questions need to be asked: Is the diplopia monocular or binocular? With or without spectacles? Constant or intermittent? Present under what circumstances? Time and type of onset, rapid or gradual? Separation distance and direction? Associated general health, neurologic, and ocular health signs and symptoms? The diagnosis often requires an accurate refraction and visual acuity assessment, a complete ocular motor evaluation, and thorough visual and general health examination.

Intractable diplopia presents a challenge to the clinician to manage successfully. It occurs when there is some insurmountable obstacle to sensory and motor fusion and lack of suppression to prevent diplopia. Fusion may not be established by conventional therapy methods: refractive error correction, prism compensation, vision training, or surgery; however, these methods for reestablishing single, clear, and comfortable binocular should be tried or at least considered before other means are tried to eliminate one of the diplopic images. Intractable diplopia can occur from several causes, such as: (1) a change in the angle of deviation in a developmental strabismus associated with ARC; (2) nonfusible metamorphopsia; (3) bilateral superior oblique palsy, and (4) sensory fusion disruption syndrome. Fortunately, these cases are somewhat rare, but most clinicians will eventually be called upon to manage or refer a case for definitive treatment. Each of these causes will be discussed along with therapeutic implications.

In some individuals having a constant strabismus in early childhood, ARC becomes adapted permanently to a particular angle of deviation. Unlike most cases with ARC in which this sensory adaptation shows considerably variability (e.g., covariation), a few patients show little or no variation in their angle of anomaly when the angle of deviation changes, for some reason later in life. The strabismic angle may change during life for any number of reasons and intractable diplopia may occur due to cosmetic strabismus surgery,[6] injury, disease, vision training (particularly inappropriate antisuppression training), growth, and idiopathic causes. Suppression is not deep in these cases, so the change in the angle of deviation may be accompanied by diplopia. We have seen cases in which the diplopia is present only when the patient's attention is directed to the second image or under certain testing conditions; otherwise, the second image is usually suspended from perception. In one case, testing revealed central horror fusionis; the images could not be fused in real space or in a major amblyoscope. The patient was reassured that the diplopia represents only a potential problem requiring no treatment at that time. The patient was counseled to continue to ignore the double image and not to look intentionally for it.

Some early onset strabismic patients experience "fixation switch diplopia."[7,8] When these patients fixate with the preferred eye, they have no diplopia due to suppression or ARC. When fixating with the nonpreferred strabismic eye, however, they notice diplopia. Fixation switch seems to occur primarily in cases of good visual acuity in the nonpreferred eye and cases in which patching of the dominant eye has occurred for an extended time, as when treating amblyopia. If there is spontaneous alternate fixation, and the resulting diplopia is bothersome, the patient needs reassurance and treatment. The patient can be taught to eliminate the diplopia by blinking the nonpreferred eye to switch fixation back to the preferred eye. If this simple measure is not sufficient, the vision of the strabismic eye can be optically blurred to discourage fixation.[9] A careful diagnosis is necessary before treating the patient on a symptomatic basis. It is possible that when the patient switches fixation to the nonpreferred eye, causing diplopia, the patient may have changed to NRC localization.[10] If this is so, fusion may indeed be possible and the graded occlusion method by Revell could be used to establish normal fusion. (See Chapter 11.)

Metamorphopsia refers to distortions of an image in one or both eyes, but our concern here is a distortion great enough to present an obstacle to sensory fusion. Some patients have these distortions due to macular damage originating from a number of sources, e.g., age-related maculopathy, diabetic retinopathy, solar or laser lesions, and central serous retinopathy. In these cases, the peripheral fields usually remain fused, but the patient may notice diplopia centrally. Diagnosis can be established by having the patient draw his perception of an Amsler grid pattern while fixating with the affected eye. Fusion training can be attempted in cases of central metamorphopsia, but often without success. We have found the most acceptable solution in these cases is central field occlusion, described in the next section.

Extreme aniseikonia is another form of visual field distortion that may preclude sensory fusion. Since this condition is usually associated with large degrees of anisometropia and occurs when the refractive error is optically corrected, a solution lies in not correcting the more ametropic eye and prescribing merely a "balance" lens. Careful evaluation, however, needs to be done before the clinician jumps to this solution. We have seen several patients adapt well and experience full binocular vision and a high degree of stereopsis with as much as six diopters of corrected anisometropia. Some patients having higher degrees of anisometropia may show peripheral fusion with central suppression with contact lenses or spectacles; therefore, they may have benefit and comfort from full optical correction.

In cases of closed head trauma and systemic disease (e.g., diabetes, multiple sclerosis), some patients have a bilateral palsy of the superior obliques muscles (a bilateral 4th nerve involvement). Von Noorden reported that 21% of fourth-nerve trauma cases are bilateral, but other observers found even higher prevalence.[11] This bilateral palsy can result in severe excyclo deviation of each eye, particularly at near; this can be an insurmountable obstacle to sensory fusion. Prism compensation is not effective, but patching and vision training may help to advance the healing process. These patients can fuse readily in a major amblyoscope set to the subjective angle of deviation with the torsional component included. If the condition does not resolve within 8 months from the time of onset, surgery is often required. Sometimes, however, it will be necessary to implement a permanent management scheme for intractable diplopia. For such an event, in which acuities are usually normal and equal, a monovision solution may be attempted.

Closed head trauma followed by coma can result in a total or partial loss of the capacity for sensory and motor fusion. This condition is referred to as *sensory fusion disruption syndrome.*[12] Worth[13] first proposed the idea of a "central fusion faculty." Several rare cases reported in the literature[12,14] appear to support this notion and they also suggest a midbrain site for a sensory fusion center. Most patients with this affliction and a history of normal binocular vision, and having had "successful" surgery or prism compensation, still show no ability to join the two overlapping images. This would occur even if there is "orthotropia." London and Scott,[12] however, described one 17-year-old patient who eventually regained fusion following a bicycle accident rendering her comatose for 3 weeks. They neutralized the esotropic-hypertropic strabismus with Fresnel prisms, which superimposed the images for 4 months before the patient reported the recovery of sensory fusion. She gradually regained fusion without the necessity of prisms and demonstrated 50 seconds of stereopsis. This impressive result is not typical, unfortunately. If the patient can tolerate superimposition of images, perhaps it is prudent to attempt a functional cure in such cases. Those who do not readily regain fusion need further management for their intractable diplopia, using principally an occlusion approach.

When a patient has a persistent complaint of diplopia and single, clear, comfortable, binocular vision cannot be successfully re-established, we usually recommend one of three management approaches: some form of occlusion, prism displacement, or hypnotherapy. (Table 15-2).

Occlusion Strategies

Some patients who experience intractable diplopia can tolerate the condition under certain circumstances but not others. They occlude their nondominant eye only when critical viewing is needed, e.g., when driving or reading. Other patients find diplopia intolerable at all times and prefer constant occlusion. In these latter cases, one acceptable solution may be wearing an occluder contact lens or even a plastic clip-on occluder over one spectacle lens. When an opaque soft contact lens is used, Burger and

---

TABLE 15-2. *Management Approaches for Intractable Diplopia*

Occlusion Strategies:

1. Total, opaque occlusion
   A. Bandage or tie-on occluder. Recommended only as a temporary solution.
   B. Wearing an opaque soft contact lens can be an acceptable long term solution.
2. Monovision optical prescription using contact lenses or single vision spectacles. This is our preferred treatment approach.
3. Central field occlusion: small central translucent or opaque spot; stippled clear nail polish.

Prism Displacement: Increased separation of diplopic images.

Hypnotherapy: The patient is given a post-hypnotic suggestion to ignore the diplopic image and experience less anxiety. (Formal hypnosis is given by a professionally trained psychological counselor.)

London[15] recommend incorporating a fogging element in the prescription (+2.00 to +4.00 D greater than the manifest) since all opaque contact lenses transmit some light. We usually attempt to avoid total constant occlusion since the field of view is reduced. The two techniques we have found most effective are monovision and central field occlusion.

The patient may find that a monovision correction, with spectacles or contact lenses, provides adequate diminution of binocular vision to alleviate diplopia awareness under most circumstances while allowing the perception of movement in the retinal periphery of both eyes. London[16] reported a series of intractable diplopia cases managed successfully with monovision prescriptions. He recommended correcting a strongly dominant eye for near using the plus-add in single vision spectacles or contract lenses. Otherwise, the dominant eye tends to be used for both far and near. The amount of plus-add is determined empirically in each case, but we have found +2.00 D to +2.50 D to be optimum in most cases we have managed. Monovision is our preferred treat-

ment option in cases of intractable diplopia or even with patients having long-term uncomfortable binocular vision than cannot be resolved using conventional treatment.

Central field occluders can also be tried to determine which is the most appropriate approach for a particular patient.[17] This approach can be achieved in various ways as follows: (1) a translucent cellophane tape or contact paper button cut to about the side of a dime; (2) a central opaque dot, or (3) a central spot of clear nail polish that has been stippled to appear like shower glass. This approach allows for clear, full-field, peripheral binocular vision, an advantage in some cases of central metamorphopsia, for example. Unfortunately, the poor cosmesis of the occluder may eventually be unacceptable to some patients.

Prism Displacement

Most patients with intractable diplopia do not respond well to compensatory prisms. For cases of horror fusionis and sensory fusion disruption syndrome[12] in which the images are closely aligned or overlapped with prisms but fusion does not occur, patients may find the diplopia more annoying than if the images are greatly separate. Also, in cases of ARC, compensatory prisms are not recommended for long-term management, because the angle of deviation may increase as a result of prism adaptation. Even some patients with NRC and acquired noncomitant strabismus show prism adaptation to horizontal prisms.[16] In such cases, however, vertical prism displacement may provide some improvement in the management of diplopia. A 10^Δ to 15^Δ base-down Fresnel prism can be tried on a trial basis before the nonpreferred eye to see if the diplopic image is easier to ignore or, at least, interferes less under critical viewing conditions. Base-up Fresnel prisms are not well accepted by most patients; the small ridges reflect overhead lights into the eyes causing glare. If the patient does find vertical prism helpful after 1 or 2 weeks of trial wear, spectacle prisms can be ground-in and the power split between the eyes to distribute the weight and thickness. Prism displacement may not be successful in some cases if there is confusion (i.e., two different images in the same place). However, we have had limited success using inverse prisms to separate the images in several cases of intractable diplopia.

Hypnotherapy

We have recommended hypnosis as a "last ditch" therapy for cases of intractable diplopia in which nothing else has worked. These unhappy patients were referred to a professional (e.g., clinical psychologist) skilled in hypnotherapy. The hypnotherapist evaluates and counsels the patient regarding his emotions surrounding the condition and sets specific goals for hypnotherapy. If the patient is a good hypnosis candidate, and not everyone is, he is given a post-hypnotic suggestion to ignore the double image and to experience less anxiety about the problem. Several sessions may be required, but some patients benefit greatly from this approach.

CONGENITAL NYSTAGMUS

Diagnosis

Nystagmus, affecting about 0.4% of the population,[18] is a "red flag" for a neurologic disorder. Most cases, however, are congenital, static, and of long duration. The cause of congenital afferent nystagmus may be easily identified, e.g., optic atrophy, ocular albinism, congenital cataracts. Etiology can be subtle in congenital efferent nystagmus due to obscure lesions in the brain stem. An effort should be made to determine the cause and characteristics in every nystagmus case.[19] (Refer to Chapter 8.) If there are signs of some underlying active pathological process, referral and medical treatment are indicated.

For cases of congenital nystagmus in which there are no indicators of active disease, several palliative forms of vision therapy should be tried to see if: (1) control of the nystagmus can be improved, (2) a cosmetically noticeable head turn can be minimized, and (3) increase of binocular visual acuity is possible. Therapeutic options that are potentially available are listed in Table 15-3. These options, other than surgery, can and should be implemented on a trial basis to see what helps and what does not. The

TABLE 15-3. Management of Congenital Nystagmus: Therapeutic Options

- Full correction of the refractive error, spectacles, or contact lenses.
- Trial fit with rigid gas-permeable contact lenses.
- Prisms and added lenses to promote sensory fusion.
- Yoked prisms to treat under 15° of abnormal head posture.
- Standard vision training techniques to increase sensory and motor fusion, if present.
- Afterimage tag techniques to provide visual feedback of nystagmoid eye movements.
- Mallett's technique of intermittent photopic stimulation with the major amblyoscope to increase motor control and visual acuity.
- Auditory biofeedback to build conscious control of nystagmoid eye movements, at least for short periods.
- Medications to relieve oscillopsia, if associated.
- Galilean telescope system to relieve oscillopsia, if needed.
- Strabismus surgery, if indicated, to promote sensory and motor fusion, especially in cases of nystagmus blockage syndrome.
- Surgical procedures, e.g., Kestenbaum operation, to correct large head turns, greater than 15°.

sequence is flexible and must be varied for each patient. Sometimes the effect with each option can be dramatic, long lasting, and deeply appreciated by the patient. Unfortunately, there are few indicators that predict the outcome. The doctor and patient must explore the possibilities together.

Optical Management

In treating binocular anomalies, we have consistently emphasized the importance of fully correcting any significant refractive error and in the case of congenital nystagmus, this principle applies, even more so. Refracting, however, is not easy in nystagmus cases for obvious reasons. The prescription needs to be frequently refined through repetition. Binocular visual acuity may be improved and nystagmic eye movements lessened with the wearing of an appropriate spectacle or contact lens correction in both afferent and efferent types of nystagmus.

In cases of significant refractive error, a trial fit with rigid gas permeable contact lenses should be evaluated and seriously considered as a treatment option. In some cases, contact lenses have resulted in immediate improvements of nystagmus and visual acuity, whereas other patients improve over time. Many patients, however, show no improvement, but this cannot be accurately predicted before a trial fit. The improvements, if they occur, may be attributed to previously undetected and uncorrected astigmatism that is often associated with congenital nystagmus. Another possible explanation is that the lenses cause subtle lid sensations of the nystagmic eye movements; the patient may learn some degree of nystagmus control using this form of tactile sensory feedback.

Prism can be used in some cases of congenital nystagmus to lessen the oscillations. One common observation is that the frequency and magnitude of nystagmus decrease with convergence.[20] If, for example, the patient has an exophoria, the clinician should evaluate the effect of base-out prisms or plus-adds on the control of nystagmus. Metzger[21] reported a case of a 10-year-old highly myopic male who was given prisms of 6^Δ BO; his binocular visual acuity improved from 10/100 to 10/40 and reading became comfortable.

If the binocular status can be improved in cases of esotropia, there often is an improvement in the characteristics of nystagmus. (See Case Five: Congenital Nystagmus.) The amount of prism necessary to reduce the nystagmus by placing the eyes in a fused converged position varies depending on the specifics of each case; the total amount generally ranges between 6^Δ and 20^Δ base-out. Fresnel prisms may be necessary for the higher prescriptions. Metzger[21] described an albino girl with congenital nystagmus, high myopia and astigmatism, a hearing impairment, latent nystagmus, and an alternating esotropia. Prisms of 15^Δ base-out were prescribed and gave immediate improvement of the nystagmus oscillations and visual acuity.

Minus-add lenses have also been used to attempt to reduce the nystagmus, but this approach may be undesirable in some cases.[20] The primary problem with minus adds is that an esophoria at near may be produced making reading or other sustained close viewing activities uncomfortable.

Yoked prisms may be used as a means of treating an abnormal head posture associated with congenital nystagmus. As an example, consider the patient with a left head turn and a quiet zone in right gaze. A base-in prism over the left eye and an equal base-out prism over the right eye will shift both eyes and the null point to the left toward primary position, partially relieving the head turn. Small to moderate amounts of head turn (to about 15°) can be managed in this way. The prisms required for larger amounts are often unacceptable to the patient due to distortion and cosmesis. Through the prisms, the eyes appear deviated to an observer and one cosmetic problem is merely substituted for another. It seems that yoked prisms have a role to play, but only in borderline cases of abnormal head posture. For example, if a patient has a 15° head turn to the left, 10^Δ yoked prism bases right would reduce the head turn by about 5°, making the remaining head turn cosmetically acceptable. This amount of prism can be ground into spectacle lenses with an acceptable edge thickness, if the eye-size and lens power are relatively small.

Vision Training

Several vision training procedures may be attempted to help lessen or eliminate nystagmus in congenital cases. A consistent clinical observation regarding nystagmus intensity is that it lessens as binocular vision is enhanced. If a patient has insufficient sensory or motor fusion, the nystagmus seems to have larger amplitude and higher frequency. Because of these observations, various methods have been attempted to improve sensory and motor fusion.[22] Antisuppression and fusional vergence training can be administered using most of the instruments and techniques discussed in the other chapters. This form of therapy seems to have a beneficial effect in heterophoric cases for which there is already some normal peripheral sensory fusion, but it has seldom been attempted in nystagmus cases complicated by esotropia. Three training methods that have been particularly effective in the management of congenital nystagmus are afterimage tag techniques, intermittent photopic stimulation, and auditory biofeedback.

Afterimage Tag Techniques T15.3

The use of afterimages is a practical training technique for improving steadiness of fixation and reducing a compensatory head turn. The afterimage gives the patient visual feedback regarding the intensity of nystagmic oscillations. A binocular afterimage is applied using a strobe flash generator (Figure 5-40a) from a distance of about 50 cm while the patient holds his eyes as steady as possible at the null point, if present. The patient observes the movement of the afterimage as a blank screen is viewed with a blinking light in the background to intensify its perception. As targets of threshold size are gradually introduced into the visual field, the patient attempts consciously to reduce the intensity of the afterimage movements and to resolve the detail of the targets. The goal of this technique is to develop the patient's conscious control of the nystagmic eye movements so he can dampen the oscillations at will, under social circumstances or when maximum visual acuity is required. Expanding the null region to the primary position also can be attempted by having the patient first adjust the head posture to reduce the oscillations (the null position) and then slowly moving the head toward the primary field of gaze while attempting to maintain the dampened oscillations.[23]

Intermittent Photopic Stimulation T15.4

Mallett[24] adapted an amblyopia training technique using a Synoptophore in congenital nystagmus cases. He presented a series of 54 patients showing significant improvements in nystagmus control, visual acuity, and stereopsis. This clinical series included successful treatment of patients ranging in age from 6 to 49 years. Another encouraging result was the relatively small number of training sessions (average of 12) needed to achieve the optimum response. All patients applying for treatment were accepted except those individuals who

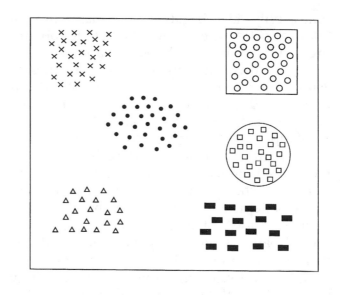

FIGURE 15-5—Example of a Synoptophore slide, modified from Mallett,[24] that can be used in intermittent photic stimulation. The slide is covered with a red filter and the patient is instructed to count the critical detail, e.g., number of triangles.

had poor concentration or were epileptic (possibly sensitive to flashing lights).

The therapy method consists of monocularly stimulating each eye in turn, 15 to 20 minutes per session, using a Synoptophore flashing at a frequency of 3 to 4 Hz. This frequency was chosen because of success in cases of amblyopia, suppression, and anomalous correspondence. Mallett[24] noted that binocular stimulation may be even more effective, but this was not attempted. The patient's task is to identify and count detailed targets on slides such as groups of dots or triangles (Figure 15-5). All slides have a red filter background because that tends to promote foveal fixation in amblyopic and nystagmus cases.[23,25] Therapy sessions lasted 30 to 40 minutes. Patients initially experienced considerable difficulty moving fixation within patches of detail, but with practice on a large variety of targets, precision of fixation and visual acuity both improved. To prevent regression of learned skills, Mallett[24] recommended that patients train for an additional six sessions after maximum acuity is attained.

The results of photic stimulation were consistently good with both heterophoric and strabismic patients. Of the 54 patients in this series, only 43% began with visual acuity of 20/40 or better, the current standard for obtaining a driver's license; however, after therapy, 83% met this criterion. At least two lines of acuity improvement could be expected. In those tested, contrast sensitivity also improved after treatment sessions. Mallett[24] noted that amblyopic eyes also increased in acuity, which is not surprising because the technique originally was designed for this anomaly. The amplitude of nystagmus diminished appreciably in many patients and was completely neutralized in a few cases. Stereopsis was established in several patients previously without it and was increased in others. Little regression of visual acuity was found in progress checks. Only about 10% of the patients lost acuity of a line or more on the Snellen chart; however, this was quickly regained after a few therapy sessions. Although not a panacea for congenital nystagmus, photic stimulation does appear to result in some impressive and appreciated benefits. It seems appropriate to attempt this technique at some point in the long-term management of congenital nystagmus, ideally during the early school-age years.

Auditory Biofeedback T15.5

There have been several encouraging case reports and patient series reporting the use of auditory biofeedback in the management of congenital nystagmus. Ordinarily, a nystagmus patient has no sensation, impression, or perception that the eyes are oscillating. Their visual world appears stable without apparent image movement (oscillopsia) except in a few rare cases. With auditory biofeedback, the patient's eye position and movements are measured using an infrared eye monitor and the signal is converted into an audible tone. The patient literally hears his nystagmus. Some systems provide a continuous tone at which the pitch changes as the eyes oscillate.[26,27] Other systems provide a "dead zone" when the eyes fall on target, and a signal tone when fixation moves off.[28] The patient attempts to turn the tone off by keeping the eyes steadily on the target. Using this feedback, the patient can consciously (and later unconsciously) learn to alter the motor output to stabilize the eyes. The specific mechanism for doing this, however, is not well understood. Mezawa et al.[29] found that during voluntary suppression of nystagmus following training, there was increased muscle tension in the lids as well as changes in the tonicity of the laryngeal or pharyngeal muscles. Embryologically, these nerves develop from the same branchiogenic nerve. They suggest that biofeedback training possibly makes use of these common pathways, which may still exist after birth.[29]

It is surprising how rapidly many patients can learn to lessen the amplitude of their nystagmus. Ciuffreda et al.[27] reported five subjects who learned to reduce nystagmus amplitude, decrease peak slow-wave velocity, and reduce frequency with less than 1 hour of auditory biofeedback training (Figure 15-6). Kirschen[28] demonstrated reductions of nystagmus amplitude in three subjects ranging from 41% to 73% within the first hour of training. Frequency, however, appeared to be less affected by training. He attributed the speedy and large effect on amplitude to the specific type of auditory feedback using the "dead zone" approach.

Presently, there are no objective longitudinal reports of the efficacy of biofeedback training for nystagmus. Some authors have noted that most subjects after biofeedback training were able to dampen the amplitude and frequency of nystagmus on command or with conscious intent and increase foveation time; however, there does not seem to be a permanent, complete cure of nystagmus. In a detailed study of seven young subjects, aged 7 to 20 years, Mezawa et al.[29] reported an average of 40% reduction in nystagmus intensity and the foveation time increased about 190%.

In general, patients have reported subjective benefits from therapy. These benefits include: (1) cosmetic lessening of the nystagmus in face-to-face social situations; (2) better visual acuity when looking at street signs or watching TV; and (3) improved psychological adjustment to the presence of nystagmus and personal satisfaction by gaining some control. The persistence of these perceived benefits for 1 year after training has been reported by Ishikawa[30] in

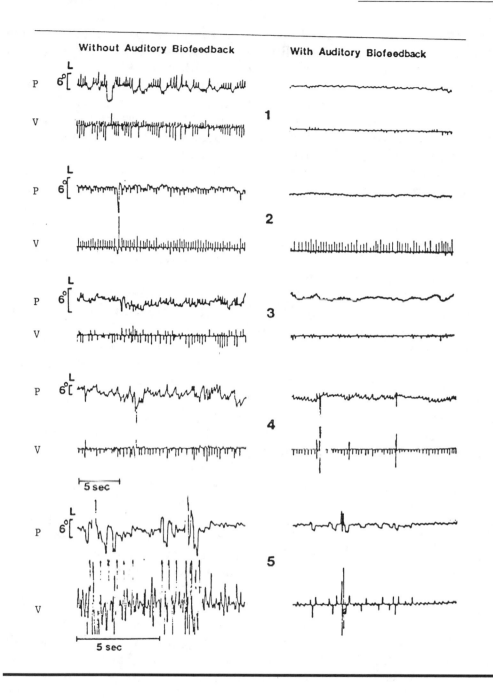

Without Auditory Biofeedback   With Auditory Biofeedback

FIGURE 15-6—Control of nystagmus in five patients using auditory biofeedback. Eye position (P) and velocity (V) as a function of time with and without auditory biofeedback. Reduction of nystagmus is evident in each patient with addition of auditory biofeedback. L = leftward eye movements. (Reprinted with permission from Ciuffreda et al. 1982.)

one-third of his 29 patients. Another one-third reported moderate long-term improvement, and the remainder complained of poor results.

The potential appears good for application of auditory biofeedback techniques in children afflicted with congenital nystagmus. Ciuffreda et al.[27] reported working with one 4-year-old child and obtaining encouraging results. The patient could reduce her nystagmus for brief periods at the initial training session. Unfortunately, there is no clinical biofeedback system commercially available as a package. The doctor must purchase an eye movement monitor system, a computer, a data acquisition board, and a speaker and must do some computer programming. It is hoped that further positive experimental reports will stimulate commercial development of such instrumentation.

Surgical Management

One of the cosmetic consequences in many cases of congenital nystagmus is a disfiguring head posture. The patient naturally prefers a peripheral field of gaze where the nystagmus oscillations lessen and visual acuity improves. Kestenbaum[31] introduced a surgical procedure designed to move the null point to the primary position, obviating the need for a head turn. All four horizontal rectus muscles were operated on to rotate both eyes away from the eccentric null point. Resection and recession procedures were recommended for yoke muscles in each eye with an identical amount of adjustment done to each. For example, to move the null point from left gaze, resections of the RLR and LMR are required along with recessions of the RMR and LLR. Several modifications of the Kestenbaum procedure have been recommended by various surgeons and results of the surgery have improved. The benefits to the patient often are more than cosmetic. There are objective reports of increased visual acuity with the null point in the primary position, an overall lessening of the nystagmus intensity, and a spreading of the null point over a wide range of gaze angles.[32,33] For the rare patient who has an abnormal vertical head posture, all four vertical rectus muscles may require surgery. Parks[34] reported this procedure for a patient showing 25° of chin depression.

Surgical management of head turns caused by nystagmus seems promising. In one series of 38 patients, five different modifications of the Kestenbaum procedure were compared.[35] In this series, the mean age at the time of surgery was 7 years, ranging from 1 to 35 years old, and the average amount of head turn was about 40°. A head turn of 15° was considered cosmetically acceptable, and using this criterion, an 82% success rate was reported. Overcorrection of more than 15° occurred in only one case. All but one procedure were found equally effective over a follow-up period of about 3 years. These are encouraging results that confirm the results of an earlier clinical series.[36]

Several recommendations can be made regarding the appropriateness and expectations of surgical intervention for a head turn secondary to congenital nystagmus. First, most authorities do not recommend surgery for a 15° head turn or less.[34,37] An attempt is made to manage these cases with yoked prisms if there is a small cosmetic head turn. Second, the best surgical results have been reported in children aged 4 years and older. Many cases of overcorrection have occurred in children younger than 4 years. Moreover, some patients before age 4 have spontaneous remission of their head turn. Third, a different surgical approach from the Kestenbaum procedure is taken when the nystagmus is complicated by the presence of a strabismus. In these cases, surgery usually is performed solely on the dominant eye to correct for the head turn because any change in head position will be mediated by the fixating eye.

Treatment of esotropia in nystagmus blockage syndrome (NBS) during childhood usually requires an operation after a period of alternate occlusion to eliminate amblyopia and to promote full motility of each eye. The Faden operation together with a small recession of the involved medial rectus may be sufficient, but frequently a bimedial rectus recession is required. The results of surgery generally are not as good as those found in cases of congenital esotropia alone. For example, von Noorden and Wong[38] reported a clinical series of 64 patients with NBS whose results were compared to that of a control group of 85 infantile esotropia cases without nystagmus. More than one-half of the NBS patients required at least one additional operation. No functional cures were reported in this series; however, 26% of the NBS cases resulted in a microtropia with some binocular vision. These results also suggest a fair cosmetic prognosis (about 50%) for children having nystagmus blockage syndrome with apparent alignment of the eyes in the primary position of gaze.

In cases of strabismus with nystagmus that increases with monocular occlusion (latent component) and if binocular vision can be reestablished by surgical and optical means, the nystagmus is frequently converted to merely the latent form. Binocular visual acuity consequently improves.[39] In these cases, the possibility of converting manifest nystagmus to latent by strabismus surgery is a reasonable goal.

ACQUIRED NYSTAGMUS

Diagnosis

When a patient presents with acquired nystagmus, the presumption is that the cause is a disease process of some type affecting oculomotor neurology. A differential diagnosis must be established so the underlying cause can be treated. When the cause is successfully treated, the nystagmus usually disappears. (Refer to Tables 8-15 and 8-16 for a description of several acquired and, fortunately, rare types of nystagmus.) When the cause is not readily apparent, computer tomography (CT) and magnetic resonance imagery (MRI) studies are often indicated. If the etiology of nystagmus is attributable to an infectious process, a vascular disorder, or a metabolic or toxic imbalance, appropriate medications are an indispensable part of the medical management of the underlying condition. Description of the many possible alternatives is beyond the scope of this text.

Management

A few medications have been effective in the symptomatic relief of oscillopsia and vertigo association with vestibular nystagmus, downbeat nystagmus, and, on rare occasions, congenital nystagmus. The illusory sensation of movement of an object or the environment is a particularly distressing and debilitating symptom. When this symptom occurs, it is nearly impossible to read comfortably or sustain any demanding visual activity. Symptomatic relief from an oscillating world, even for a short time, is a desired goal of all afflicted patients.

Currie and Matsuo[40] reported a series of ten patients whose vertical oscillopsia associated with downbeat jerk nystagmus was successfully reduced or eliminated with the administration of a 1 to 2 mg dose of clonazepam. The nystagmus in these cases had various etiologies:

Arnold-Chiari malformation, cerebellar hemangioblastoma, cerebellar infarction, and multiple sclerosis. The nystagmus and oscillopsia were lessened or eliminated for 2 to 6 hours per dose, and one patient experienced relief for 72 hours per dose. In 7 of the 10 cases, visual acuity improved during the treatment period. The side effects of this medication are drowsiness and sedation. These symptoms limit the long-term benefit of the medication in some cases, and vary considerably between individuals. The primary mode of action of clonazepam on the central nervous system appears to be through enhancement of the inhibitory GABAergic system. It primarily reduces the slow-phase velocity of the jerk nystagmus.

Another drug showing promising results in reducing oscillopsia and nystagmus amplitude is Baclofen; this inhibits the excitatory neurotransmitter system (glutamate). It has been useful in some cases of congenital nystagmus, periodic alternating nystagmus (PAN), and seesaw nystagmus.[41] The reported side effects include drowsiness, dizziness, weakness, hypotension, and nausea. Furthermore, Baclofen is expensive.

An optical device, similar to a Galilean telescope, that produces partial retinal image stabilization in cases of acquired nystagmus and oscillopsia has been described by Yaniglos and Leigh.[42] This device consists of a high-plus spectacle lens and is used in combination with a high-minus, rigid gas-permeable (RGP) contact lens. A patient with multiple sclerosis achieved 30 to 90 minutes of relief from oscillopsia and improved visual acuity by wearing a monocular spectacle/contact lens combination, +17 D and −28 D respectively. The device has limited depth of field and cannot be tolerated for long periods of time due to discomfort, but patients appreciate the periods of stabilized imagery for specific activities such as watching television.

Some cases of persistent acquired nystagmus and debilitating oscillopsia that have not responded to conservative therapy, have benefited by retrobulbar injections of botulinum toxin. In one series of 12 patients, eight demonstrated an increase in visual acuity.[43] Injections were repeated at 3- to 4-month intervals as long as patients noted an improvement in their quality of life.

CASE EXAMPLES

Case One: Duane Retraction Syndrome

Griffin and Carlson[44] reported successful results with vision therapy in a 10-year-old male with Duane retraction syndrome. (Refer to Chapter 8.) The patient presented with complaints of discomfort, fatigue, and pain when reading. He also was aware of occasional diplopia in secondary and tertiary positions of gaze and relied on head turning for compensation. Duane retraction syndrome (DRS) was first diagnosed at age 3 years old by a pediatric ophthalmologist.

Clinical findings were as follows. Refraction and acuities were:

OD plano 20/20 (6/6)

OS +0.25 −0.25 x 105 20/20 (6/6)

Type III DRS was indicated as ductions were restricted in each eye: OD 25 degrees abduction, 15 degrees adduction; OS 50 degrees abduction, 35 degrees adduction. Retraction of each eye was observed on adduction. Cover testing in the primary position of gaze revealed 2^Δ exophoria at far and 10^Δ exophoria at near. The nearpoint of convergence was remote, 30 cm, but improved to 12 cm with left head turn. Relative fusional vergences were fair except for 6^Δ BO recovery at near. Vergence facility was poor at far and near. Accommodative amplitudes and facility were normal monocularly but marginally adequate with binocular viewing. NRA and PRA were normal. Fixation in the primary position was normal, monocularly and binocularly. Pursuits were: OD slightly jerky and restricted with narrowing of the palpebral fissure on adduction: OS smooth but greatly restricted on adduction with narrowing of the palpebral fissure. Saccades were: OD restricted with narrowing of the palpebral fissure on adduction; OS normal but slightly restricted on adduction with narrowing of the palpebral fissure; binocular testing revealed significant restrictions (Figure 15-7). Binocular fusion test-ing, using a tangent screen at 1 m with a penlight target to plot the area of fusion, revealed a horizontal extent of 4° on left gaze and 8° on right gaze for a total of 12° of bifixation without head turning.

Because of complaints with reading, the King-Devick test (Chapter 2) was given and reading saccades were normal. Also, The Dyslexia Screener (TDS)[45] was administered; the patient scored above normal on phonetic and eidetic coding, thus ruling out dyslexia as a cause of reading problems.

The case was comanaged with the patient's pediatric ophthalmologist. The ophthalmologist agreed that there was no strabismus in the primary position of gaze and a slightly abnormal head posture, but of no great concern to the patient. The ophthalmologist thought that forced duction testing need not be repeated; extraocular muscle surgery was not a feasible option. The principal problem was that of gross convergence insufficiency; a secondary problem was poor binocular accommodative facility. The symptoms associated with prolonged reading were probably due to these binocular anomalies. The management plan in vision therapy was: (1) No spectacle lenses were necessary but yoked prisms could be tried to eliminate the head turn. They were applied for 30 minutes in the office with no beneficial effect. (2) Vision training was prescribed to improve positive fusional vergence, gross convergence and accommodative facility. Vision training for improving the restricted motility is usually ineffective, although fusional vergence training can be attempted.[5] Vision training was done only at home using Minivectograms and pencil pushups in all positions of gaze.

After a 2-month period of home vision training, most of the restrictions of Duane retraction syndrome remained; however, the patient's base-out recovery at near had improved from 6^Δ to 14^Δ and binocular accommodative facility had improved to 6 c/m. Recovery speed was noticeably improved in all BI and BO testing. Also, the patient's speed on the King-Devick test improved from 77 to 59 seconds. These improvements were probably responsible for the patient's reporting that comfort and efficiency of visual tasks at near,

a.

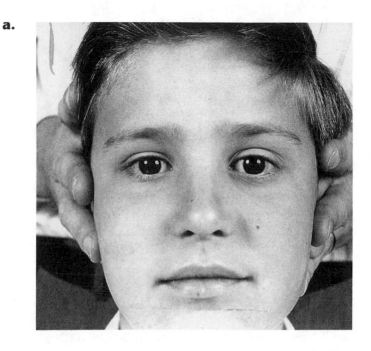

b.   **c.**

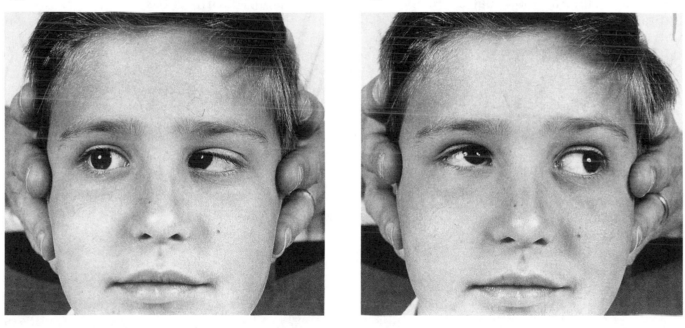

FIGURE 15-7—Binocular saccades in Duane retraction syndrome. (a) Patient fusing in the primary position of gaze. (b) Esotropia on dextroversion due to restriction of abduction of the right eye. There is narrowing of the left palpebral fissure, which is made more obvious by the vertical strabismus in this position of gaze. The appearance is that of a left hypertropia, but the left eye was the fixating eye; therefore, the right eye was hypotropic, and esotropic, in this position of gaze. (c) Exotropia on levoversion due to restriction of adduction of the right eye. There is narrowing of the right palpebral fissure that is made more obvious by the right hypertropia in this position of gaze.

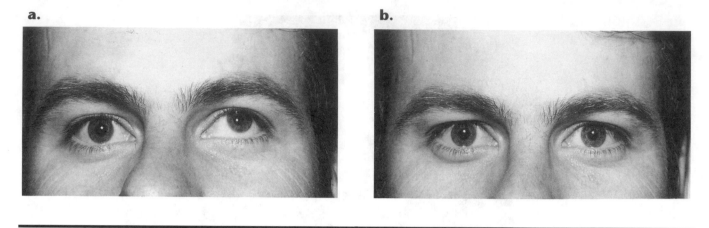

FIGURE 15-8—Left hyperdeviation of 52$^\Delta$: (a) manifest deviation; (b) patient fusing.

particularly when reading, had improved. The patient was advised to continue the home vision training and return in 1 year. Follow-up history indicated that the patient is doing well except for occasional fatigue during reading and not being a good batter in baseball, although a good pitcher. The patient and parents expressed gratitude that vision therapy was done and significant improvement of binocular status was achieved.

Case Two: Noncomitant Intermittent Hypertropia

Bergin et al.[46] reported a case of hyperphoria of large magnitude with mild noncomitancy. The patient was a 27-year-old male who presented with no symptoms other than noticing momentary diplopia when tired and having a dislike for reading, especially when fatigued with prolonged reading. These symptoms had been noticed for many years. His lens prescription and acuities were as follows:

OD −3.50 −0.75 x 140   20/15 (6/4.5)

OS −3.75 −0.75 x 020   20/15 (6/4.5)

Alternate cover testing showed a small exophoria, approximately 10$^\Delta$ at far and near with a hyper deviation of the left eye upon continuous testing. Base-down prism before the left eye was gradually introduced in increasing amounts as the vertical deviation increased, ultimately stopping with 50$^\Delta$ base-down.

The left eye was patched and the patient was allowed to rest for 30 minutes. When the patched was removed, the left hyperdeviation was 26$^\Delta$. As greater power of base-down prism was given as he maintained fusion, the deviation stabilized with 52$^\Delta$ base-down after 10 minutes, presumably through prism adaptation (Figure 15-8a). When the vertical prism was removed, he quickly regained fusion; this was objectively observable and the patient reported the merging of the momentarily seen diplopic images (Figure 15-8b). Other testing indicated that the right eye was the dominant eye and there was intermittent central suppression of the left eye. The Hess-Lancaster test suggested a mild paresis of the left inferior rectus and possibly of the right inferior oblique. Pursuit movements were normal but the patient showed frequent regressions on reading tasks. Nearpoint of convergence was normal. Stereoacuity was 30 seconds of arc and BI and BO motor fusion ranges were fair but slightly limited. Fixation disparity testing revealed a left hyper fixation disparity with neutralization varying from 5$^\Delta$ to 20$^\Delta$.

To summarize briefly, a vision training program was designed to increase BI and BO fusion ranges over a period of several weeks, mostly at home. They were sufficiently increased to provide the patient with more comfort with reading tasks. As he was a college student, this was greatly appreciated. There was little vertical vergence training; expanding horizontal vergences was emphasized. The vergence techniques for home training included the use of Vectograms, Aperture Rule Trainer, Brock string and beads, and chiastopic fusion cards. A major amblyoscope was also utilized in a few office training sessions.

Because of the absence of past-pointing and an unremarkable case history, no other treatment was recommended. Prism compensation was not recommended because of the prism adaptation that occurred in this case. Extraocular muscle surgery was not elected by the patient as a viable treatment option. It was also contraindicated because of the prism adaptation; besides, the patient always had fusion under ordinary seeing conditions and fusional vergences had been normalized with vision training. Vision training appeared to be the best choice of treatment for this patient; the results were successful. An important point is that vertical deviations can sometimes be managed successfully by improving horizontal deviations. Another important point exemplified by this case is that latent deviations need to be brought out with time; the clinician should do a prolonged occlusion test to reveal the full deviation that is responsible for the patient's symptoms.

Case Three: Acquired Third Nerve Palsy

A 53-year-old female complained of constant vertical diplopia in the primary position and the necessity of using extreme chin elevation to achieve binocular fusion. Two years previously, she had suffered from a basilar artery aneurysm resulting in a bilateral third nerve paresis, left facial palsy, and balance problems. Neurovascular surgery at the time saved her life. With healing, she regained some of the lost functions, her balance improved as did the facial palsy, but she presented with a stable bilateral restriction of up-gaze (−3), a constant, noncomitant, unilateral, left 11^Δ hypertropia decreasing in down-gaze, and horizontal jerk nystagmus on attempted up-gaze. She could fuse in down and left gaze and therefore adopted an elevated head (chin) position of 30° and head turn 10° to the right. The patient was wearing bifocal spectacles without any prism that gave her adequate visual acuity and fusion for reading in down-gaze.

The initial therapy approach was to prescribe yoked vertical prisms (base-up) in an attempt to reduce the chin elevation and the left hypertropia. The single vision distance prescription that optimally accomplished these goals and provided acceptable visual acuity was:

OD: +0.75 −1.00 X 023 15^Δ BU 20/20−

OS: −1.75 −1.50 X 168 8^Δ BU 20/20−

After wearing this correction for 2 weeks, the patient presented with only 10° of chin elevation and had binocular fusion for distance viewing. This amount of elevation was acceptable to the patient and not cosmetically noticeable. Having learned to turn her head more than her eyes, the patient experienced fusion most of the day with these spectacles, except in down-gaze. A second pair of spectacles for reading without incorporating prism was prescribed, because at about 30° in down-gaze, she showed no vertical deviation and only a small exophoria. The single vision reading prescription was:

OD: +3.25 −1.00 X 023

OS: +0.75 DS −1.50 X 168

This reading prescription gave her good vision and binocular fusion for most nearpoint activities, but she also noticed that she could only move her eyes about 15° before she saw an intermittent diplopic image. There was significant horizontal noncomitancy of the deviation leaving her fusion field restricted.

The patient was given two vision training procedures with goals of strengthening her horizontal fusional vergence ranges (which were deficient) and expanding her field of binocular fusion. She did base-in and base-out sliding vergence training about 20 minutes per day using either a Mini-Tranaglyph (Figure 16-6) or a Minivectogram. Each has a stereopsis target for fusional lock. Also, several times a day for about 5 minutes, she attempted to expand her field of fusion in all directions, particularly horizontal. She would attempt to maintain a stereo fusion lock on the Minivectogram as she slowly moved it into secondary and tertiary fields of gaze (T15.1). After 2 months of training, she had doubled her near vergence ranges; they were BI: X/21/13 and BO: X/24/14. The horizontal fusion field had increased to 35°. Although there was no improvement with the superior gaze palsy, she felt gratified with the results of the prism spectacles and vision training and was released from therapy. The patient was advised to continue these training procedures on a periodic basis indefinitely, once per week, to prevent regression. She was placed on a yearly recall for primary care vision examinations.

Case Four: Intractable Diplopia

A 67-year-old female presented with a 4-year history of Graves' disease (thyroid ophthalmopathy). This patient complained of constant diplopia and visual confusion (overlapping images) at far and near during this period of time; she wore a patch over her left eye for driving. The hyperthyroid condition was being medically managed and was reported to be stable. By gross inspection, her eyes appeared slightly proptotic, left more than the right, with slight lid retraction revealing a small portion of sclera superiorly (Dalrymple's sign), but the corneas were not constantly exposed. She was not concerned about cosmesis, only the diplopia.

The clinical findings were as follows: Refraction and acuities:

OD −1.50 −0.25 X 095 20/20 +2.50 add .4 M

OS −1.25 −0.50 X 088 20/20 +2.50 add .4 M

Oculomotility and binocular vision: noncomitant, constant, unilateral, left 7^Δ hypotropia and 3^Δ exotropia at far; constant, left 3^Δ hypotropia and 12^Δ exotropia at near; subjective testing with the double Maddox technique indicated a left 6° excyclotropia that changed with field of gaze. Motility was restricted in up-gaze: −2 right eye, -3 left eye, presumably due to contracture of the inferior recti muscles. Fusional evaluation on the major amblyoscope indicated second-degree fusion at the subjective angle, but very limited fusional vergence ranges in BI and BO directions, due primarily to the variable hyper and cyclodeviation.

Vision therapy: Prism compensation was attempted at both far and near without success; superimposition of the images was possible, but sensory fusion did not occur or was unstable. Vision training was considered as a treatment option, but rejected due to the noncomitant torsional nature of the deviation and the impracticality of an in-office training program in this case. Vertical and horizontal prism displacement was tried to see if suppression would be easier for the patient. It was not. The patient's main problem was visual confusion. Since the patient had good visual acuity in each eye, a monovision spectacle correction was evaluated using a trial frame. The patient's far-point correction was placed before the right eye and the near correction before the left since that eye was hypotropic, already in down-gaze. The patient's initial response was the report of diplopia, but now with one clear image and the other blurred. With a little practice, she was able to alternate fixation easily between far and near. The following prescription was given for a trial period of wear:

OD −1.25 −0.50 X 095   20/20

OS +1.00 −0.25 X 088   .4M

The patient was instructed to wear the monovision correction as much time as she could during a trial period of 2 weeks. At the progress check, she reported that the monovision correction seemed to be a major improvement. She had learned to ignore the blurred image even during critical viewing such as television and reading. Diplopia was noted less frequently as she gained experience with monovision spectacles. At a 6-month progress check, the deviation had not changed significantly, but she was essentially symptom free, except for high contrast situations such as when viewing street lights at night.

Case Five: Congenital Nystagmus

A 13-month-old male child was brought in by his parents for his first complete eye examination. His parents had the following questions: Why did the child have nystagmus? How well did he see? What could be done for him? The mother had a normal prenatal history and a relatively easy delivery, only 6 hours of labor. The full-term child weighed 8 lbs 6 oz at birth. There was fetal distress, however, due to anoxia. The infant had a ductus arteriosus shunt, an abnormal connecting tube between the aorta and a pulmonary artery. This shunt closed by itself within 24 hours. Thereafter, the child experienced good health and normal development until age 2 months when nystagmus was first noticed. A left head turn developed at age 4 months and a left esotropia was seen at 10 months of age. There was no family history of nystagmus, strabismus, or severe vision disorders.

Clinical Findings: Cycloplegic retinoscopy (1% Cyclogyl) revealed a small amount of hyperopia: OD +1.00 DS; OS +0.75 DS. Visual acuity was assessed by visually evoked potential (VEP) and indicated a significant difference between the eyes: OD 20/55; OS 20/130. Cover test showed the presence of a noncomitant, intermittent, unilateral, left 35$^\Delta$ esotropia at farpoint and near. The child apparently fused in right gaze and therefore had an habitual 25° left head turn. The noncomitancy pattern suggested a paresis of the left lateral rectus (LLR), a slight limitation of abduction of the left eye, and a mild V pattern (Figure 15-9). The Bielschowsky head tilt test was negative. The nystagmus appeared constant, pendular, conjugate, with equal amplitude in each eye, variable frequency and amplitude, which decreased on convergence and increased in left gaze. No latent component to the nystagmus was seen. The ocular health seemed unremarkable, except that the fundi appeared to lack pigment. An ERG was done to rule out the possible etiology of ocular albinism; this proved to be negative. The child was diagnosed as having efferent congenital nystagmus, possibly related to anoxia at the time of birth, LLR paresis, and amblyopia of the left eye.

Vision Therapy: No spectacles were recommended because of the insignificant refractive error. In an attempt to cure the amblyopia, 4 hours per day of direct occlusion using a bandage occluder was prescribed. Fortunately, the nystagmus did not worsen with patching. (If latent nystagmus had been present, the right

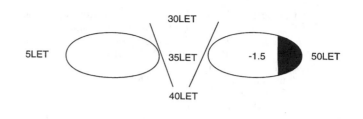

FIGURE 15-9—Diagram illustrating noncomitant esotropia with V pattern.

eye would have to be fogged rather than totally occluded to promote fixation with the amblyopic eye.) Ocular calisthenics were prescribed intermittently to improve the restriction of abduction of the left eye while the right eye was patched. After 2 months of this regimen, there was no restriction of abduction, the VEP acuity of the left eye equaled that of the right, 20/50, and there was less nystagmus than before in the left field of gaze. Strabismus surgery was performed at age 18 month, a recession-resection operation of the left eye, resulting in an intermittent 12$^\Delta$ left esotropia and improved horizontal comitancy. The head turn reduced to about 10° left. Spectacle lenses with base-out prisms were then prescribed (OD 3$^\Delta$ BO; OS 6$^\Delta$ BO). These prisms improved the child's fusion in the primary position, further reduced the head turn, and dampened the nystagmus. Although initially resistant to wearing the prism spectacles, the child eventually accepted them over a 2-month period; the binocular acuity improved to 20/30. The patient was scheduled for progress checks every 6 months and released. The parents were pleased with these results: minimal nystagmus, adequate acuity in each eye, no strabismus in the primary position, and no apparent head turn. This case illustrates that vision therapy can help reduce congenital nystagmus.

REFERENCES

1. Burian H, von Noorden GK. *Binocular Vision and Ocular Motility.* 2nd ed. St. Louis: CV Mosby Co; 1974:363.
2. Erickson GB, Caloroso EE. Vertical diplopia onset with first-time bifocal. *Optom Vis Sci.* 1992;69: 645-651.

3. Wick B. Vision therapy for cyclovertical heterophoria. In: *Problems in Optometry: Ocular Vertical and cyclovertical Deviations*. Philadelphia: Lippincott; 1992;4:663.

4. Iwasaki Y, Wanaka Y, Ikeda N, Uyama J, Mimura O. Treatment and prognosis of diplopia. Nipon Ganka Gakkai Zasshi. *Acta Soc Ophthalmol Japonicae*. 1993;97:815-850.

5. Rutstein RP. Evaluation and treatment of incomitant deviations in children. In: Scheiman MM, ed. *Problems in Optometry: Pediatric Optometry*. Philadelphia: Lippincott: 1990;2:528-561.

6. Eskridge JB. Persistent diplopia associated with strabismus surgery. *Optom Vis Sci*. 1993;70:849-853.

7. Boyd TAS, Karas Y, Budd GE, et al. Fixation switch diplopia. *Can J Ophthalmol*. 1974;9:310-315.

8. Karas Y, Budd GE, Boyd TAS. Late onset diplopia in childhood onset strabismus. *J Pediatr Ophthalmol*. 1974;11:135-136.

9. Maraining SM. Anomalous retinal correspondence and monolateral squint. *Ophthalmologica*. 1967;153:179-183.

10. Revell MJ. Anomalous retinal correspondence: A refractive treatment. *The Ophthalmic Optician*. 1971;2:110-112

11. Von Noorden GK. *Binocular Vision and Ocular Motility*. 4th ed. St. Louis: CV Mosby Co; 1990:387.

12. London R, Scott SH. Sensory fusion disruption syndrome. *J Am Optom Assoc*. 1987;58:544-546.

13. Worth C. *Squint: Its Causes, Pathology, and Treatment*. Philadelphia: P Blakiston's Son and Co; 1921.

14. Pratt-Johnson JA, Tillson G. Acquired central distruption of fusional amplitude. *Opthalmol*. 1979;86:2140-2142.

15. Burger DS, London R. Soft opaque contact lenses in binocular vision problems. *J Amer Optom Assoc*. 1993;64:176-180.

16. London R. Monovision correction for diplopia. *J Am Optom Assoc*. 1987;58:568-570.

17. Kirschen D, Flom MC. Monocular central-field occlusion for intractable diplopia. *Am J Optom Physiol Optics*. 1977;54:325-331.

18. Anderson JR. Latent nystagmus and alternating hyperphoria. *Br J Ophthalmol*. 1954;38:217-231.

19. Grisham D. Management of nystagmus in young children. In: Scheiman MM, ed. *Problems in Optometry: Pediatric Optometry*. Philadelphia: Lippincott; 1990;2:496-527.

20. Dickinson CM. The elucidation and use of the effect of near fixation in congenital nystagmus. *Ophthalmic Physiol Opt*. 1986;6:303-311.

21. Metzger EL. Correction of congenital nystagmus. *Am J Ophthalmol*. 1950;33:1796.

22. Healy E. Nystagmus treatment by orthoptics. *Am Orthopt J*. 1952;2:53-55.

23. Stegall FW. Orthoptic aspects of nystagmus. Symposium on nystagmus. *Am Orthoptic J*. 1973;23:30-34.

24. Mallett RFJ. The treatment of congenital idiopathic nystagmus by intermittent photic stimulation. *Ophthalmol Physiol Optics*. 1983;3:341-356.

25. Brinker WR, Katz SL. A new and practical treatment of eccentric fixation. *Am J Ophthalmol*. 1963;55:1033-1035.

26. Abadi RV, Carden D, Simpson J. A new treatment for congenital nystagmus. *Br J Ophthalmol*. 1980;64:2-6.

27. Ciuffreda KJ, Goldrich SG, Neary C. Use of eye movement auditory biofeedback in the control of nystagmus. *Amer J Optom Physiol Optics*. 1982;59:396-409.

28. Kirschen DG. Auditory feedback in the control of congenital nystagmus. *Am J Optom Physiol Optics*. 1983;60:364-368.

29. Mezawa M, Ishikawa S, Ukai K. Changes in waveform of congenital nystagmus associated with biofeedback treatment. *Brit J Ophthalmol*. 1990;74:472-474.

30. Ishikawa S, Tanakadate A, Nabatame K, Ishii M. Biofeedback treatment of congenital nystagmus. *Neuroophthamology*. 1985;2:58-65.

31. Kestenbaum A. Nouvelle operation de nystagmus. *Bull Soc Ophthalmol Fr*. 1953;6:599.

32. Dell'Osso LF, Flynn JT. Congenital nystagmus surgery: a quantitative evaluation of the effects. *Arch Ophthalmol* 1979;97:462-469.

33. Flynn JT, Dell'Osso LF. The effects of congenital nystagmus surgery. *Ophthalmology*. 1979;86:1414-14127.

34. Parks MM. Congenital nystagmus surgery. *Am Orthopt J*. 1973;23:35.

35. Mitchell PR, Wheeler MB, Parks MM. Kestenbaum surgical procedure for torticollis secondary to congenital nystagmus. *J Ped Ophthalmol Strabismus*. 1987;24:87-93.

36. Scott WE, Kraft SP. Surgical treatment of compensatory head position in congenital nystagmus. *J Ped Ophthalmol Strabismus*. 1984;21:85-95.

37. Nelson LB, Wagner RS, Harley RD. Congenital nystagmus surgery. *Int Ophthalmol Clin*. 1985;25:133-138.

38. Von Noorden GK, Wong SY. Surgical results in nystagmus blockage syndrome. *Ophthalmology*. 1986;93:1028-1031.

39. Zubcov AA, Reinecke RD, Gottlob I, Manley DR, Calhoun JH. Treatment of manifest latent nystagmus. *Am J Ophthalmology*. 1990;110:160-167.

40. Currie JN, Matsuo V. The use of clonazepam in the treatment of nystagmus-induced oscillopsia. *Ophthalmology*. 1986:93:924-932.

41. Yee RD, Baloh RW, Honrubia V. Effect of baclofen on congenital nystagmus. In: Lennerstrad G, Zee DS, Keller EL, eds. *Functional Basis of Ocular Motility Disorders*. Oxford: Pergamon; 1982:151-157

42. Yaniglos SS, Leigh RJ. Refinement of an optical device that stabilizes vision in patients with nystagmus. *Optom Vis Sci* 1992;69:447-450.

43. Ruben ST, Lee JP, O'Neil D, Dunlop I, Elston JS. The use of botulinum toxin for treatment of acquired nystagmus and oscillopsia. *Ophthalmology*. 1994;101:783-787.

44. Griffin JR, Carlson GP. Duane retraction syndrome and vision therapy: a case report. *J Am Optom Assoc*. 1991;62:318-321.

45. Griffin JR, Walton HN, Christenson GN. *The Dyslexia Screener (TDS)*. Culver City, Calif: Reading and Perception Therapy Center; 1988.

46. Bergin D, Griffin J, Levin M. Hyperphoria of large magnitude: a case report. *Am J Optom Arch Am Acad Optom*. 1972;49:947-950.

Chapter 16 / Therapy for Vision Efficiency Skills

Visual Comfort and Performance   462
Aniseikonia   462
Monovision   465
Saccadic Eye Movements   466
   General Approaches to Training   466
   Specific Techniques   469
      Picking Up Objects T16.1   469
      Toothpick in Straw T16.2   469
      Pegboard Games T16.3   469
      Wall Fixations T16.4   469
      Wall Fixations with an Afterimage
         T16.5   469
      Continuous Motion Saccades
         T16.6   469
      Prism Steps T16.7   469
      Dot-to-dot Games I16.8   469
      Filling Os T16.9   469
      Sequential Fixations with Nonlinguistic
         Symbols T16.10   469
      Saccades with Letters and Words
         T16.11   469
      Computerized Programs T16.12   469
Pursuit Eye Movements   471
   General Approaches to Training   471
   Specific Techniques   473
      Automatic Rotating Devices
         T16.13   474
      Swinging Ball T16.14   474
      Penlight Pursuits T16.15   474
      Pie Pan Pursuits T16.16   474
      Flashlight Spot Chasing T16.17   474
      Minivectogram and Mini-Tranaglyph
         Pursuits T16.18   474

      Computerized Pursuits T16.19   474
Accommodation   474
   General Training Approaches   474
   Optical Management   476
      Plus-Lens Additions   476
      Plus-Lens-Acceptance Training
         T16.20   476
   Specific Training Techniques   476
      Accommodative Tromboning
         T16.21   477
      Jump Focus Rock T16.22   477
      Lens Rock T16.23   477
      Other Considerations   478
Vergences   478
   Finishing Concepts in
      Heterophoria   478
   Hyperphoria   479
      Vertical Step Vergence T16.24   479
      Variations on Vertical Vergence
         Training T16.25   479
   Cyclophoria   479
   Symptomatic Orthophoria   480
Stereopsis   480
   Vectogram® Stereo Enhancement
      T16.26   480
   Computer Stereo Enhancement
      T16.27   481
Case Examples   482
Future Directions in Binocular Vision
   Therapy   485

VISUAL COMFORT AND PERFORMANCE

Vision efficiency is a modern concept. This concept, however, continues to be irrelevant to the majority of people subsisting in a third-world agrarian culture. The farmer guiding a water buffalo does not have as high a level of visual requirements as a technical worker who is expected to succeed in 12 to 20 years of formal education; this is just a prerequisite for his or her occupation. Vision efficiency refers to ocular comfort with high performance over time. Many workers who must look at a computer display for 7 or 8 hours a day experience severe symptoms of ocular discomfort. The causes of these disturbing symptoms may be binocular anomalies such as poor vergence or accommodative skills, and they are intensified if there is a mismatch between that individual's particular oculomotor physiology and psychological disposition with the visual job requirements. This chapter is based on the premise that inefficient visual skills can be remedied when it is in the patient's interest to do so. Over the years, we have seen an increasing number office workers, computer operators, machinists, lawyers, athletes, and others seeking improvement in visual comfort and performance. Unless world culture takes an unexpected turn in its evolution, this trend toward the necessity of higher vision efficiency will continue to accelerate.

The rise in world literacy is a fundamental part of cultural and economic development. The printing press, invented approximately 400 years ago, made possible the distribution of books to the public at large. Now we find there are many ocular conditions that compromise reading comfort and performance. Clinical experience and studies have shown there is a higher prevalence of certain visual problems among poor readers compared with skilled readers. Uncorrected hyperopia and anisometropia, excessive exophoria and fusional vergence deficiency, hyperphoria, and accommodative infacility have all been implicated by association.[1] The computer age has burgeoned into mass markets during the last few decades and this genie will not be put back into the bottle. A large number of computer operators show deficiencies in vergence and accommodation over time.[2] Many symptomatic individuals respond to the increasing visual requirements in inefficient ways. Some lose interest and avoid the noxious stimulus altogether whereas many individuals put up with the discomfort but reduce their work output. Others rightfully complain to the eye doctor and hopefully, appropriate vision therapy is prescribed to ameliorate the patient's signs and symptoms of dysfunction.

Vision therapy techniques and considerations discussed in this chapter are appropriate for those patients who have specific skill deficiencies, with associated signs and symptoms, and for those individuals seeking enhancement of their visual performance in school, work, and play. These techniques are also appropriate for the strabismic patient who has made progress in a vision therapy program, but has not yet achieved the highest level of vision efficiency.

ANISEIKONIA

Aniseikonia is an often overlooked condition that is a barrier to efficient binocular vision. Unexplained binocular symptoms may be due to aniseikonia. This condition is one in which the ocular image size of one eye is different from the other. This problem is often produced by anisometropic corrective lenses if the power difference is significantly large between the two eyes. Contact lenses may be a remedy in certain cases, particularly if the anisometropia is "refractive," meaning that the corneal curvatures of each eye are greatly different. If, however, the anisometropia is due to difference in eyeball length ("axial"), then a spectacle lens correction may be preferable to contact lenses. There are exceptions, however, that show inconsistencies in Knapp's Law.[3] This may be due to the fact that aniseikonia can result from a difference in distribution of the retinal elements as well as a difference in the size of the dioptric images formed on the retinas. The clinician must, therefore, evaluate each patient and not always adhere strictly to Knapp's law. In some cases of axial anisometropia, contact lenses may be the preferred prescription. When the difference in ocular image size is very small (e.g., less than 1%), symptoms are usually not produced. As the size difference increases, symptoms may result. If the aniseikonia is greater than 5%, this obstacle to fusion may make it impossible for the individual to have central fusion.

Many of the symptoms reported by patients with aniseikonia do not differ significantly from symptoms of ametropia, heterophoria, and intermittent strabismus, e.g., headaches, asthenopia, reading difficulties, and diplopia.[4] Other symptoms associated with aniseikonia are photophobia, nausea, nervousness, dizziness, vertigo, and general fatigue. When ametropia and binocular anomalies are eliminated, the persistence of such symptoms may indicate aniseikonia, providing the patient is in sound physical and mental health. Aniseikonic symptoms are generally of long standing and are not relieved by conventional prescription lenses or vision training.

Unfortunately the Space Eikonometer is no longer available for the precise measurement of the magnitude of aniseikonia. Two other methods remain for the clinician. A clinician can estimate the magnitude of aniseikonia from the refractive correction of anisometropia. Ogle[5] suggested that aniseikonia of 1.5% to 2.0% is induced by every diopter of anisometropia that is corrected with spectacle lenses. Others have disagreed with Ogle's estimate and indicate that 1% per diopter is a more realistic value.[6,7] Most clinicians use the 1% per diopter as a clinical guideline. The other method is direct comparison of the two images. There are several ways images can be dissociated for direct comparison, e.g., vertical prism dissociation, stereograms, and vectographic methods. We recommend using a Maddox rod and two penlights (Figure 16-1). The lights are held by the clinician, one above the other (separation of 15 to 20 cm), and the patient fixates the lights from a distance of approximately 2 meters. The Maddox rod is oriented with its axis 90 degrees, so the patient should see two horizontal streaks with that eye. The other eye does not have a Maddox rod before it, but looks directly at the lights. If there is no aniseikonia, the patient should report the streaks going through the lights (Figure 16-1b).

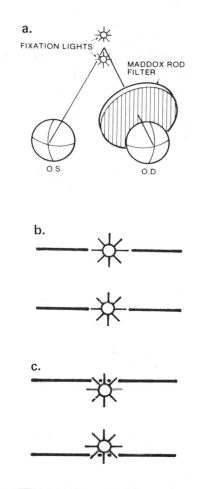

FIGURE 16-1—Direct method to detect aniseikonia: (a) Diagram showing the right eye looking through a Maddox rod and the left eye seeing the penlights; (b) patient's perception if there is no aniseikonia; and (c) perception if there is aniseikonia.

With a significant degree of aniseikonia, the distance between the streaks will be different from the distance between the lights (Figure 16-1c). Iseikonic size lenses are introduced before each eye in an attempt to equalize the size of ocular images in the vertical meridian. To test other meridians, the orientation of lights and the Maddox rod are rotated by the same amount to axes of 180, 45, and 135 degrees. Any horizontal or vertical phoria or tropia, however, must be neutralized with prism before these aniseikonic measurements can be made.

The correction of overall, meridional, or compound (both types) aniseikonia is accomplished by magnifying the smaller image in the appropriate meridian(s) until a reasonable size

TABLE 16-1. *Magnification of Trial Lenses Based on Curvature and Thickness of Crown Glass Lenses with Index of Refraction of Approximately 1.53*

Magnification	Front Surf. (D)	Back Surf. (D)	Thickness (mm)
1%	+ 6.75	− 6.87	2.2
2%	+11.25	−11.50	2.7
3%	+12.00	−12.37	3.7
4%	+12.00	−12.50	4.9
5%	+12.00	−12.62	6.1
7%	+16.50	−17.62	6.1
9%	+20.75	−22.62	6.1
11%	+25.00	−27.75	6.1

TABLE 16-2. *Magnification of Trial Lenses Based on Curvatures and Thickness of Plastic Lenses (CR-39) with Index of Refraction of Approximately 1.50*

Magnification	Front Surf. (D)	Back Surf. (D)	Thickness (mm)
1%	+ 5.00	− 5.00	2.2
2%	+ 7.50	− 7.62	3.9
3%	+ 9.00	− 9.25	4.9
4%	+10.00	−10.37	5.8
5%	+12.50	−13.12	5.7
7%	+16.37	−17.50	6.0
9%	+20.62	−22.50	6.0
11%	+24.75	−27.50	6.0

match for the patient's eyes is achieved, which is the tentative size-lens prescription. Overall magnification trial lenses can be used to measure separate meridians. Kleinstein[8] suggested using custom made trial lenses. Calculations for glass and plastic lenses were made by Dr. Richard Hemenger, of the Southern California College of Optometry, for optical parameters of an afocal aniseikonic trial lens set (Tables 16-1 and 16-2). Local optical laboratories can fabricate a trial lens set such as this, either in glass or plastic.

When the amount of needed magnification has been estimated, the doctor can prescribe iseikonic lenses by manipulating the lens parameters of the least-magnified eye through trial and error, if necessary, to increase its magnification to compensate for the patient's aniseikonia. Our recommended technique is that of actually measuring the patient's image size difference and then compensating for that difference with optics to provide a level of control needed to help many symptomatic aniseikonic patients. A rough clinical guideline for lens design is to equalize the base curve and thickness of the least-powered lens to that of the greater.

A certain percentage of undercorrection (e.g., 0.5%) is acceptable due to presumed patient tolerance. Spectacle magnification can be accomplished by appropriate modification of the *shape* factor of an ophthalmic lens (which is dependent on the front base curve and thickness of the lens) and/or the *power* factor (which is dependent on the vertex power and vertex distance of the lens). Since the power factor can be modified only slightly without undercorrecting or overcorrecting the ametropia, the shape factor is the variable that is most often considered to create the desired magnification. Kleinstein[8] gave the magnification formula for the shape factor as follows:

$$M = \left(\frac{1}{1 - ZF_V} \right)\left(\frac{1}{1 - CF_1} \right)$$

Where M = Magnification

Z   = Vertex distance in meters, e.g., 0.013

Fv   = Vertex power in diopters, e.g., +3.00

C   = Thickness of lens (in meters) divided by the index of refraction, e.g., 0.002/1.53

F1   = Front surface power in diopters, e.g., +9.00

Using this formula and calculating with the numbers in the example, M= 1.05, or 5 % magnification for one eye, e.g., right eye. If a lens for the left eye has the following specifications:

Fv = +5.00

C   = 0.003/1.53   (i.e., thicker lens).

F   = +11.00

$$M = \left(\frac{1}{1-0.013(5)}\right)\left(\frac{1}{1-0.003/1.53(11)}\right)$$

= 1.09, or 9% spectacle magnification

Predicted aniseikonia = M left eye – M right eye

= 9% – 5%

= 4%

If the thickness of the lens of the right eye were 5 mm and the front surface power were increased to = +11.00 D, then M would be calculated as 1.08, or 8% spectacle magnification. Predicted aniseikonia would then be :

M left eye – M right eye = 9% – 8%

= 1%

This 1% difference of ocular image size would be more tolerable to the patient than the 4% difference. Note that this example applies to overall aniseikonia. Meridional aniseikonia would require direct comparison and calculations of various meridians for toric iseikonic prescription lenses. In summary, aniseikonia is a binocular anomaly and should be considered and testing given for it when there are unaccounted for symptoms. There are some patients who need iseikonic correction for comfortable and efficient binocular vision. We recommend direct measurement of image size difference between the eyes and manipulation of the shape factor in ophthalmic lens design to reduce aniseikonia to within tolerable limits.

MONOVISION

Some presbyopic patients, particularly successful contact lens wearers, prefer a monovision contact lens prescription rather than the traditional solution of spectacle bifocals. Because these patients usually have normal binocular vision, they choose to disrupt their binocularity by wearing a contact lens correcting the distance ametropia on the dominant eye and a contact lens add on the nondominant eye for nearpoint viewing. The primary advantage of monovision contact lenses is self evident—no need for spectacles. In addition, monovision can provide far and near vision independent of field of gaze. Unlike bifocals, they do not often present vision problems while the individual is walking or climbing stairs. However, monovision is accurately described as optically induced anisometropia. When a monovision patient is carefully tested, foveal suppression will often be found. In monovision patients, stereopsis measures, on average, 60 to 90 seconds of arc.[9,10] This represents a small reduction, but monovision contact lens wear does affect accuracy in some occupational tasks.[11] Monovision also compromises visual resolution under low contrast viewing conditions, especially for adds beyond 1.50 D.[12] This means that contrast sensitivity for night driving, for example, can be significantly reduced.

Whether or not monovision contact lens wear is in the patient's best interest is a decision that must be carefully made by the patient in consultation with the doctor. What must be seriously considered is the patient's need for binocular vision efficiency and the chances of producing symptoms. We generally do not recommend monovision contact lenses to presbyopic patients who have high vision requirements, e.g., commercial drivers, pilots, surgeons, lawyers, or computer operators. These patients are often not successful in making the adaptation. Drivers at night can experience an annoying glare;[13] depth perception and resolution can be reduced for critical nearpoint work;[11] degraded binocularity can result in asthenopia with prolonged reading demands.[14]

Based on our experience, we do not recommend the monovision approach to patients whose binocular status is fragile or poor. Lebow and Goldberg reported that 20% of their monovision patients were unable to achieve second-degree fusion.[15] We consider, for example, the intermittent exotrope to be a poor candidate for a monovision prescription. If such a patient insists on wearing monovision contact lenses, the doctor should, in response, recommend vision training to improve fusional skills. This training could possibly counteract the adverse effects of monovision contact lens

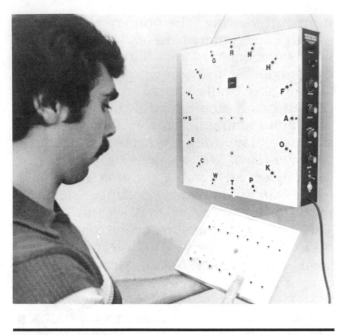

FIGURE 16-2—Continuous motion game. This can be custom made and varied for out-of-office therapy. The patient is instructed to draw a continuous line to connect the numbers in proper sequence.

wear. On the other hand, we do use a monovision approach in some cases of binocular anomalies, e.g., the amblyopic patient who is managed with optical penalization (Chapter 10) and in some cases of intractable diplopia.

SACCADIC EYE MOVEMENTS

Some patients have deficient control of their saccadic eye movements and may benefit from vision training. Amblyopic patients are the most common example, but some unilateral strabismic patients who are nonamblyopic have poor saccadic skills with the deviating eye. Some school-aged children with reading disabilities also have fine- and gross-motor immaturity, which may be reflected in their control of saccadic eye movements. Other children, independent of a learning disability, have poor saccades and eye-hand coordination, which may limit sports performance and cause inefficiency in other activities in school, work, and play. All these patients may benefit by participating in a vision therapy program although it is often not clear what part maturation plays in the outcome. Nevertheless, testing of saccades (Chapter 2) should be done when a child has behavioral and

performance problems in school; vision therapy in deficient cases is usually successful.

General Approaches to Training

It is best to begin with monocular saccadic training, right eye or left eye alone. After each eye is shown to perform equally well, proceed to binocular training. Table 16-3 lists general approaches to training for saccadic eye movement dysfunction. Either sophisticated instruments such as the Saccadic Fixator (Figure 16-2) or simple devices can be used.

Step One

The first step in vision training for good saccadic eye movements is to ensure good fixation ability of each eye. Position maintenance (fixation) probably involves all four of the eye-movement systems, i.e., saccades, pursuits, vergences, and nonoptic (e.g., vestibular). If fixation ability is reasonably good, then move on to step two for saccadic training. In cases of amblyopia, this anomaly would need to be treated initially (Chapter 10). As is customary, binocular saccadic training would follow only after the improvement of visual acuity.

Step Two

In step two, the patient practices accuracy of saccades, progressing from large to small eye movement. The large saccades are mostly voluntary and can generally be improved with concentrated effort by the patient. Fine saccades, as used in reading, tend to be reflexive; they are more difficult to train initially. Training procedures would go, for example, from the patient practicing wall fixations (gross) to working with Ann Arbor (Michigan) Tracking materials (fine). (Refer to T10.7 in Chapter 10.) Table 16-4 lists some specific training techniques that are arranged in an easy-to-difficult progressive sequence. Most of these can be performed at home and the principles listed in Table 16-3 can be applied.

Step Three

Step three introduces the element of speed for various sizes of saccades. A useful instrument for improving the speed of gross saccades is the

---

TABLE 16-3. General Training Approaches for Saccadic Eye Movement Dysfunction

1. Ensure good position maintenance (steady fixation on a stationary target)
2. Go from gross (large) saccades to fine (small saccades, as in reading)
3. Go from slow to fast (timing of several cycles)
4. Develop good eye-hand coordination during saccadic demands, and then go without hand as support (e.g., no finger reading)
5. Train until each eye has equal skills
6. Go from monocular (duction) to binocular (version) saccades
7. Eliminate any head movement
8. Introduce motor sequencing with metronome (auditory-visual integration) and ensure good left-to-right sequencing of saccades, as reading in the English language
9. Develop automated saccades (simple cognitive demands during saccades should not have an adverse effect on the quality of eye movements)
10. Eliminate (if possible) any significant overshoots, undershoots, regressions, or inefficient return sweeps.

Wayne Saccadic Fixator (Figure 16-2). Most patients enjoy working on this electronic instrument, which has an automatic timer. This instrument is similar to the more advanced DynaVision 2000 electronic fixation instrument (see Figure 10-8 in Chapter 10). Later emphasis can be placed on increased speed for fine saccades, as in timing activities using Ann Arbor Tracking booklets (see Figure 10-12).

Step Four

Good eye-hand coordination during saccadic tasks should be ensured. The goal in this phase, once good eye-hand coordination is achieved, is to discontinue the hand as a support. (It is very interesting to see how the finger is used, even by adults, as a "support" under certain stressful situations such as when reading a legal document on which a signature is required.) Usually the patient with poor saccadic ability performs better if he can point to the numbers, letters, or words, than if he has to locate them accurately by visual means alone. Since it is inefficient to point to each fixated object of regard, the hand/finger support must be discouraged as soon as possible in the therapy program.

Step Five

Saccadic training should be given for each eye separately until performance is equal or approximately so. This goal is not always possible to achieve, but an attempt should be made to reach it.

Step Six

When the eyes are approximately equal in ability, proceed to binocular saccadic eye movements (versions). Steps one through four should be repeated under binocular conditions.

Step Seven

This step in therapy is for the purpose of eliminating any unnecessary head movements during fine to moderately large saccades. The finely tuned extraocular muscles are much more efficient and accurate for saccades than are the relatively gross neck and body muscles. Most patients (even those with neurological soft signs) can voluntarily learn to control their head movements when making saccadic eye movements. Reading efficiency may improve as a result. Head movements are normally made, however, for large saccadic eye movements beyond 15 degrees.[16] An effective means of reducing head movements during saccadic training is to require the patient to balance an object (e.g., small wooden block) on his head.

Step Eight

Auditory stimuli can be introduced into the saccadic visual task and ensure that the patient is able to sequence in a left-to-right fashion, as

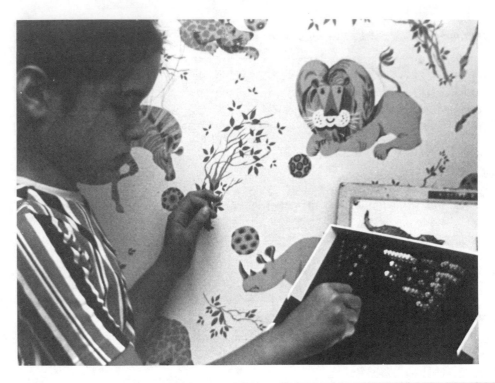

FIGURE 16-3—Example of Rosner TVAS training. (with permission from Rosner J. *Helping Children Overcome Learning Difficulties.* New York: Walker and Co; 1993.)

in written English. The patient should be able to develop the ability to keep up with the rhythm of a metronome. To proceed from less difficult to more difficult, speed is increased from slow to fast. One good method for building accurate rhythmic saccades is to combine wall fixations with a foveal afterimage. The patient moves the afterimage by fixating different objects on a wall to the beat of a metronome. (Refer to Chapter 10 on foveal tags with afterimages.) Toys, such as the Lite-Brite (Figure 16-3), can similarly be used. The Lite-Brite is relatively inexpensive and suitable for home training of children.

Step Nine

The development of automated reflexive saccades is involved in this step. The patient should be able to cope with cognitive demands (commensurate with mental ability) so he will not be distracted when making accurate eye movements. (Refer to Chpater 2 regarding automated saccades.) This is absolutely essential for good reading ability, good work performance, and effective and enjoyable play. Much of this

type of training can be done at home and, it is hoped, at school. However, close supervision must be provided to ensure proper saccadic responses for successful vision therapy. Moreover, patients who are unable to achieve step nine may be no better off than if no saccadic vision therapy was done. The importance of establishing automated responses cannot be overemphasized.

Step Ten

The final step in this sequence is the finishing process in which significant overshoots, undershoots, or regressions are eliminated. If there are neurological "soft signs," the patient may not be completely able to overcome these inaccurate eye movements. However, we have been amazed at the progress made in such cases in which saccades were very inaccurate at the beginning of therapy but improved accuracy was found afterwards. If speed can be increased, good left-to-right sequencing developed, motor planning with rhythm achieved, and unnecessary head movements eliminated, the patient is better off than before vision therapy, even if

TABLE 16-4. *Specific Techniques for Saccadic Dysfunction*

T16.1   Fixating and picking up objects on a table top (e.g., toys, raisins, peanuts, cookie sprinkles, Indian beads). All ten principles apply.

T16.2   Placing toothpicks in a soda straw that is moved from one location to another by the therapist. If the patient consistently misses, he can use his other hand to locate the straw, giving tactile-kinesthetic support. The goals are accuracy and speed of eye-hand coordination.

T16.3   Pegboard games (e.g., Lite-Brite, geoboards). The patient is instructed to place the pegs in the appropriate holes as quickly and accurately as possible. (*See* Figure 16-3 showing a Lite-Brite)

T16.4   Wall fixations. The patient fixates randomly placed pictures or objects on a wall on command by the therapist. All ten principles apply. Also, a large picture of a baseball diamond can be hung on the wall. The patient fixates certain bases on command simulating a baseball game.

T16.5   Fixations with an afterimage. This provides good feedback as to accuracy of eye movements and fixations and can be applied to most other specific training techniques.

T16.6   Continuous motion tasks. Numbers 1 through 15 are randomly drawn on a page and the patient has to find and mark each number in ascending order upon command. Also, the patient is instructed to draw a continuous line to connect the numbers in proper sequence (Figure 16-4). Speed is the primary goal with this technique.

T16.7   Loose prism steps. Prisms of various powers can be used, sequenced from large to small. The goal is for the patient to perceive image displacement and make fine saccades as small as 1/2 prism diopters. This is done monocularly with the other eye being occluded.

T16.8   Dot-to-dot games. Many games can be purchased in department stores and at newsstands for these activities. The patient is instructed to connect a series of dots by drawing a continuous line from one dot to the next, which usually completes a picture that is eventually revealed once the sequence is completed. The Rosner TVAS and training materials are excellent for many purposes, including training accuracy and speed of saccades (Figure 16-5).

T16.9   Filling Os or other designated letters. The patient is instructed to fill in each letter "O" on a page of a newspaper. The emphasis is on accuracy, eye-hand coordination, and, eventually, speed.

T16.10 Sequential fixation sheets (see Figures 2-7 and 2-8). Marks involving very little cognition, such as dots, dashes, and asterisks, are printed on a page and the patient is instructed to fixate each in a specified sequence without hand support. The goal is speed and accuracy of saccades.

T16.11 Symbols demanding cognition. Letters, numbers, and words are used in a similar manner as in T16.10 with the difference that quick and accurate saccades are required with relatively complex cognition.

T16.12 Computerized Programs. Many video games involving eye-hand coordination are available and have training value, e.g., Nintendo. Smart Eyes is a program for the Macintosh that teaches speed reading strategies with an empahsis on saccadic training. Also, the available vision therapy computerized programs all have tasks dedicated to building ocular motility.

the full goals of speed and accuracy are not attained.

Specific Techniques T16.1- T16.12.

Many types of fixation targets can be used for saccadic training techniques. The 12 exemplary techniques listed in Table 16-4 can be applied to the above general training approaches in Table 16-3. Using ordinary objects as in T16.1, the first step is for the patient to fixate an object, such as a peanut, monocularly and steadily for several seconds. The therapist observes the patient's eye and provides feedback for the patient, whether there is steady fixation. The use of an afterimage for the patient's subjective feedback as to accuracy of fixation can also be used. In the second step, peanuts can be widely dispersed on a table top for gross saccadic training. With improved performance, the peanuts can be placed more closely together for fine saccadic training. In step three, the patient is encouraged to look from one peanut

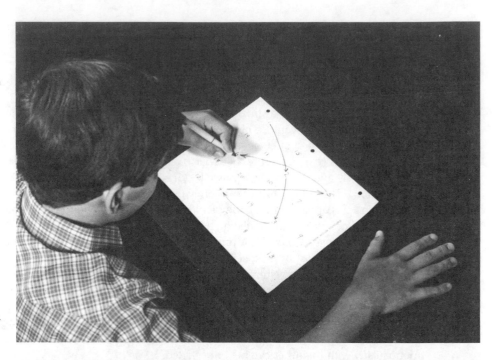

FIGURE 16-4—Saccadic Fixator. (Courtesy Wayne Engineering.)

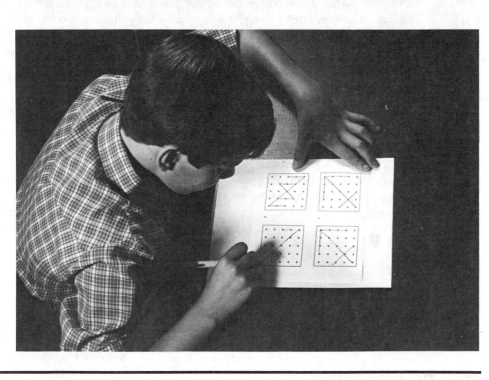

FIGURE 16-5—Lite-Brite game for saccadic eye movement training.

to the next as quickly as possible. The performance can be timed as the therapist closely watches the patient's eyes. In step four, the goal is to ensure good eye-hand coordination. The patient picks up each peanut in turn as accurately and quickly as possible. The patient's reward, of course, can be eating the peanuts. In step five, each eye is given training until there is equal ability. In step six, the patient views the peanuts with both eyes, repeating steps one through four. An afterimage tag gives important visual feedback to the patient and can be used at each step in this sequence. In step seven, the patient is instructed to eliminate head movements (with an object balanced on the head) when looking at and picking up the peanuts. In step eight, hand clapping or a metronome can be used as the patient picks up peanuts in rhythm to the auditory stimulus. In step nine, the patient attempts to pick up the peanuts while simultaneously trying to answer questions asked by the therapist. This is a cognitive loading procedure. In step ten, the therapist provides feedback to the patient as to any remaining inaccuracies in saccadic eye movements.

The specific training techniques T16.2 through T16.12 should be applied to the general training approaches listed in Table 16-3. Every training device and technique may not apply to every general approach. Sophisticated instruments (e.g., computerized programs) are available for special uses to motivate the patient, but techniques utilizing simple objects usually suffice for effective office and home vision training to improve saccadic eye movements.

PURSUIT EYE MOVEMENTS

General Approaches to Training

Many clinicians recognize a close relation between poor pursuits and poor performance in school, work, and athletics. Yet, there is little research to verify positive results from therapy. We believe, however, that it is beneficial to have smooth and accurate pursuit eye movements. If pursuits are deficient or immature, vision training can often improve tracking skills. Pursuit training is particularly useful to increase excursions when there is restricted motility in cases of noncomitancy. This is also important in amblyopia therapy to promote foveal fixation. The following therapy approaches[17] follow an easy-to-difficult sequence. General approaches to improve pursuit eye movements are listed in Table 16-5.

Step One

The goal in step one is to ensure that the patient has adequate position maintenance of a stationary target. Establishing central steady fixation of each eye is prerequisite to effective

TABLE 16-5. *General Approaches to Improvement of Pursuit Eye Movements*

1. Steady position maintenance of stationary target
2. Voluntary to reflexive responses
3. Eye-hand coordination to no eye-hand support
4. Small to large excursions
5. Slow to fast speed of pursuits
6. Jerky to smooth movements
7. Head movement to no head movement
8. Unequalness to equalness of right eye and left eye
9. Monocular to binocular pursuits
10. Simple to complex cognitive demands
11. Sitting to standing position
12. No vergence demand to prismatic demands
13. Combinations of less stress to more stress

pursuit training and should be the primary step when evaluating any of the eye movement systems.

Step Two

Step two is to proceed from voluntary to reflexive responses. The concept of "mental effort" is useful. The patient's attention must be actively engaged in the particular pursuit task. Initially, the tracking responses may be a combination of pursuit and saccadic eye movements. Even a person with good pursuits will break down and begin using saccades as the velocity of the target is greatly increased (more than 30 degrees per second). The patient attempts to coordinate saccadic and pursuit movements to maintain fixation on the moving target. The patient is encouraged to use all the volition possible to follow the target, whether it be a swinging Marsden ball, a moving handheld penlight, an afterimage on the hubcap of a passing car, or whatever. Volition will be important in the rest of the steps to follow, particularly in controlling head movement.

Step Three

In step three, eye-hand coordination is trained. The patient should practice correctly pointing to the moving target. The act of pointing provides visual-kinesthetic support for proper eye fixation and tracking. Many of the techniques for amblyopia therapy presented in Chapter 10 apply here. In time, after good eye-hand coordination is achieved, pointing should be discontinued so that pursuits can be practiced and improved without this support.

Additional eye-hand procedures may be introduced for variety. One that most children are fond of is the "Talking Pen" (Figure 10-10). The pen has an infrared light sensor in its tip. When the tip of the pen is exactly on a dark line, no sound is emitted. But when the tip falls off the dark line onto a bright portion of the paper, a buzzing sound results. The sound is louder and higher in pitch as the tip moves from a darker to lighter area. Later when auditory feedback is not essential, the pursuit tracing can be strictly visual.

Step Four

Step four involves progressing from small to large excursions, as large as possible. (Note that the progression in saccadic therapy is different; the training proceeds from gross to fine movements, because larger saccades are easier to control than smaller ones, e.g., reading saccades.) Pursuit training begins within a range where success comes easily, then ends with large excursions. The range of movement is naturally limited, being smaller for up-gaze (about 30 degrees) compared with other directions. The rotation range with a swinging Marsden ball as a target, for example, can be increased by simply having the patient move closer to the target.

Step Five

Speed is emphasized in step five. Fast pursuits are normally more difficult than slow pursuits. Therefore, it is best to start pursuit training at a slow speed within the patient's ability to perform and progressively increase the target speed. On a training task such as a buzzing pen, the patient is encouraged to finish the task more quickly while maintaining accuracy.

Step Six

Smooth movements can be strived for by giving the patient feedback regarding the accuracy of pursuits. Two types of feedback are available. The therapist can directly observe the patient's pursuit movements and report inaccuracies as they occur. Subjectively, the patient can observe pursuit inaccuracies with a foveal afterimage tag. This step is one of the most effective in building accurate pursuits. Some form of feedback is critical in all stages of vision therapy.

If jerky pursuits are due to functional causes, such as attention problems, the prognosis for achieving smoothness is good. We consider the prognosis for maturational delays in fine-motor coordination to be fair; training can improve pursuit movements in most of these cases. Nystagmus and other neurological disorders, however, presents a formidable obstacle in this regard. Nevertheless, we have seen some patients with nystagmus improve their pursuits, particularly after successful results with accommodation and vergence therapy.

Step Seven

In step seven the patient must become aware of unnecessary head movements during pursuits and exert voluntary control to stop them. Positive feedback to the patient is important. A convenient adjunct in therapy is to have the patient "wear a book" on his head. When it falls off, he knows head motion was the cause.

Step Eight

If monocular training of each eye has been effective up to this point, the pursuit skill of the right and left eyes should be approximately the same. If not, further training for the deficient eye is indicated. On occasion, it is impossible to achieve equality.

Step Nine

Binocular pursuits should be trained to the same level as monocular pursuits. Usually the patient has no problem making the transition from ductions to versions. An exception occurs when there is a vergence anomaly. For example, an intermittent exotropic patient may have difficulty in going from monocular to binocular pursuit training because of the voluntary effort required to maintain bifixation on the target.

Considerable vergence and binocular pursuit training may be needed in this step.

Step Ten

Cognitive demands are introduced, proceeding from simple to complex. Some adults can calculate numbers while maintaining fixation on a moving target. However, such complex tasks exceed what is normally expected of younger patients in vision therapy. Cognitive demands for children must be appropriate to their ability. Children can be asked, for example, to sing a song, count from one to ten, or state the names of friends and relatives.

Step Eleven

Pursuit eye movements need to be integrated with general body posture, movements, and balance. The vestibular ocular response (VOR) system involves the otolith organs, semicircular canals, and neck receptors. This system integrates eye and body movements and is increasingly involved when the individual changes posture requiring dynamic balance, as in skiing. This is so when a patient is asked to stand on a balance board or to move forward and backward on a walking rail while performing accurate pursuit eye movements. At first, there is a stimulus "overloading" for the patient; he will not be able to balance and maintain good pursuit eye movements as well as when in a sitting position. If there are no neurologic defects in the VOR and pursuit systems, most patients can eventually learn to cope with these demands and perform pursuits accurately.

Step Twelve

A stimulus "overloading" can also be accomplished by bringing in the vergence system. Base-out loose prisms can be placed before the patient's eyes to create a convergence demand while the patient views a moving target, e.g., a hand-held moving penlight. Conversely, a divergence demand can be created by placing base-in loose prism before the patient's eyes. If the patient can overcome the prismatic demand and continue to perform pursuits well, he is ready to go on to more stressful demands.

Step Thirteen

Increased stimulus "overloading" can be accomplished in many ways. There are many permutations and variations using the previous 12 steps. For example, the patient may be asked to follow a moving target while balancing a book on the top of his head, counting backward by 3's from 100, balancing on a balance board, and wearing 15^Δ base-out. The purpose of such combinations is to increase stress to a maximum. This level of training may be particularly useful for certain patients who require a high standard of performance in athletic events.

Specific Techniques T16.13 - T16.19

Most of the above general approaches listed in Table 16-5 can be applied to the five specific techniques listed in Table 16-6. An automatic rotating device such as a Bernell Rotator can serve as an example (see Figure 2-14). Once steady position maintenance of a stationary target is established, the patient is asked to follow a target on the rotating disk. The patient may have to resort to voluntary saccades before reflexive pursuits can be made to follow the moving target. An afterimage tag gives visual feedback to the patient regarding accuracy. The patient can also point to the target for eye-hand support. Next, the size of excursions can be increased by moving the patient closer to the instrument. The speed of the target can be increased. Accuracy and smoothness of pursuits are emphasized. It is important to give the patient adequate feedback on how well he is doing in all steps, but particularly when working on accuracy. Also, the patient should not make unnecessary head movements during pursuit training. Each eye is trained independently until performance is equal. Binocular pursuits are then trained. Cognitive demands (e.g., counting numbers aloud while doing pursuits) are presented. The patient stands up and balances to help integrate pursuits with the VOR system. Prismatic demands for fusional vergences are introduced. Higher levels of performance can be achieved by combining the above steps in various ways.

TABLE 16-6. Specific Vision Training Techniques for Pursuits

T16.13   Automatic rotating disks, e.g., Bernell Rotator (office). The speed of the rotation can be changed from slow to fast; the direction can be switched from clockwise to counterclockwise; and the size of excursions can be increased by having the patient move closer to the target.

T16.14   Swinging ball, e.g., Marsden ball (office or home). The ball is suspended from the ceiling and set in a swinging motion. The patient can look at the target at eye level for horizontal pursuit training or from below while lying supine for circular pursuits.

T16.15   Penlight pursuits (office or home). In the office the therapist moves the penlight target in various directions while the patient attempts to follow it smoothly and accurately. At home the helper (e.g., mother, sibling, friend) acts at a therapist to provide the target movements.

T16.16   Pie-pan pursuits (home). The patient is instructed to view a marble in a pie pan or similar dish, and move the pan so that the marble rolls around the edge, either in a clockwise or counterclockwise direction.

T16.17   Flashlight spot chasing (office or home). The therapist, or helper, shines a spot on the wall or ceiling from a flashlight while the patient holds another flashlight. The patient's task is to follow the therapist's spot with his, attempting to superimpose both spots of light. The therapist moves the spot slowly but as training progresses, the speed and extent of the movements are increased.

T16.18   Minivectogram and Mini-Tranaglyph (T16-7) vergence and pursuit training (office and home). Sensory fusion can be monitored while base-in and base-out demands are presented. The target can be moved by hand into various fields of gaze for pursuit training while sensory-motor fusion is monitored and trained.

T16.19   Computerized pursuits (office and home). Sophisticated programs for pursuits are available for office vision training, e.g., Teletherapy, Inc., Learning Frontiers, Inc., and Bernell Computer Software. Various video and computer games can be applied to pursuit training for home use, e.g., Nintendo. Tetris® is a popular computer game that trains smooth pursuits and visual perceptual skills.

ACCOMMODATION

In this section, vision therapy is discussed for accommodative excess, insufficiency, infacility, lag, and poor stamina. These dysfunctions and their diagnoses are discussed in detail in Chapter 2.

General Training Approaches

Eight steps of active vision training are listed in our recommended sequential order for the improvement of accommodative functions (Table 16-7). Clinicians, however, may wish to vary this sequence depending on the particular needs of their patients.

Step One

The goal is to increase the patient's monocular accommodative amplitude to its maximum. Our preferred techniques include accommodative pushups (T16.21) and jump focus exercises (T16.22). This step is omitted if the patient initially has sufficient amplitude. Also, presbyopic patients and those having organic lesions limiting accommodation are excluded from this type of therapy. Speed is not an important consideration in this step, but amplitude and accuracy of focus are. A training goal should be an accommodative amplitude commensurate with the mean for the patient's age (Chapter 2).

Step Two

Accommodative facility and stamina are improved by changing the accommodative stimulus demand beginning with small steps and proceeding to large. For example, using monocular accommodative flippers (T16.23), training proceeds from small to large lens powers, e.g., from ±0.50 to ±2.50 D. Training is similar to the testing procedure described in Chapter 2. Note that ±2.00 D is the standard power for testing young patients but training beyond that criterion is recommended. (With nonpresbyopic adults less power may be appropriate, e.g., ±1.50 D flippers.) This lens-rock procedure

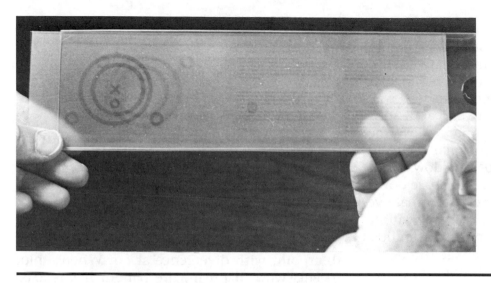

FIGURE 16-6—Mini-Tranaglyph. The patient wears red and green filters while trying to fuse split targets with variable demands on fusional vergence. The device can be moved into various fields of gaze for pursuit eye movements simultaneously with motor fusion and appreciation of stereopsis. This is an excellent home training procedure.

assumes the patient has the full refractive correction (CAMP lenses) in place, particularly a myopic patient. The target should be detailed nearpoint print. The patient alternately clears the print as quickly as possible with each flip of the lenses. Training progress can be recorded in two different ways. The time can be recorded for a given number of lens flips (or cycles); or conversely, the number of flips (cycles) is noted within a certain time limit. Out-of-office flipper training can be conveniently done because very little equipment is necessary.

Step Three

Speed rather than the amplitude is emphasized in this step. The ideal goal is to have the patient achieve 20 cycles per minute on accommodative rock. Using accommodative flippers (T16.23), for example, once adequate speed is achieved with low power lenses, use higher powers until the ideal range of clear vision (if possible for a particular patient) of ±2.50 D is achieved with a speed of 20 cycles per minute.

Step Four

The stimulatory and inhibitory phases of jump focus (near-far-near rock) or accommodative flipper (lens rock) training should be equalized. If the patient has trouble clearing the target through plus lenses in flipper training, for example, this problem should be worked on both in-office and at home. When equality is

TABLE 16-7. *Approaches to Accommodative Training*

1. Achieve sufficient accommodative amplitude, monocularly
2. Monocularly, achieve a range of +2.50D, untimed; proceed from small to large ranges
3. Achieve 20 cycles per minute, monocularly; proceed from slow to fast
4. Stimulatory and inhibitory phases should be quick
5. Facility of the right eye and left eye should be equal
6. Introduce bi-ocular rock
7. Introduce binocular rock, achieving goals in steps one through four
8. Introduce base-in and base-out prism demands during binocular rock

achieved for plus and minus lenses, the patient moves on to the next step.

Step Five

The accommodative skills of each eye should be approximately equal. Sometimes achieving this goal is not possible for many reasons, e.g., ocular pathology or incurable amblyopia. However, most patients are able to achieve good monocular accommodative skills in each eye even though one eye has strong ocular dominance.

Step Six

Bi-ocular rock exercises are another way to train and equalize monocular accommodative skills. This is a transition phase between monocular and binocular training. The most practical way to set this up is to introduce a vertical dissociating prism before one eye. Simply remove the occluder that was used in monocular rock and replace it with a prism, e.g., 10^Δ base-down. This should create vertical diplopia. If the base-down prism is placed before the left eye and that eye views through a minus lens, the image will be higher and will be an accommodative stimulus. The right eye views the lower image through a plus lens, which requires inhibition of accommodation for clarity. The patient alternately fixates the targets with increasing speed. The power of the lenses can be increased as training progresses.

Step Seven

Binocular accommodative rock is introduced in this step. Training is similar to testing procedures (Chapter 2). The same goals of range and speed in the first six steps also apply to binocular rock. Training techniques include near-far-near jumps (T16.22) and lens rock with flippers (T16.23). The ideal goal is 20 cycles per minute using ±2.50 D flippers.

Optical Management

Plus-Lens Additions

Plus-addition lenses are usually associated with the correction of presbyopia. They are sometimes prescribed for children and young adults, although not without controversy.[18-20] We have seen certain young patients with accommodative problems improve in reading and other nearpoint tasks when wearing plus-addition lenses (either single vision reading lenses or bifocals). Plus-addition lenses may be considered when there is a large accommodative lag; also if there is accommodative excess (Chapter 2). We recommend lending plus-lens spectacles to patients having accommodative problems to provide immediate relief of symptoms; they are particularly useful to relax functional spasm of accommodation as found in latent hyperopia, pseudomyopia, and accommodative excess. These lenses also help modify imbalances in the AC/A and CA/C crosslinks (Chapter 3).

Plus-Lens-Acceptance Training T16.20

Wearing of plus lenses is a passive form of vision therapy to help the patient relax the accommodative mechanism. Active vision training techniques to accomplish this result is done at far (Peckham method) and at near (modified Updegrave method). The Peckham method works best when the patient shows a blurpoint with divergence at far. When a blur occurs with BI prism, the patient has relaxed accommodation and is underfocused for the target. Plus power (or less minus) can then be added to clear the image. The process is repeated until the maximum plus power is accepted. This is an effective procedure to treat latent hyperopia and pseudomyopia.

The modified Updegrave technique is done at 40 cm. The patient is trained to accept plus lenses to the maximum without blur. The NRA is determined with the CAMP lenses in place. The NRA lenses are placed in a trial frame. A +0.50 D lens addition is combined with the NRA finding and the patient tries to push-away reading material while maintaining clarity. When material is clear beyond 40 cm, another +0.50 D addition is introduced. The process is repeated until maximum plus is accepted at 40 cm; then the NRA is subtracted and the remainder possibly represents the amount of the patient's latent hyperopia or pseudomyopia. The goal is to relax accommodation by slowly forcing the patient to accept the most plus power that allows for clear, single, binocular vision at near.

Specific Training Techniques

Functional training procedures are prescribed in many cases of accommodative insufficiency, excess, infacility, and ill-sustained accommodation. Two basic vision training methods generally apply to all these accommodative anomalies; they are accommodative tromboning (pushups) and accommodative rock. Tromboning builds amplitude, and stamina accuracy of accommodation. The two principal techniques for accommodative rock are near-far-near jumps (T16.22) and lens rock with flippers (T16.23). These rock techniques improve accommodative accuracy, facility, and stamina.

Accommodative Tromboning T16.21

The patient selects a good book or some interesting reading material. Holding the book at arm's length, the patient reads the selection for meaning while pulling it closer. The book is advanced to the binocular nearpoint of accommodation and then slowly pushed away to arm's length again. This process is continued for a 10-minute training period or for some other appropriate duration depending on the patient's abilities. Initially, the patient may have difficulty comprehending the material because the focus of attention is on the movement of the book; but with practice, the movement becomes a background activity and comprehension increases. This technique improves amplitude, accuracy, and stamina of accommodation in an entertaining manner.

Jump Focus Rock T16.22

The most popular jump focus procedure for accommodative rock is with the use of Hart Charts, discussed in Chapter 10 (Refer to T10.8 and Figure 10-13). Many variations of near-far-near rock are suitable for home training. A procedure referred to as "calendar rock" is good for improving accommodative facility, as well as working on other accommodative dysfunctions. In calendar rock, for example, the patient is instructed to look at newsprint at his absolute nearpoint of accommodation, monocularly. This helps train accommodative insufficiency in cases of low amplitude of accommodation. After focusing on a small letter at the limit of his accommodation, the patient is instructed to focus at far on a large number on a wall calendar; then the patient is to look back to the newsprint, and so on. This is training to improve accommodative facility. This can be done for 1-to-2 minutes several times a day. If there is a lag, the patient must learn to focus accurately to eliminate accommodative insufficiency at near. If there is blurring, either at near

of far, the patient must learn to focus accurately to achieve clear vision with each alternation of fixation distance. Speed of focus is then emphasized. When the technique can be done successfully for short periods, longer training times can be instituted to work on stamina and eliminate any problem of ill-sustained accommodation. The goal in this technique is 20 cycles per minute with clear and comfortable binocular vision for at least 3 minutes. When successful results are achieved monocularly, the patient repeats the regimen with both eyes open to work on binocular accommodative infacility, insufficiency, excess, and poor stamina.

Lens Rock T16.23

The use of flipper lenses for accommodative rock can be done either at home or in the office (see Figure 2-18). The technique is usually introduced monocularly with the goal of maximally increasing accommodative facility of each eye. Monocular accommodative rock with flipper lenses is particularly effective. Flipper lenses are available in powers of ±0.50 D to ±2.50 D so they can be selected to match the patient's skill level. The patient views a watch that has a second hand (or a digital watch is good) and records the number of cycles that can be completed within 1 or 2 minutes, whichever is assigned. The patient completes as many sets as possible within a 10-minute training period.

Another variation that is more entertaining for the patient is called flipper reading. The patient reads the newspaper, or other material printed in columns, for a 10-minute period. At the end of each line in the column, the lenses are flipped as the patient continues reading for comprehension. This technique builds reflex accommodative facility. AS a goal, no conscious effort to clear the print with each flip should be required.

Binocular accommodative training should always include monitoring of suppression, e.g., with vectographic targets, as in the testing procedure discussed in Chapter 2 (see Figure 2-19). Binocular accommodative rock is also discussed in T13.11 and T14.15.

Vision training with this technique is applicable to all seven steps discussed previously. The patient progresses through the steps by developing sufficient monocular amplitude, a large plus and minus range, adequate speed, quick stimulation and inhibitory phases, monocular functions being equal for each eye, ability to do bi-ocular rock, normal binocular facility, and with the ability to meet base-in and base-out vergence demands.

Other Considerations

We have found that most patients with functional accommodative deficiency can be trained successfully within 5 or 6 weeks, assuming there is good compliance. This guideline applies if no significant vergence anomalies exist. Accommodative excess, however, can vary considerably in the strength of the spasm; training time varies accordingly.

Vergence and accommodation are part of a reciprocal neurologic system. Vergence problems can have a profound effect on binocular accommodative facility. Take, for example, an esophoric patient. When minus lenses are introduced binocularly, accommodation causes accommodative convergence to increase. The patient offsets this increased convergence by exerting extra fusional divergence. If he has a sufficiently large fusional divergence range, he can keep the target clear and single. But suppose the patient's fusional divergence is less than adequate for this particular demand. To diverge his eyes enough to keep the target single, the patient will have to give up some accommodative convergence. In doing so, the accommodative response is reduced and the target appears blurred. A similar explanation can be made for the exophoric patient who has trouble keeping the target clear and single when plus lenses are introduced binocularly. The excessive accommodation results in blurring of the target. Patients during binocular accommodative rock may resort to blur, because the desire to keep the target single is so great that they will sacrifice clarity for singleness. Vision training of accommodation helps vergences and vision training of vergences helps accommodation. Successful results may depend on vergence therapy (Chapters 13 and 14) to achieve ideal binocular accommodative functions.

VERGENCES

Techniques for improving vergence ranges in cases of eso deviations were extensively discussed in Chapter 13, and for exo deviations in Chapter 14. Finishing concepts of training in cases of esophoria and exophoria are discussed in this section as well as vision therapy for hyperphoria and cyclophoria.

Finishing Concepts in Heterophoria

Fusional vergence ranges are expanded with vision training with five basic methods of presenting vergence demands: sliding, stepping, tromboning, jumping, and isometrically bifixating (see Table 9-4). Any or all of these may be necessary for a patient to achieve *adequate* vergence ranges. Better yet, the patient should be given the opportunity for *enhancement* vision therapy so that the vergence skills improve from being just adequate with a score of *3*, to being very strong with a score of *5* (Chapter 2). Moreover, the ideal is for the patient to achieve good vergence ranges *without* suppression, blur, diplopia, diminished stereopsis, fixation disparity, discomfort, infacility, or lack of stamina.

Another concept in the finishing phase of vision therapy is the visualization of a four-dimensional model of binocular vision, i.e., accommodation, vergence, fixation disparity, and time (Chapter 3). The first two dimensions in this model apply to clarity and singleness of binocular vision as in classical graphical analysis. The third dimension of fixation disparity relates to the comfort factor. The fourth dimension of time implies the concept of vision efficiency. Furthermore, vision therapy results need to be lasting. Objective evidence shows that these goals need to be met to prevent regression.[21-23] Also, an important concept in the finishing process is that vergence ranges in both horizontal directions should be very strong. Vision training should optimize the four-dimensional zone of clear, single, comfortable, and efficient binocular vision.

Hyperphoria

Many of the training techniques for eso deviations (Chapter 13) and exo deviations (Chapter 14) can be applied to training in cases of hyperphoria. During chiastopic fusion, for example, Keystone Eccentric Circles (T13.15 and T14.14) can be separated vertically by a slight amount to induce a disparity stimulus for vertical vergence. This procedure is not easy for the patient to do and should be introduced as one of the last training procedures. We have, however, seen several patients increase the vertical vergence by as much as 12^Δ with these procedures.

Vertical Step Vergence T16.24.

Bernell has a series of vertical step Tranaglyphs that introduces disparities in 0.25^Δ increments up to 3^Δ (Figure 16-7). This range can be extended with the use of loose vertical prisms. The patient fuses each of the four targets in turn working to improve speed and accuracy of step vergence while monitoring suppression and stereo perception. To train sliding vergence, we recommend rotating the targets 90 degrees so there is no demand on vertical vergence. When the red and green images are fused, slowly rotate the target to its original position of maximum vertical demand. A very gradual increase in vertical demand can be smoothly made to the maximum limit of fusion. This is possible since red and green filters are used rather than a vectographic system that would not allow for rotation of the target.

Variations on Vertical Vergence Training T16.25

For other targets without built-in vertical disparities, the clinician can use a small base-up or base-down prism (whichever is appropriate for the patient) to create a vertical fusion demand. Again, speed of step vergence is increased. If a loose prism is quickly flipped from base-up to base-down, facility and stamina can be trained. Also, vertical clip-on or Fresnel prisms can be placed on the patient's spectacle lenses as an isometric method. Most standard fixation disparity targets are excellent for training vertical vergences in this manner. As vertical prism demand is increased, suppression and fixation disparity can be evaluated. The ultimate vertical ranges may be quite small, perhaps only several prism diopters; nevertheless, vision training may help the patient cope with a problem caused by hyperphoria.

Improvement of horizontal vergence efficiency usually helps the patient cope with a vertical deviation. (Refer to the case example in Chapter 15 of the patient with a hyperphoria of 52^Δ.) Once the horizontal ranges begin to expand, introduce a vertical demand, e.g., a loose base-down prism along with base-in and base-out demands.

Vertical vergence training has limits, however, and the patient may have to rely on the compensatory effect of a prescribed vertical prism. This is particularly true when the prism neutralizes a vertical fixation disparity, i.e. measuring the associated phoria, as with the Mallett unit. The criterion of clinical wisdom calls for total compensation in hyperphoria (see Table 3-5). When prescribing any prism, the clinician is advised to do the prism confirmation procedure discussed in Chapter 3. Only when a vertical deviation exceeds 10^Δ should extraocular muscle surgery be seriously considered in cases of heterophoria.

Cyclophoria

Much of what was said for functional training for vertical deviations can be said for cyclotorsional deviations since they are usually associated. Prism compensation, however, is not feasible for cyclophoria. Vision training is the best and often the only option. Many targets can be used in this manner. For example, Keystone Eccentric Circles can be rotated during orthopic (T13.15) or chiastopic (T14.14) fusion to stimulate incyclovergence or excyclovergence. The major amblyoscope is the most ideal instrument for this type of training. Torsional amplitudes can be increased for some patients, in our experience, up to 25°. Besides vision training procedures, surgery is the only other method of treatment for these problems. However, it is not advisable in most heterophoric cases. Fortunately, cyclophoric problems are often allevi-

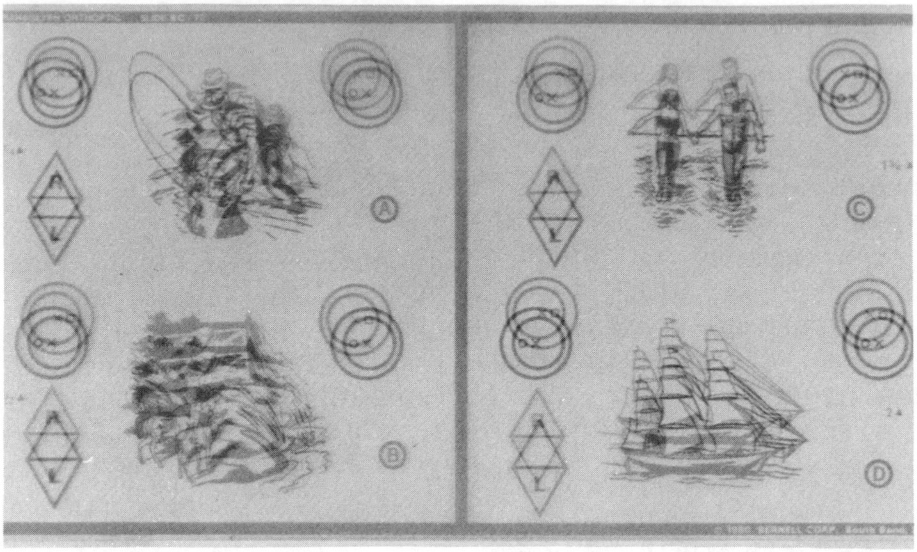

FIGURE 16-7—Vertical Tranaglyph for the training of vertical fusional vergence in cases of hyperphoria.

ated after horizontal and vertical vergences become efficient by means of vision therapy.

Symptomatic Orthophoria

Vergence efficiency therapy is sometimes important for the orthophoric patient. This is particularly true if the fusional vergence range is decreased and vergence facility and stamina are poor. Clinicians may wonder why a patient who is orthophoric at far and near has symptoms pathognomonic of vergence anomalies. Testing with the alternate cover test in conjunction with pencil pushups can sometimes answer this enigmatic question. This testing procedure is called the *kinetic* cover test, as opposed to a regular *static* cover test. An orthophoric patient (found with usual testing procedures) is only orthophoric under static viewing conditions. People, however, live under dynamic viewing conditions and not in a static world. The kinetic cover test reveals how an orthophoric patient will momentarily have an exo deviation as fixation is changed from far to near, and an eso deviation when fixation changes from near to far. An orthophoric patient may have binocular symptoms if there are inadequate vergence ranges (see Figure 3-20). All vergence and accommodative ranges, including facility and stamina, should be expanded with vision training in these cases of a "tight" zone of clear, single, binocular vision.

STEREOPSIS

Stereopsis represents the highest level of binocular vision. There is little doubt in the minds of experienced clinicians that stereoacuity can be improved with vision therapy. Improvement can be due to the successful results of antisuppression training, cure of amblyopia, elimination of ARC, reduction or elimination of fixation disparity, and increased perceptual awareness of binocular depth. Wittenberg[24] reported a study done with the late Dr. Frederick Brock and indicated that "stereoscopic acuity had definitely improved in the trained group." Before a patient is released from a vision therapy program, stereoacuity should be maximally enhanced if it remains deficient.

Vectogram Stereo Enhancement T16.26

A number of Vectograms are beautifully designed for enhancing the patient's sense of stereopsis. The Spirangle is one of our favorite targets for this purpose (see Figure 13-10b). The figure has an overall disparity of 6^Δ at 40 cm. When the central windows are aligned, the peripherally fused window appears to float forward. The first step is for the patient to track along the spiral as quickly as possible from the central window to the peripheral window and back again several times. The suppression controls in the windows should be monitored. The goal is to develop the most vivid sense of depth of the target so that it floats maximally from the plane of the instrument. Continuing to move the eyes, the patient walks away from the target, noting the degree of depth, and then walks toward the target. If a foveal clue ever disappears, the patient immediately breaks the suppression before proceeding, by blinking, flashing, pointing, and increasing the target illumination when feasible. This process continues with varying BO and BI vergence demands. The patient should try to improved his sense of depth at various distances and vergence demands over a 10-minute period. A second step requires the patient to report the subtle depth clues of each letter along the spiral figure. Each letter should be perceived either nearer, farther, or at the plane of the target. This sense of subtle stereopsis is trained by increasing response speed and accuracy, target distance, and vergence demands. A third step would be to project the Spirangle at far on a metallic (or vinyl) screen and repeat the previous steps.

Another effective vectographic technique for enhancing stereopsis utilizes the combination of the Acuity-suppression slide (nonvariable) with the Quoits slides (variable) (see Figures 13-10h and 13-10a). Both Vectograms are placed together in a transparent slide holder held by the therapist. The patient views these targets through polarized filters from a distance of about two meters. Quoits slides are slowly disparated in the BO direction by a slight amount. The patient always bifixates the suppression controls on the nonvariable slide and notes the distance the fused Quoits appears to float forward in space. The stereo percept can be quite dramatic. The therapist continues to introduce BO and BI demands slowly without the Quoits doubling. The patient estimates the maximum distance the image appears to float in both fore and aft directions at a particular distance from the targets. Both the patient and therapist work together to increase the distance the Quoits target appears to float off the plane of the holder. This stereo awareness technique should be tried at various distances from the target holder. For isometric vergence training,

different loose prism demands can be attached to the patient's spectacles.

An interesting variation of the above procedure with Quoits is as follows. Have the patient look through the center of the Quoits while holding them in a clear slide holder. The Vectogram is at arm's length and the patient fixates a Marsden ball 1 or 2 meters away with the ball being seen in the center of the fused Quoits. The therapist next disparates the Quoits about 2^Δ in the base-in direction. This creates an uncrossed disparity on Panum's area when the patient bifixates the ball. The fused Quoits should appear floating away, back to the plane of the Marsden ball with exact disparity conditions. The therapist then swings the ball in a fore and aft direction. The patient should be able to perceive the ball "going through the Quoits" toward him and then see it swing back through them as it travels farther away. This is fascinating to children, as well as adults, as though something magic is happening. The swinging ball is a form of tromboning exercise in this instance. For combining this accommodative training procedure with pursuit training, the ball can be swung in a circular fashion so the patient has to move the handheld Quoits in synchrony with the ball to keep it centered in the Vectogram. Besides tromboning for accommodation and following the ball for pursuits, prism can be worn for vergence training while the patient is experiencing this novel procedure for enhanced awareness of stereopsis.

Computer Stereo Enhancement T16.27

Computer Orthoptics by Cooper utilizes random dot stereograms to generate stereo perception in a game format (T13.16 and T14.20). The stereoscopic target can be seen in only one of four random positions on the screen: up, down, left, and right. The patient indicates its position by rapidly moving a joystick in the appropriate direction. Initially, without BI or BO demand, the patient builds speed of stereo perception. The next step is to change fixation distance by walking away, holding the joystick, and continues the process. Next, the targets are disparated BI and BO within the patient's range of fusional vergence at various speeds. The therapist programs these parameters into the computer. The computer gives an analysis of the "hit rate" for each task so that progress can be charted.

Improved stereoacuity often results when sensory and motor fusion improve with vision therapy. All treatment procedures discussed in the previous chapters should be considered and used as needed. Furthermore, good stereoacuity is an indicator of success in vision therapy for persons with binocular anomalies. Poor stereoacuity (or possibly none) in the strabismic patient can be transformed into good stereoacuity when the strabismus is cured in many, but not all cases. In heterophoria cases, superior stereoacuity represents the touchstone of success when efficient visual skills have been achieved.

CASE EXAMPLES

Case One: Eye Movement Dysfunctions

This is a case of an 18-year-old female presented with the complaints of sharp pain in her left eye and headaches.[25] She had noticed these symptoms for many months. They were consistent in that they would begin after approximately 15 minutes of reading. The symptoms subsided, however, in about 30 minutes after cessation of reading. She also reported skipping lines and losing her place while reading. The patient was a freshman in college with a history of being an excellent reader in the past, but not recently because of her symptoms. She mentioned that she was able to read on a college level when she was in junior high school.

At the first visit further history indicated that the patient had an eye examination 1 year previously. Accommodative rock training was recommended at that time but this was never carried out. She reported that her mother has intermittent exotropia. There was no other remarkable eye or health history in her family.

Subjective refraction was:

OD plano –0.25 x 180   20/15(6/4.5)
OS Plano   20/15 (6/4.5)

The patient had $1/2^\Delta$ exophoria at far and 5^Δ exophoria at near. Base-in to break at 6 m was 5^Δ, recover 3^Δ; base-in to blur at 40 cm was 10^Δ, break 16^Δ, and recover 4^Δ. Base-out to blur at 6 m was 4^Δ, break 9^Δ, and recover 8^Δ; Base-out to blur at 40 cm was 12^Δ, break 18^Δ, and recover 6^Δ. Fusional vergence ranges were considered to be slightly below normal. Her nearpoint of convergence was normal, about 2 cm from the bridge of the nose.

Accommodative amplitude of the right eye was 11.00 D, but was only 8.50 D for the left eye. NRA was +1.75 D, and PRA –5.25 D. Accommodative facility with ±2.00 D was 15 cycles per minute, OD, OS, and binocularly. Accommodative skills were considered fairly normal with the exception of insufficient amplitude of the left eye. The cause of less accommodative amplitude of the left eye could not be explained on any organic basis.

The patient had problems with saccadic eye movements. She scored an equivalent age of 10 years on the Pierce Saccade Test (Chapter 2). Problems with position maintenance and saccadic eye movements could be seen on results of Eye-Trac® testing (Figure 16-8).

To summarize, on the first visit the patient seemed to have a significant problem with saccadic eye movements, possible accommodative insufficiency of the left eye, and reduced fusional vergence ranges. Prescribed home vision therapy consisted of accommodative tromboning, e.g., monocular pencil pushups to work on accommodative amplitude, for 5 minutes a day.

The second visit was approximately 2 months later. Accommodative facility was tested and found to be 21 c/m OD, 19 c/m OS, and 17 c/m binocularly, using ±2.50 D lenses. Base-out to blur on the Vodnoy Aperture-Rule Trainer was 20^Δ. Home training was prescribed as follows: (1) Monocular pencil pushups, each eye, 5 minutes a day; (2) binocular pencil pushups, 5 minutes a day; (3) accommodative rock using ±2.50 D, OD, OS, and binocularly, 5 minutes a day; and (4) Landolt C charts for identification of the direction of open portion of C's and star-like charts for saccadic eye movement training, for 5 minutes a day (Figure 16-9).

The third visit was 1 week later, and the patient reported doing her home training faithfully, with no problems doing the tasks except for occasionally having trouble seeing clearly with the plus lenses during accommodative rock. She was able to converge more than 33$^\Delta$ with clear single vision on the Aperture-Rule Trainer, and she could diverge 16$^\Delta$ with clear single vision with Vectograms. Saccadic eye movements were normal on the Pierce Saccade Test. Prescribed home training consisted of the following: (1) Keystone Eccentric Circles combined with farpoint Hart chart for 5 minutes a day; this was for chiastopic fusion at near with jump vergences to the Hart chart for saccadic training; (2) Michigan tracking for saccadic training, for 5 minutes a day; (3) Circling vowels in newspaper print along with "dive bombing" them with a pencil from above, i.e., fast pointing.

The patient reported on the fourth visit that she noticed better performance during home training. Office training included saccadic and fusional vergence training. She was able to fuse with clearness and singleness on the Aperture-Rule Trainer over 30$^\Delta$ base-out and 22$^\Delta$ base-in. The patient showed excellent compliance with home and office training and had high motivation. Home training was prescribed as follows: (1) Orthopic and chiastopic fusion for vergence rock in free space, 5 minutes a day; the purpose of this was to improve vergence ranges and facility. (2) The first procedure was combined with shifts of fixation to a farpoint Hart Chart, 5 minutes a day. (3) Combination of the first procedure with Landolt C and star-like charts, 5 minutes a day. (4) Michigan tracking activities, 5 minutes a day.

The fifth visit was 3 weeks later. Using the SOAP (subjective, objective, analysis, plan) format the results on this progress evaluation visit were:

S. There were no subjective complaints. The patient was doing a great deal of reading in college and was not experiencing any headaches or pain in the eye. She reported "noticing a greatly increased reading speed."

O. Phorometry indicated orthophoria at far and 5$^\Delta$ exophoria at near. Base-in at far

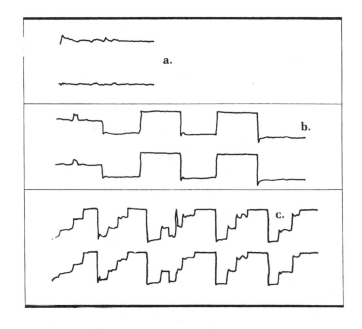

FIGURE 16-8—Eye movement testing results *before* vision therapy: (a) Position maintenance; (b) gross saccades; and (c) fine saccades, on card with 5 dots per row (Figure 2-3).

was X/5/4, and 20/24/18 at near. Base-out at far was 14/24/12 and 18/24/18 at near. Accommodative amplitude was 11.00 D, OD and 11.00 D, OS. Keystone Eccentric Circles, 55$^\Delta$ BO chiastopic and 37$^\Delta$ BI orthopic fusion. The Eye-Trac showed improvement in fixation and eye movements with fewer regressions during saccades, and better return sweeps (Figure 16-10).

A. All subjective and objective problems were abated.

P. The patient was dismissed for 6 months and put on a maintenance program with the following home vision training prescribed: pencil pushups, monocular and binocular, 5 minutes a week; binocular pencil saccades (two pencils), 5 minutes a week; and Keystone Eccentric Circles for orthopic-chiastopic vergence rock with fixation shifts to a farpoint Hart chart, 5 minutes a week. The patient was advised to have a progress evaluation in 6 months.

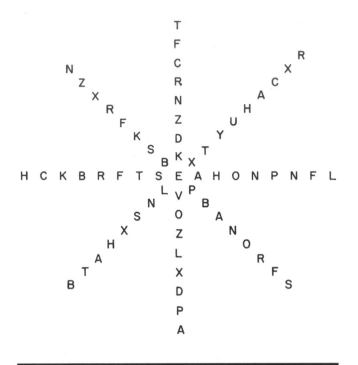

FIGURE 16-9—Example of starlike configuration of rows of letters for saccadic training (also useful as a target for near-far-near accommodative and other vision training).

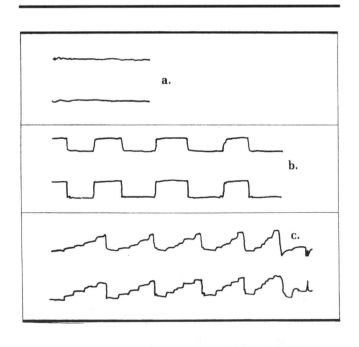

FIGURE 16-10—Eye movement testing results *after* vision therapy: (a) Position maintenance; (b) gross saccades; and (c) fine saccades.

Case Two: Accommodative Dysfunctions

This is a case report of a patient with accommodative insufficiency and infacility.[26] A 30-year-old female college student presented with frequent headaches and burning of the eyes after an hour of concentrated reading. She would sometimes become dizzy when shifting focus abruptly from the chalkboard to her notebook. Onset of symptoms coincided with entrance into college 6 months previously. Her history was unremarkable and the patient had never worn any spectacle or contact lenses.

There was no significant refractive error, and unaided visual acuities were 20/15 (6/4.5) each eye. The patient had 1^Δ exophoria at far and 5^Δ exophoria at near. Fusional convergence at far was slightly restricted, 4/12/10. The nearpoint of convergence was normal, 7 cm. Monocular accommodative amplitude, however, was markedly reduced for her age, 6 diopters. Also, accommodative facility using ±1.50 D lens flippers was only 2 cycles in a period of 90 seconds.

A home vision training program of 20 minutes a day was initiated to build accommodative facility, working on speed, accuracy, and sustaining ability. Vision training prescribed included pencil pushups, jump vergences, accommodative lens rock with flippers, Brock string and beads, and monocular jump focusing. The patient used home instruction sheets for each of the above and faithfully followed the program for 5 weeks. She returned once a week for a progress check. The patient's accommodative amplitude and facility improved quickly to almost normal levels after only 2 weeks of training. By week 3 the lens flipper rate was 25 cycles in 90 seconds (Figure 16-11). Reduction of symptoms paralleled the increase in skills. Headaches, dizziness, and asthenopia with reading decreased noticeably after week 2 of training; they were completely eliminated by the fifth week.

Patients with accommodative insufficiency and infacility often respond quickly and dramatically to a short term vision training program. If not, then other possible causes should be reinvestigated. Prescribing plus-add reading lenses also often helps to relieve symptoms.

FUTURE DIRECTIONS IN BINOCULAR VISION THERAPY

Binocular anomalies, particularly heterophoria and vision efficiency dysfunctions, can cause visual discomfort and inefficiency at school, work, and play. In the past two decades, we have seen a rising number of heterophoric and vision efficiency patients needing and wanting vision therapy. Although the prevalence of strabismus and amblyopia will probably remain constant, at least in the foreseeable future, we believe there will be an ever-increasing demand for binocular vision therapy services. At least three cultural movements provide the impetus: (1) a movement toward lifelong education, (2) the emergence of "high tech" industries as the basis of modern economies, and (3) a movement toward universal physical fitness with increasing participation in sports.

One recurring theme in this text has been the relation between binocular vision symptoms and reading problems. In their investigation of this issue, Grisham et al.[27] reported that poor readers (defined by standardized testing) generally experience more visual symptoms than good readers. They also found a low but significant correlation between reading achievement and the number of visual symptoms reported during the act of reading; this is a surprising result since reading achievement is influenced by many factors, e.g., I.Q. There is, however, a preponderance of evidence in the literature that shows that heterophoric, fusional vergence, and accommodative problems occur more frequently among poor readers compared with peers who read normally.[27,28,29] There is one particularly interesting ophthalmological report regarding improvement in reading performance following vision training. This clinical series, by Haddad et al.,[30] consisted of 73 children referred for vision examinations because of reading difficulties. Fifty-eight percent of the total group were considered to have "dyslexia" since they complained of excessive reversal confusion on letters and small words. This is not a rigorous definition of dyslexia, in our opinion, and more formal testing[31] is recommended for future investigations regarding dyslexia. Never-

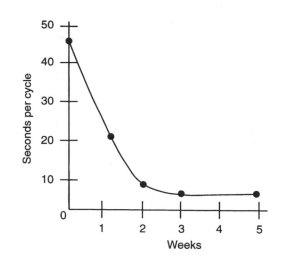

FIGURE 16-11—Graphical representation showing improvement in accommodative facility with vision training.

theless, more than half of the "dyslexic" children had deficient fusional amplitudes by clinical testing. A vision training program designed to increase fusional vergences, improve the nearpoint of convergence, and break suppression was initiated in cases of fusional deficiency. Improvements in attention and reading performance (length of time of uninterrupted reading) were reported following resolution of the fusional deficiency in both the "dyslexic" and "nondyslexic" children. These authors concluded that the vision training did not cure the "dyslexic" students' perceptual problems but did improve their reading performance.

We frequently see students who suddenly have reading improvement following a vision therapy program for inefficient visual skills. We believe these clinical observations will eventually be confirmed by formal, properly controlled, clinical trials. Then, students of all ages will likely be referred for evaluation of vision efficiency skills when reading performance does not meet the expectations of parents and teachers. As the visual demands associated with lifelong education increase, we anticipate a commensurate increase in the number of patients needing and wanting vision therapy.

Many "high tech" industries place intense visual demands on their workers. Quality control of microchips, for example, requires workers to develop new levels of visual skills, c.g., increased attention and critical viewing for long periods of time. Microcomputers are now found on most office desks and in an increasing number of homes. Accompanying these technological advances are some undesirable problems, one of which is visual asthenopia in the work place. Certain aspects of work performance, particularly those utilizing depth perception, are facilitated by normal binocular vision.[32] On the other hand, more than half of the computer-related complaints of eye-care patients stem from deficiencies in accommodation and convergence.[2] The need for high quality binocular skills is evident in these visual environments. Nearpoint lenses for computer use, and often vision training, usually resolve patient complaints. It seems realistic to say that the joint influences of "high tech" industries and the drive toward universal usage of computers will continue to generate increasing demands for binocular vision services. This technological revolution has inspired the collaboration of vision scientists and optometric practitioners to solve new problems regarding visual comfort and efficiency. Many optometry schools and private practices offer some form of video display terminal assessment, and vision therapy and the need is growing.

Binocular vision therapy is an integral part of the emerging specialty of sports vision. Several binocular vision skills have been reported to be superior in athletes, particularly players of ball games: these include speed and accuracy of ocular motility,[33] farpoint vergence facility,[34] static depth perception,[35,36] and dynamic stereopsis.[37] Studies have shown that all these skills can be trained to higher levels of performance.[38] Most outstanding athletes do not have significant visual dysfunctions, but when an athlete does have them, doctors render care with the hope that athletic performance will improve.

Clinical application in sports vision also goes beyond the classical concept of vision therapy, i.e., from remediation to visual enhancement. A growing number of optometrists provide enhancement programs in vision therapy. They train amateur and professional athletes having normal binocular vision and perceptual-motor skills and help them attain superior levels with the intent that this training will facilitate increased on-the-field sports performance. The glamour aside, this new direction does indeed have a serious basis—that of helping individuals overcome their limitations and achieve their dreams. Controlled studies of vision training and athletic skills are needed to confirm the hopes of many fledgling athletes and of sports vision doctors.

Visual rehabilitation fits comfortably within the primary-health-care model of practice. Rehabilitation has been a part of traditional health care from its inception. The concept of prevention was later emphasized. Modern health-care management, however, promotes the concept of enhanced performance in school, work, and play. This evolution also applies to vision therapy.

The ultimate goal for any patient being treated for binocular anomalies, is the achievement of clear, single, comfortable, and efficient binocular vision. This simple statement represents an evolving model of vision care that continues to change. Practitioners in the 19th century were concerned almost exclusively with clarity of eyesight. They prescribed spectacle lenses to correct blurred vision. Clear and single binocular vision became the issue with the advent of orthoptics. Effective therapeutic regimens for strabismus were introduced by Javal, Worth, and Maddox. Astute clinicians in the first half of the 20th century became aware of the relation between accommodation and convergence. Knowledge of the zone of clear, single, comfortable, binocular vision was gained through various models of vision, such as graphical analysis and fixation disparity. As a result, practitioners (Brock and many others) extended vision training to the treatment of nonstrabismic binocular anomalies. There has been an increasing emphasis on efficiency of vision in the latter half of the 20th century. There is growing awareness that efficient (i.e., accurate, sustained, and integrated) visual skills are related to good scholastic progress, to occupational production, and to achievement in sports.

The model of vision care and clinical practice continues to change. More and more doctors of optometry consider themselves primary eye care providers, and most optometry schools embrace this perspective. "Primary eye care" is a metaphor signifying, in part, the taking of responsibility as a full member of the health care team. Optometrists are taking responsibility for the diagnosis and management of eye disease and injury within the limits of law and standards of practice. It is time to make explicit another concept in our approach to binocular vision therapy that has always been implicit; this is oculomotor and binocular vision *health* management. Optometrists are dedicated to meeting all vision care needs of their patients. Within this context, they help their patients achieve clear, single, comfortable, and efficient binocular vision.

REFERENCES

1. Grisham D, Simons H. Perspectives on reading disabilities. In: Rosenbloom AA, Morgan MW, eds. *Pediatric Optometry*. Philadelphia: Lippincott; 1990: 518-559.
2. Sheedy JE, Parsons SD. The video display terminal eye clinic: Clinical report. *Optom Vision Sci.* 1990;67: 622-626.
3. Mets M, Price RL. Contact lenses in the management of myopic anisometropic amblyopia. *Am J Ophthalmol.* 1981;91:484-489.
4. Bannon RE. *Clinical Manual on Aniseikonia*. Buffalo, NY: American Optical Co; 1976.
5. Ogle, KN. *Researchs in Binocular Vision*. Philadelphia: WB Saunders Co; 1950:264.
6. Polasky M. *Aniseikonia Cookbook*. Columbus, Ohio: The Ohio State University School of Optometry; 1974.
7. Ryan VI. Predicting aniseikonia in anisometropia. *Am J Optom.* 1975;52:96-105.
8. Kleinstein RN. Iseikonic trial lenses: an aid to diagnosing aniseikonia. *Optom Monthly.* 1978;69:132-137.
9. Koetting RA. Stereopsis in presbyopes fitted with single vision contact lenses. *Am J Optom Arch Am Acad Optom.* 1970;47:557-561.
10. Emmes AB. A statistical study of clinical scores obtained in the Wirt stereopsis test. *Am J Optom Arch Am Acad Optom.* 1961;38:298-400.
11. Sheedy JE, Harris MG, Busby L, et al. Monovision contact lens wear and occupational task performance. *Am J Optom Physiol Opt.* 1988;65:14-18.
12. Josephson JE, Erickson P, Back A, et al. Monovision. *J Am Optom Assoc.* 1990;61:820-826.
13. Schor C, Carson M, et al. Effects of interocular blur suppression ability on monovision tasks performance. *J Am Optom Assoc.* 1989;60:188-192.
14. Josephson JE, Caffery BE. Monovision vs. bifocal contact lenses. A crossover study. *J Am Optom Assoc.* 1987;58:652-654.
15. Lebow KA, Goldberg JB. Characteristics of binocular vision found for presbyopic patients wearing single vision contact lenses. *J Am Optom Assoc.* 1975;46: 1116-1123.
16. Bahill, AT, Adler D, Stark L. Most naturally occurring human saccades have magnitudes of 15 degrees or less. *Invest Ophthalmol.* 1975;14:468-469.
17. Griffin JR. Pursuit fixations: an overview of training procedures. *Optom Weekly.* 1976:534-537.
18. Keller JT, Amos JF. Low plus lenses and visual performance: a critical review. *J Am Optom Assoc.* 1979; 50:1005-1011.
19. Greenspan SB. Behavioral effects of children's near-point lenses. *J Am Optom Assoc.* 1975;46: 1031-1036.
20. Pierce JR. A response to low plus lenses and visual performance: a critical review. *J Am Optom Assoc.* 1980;51:453-459.
21. Grisham JD, Bowman MC, Owyang LA, Chan CL. Vergence orthoptics: validity and persistence of the training effect. *Optom Vision Sci.* 1991;68: 441-451.
22. Patano F. Orthoptic treatment of convergence insufficiency: a two-year follow-up report. *Am Orthopt J.* 1982;32:73-80.
23. Griffin JR, Bui K, Ko C. *Durability of vision therapy*. M.B. Ketchum Library, Southern California College of Optometry, Fullerton; 1991.
24. Wittenberg S. Brock's research in stereopsis. *Am J Optom.* 1981;58:663-666.
25. Camuccio D, Griffin JR. Visual skills therapy: a case report. *Optom Monthly.* 1982;73:94-96.
26. Grisham JD. A short program for accommodative insufficiency. *Rev Optom.* 1978;115:35.
27. Grisham JD, Sheppard MM, Tran WU. Visual symptoms and reading performance. *Optom Vis Sci.* 1993;70:384-391.
28. Flax N. The contribution of visual problems to learning disability. *J Am Optom Assoc.* 1970;41:841-845.
29. Simons HD, Gassler PA. Vision anomalies and reading skill: A meta-analysis of the literature. *Am J Optom Physiol Opt.* 1988;65:893.
30. Haddad HM, Isaacs NS, Onghena K, Mazor A. The use of orthoptics in dyslexia. *J Learn Disabil.* 1984;17: 142-144.
31. Griffin JR. Office testing for dyslexia. *Current Opinion in Ophthalmol.* 1992;3:35-9.
32. Sheedy JE, Bailey IL, Muri M., Bass F. Binocular vs. monocular task performance, *Amer J Optom Physiol Opt.* 1986; 63;10:839-846.
33. Trachtman JN. The relationship between ocular motilities and batting averages in little leaguers. *Am J Optom Arch Acad Optom.* 1973;50:914-919.
34. Christenson GN, Winkelstein AM. Visual skills of athletes versus non-athletes: development of sports vision battery. *J Am Optom Assoc.* 1988;59:666-675.
35. Melcher MH, Lund DR. Sports vision and the high school student athlete. *J Am Optom Assoc.* 1992;63: 466-474.
36. Ridini LM. Relationship between psychological functions tests and selected sports skills of boys in junior high school. *Res Q Am Health Phy Ed.* 1968;39:674-683.
37. Solomon H, Zinn WJ, Vacroux A. Dynamic stereoacuity: A test for hitting a baseball? *J Am Optom Assoc.* 1988;59:522-526.
38. Stein CD, Arterburn MR, Stern NS. Vision and sports: a review of the literature. *J Am Optom Assoc.* 1982;53:627-633.

APPENDIXES

APPENDIX A

Conversions of Prism Diopters and Degrees

Prism diopters	Degrees	Degrees	Prism diopters
1	0° 34'	1	1.75
2	1° 9'	2	3.49
3	1° 43'	3	5.24
4	2° 17'	4	6.99
5	2° 51'	5	8.75
6	3° 26'	6	10.51
7	4° 0'	7	12.29
8	4° 34'	8	14.05
9	5° 9'	9	15.84
10	5° 43'	10	17.63
15	8° 32'	15	26.80
20	11° 19'	20	36.40

APPENDIX B

Visual Acuity and Visual Efficiency

Snellen Acuity	Angle of Resolution	Visual Efficiency in Percent	Percentage Loss of Vision
20/20 (6/6)	1.0'	100.0	0
20/25 (6/7.5)	1.25'	95.6	4.4
20/30 (6/9)	1.50'	91.4	8.6
20/40 (6/12)	2'	83.6	16.4
20/50 (6/15)	2.5'	76.5	23.5
20/60 (6/18)	3'	69.9	30.1
20/70 (6/21)	3.5'	63.8	36.2
20/80 (6/24)	4'	58.5	41.5
20/100 (6/30)	5'	48.9	51.1
20/200 (6/60)	10'	20.0	80.0
20/300 (6/90)	15'	8.2	91.8
20/400 (6/120)	20'	3.3	96.7
20/800 (6/240)	40'	0.1	99.9

APPENDIX C

Stereoacuity Calculations

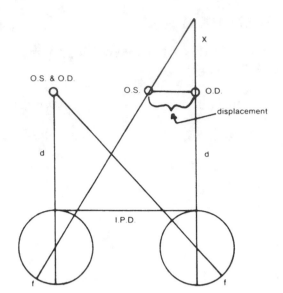

To determine the stereoacuity when lateral displacement is known, first this must be expressed in terms of a theoretical value that represents the apparent linear displacement. This is the x value in the formula:

$$\text{Eta} = \frac{\text{I.P.D. } (x)}{d^2} (206{,}000).$$

Assume, for instance, the eyes are bifixating a circle by means of polarization. Another target (such as the disparate circles in the Wirt rings test) is designed so that each can be seen by only one eye. Assume: The lateral displacement is 1mm for this particular stereoscopic test, the I.P.D. is 60 mm, and the testing distance (d) is 40 cm (400 mm). Find x from the formula:

$$\frac{x}{\text{displacement}} = \frac{x + d}{\text{I.P.D}}$$

$$\frac{x}{1} = \frac{x + 400}{60}$$

$$59x = 400$$

$$x = 6.78 \text{ mm}$$

Now substituting into the linear formula for stereoacuity,

$$\text{Eta} = \frac{60 \, (6.78)}{(400)^2} (206{,}000)$$

$$\text{Eta} = 524 \text{ seconds of arc}$$

APPENDIX D

Visual Skills Efficiency Evaluation (Testing Outline)

Visual Skills Efficiency Evaluation (Testing Outline)   Date: _____

Patient _____   Age ____   Reason for Exam _____

  1. VISUAL ACUITY: @Farpoint   @Nearpoint
      Lenses Worn   VA $\overline{SC}$ $\vee$ OD $\overline{SC}$ $\vee$ OD
      OD   OS   OS
      OS $\overline{CC}$ $\vee$ OD
                                                                   OS

      Refractive data: OD   Comments
                            OS
  2. SACCADIC EYE MOVEMENTS:
      Results:
  3. PURSUIT EYE MOVEMENTS:
      Results:
  4. ACCOMMODATION: e.g., Insufficiency, excess, infacility, ill-sustained
      Testing Results
  5. VERGENCES:
      Ranges: Far BI   Far BO   Near BI   Near BO
      Facility:
      Stamina:
      Phoria/tropia data:
      Nearpoint of Convergence (in centimeters)
        Results: (one trial and after 5 trials):
      Fixation Disparity
        Results.
  6. SENSORY FUSION (ortho demand) @ Farpoint and @ Nearpoint
      Flat Fusion $\overline{s}$ suppression:
      Stereoacuity (specify tests used):
  7. OTHER SENSORY-MOTOR FUSION RANGES: e.g., $\overline{s}$ suppression, $\overline{s}$ loss of stereoacuity,
        $\overline{s}$ fixation disparity, $\overline{s}$ discomfort
      Results:
  8. DIAGNOSIS:
  9. PROGNOSIS:
 10. RECOMMENDATIONS AND ADVICE GIVEN:

APPENDIX E

Strabismus Examination Record

Name		Examiner	Date
Address		Recorder	Birth
City	Phone	Referred by	Report Rec'd

HISTORY

What is the main vision problem?

Has there ever been an eye-turn?   Is there now?   Age when first noticed?

How often and under what conditions does the eye turn?   Have you ever seen a single object as two?

To what extent is the eye-turn apparent to others?   Do you have a relative with an eye-turn?

Any previous treatment?   Glasses?   Patching?   Excercises?   Surgery?

        Ages?

        Type?

        Results?

Other pertinent history?

AMETROPIA AND GLASSES

a. Latest retinoscopy	RE	LE	Date	By
b. Latest subjective	RE	LE	Date	By
c. Present glasses (major lens)	RE	LE	Date	By
d. Other (Eg. add)	RE	LE	Date	By

ACUITY

Rx a b c d (circle one)	RE	LE	Method
Rx a b c d (circle one)	RE	LE	Method

CONFRONTATION

Angle kappa and steadiness	RE	LE	Suggests
Hirschberg, primary gaze, Rx _____	RE	LE	Suggests

Hirschberg, cardinal fields:

Observations and remarks: epicanthus, facial asymmetries, ptosis, torticollis, etc.

NPC conv. (cm):   IPD:

OBJECTIVE COVER TEST

Rx _____ at ___ M.

UNILATERAL Cover RE, LE moves:

Cover LE, RE moves:

ALTERNATE RE fixating:

LE fixating:

(UNILATERAL NEUTRALIZATION):

(LOOSE PRISM TEST):

[AC/A = _____ Δ/1.00 D]

ADDITIONAL TEST RESULTS

Comitance	Monocular Fixation and Amblyopia
Retinal Correspondence (without bifixation)	Sensory and Motor Fusion, and Suppression
Other Results	

DIAGNOSIS

Oculomotor Deviation with following Rx: RE   LE

At ___ M: Magnitude Direction	At ___ M: Magnitude Direction
Laterality Freq of Strabismus	Laterality Freq of Strabismus
Comitance	

ASSOCIATED CONDITIONS

Monocular Fixation	Amblyopia
Retinal Correspondence	Suppression
Fusion	Ametropia
Other Relevant Conditions	

IMPRESSIONS AND RECOMMENDATIONS

Impressions (including frequency of squint, cosmesis, and prognosis)
Recommendations

Instructor's Signature

Modified from form used at the School of Optometry, University of California, Berkeley 94720.

APPENDIX F

Suppliers and Equipment (partial list)

Allbee Optometric Printers
224 West Park Avenue
P.O. Box 177
Waterloo, IA 50704
  3-dot card
  Root Rings

Ann Arbor Publications
P.O. Box 7249
Naples, FL 33940
  Michigan Tracking

Bernell Corporation
750 Lincolnway East
P.O. Box 4637
South Bend, IN 46634
  Bernell Computer Software for Vision
    Skills, computerized vision training
  Dual Polachrome Illuminated Trainer,
    Vectograms® and Tranaglyphs
  Television Trainer
  Aperture-Rule Trainer
  Mirror Stereoscope (Wheatstone)
  Flippers, prisms, and lenses
  Accommodative Rock Cards (Terranova)
  Hart Charts
  Macula Integrity Tester (MIT)
  Single Oblique Stereoscope
  Rotation Trainer
  Test Lantern for Fixation Disparity
  King-Devick Test
  Developmental Eye Movement Test (DEM)
  Broken Wheel Test (visual acuity)
  Prisms
  OKN Prism
  Flipper Trial lens/prism holder
  Striated (Bagolini) lenses
  Other equipment for binocular testing and
    training

Clement Clarke, Inc.
3128 East 17th Avenue, Suite D
Columbus, OH 43219
  Synoptophone, and Slides

Efficient Seeing Publications
7510 Soquel Drive, Box 28
Aptos, CA 95003
  Alphabet Pencils

Fresnel Prisms and Lens Co.
Route 1, Box 298-3
Siren, WI 54872
  Fresnel Prisms and Lenses

GTVT
18807 10th Place West
Lynwood, WA 98036
  Filtered Strips for bar reading

Keystone View
Division of Mast/Keystone, Inc.
4673 Aircenter Circle
Reno, NV 89502
  Eccentric circles (opaque and transparent)
  "Lifesaver" Colored Circles (opaque and
    transparent)
  Sherman TV Trainer for Amblyopia and
    Strabismus
  Telebinocular and other Brewster stereo-
    scopes
  VT Playing Cards

Learning Frontiers, Inc.
190 Admiral Cochran Drive, #180
Annapolis, MD 21401
  The Optimum System (Ludlam), computer-
    ized vision training

Light House Low Vision Services
New York Association for the Blind
111 East 59th Street
New York, NY 10022
  Light House Charts

Manico/Bloomington
418 East 17th Street, Suite 2
Bloomington, IN 47408
  Rotating Pegboard Trainer
  Translid Binocular Interactor (TBI)

Midwest Vision Therapy Equipment
  Company, Inc.
P.O. Box 949
Ciceno, IN 46034
  Accommodative Flippers
  Anti-Suppression Bar Reader
  Near-Far Accommodation Charts
  Polarized Glasses
  Variable and Non-variable
    Vectograms

Ocular Instruments Co.
c/o Dr. Benjamin Nehenberg
P.O. Box 1781
Los Gatos, CA 95031

Halberg Clips
Mallett Unit
Near Fixation Targets

OEP Foundation Inc.
1921 E. Carnegie Ave., Suite 3-L
Santa Ana, CA 92705
  Wayne Computerized Saccadic Fixator
  Wayne Afterimage Strobe Flasher
  The Talking Pen
  Ann Arbor Tracking ("Michigan Tracking")
  Super Stereoacuity Timed Tester
  Wesson Fixation Disparity Card
  Rotation Pegboard Machine

Optical Technology Corporation
515 East 22nd Terrace
Lawrence, KS 66046
  Infant Vision Tester (Preferential looking
    instrument)

Performance Enterprises
88 Liebeck Crescent
Unionville, Ontario L3R 1Y5
CANADA
  Dyna Vision 2000

Dr. John R. Pierce
University of Alabama
School of Optometry
Birmingham, AL 35294
  MEM
  Pierce Saccade Test

School of Optometry
University of California
Berkeley, CA 94720
  Bailey-Hall Cereal Test, c/o Center for the
    Study of Visual Impairment
  Bailey-Lovie Chart, c/o Center for the
    Study of Visual Impairment
  Tumbling E's, c/o Optometry Alumni
    Association

Stereo Optical Co., Inc.
3539 N. Kenton Avenue
Chicago, IL 60641
  Various polarizing tests for stereopsis

Taylor Associates
200-2 E. 2nd Street
Huntington Station
New York, NY 11746
  Ober 2: Visagraph, Eye-Movement
    Recording System

Teletherapy, Inc.
P.O. Box 50935
Indianapolis, IN 46256
  Computer Orthoptics (Cooper),
    Computerized Vision Training

Vision Analysis
136 Hillcroft Way
Walnut Creek, CA 94596
  Disparometer (Sheedy)

Wayne Engineering
1825 Willow Road
Northfield, IL 60093
  Perceptuomotor Pen (Talking Pen)
  Saccadic Fixator
  Wayne Afterimage Strobe Flasher

Dr. Michael Wesson
University of Alabama
School of Optometry
Medical Center
Birmingham, AL 35294
  Wesson Card (Fixation disparity and other
    tests)
  Wesson Psychomotor Chart (S-chart for vis-
    ual acuity)

GLOSSARY

This glossary is intended to provide brief definitions of terms and to clarify some of the abbreviations used in this text.

Abduction Outward horizontal movement of the eye.

Abnormal fixation Fixation in which the fovea is not used and/or the fixation is unsteady.

AC/A The accommodative-convergence to accommodation ratio.

Adduction Inward horizontal movement of the eye.

AI Afterimage.

Alpha rhythm Intermittent photic stimulation of 7 to 10 cycles per second.

Angle A (angle of anomaly) In the deviating eye this is represented by the distance from point "a" to the center of the fovea.

Angle E (angle of eccentric fixation) Magnitude of the angle of eccentric fixation, which is represented by the distance on the retina from point "e" to the center of the fovea.

Angle eta Designation for stereoacuity.

Angle F Angle of fixation disparity.

Angle H Horizontal angle of deviation of the visual axes measured by objective testing methods.

Angle K (angle kappa) Angle subtended by the visual axis and the pupillary axis at the nodal point; see angle lambda.

Angle lambda Angle subtended at the center of the entrance pupil of the eye by the intersection of the pupillary axis and the visual axis; this angle is inappropriately referred to as "angle kappa" in clinical testing; angle kappa testing actually determines angle lambda, not angle kappa.

Angle S Subjective angle of directionalization; it should be the same as angle H if there is NRC, but different if there is ARC.

ARC (anomalous retinal correspondence) Condition in which the two foveas do not correspond (theoretically more correctly referred to as "anomalous correspondence," since correspondence is cortical rather than retinal).

Associated phoria This is determined by the amount of compensatory prism needed to reduce angle F to zero.

Attenuation A form of occlusion in which the transmission of light is altered by means of certain filters and/or lenses (sometimes referred to as graded occlusion).

Bifixation Implication of central fusion in which the center of the fovea of each eye participates in viewing a fixated object.

Bifoveal test of Cüppers (maculo-macular test) Estimate of angle A by means of visuoscopy when the patient is seeing under binocular conditions.

Concomitancy Condition in which the measurement of the angle of deviation is approximately the same magnitude in all positions of gaze. Clinically most often referred to as "comitancy."

Contracture Inability of an extraocular muscle to relax, which may result in permanent structural changes with the inelasticity becoming irreversible.

Covariation Intermittency of ARC and NRC in the case of intermittent strabismus, particularly in exotropia.

DAF (diagnostic action field) Six positions of gaze used to evaluate the action of the six extraocular muscles of each eye.

Eccentric fixation Fixation (designated by point "e") not employing the center of the fovea; it may vary in magnitude and/or direction from moment to moment or day to day and may be relatively steady or unsteady.

ET Esotropia at far.

ET' Esotropia at near.

First-degree fusion Term used interchangeably with "superimposition."

Fixation disparity A slight error of vergence in cases of heterophoria; the limit of the magnitude of the angle of fixation disparity (angle F) is considered to be less than 30 minutes of arc.

Free space Patient is directly viewing a fixation object that is not housed inside an instrument, such as a stereoscope, or that is not viewed through any optical system in which the apparent position of the object is not being altered (see true space). Also clinically referred to as "open environment."

Functional amblyopia Central visual acuity reduction that is not attributable to pathological causes but to functional causes (e.g., refractive, strabismic, and hysterical).

Functional cure Criteria used in strabismus are: single, clear, comfortable, binocular vision at all distances from the far-point to a normal NPC with normal stereoacuity and with no central suppression. The criterion of *efficiency* may also be included.

HB (Haidinger's brushes) Entoptic phenomenon used to tag the projected location of the center of the macula.

Heterophoria A latent deviation of the visual axes from the ortho position that requires vergence for bifixation to be maintained; (the direction of the deviation may be horizontal, vertical, or torsional).

IPD Abbreviation for interpupillary distance; clinically, but inappropriately, referred to as the pupillary distance (P.D.).

KCT (kinetic cover test) A test for estimating angle H by means of a moving fixation target and alternate occlusion.

Maddox cross A graduated vertical and horizontal ruler in the form of a cross with a light source placed at the intersection for the purpose of subjectively measuring vertical and horizontal angles of directionalization; also called "Maddox scale."

Mental effort An attempt by the patient to make vergence movements by imaging fixation above or below the horizon or the use of other willful means to produce voluntary vergence, or control other visual functions.

MITT Macula Integrity Tester-Trainer of Bernell (instrument used to produce the entoptic phenomena of Haidinger's brushes). Also called *MIT*.

M.S. (Maxwell's spot) Entoptic phenomena used to tag the projected location of the center of the macula.

Negative fusional vergence The ability to diverge the visual axes behind the object of regard without blurring (this is stimulated by base-in prism).

Nonvariable eccentric fixation A condition in which point "e" has a fixed site, although fixation may be unsteady as to the point used for fixation.

NPC (nearpoint of convergence) Single vision with bifixation, but not necessarily clear vision, normally expected to be about 3 cm from the bridge of the nose as an ideal

Organic amblyopia Central visual acuity loss, attributable to pathological causes that are not obvious by means of ophthalmoscopy.

Partial occlusion Less than the full visual field of an eye is occluded.

Past pointing The demonstration of faulty eye-hand localization ability by inaccurately pointing to one side or the other of a fixated object (commonly found in cases of amblyopia with eccentric fixation and in cases of extraocular muscle paresis of recent onset).

PAT (prism adaptation test) A prognostic test in cases of esotropia to determine if base-out prism causes angle H to increase.

Pathological diplopia Perception of a doubled image of a fixated target.

Physiological diplopia Perception of a doubled image of a nonfixated target.

Point "a" The place on the retina of the deviating eye corresponding to the fovea of the nondeviating eye.

Point "e" The time-averaged point used for fixation under monocular conditions in eccentric fixation.

Point "f" The center of the fovea of an eye.

Positive fusional vergence The ability to converge the visual axes in front of the object of regard without blurring (stimulated by base-out prism).

Secondary angle of deviation The measured angle of deviation found with the paretic eye fixating.

Second-degree fusion Term used interchangeably with "flat fusion."

Steady fixation The condition determined on visuoscopy in which the point on the retina used for fixation (either "f" or "e") appears relatively stationary as the patient fixates the nonmoving target of a visuoscopic instrument.

TBI Translid Binocular Interaction Trainer.

Third-degree fusion Term used interchangeably with "stereopsis" and in reference to stereoacuity.

True space Viewing conditions in which the patient is directly looking at a fixation object without intervening optics that cause reflection or refraction; in clinical usage, filters may be used (e.g., polarizing) with this definition being satisfied; see free space.

Unsteady fixation In central fixation, point "f" appears on visuoscopy to be moving rapidly in a nystagmoid manner around and about the center of the star; in eccentric fixation, this rapid movement would be seen around and about point "e" during visuoscopy.

Variable eccentric fixation The condition in which the time-averaged point "e" changes site from one measurement to the next on visuoscopy, although fixation may be relatively steady at any particular moment; also called "wandering eccentric fixation."

VER (visual evoked response or visually evoked response) The same as VECP (visually evoked cortical potential) or VEP (visually evoked potential).

Vergence Disjunctive movement of the eyes.

Version Conjugate movement of the eyes.

Visual axis The line of sight that extends from the fixated target through the nodal point to the center of the fovea.

XT Exotropia at far.

XT' Exotropia at near.

Zero point The point on the retina of the strabismic eye representing no vergence demand. When there is bifixation, point "zero" is at point "f," the center of the fovea.

INDEX

A

A and V patterns, 224–226
  characteristics, 224–225
  etiology of, 224–225
  management, 225–226
Abduction nystagmus, 245
Aberrant regeneration, 236–237
Abnormal head posture, 116–117, 234, 448
Abraham, S.V., 201
Absolute accommodation, 35–36
  testing, 43–44
Absolute convergence
  developmental considerations, 46
  facility (flexibility) of, 45–46
  functions and norms for, 45–46
  nearpoint of convergence (NPC), 44, 45
  stamina of, 46
  sufficiency (amplitude) of, 45
  testing
    Hirschberg test, 45
    techniques, 44–45
AC/A, 64–67, 128, 396–397
  calculated, 65, 66, 128
  gradient, 65–67, 128, 223
  prognosis and, 190
Accommodation, 34–44
  absolute, 35–36, 43–44
  amplitude of, 35–36
  dysfunctions, case example, 484
  excess of, 34, 38–40
  functional disorders of, 34
  hyper-, 39
  hypertonic, 39
  ill-sustained, 34, 42–43
  inertia of, 40
  infacility of, 34, 35, 40–42
  insufficiency of, 34, 35–38, 367
  lag of, 37–38, 39
  maintaining or sustaining, 39
  neurology of, 6
  optical management, 476
  paresis/paralysis of, 34, 35
  reduction of, 34
  relative, 36, 43
  testing, 35–44
  unequal, 34
  vergence training, 478
  vision training, 474–478
    accommodative tromboning, 477
    general approaches, 474–476
    jump focus, 474, 477–478
    lens rock, 477
    plus-lens-acceptance training, 476
    plus-lens additions, 476
    specific techniques, 476–478

Accommodative accuracy, testing, 39–40
Accommodative amplitude
  Donder's Table of, 35, 36
  measuring, 35–36
  ranking of, 36
Accommodative esotropia, 188, 211–216, 372, 397
  nonrefractive (high AC/A)
    characteristics of, 214
    management of, 214–216
    miotics, 215–216
    optical treatment, 214
    surgery, 215–216
    vision training, 215
  refractive (normal AC/A)
    characteristics of, 212
    management of, 212–214
    optical treatment, 212–213
Accommodative excess, 34, 38–40
  ranking of, 39
  reliable diagnosis of, 39
  symptoms associated with, 39
Accommodative exotropia, 202
Accommodative facility
  norms for, 41
    developmental, 42
  ranking of, 42
  testing, 41–42
Accommodative fatigue, 71
Accommodative infacility, 36, 40–42, 192
  norm of accommodative facility, 41, 42
  testing, 40, 43
Accommodative insufficiency, 34, 36
  absolute accommodation, 35–36
  defined, 35
  relative accommodation, 36
  testing, 43
Accommodative lag, 37–38
  ranking of, 38
  tests, 37–38
    MEM Retinoscopy, 37–38, 39
    Nott Method, 37, 39
Accommodative rock. *See* Binocular accommodative rock
Accommodative spasm, 39
Accommodative stamina
  ranking of, 43
  testing, 43
Accommodative strabismus. *See* Accommodative esotropia
Accommodative tromboning, 477
Accommodative vergence, 8, 46, 50
Achromatopsia, 251
Acquired nonaccommodative esotropia, 220–221
Acquired noncomitant deviations

diagnosis, 438
management, 438–443
  occlusion, 438–440
  ocular calisthenics, 441
  prism compensation, 440–441
  surgery and follow-up, 443
sensory and motor training, 441–443
  double Maddox torsion training, 443
  fusion filed expansion, 442–443
Acquired nystagmus
  diagnosis, 453
  management, 453–454
Acquired sixth nerve paresis. *See* Sixth nerve (abducens) palsy
Acquired third nerve palsy. *See* Third nerve (oculomotor) palsy
Acute allergic suture reaction, 201
Adherence syndromes, 244
Afterimages at the centration point, 338–341
Afterimages testing, 31, 173–177
Afterimage tag techniques, 449
Afterimage transfer training, 300–301, 316
AIDS, 245
Alcohol intoxication, 249
Allen, M.J., 356
Allen Translid Binocular Interaction (TBI), 310, 356–358, 367
Alpern, M.B., 199
Alternate cover test, 104–106, 124, 480
Alternate exclusion method, 178
Alternate fixation, 288, 331–332
Alternation theory, 14–15
Amblyopia, 56, 138–163, 191
  anisometropic, 9, 140–141, 142, 143, 191, 228, 279, 281, 284, 314–321
  of arrest, 142, 191–192, 203
  case history, 144–145
  classification, 139–141
  defined, 138–139
  developmental, 142–145, 162
  eccentric fixation and, 140, 141, 144, 176, 177
  etiology of, 278
  and exotropia, 407
  of extinction, 142, 191–192
  fixation evaluation, 156–163
  image degradation, 141
  and infantile esotropia, 217
  isoametropic, 141, 279
  meridional, 141, 279
  and nystagmus, 256
  onset of, 145, 146, 192
  organic, 140

prognosis and, 192, 203
psychogenic, 140
saccadic and pursuit eye movements in, 144
strabismic, 9, 140, 143, 191, 284, 286, 319
suppression with, 310
testing, 161–163
    neutral density filters testing, 162
    ophthalmoscopy, 161
    retinal function testing, 162–163
    visual field, 161–162
therapy (*see* Amblyopia therapy)
visual acuity testing, 145–156
Amblyopia therapy, 197, 277–321, 471
antisuppression techniques, 367
    bar reading and tracking, 312, 367
    red filter and red print, 311, 367
    visual tracking with a Brewster stereoscope, 311, 367
binocular therapy, 309–312
    antisuppression techniques, 310–312
    ARC considerations, 310
    recommendations for, 312–313
    suppression with amblyopia, 310
case examples
    anisometropic amblyopia, 314–319
    anisometropic and strabismic amblyopia, 319–321
fixation and ocular motility activities (without foveal tag), 292–299
    Ann Arbor tracking, 295–297
    counting small objects, 298
    Hart charts, 297–298
    monocular telescope, 299
    reading for resolution, 299
    swinging ball training, 294
    tachistoscopic training, 299
    throwing and hitting games, 293
    tracing and drawing, 293
    tracking with auditory feedback, 295
    video game tracking, 293–294
    visual tracing, 295
foveal tag techniques, 300
    afterimage transfer training, 300–301
    basic central fixation training, 301
    foveal localization (fast pointing), 303

Haidinger brush training, 300
    pursuits with tag, 303–304
    resolution practice with tag, 304–305
    saccadic movements with tag, 302
    steadiness of fixation training, 301–302
intermediate goals, 278
monocular fixation training, 292–299
    eye-hand coordination techniques, 292–297
    resolution techniques, 297–299
occlusion, 279, 280–292
    direct, 280–282
    efficacy of, 284–286
    motivation and patching management, 283–284
    patching progress, 284
    penalization, 286–290
    preventing occlusion amblyopia, 282
    prism therapy and, 290
    procedures, 280–292
    red filter therapy and, 290
    short term, 291–292
    types of occluders, 280, 282–283
optical correction, 278
pleoptics, 305–309
    Bangerter's method, 305–306
    Cüppers home pleoptics, 309
    Cüppers' method, 306–307
    efficacy of, 307–308
    practical pleoptic techniques, 308–309
    Vodnoy afterimage technique, 308
progress in, 313
refractive error management, 278–280
sequence of, 278
Amblyoscopes, 137, 138, 178–181. *See also* Major amblyoscope
Amblyoscopic convergence technique, 414
Amigo, G., 328
Ammann, E., 162
Anaglyphic fusion games, 384–385
Anesthesia, 201
Angle kappa, 102, 193–194
Aniridia, 251
Aniseikonia, 170, 171
    extreme, 445
    signs and symptoms, 462–463
    therapy for, 462–465
Anisocoria, 247
Anisometropia, 222, 406, 445

axial, 462–463
    myopic, 406
    refractive, 462
Anisometropic amblyopia, 9
    antisuppression techniques for, 367
    and astigmatism, 278
    case examples, 314–321
    classification, 140–141, 142, 143, 228
    management, 279, 281, 284
    with strabismus, 191
    without strabismus, 281
Ann Arbor tracking materials, 295–297, 466
Annulus of Zinn, 5
Anomalous correspondence therapy, 266–267, 323–347
    case examples, 344–347
        Flom Swing technique, 346–347
        prism overcorrection, 344–345
        stimulating covariation in constant exotropia, 345–346
    case management, 343–344
    exotropia with ARC, 341–343
        gross convergence for, 341–343
        theoretical considerations, 341
    major amblyoscope, 328–347
        alternate fixation, 331–332
        classical techniques, 328, 329–334
        divergence technique for esotropia (Flom Swing), 334–337
        entoptic tags, 332–334
        flashing targets at the objective angle, 329
        macular massage, 331
        open space training, 334
        vertical displacement of targets, 331
    occlusion, 325–327
        binasal, 326
        constant, total, 325–326
        graded method of Revell, 326–327
    open environment training, 337–340
        afterimages at the centration point, 338–341
        Bagolini lens technique, 340, 341
        binocular luster training, 337–338
        Haidinger brush technique, 339–341
        prism-rack afterimage technique, 339
    optical procedures, 327–328
        Ludlam's method, 328
        prism overcorrection, 327–328

precautions, 323–324

sensory and motor therapy, 324–325

surgical results in, 343

Anomalous retinal correspondence (ARC), 56, 117, 163–183

adaptation theory of, 171, 172, 324, 327

and amblyopia, 310

characteristics of, 166–173

classification of, 9, 10, 163–166

covariation, 172

defined, 163

depth of, 172

etiology of, 171–172

and exotropia, 341–343, 407

harmonious (HARC), 164, 165, 166, 181–182, 324, 339–340, 343

horopter in, 166–170

horror fusionis, 171, 192, 266, 446

motor theory of, 171, 172, 325

paradoxical type one (PARC I), 165, 167, 324

paradoxical type two (PARC II), 165–166, 168, 324

prevalence of, 173

prognosis and, 192

testing, 173–183

afterimages, 173–177

Bagolini striated lens test, 181–182

bifoveal test of Cüppers, 177–178, 179

color fusion, 182–183

dissociated red lens test, 173

major amblyoscope, 178–181

therapy (see Anomalous correspondence therapy)

unharmonious (UNHARC), 164, 181–182

Anoxia, 459

Anticholinesterase drugs, 215

Antisuppression therapy, 262, 349–368

case example, 367–368

four-step approach to, 354–356

general approach to, 351

management considerations, 366–367

occlusion, 350

specific techniques, 310–312, 356–366

for amblyopia, 310–312

bar reading and tracking, 312

red filter and red print, 311, 367

visual tracking with a Brewster stereoscope, 311

Brock string and beads, 362–364

chasing, 358

cheiroscopic games, 351, 360–361

end point suppression, 358–359

hand mirror superimposition, 359–360

illumination gradient and flashing, 358

major amblyoscope, 358–359

modified Remy Separator, 361–362

penlight and filters, 359

Pola-Mirror, 365–366, 427

reading bars, 366

television trainers, 364–365

Translid Binocular Interaction Trainer, 356–358

variables to consider, 350–354

attention, 351

auditory sense, 354

combinations, 354

intermittent stimuli, 353

tactile and kinesthetic senses, 354

target brightness, 351

target color, 352

target contrast, 351

target movement, 353–354

target size, 352–353

Aperture-Rule Trainer (ART), 391–393, 403, 419–420

Apperceptive agnosia, 246

Arruga, A., 328

Associated phoria criterion, 77–78, 86

Asthenopia, 231, 268

Astigmatism, 278, 406

Athletes, vision skills in, 19, 31, 486

Atkinson, W.F., 51

Atropine, 286, 288

Atropinization, 287

Attiah, F., 288

Auditory biofeedback, 430, 450–452

Auditory stimulation, 354

Aust, W., 191, 198

Avilla, C.W., 396

B

Baclofen, 453

Bagolini, B., 172, 327

Bagolini striated lens test, 181–182, 227, 324, 340, 341

Bailey-Lovie visual acuity chart, 147

Bajandas, F.J., 114

Bangerter, A., 305, 308

Bangerter's method, 305–306

Bar reading, 366, 367, 391, 426

Bartlett, J.D., 201

Basic central fixation training, 301

Basic esophoria (BE), 90–91, 373, 376. See also Eso deviations, vision therapy

Basic esotropia (BE), 221, 372, 373, 376, 398–401. See also Eso deviations, vision therapy

Basic exophoria (BX), 89, 430. See also Exo deviations, vision therapy

Basic exotropia (BX), 406, 415, 429–431. See also Exo deviations, vision therapy

Basic orthophoria with restricted zone, 91–92

Bedell, H.E., 143, 157

Bergin, D., 456

Bernell Dual Polachrome Illuminated Trainer, 387, 389, 418–419

Bernell Eccentric Circles, 424

Bernell Macular Integrity Tester-Trainer (MITT), 159, 160, 300, 301

Bernell Mirror Stereoscope training, 379–380, 415–416

Bernell Rotator Trainer, 31, 473

Bernell Single Oblique Stereoscope, 355

Bernell 900 Stereo Trainer, 415

Bernell System, 273

Bieber, J.C., 38

Bielschowsky, 327

Bielschowsky head tilt test, 113, 114, 236

Bifoveal test of Cüppers, 177–178, 179

Binocular accommodative rock, 390–391, 397, 425, 476, 477

Binocular accommodative training, 390–391

Binocular efficiency dysfunction, 5

Binocular luster training, 337–338

Binocular triplopia, 330, 331

Binocular vision. See Normal binocular vision

Binocular vision therapy

for amblyopia, 309–312, 316–317

ARC considerations, 310

suppression and amblyopia, 310

future directions in, 485–487

recommendations for binocular training, 312–313

see also Vision therapy

Bioengineering model, 92–94

Birnbaum, M.H., 285

Blow-in fracture, 244

Blow-out fracture, 244

Boisvert, R.P., 74

Borish, I.M., 40, 183

Botulinum toxin injections, 202, 453–454

Boyer, F., 103
Bracketing, 35
Brainstem lesions, 246
Brain tumors, 245, 443
Brewster stereoscope, 380–384
    cheiroscopic games with, 361
    isometric and step vergences, 382–383, 417–418
    tromboning, 383–384, 418
    visual tracking with, 311
Bridgeman, G.J., 263
Brinker, W.R., 290
Brock, F., 264, 480
Brock-Givner afterimage transfer test, 176–177
Brock string and beads, 362–364, 385–386, 397
Broken Wheel test, 152
Brown, H.W., 243
Brown syndrome, 242–243, 438
    characteristics of, 242–243
Brückner test, 107
Buffon, G. de, 262, 280
Burge, S., 42
Burger, D.S., 445
Burian, H.M., 162, 171, 223, 290

C

CA/C reflex, 68
Caloroso, E.E., 162, 313, 327, 336, 397, 442
Calrider, N., 408
CAMP lenses (Corrected Ametropia Most Plus), 35
Cantonnet, A., 262
Carlson, G.P., 454
Carter, D.B., 199
Cassady, J.C., 140
Cataracts, 9
    congenital, 141, 447
Central fusion faculty, 445
Central stereopsis, 13, 14
Centration point training, 374
Cereal test, 152
Cerebral palsy, 248
Char, D.H., 239, 240
Charman, W.N., 38
Chasing, break and join task, 358
Chavasse, F.B., 191–192, 230, 263, 264
Cheiroscope, 360
Cheiroscopic games, 360–361
    coloring and drawing, 360–361
    counting, 360
    point-to-point chasing, 361
    tracing, 354, 355, 361
Cheiroscopic training, 351, 354
Chiastopic fusion, 422–425, 479
Chin elevation, 240, 243, 457

Christenson, G.N., 319, 344, 430, 435
Chronic progressive external ophthalmoplegia (CPEO), 241
Chrousos, G.A., 35
Ciuffreda, K.J., 139, 142–143, 157, 250, 291, 299, 307, 450, 451
Clarke, C., 333
Cline, D., 35, 56, 171
Clinical wisdom criterion, 72, 86
Clonazepam, 453
Coffey, B., 409, 410, 411
Cogan's anterior INO, 245
Cogan's posterior INO, 245
Cogwheel pursuits, 246, 248
Cohen, A., 25
Cole, R.G., 74
Color fusion, 12, 182
    testing, 182–183
Color vision testing, monocular, 162–163
Coma, 445
Comitancy, 107–121, 189
    causes, 107–108
    criteria and terminology, 108–109
    defined, 107
    ductions, 111–112
    primary and secondary deviations, 109–111
    signs and symptoms, 116–117
        abnormal head posture, 116–117
        diplopia, 116
    testing
        single-object method, 117–118
        spatial localization, 115–116
        subjective, 117–121
        three-step method, 112–115
        two-object method, 118–121
    versions, 112
Comitant esotropia
    infantile (see Infantile esotropia)
    vision therapy sequence for
        centration point training, 374
        changing viewing distance, 376
        compensating prisms and lens additions, 373–374
        correction of refractive error, 372–373
        elimination of major sensory anomalies, 373
        follow-up care, 377
        sensory and motor fusion training, 374–376
        surgical management, 376–377
Comitant hyper deviations, 228, 229
Comitant vertical deviations, 229
Computer industries, 485–486
Computerized convergence procedures, 427

Computerized divergence procedures, 395–396
Computer Orthoptics, 273, 294, 396, 427
Computer stereopsis enhancement, 481
Computer tomography (CT), 453
Confusion, 131, 132–133
Congenital cataracts, 141, 447
Congenital esotropia, 187, 216
Congenital exotropia, 256
Congenital nystagmus, 250–252, 447–453
    afferent and efferent, 251, 447
    case example, 458–459
    characteristics of, 251
    diagnosis, 447
    incidence of strabismus in, 252
    management
        optical, 447–448
        surgical, 452–453
        therapeutic options, 447
    vision training, 448–452
        afterimage tag techniques, 449
        auditory biofeedback, 450–452
        intermittent photopic stimulation, 449–450
Congenital torticollis of the head, 234
Conjugate gaze movements, 7–8
Consecutive strabismus, 230–231
Contact lenses
    bifocal, 214
    disadvantages of, 279
    for hyperopia, 279
    monovision, 465–466
    for nystagmus, 448
    occluders, 284, 445
    soft, 213
    for strabismic amblyopia, 279
Continuous motion game, 466
Contoured tests, 187
Contour interaction, 146
Contrast sensitivity, 4
Convergence, 8. See also Vergence
Convergence excess (CE) esophoria, 91. See also Eso deviations, vision therapy
Convergence excess (CE) esotropia, 91, 214. See also Accommodative exotropia; Eso deviations, vision therapy
Convergence fatigue, 71
Convergence insufficiency (CI) exophoria, 88–92, 406, 422, 431–435. See also Exo deviations, vision therapy
Convergence insufficiency (CI) exotropia, 406. See also Exo deviations, vision therapy

Convergence training at near, 418–419
Convergence walk-aways, 419
Cook, D., 343
Cooper, E.L., 409, 411
Correct-Eye-Scope, 40
Corticosteroids, 239
Cosmesis, 130, 193–195, 194. *See also*
   Extraocular muscle surgery
Costenbader, F.D., 195
Counting small objects, 298
Crowding phenomenon, 146
Cüppers home pleopics, 308–309
Cüppers home pleoptics, 306–307
Cüppers' method, 306–307
Currie, J.N., 453
Cyclo deviations, 125, 126
Cyclopean projection, 12
Cyclophoria, vergence therapy,
   479–480
Cycloplegics, 201
Cyclovergent deviations, 443
Cyclovertical deviations, 228–230
   comitant vertical deviations,
     229
   dissociated vertical deviations
     (DVD), 230
Cysts, 215

D

Dale, R.T., 198, 220, 229
Dalrymple's sign, 239, 458
Daum, K.M., 270
Davidson, D.W., 148
Day, R.M., 239
De Decker, W., 343
Degenerative diseases, 247, 248
Delgadillo, H., 52
Demand line, 63, 73
DEM Test. *See* Developmental Eye
   Movement Test (DEM)
Depth clues, 14
Developmental Eye Movement Test
   (DEM), 26–27, 28
Dextroversion, 7
Diabetes, 235, 445
Diagnosis, 3, 185–209
   components of, 185–186
   establishing, 185–186
   normal binocular vision, 3–15
   validity of diagnostic criteria,
     81–86
   vision efficiency skills, 17–59
   see also Prognosis
Diagnostic action field (DAF), 111,
   112
Diagnostic statement, 186
Diagnostic therapy, 344
Diisopropyl fluorophosphate (DFP),
   201

Diisopropyl fluorophosphate (DFP)
   ointment, 215
Diplopia, 10–11, 12–13, 53
   fixation switch, 444
   and Graves' disease, 240
   intractable, 171, 310, 323, 343,
     443–447, 458
   and neurogenic palsies, 234, 438
   pathological, 12, 414
   physiological, 10–11, 13, 414,
     416–417
   postoperative, 200, 231, 343
   signs and symptoms, 116
   testing, 123
Direct occlusion, 280–282
Disparity vergence. *See* Fusional vergence
Disparometer (Sheedy), 75, 77, 79, 85
Dissociated red lens test, 173
Dissociated vertical deviation (DVD),
   217–219, 230, 256
Divergence, 8. *See also* Vergence
Divergence excess (DE) exophoria,
   89–90, 427
Divergence excess (DE) exotropia,
   427–429
Divergence insufficiency (DI)
   esophoria, 90, 372, 378
Divergence insufficiency (DI) eso-
   tropia, 221, 372, 373, 376,
     401
Donders, 264
Donders, F.C., 36, 63
Dorsal midbrain syndrome, 247
Double elevator palsy, 237238
Double hyper deviations, 230
Double Maddox torsion training, 443
Double pointing techniques, 361,
   362, 367
Double vision, 5, 9, 10, 443
Douse target test, 181, 331
Dowley, D., 85
Downbeat nystagmus, 254, 453
Drug intoxications, 245
Drugs, 35, 201–202
Duane, 241
Duane, A., 87
Duane cover test, 104–106
Duane retraction syndrome (DRS),
   31, 241–242, 438
   case example, 454–456
   characteristics of, 241–242
   etiologic factors, 242
Duane-White classification model,
   87–88, 92
Ductions, 111–112
DynaVision 2000 electronic fixation
   instrument, 294, 467
Dyslexia, 59, 485

Dysthyroid eye disease. *See* Graves'
   disease

E

Early acquired strabismus, 98, 188
Eason, R.G., 154
Eccentric Circles, 394–395, 424, 479
Eccentric fixation (EF), 106, 156
   and amblyopia, 140, 141, 143,
     176, 177
   causes of, 157, 303, 305
   description of, 157–158
   prognosis and, 191
   therapy, 300
Echothiophate iodide (Phospholine),
   201, 286
Edrophonium chloride (Tensilon), 238
Efficiency of vision. *See* Vision effi-
   ciency skills
Electroretinogram (ERG), 163
Elevated chin posture, 240, 243, 457
End-point suppression, 358–359
Enophthalmos, 244
Entoptic tags, 331–334
Epileptic seizures, 357
Erikson, G.B., 442
Eskridge, J.B., 103, 148
Eso deviations, vision therapy,
   371–404, 478
   with ARC, 378
   basic esotropia, 373, 376
     case example, 398–401
   case management and examples,
     396–404
   comitant esotropia, 372–377
     centration point training, 374
     changing viewing distance, 376
     compensating prisms and lens
       additions, 373–374
     correction of refractive error,
       372–373
     elimination of major sensory
       anomalies, 373
     follow-up care, 377
     sensory and motor fusion train-
       ing, 374–376
     surgical management, 376–377
   convergence excess esotropia, case
     example, 396–398
   diagnostic variables, 372
   divergence insufficiency esotropia,
     case example, 401
   esophoria
     case example, 403–404
     therapy sequence for, 377–378
   esotropia, free-space training, 262
   microesotropia, case example, 402
   specific training techniques,
     378–396

Eso deviations, vision therapy
(*continued*)
amblyoscopic divergence technique, 334–337378–379
anaglyphic fusion games, 384–385
Aperture-Rule Trainer (double aperture), 391–393
Bernell Mirror Stereoscope, 379–380, 415–416
binocular accommodative rock, 390–391
Brewster stereoscope training, 380–384
Brock string and beads, 385–386
computerized divergence procedures, 395–396
divergence training at near, 389–390
divergence walk-aways, 390
isometric and step vergences, 382–383
othopic fusion, 394–395
peripheral fusion rings training at far, 386
projected slides, 390
Remy Separator, 393–394
stereoscope tromboning, 383–384
tranaglyphs, 386
vectograms, 386
vergence rock techniques (flipper prisms), 391
Esophoria, 372
basic (BE), 90–91, 373, 376
case example, 403–404
convergence excess (CE), 91
divergence insufficiency (DI), 90, 378
Esotropia, 372
accommodative, 211–216, 372, 397
basic (BE), 221, 372, 373, 376, 398–401
comitant, 372–377
congenital, 187, 216
convergence excess (CE), 372, 374, 376, 396–398
divergence insufficiency (DI), 221, 372, 373, 376, 401
infantile (*see* Infantile esotropia)
management, 371–372
primary comitant, 220–221
prognosis, 199, 201
surgical procedures for, 377
therapy (*see* Eso deviations, vision therapy)
Essential infantile strabismus, 98
Etting, G., 187, 192
Euthyscope, 306

Exo deviations, vision therapy, 405, 478
basic exotropia, case example, 429–431
case management and examples, 427–435
comitant exotropia, 406–412
changing viewing distance, 410
compensating prisms and lens additions, 408–409
correction of refractive error, 406–407
elimination of major sensory anomalies, 407
follow-up care, 412
gross convergence training, 344, 408
sensory and motor fusion training, 409–410
surgical management, 410–412
convergence insufficiency, 431–435
diagnostic considerations, 406
divergence excess exotropia, case example, 427–429
divergence technique for (Flom Swing), 334–337, 372
exophoria, 412–413
specific training techniques, 413–427
amblyoscopic convergence technique, 414
Aperture-Rule Trainer (single aperture), 419–420
bar reader with prisms, 426
Bernell Mirror Stereoscope, 415–416
binocular accommodative rock, 425
Brewster stereoscope, 417–419
Brock string and beads, 416
chiastopic fusion, 422–425
computerized convergence procedures, 427
convergence training at near, 419
convergence walk-aways, 419
3-dot card, 416–417
framing and prisms, 426
isometric and step vergences, 417–418
pencil pushups and push-aways, 420–422
peripheral fusion rings, 415
physiological diplopia, 416–417
Pola-Mirror vergence techniques, 427
projected slides, 419
stereoscopic tromboning, 418

television trainer and prisms, 426
vectograms and tranaglyphs, 418–419
vergence rock techniques, 425–427
voluntary convergence, 413–414
Exophoria, 35, 39
accommodative deficiencies and, 413
basic (BX), 89, 406, 430
convergence insufficiency (CI), 88, 406, 422, 431–435
divergence excess (DE), 89–90, 406, 427
presbyopic, 88, 432
therapy (*see* Exo deviations, vision therapy)
Exophthalmos (proptosis), 239
Exotropia
with ARC, 341–343
basic (BX), 406, 415, 429–431
case example, 345–346
comitant, 506–412
congenital, 256
convergence insufficiency (CI), 406
divergence excess (DE), 406, 415, 427–429
primary comitant, 221–224
therapy (*see* Exo deviations, vision therapy)
External ophthalmoplegia, 237)
Extraocular muscles, 5–6, 438
Extraocular muscle surgery
adjustable suture procedure, 200
advancement of the insertion, 198
bilateral lateral rectus resection, 376–377
bimedial rectus recession, 376
general approach, 198–200
informed consent, 200
myotomy or myectomy, 198
prognosis, 194, 198–201
recession-resection, 377
reoperation, 200–201
resectioning, of muscle or tendon, 198
tenectomies, 198
tucking, 198
for turned eye, 230
see also Surgery
Eye dominancy, 129, 190–191
Eye in reserve, 4
Eye laterality, 128–129, 135, 190
Eye movements
accommodation, 6
conjugate, 7–8, 44
disjunctive, 8, 44

duction, 29
dysfunctions, case example,
    482–484
neurology of, 18, 66–8
nonoptic, 18
pursuit, 7–8
saccades, 7, 19
systems, 18, 33
vergence, 8
vestibular, 7
see also Vision efficiency skills
Eye preference, 129
Eyestrain, 5
Eye-Trac, 18, 21, 22, 24

F

Falling eye syndrome, 236
Fibrosis of the extraocular muscles,
    243–244
Field of vision, 4
Fisher, N.F., 101
Fixation, 33–34
    amblyopic, 157–158
    centricity of, classification, 158
    crossed, 217
    disparity (*see* Fixation disparity)
    eccentric, 156, 157–158
    evaluation
        and amblyopia, 156–163
        eye disease evaluation, 161–163
        Haidlinger brush testing,
            159–160
        refraction techniques, 160–161
        visuoscopy, 158–159
    foveal, 297, 300
    nystagmus and, 249
    testing, 32
        position maintainence, 33
        SCCO 4+ System, 33
    training
        basic central, 301
        monocular, 292–299
        steadiness of, 301–302
    unsteadiness of, 157–158
Fixation disparity, 12
Fixation disparity analysis, 73–81
    definition and features, 73–74
    prism prescription, 81
    prognosis, 196
    and stereopsis, 74
    testing, 75–81
Fixation disparity curve (FDC), 79, 85
    types of curves, 80–81
Flashing a target, 329, 353, 355, 357,
    358
Flat fusion, 54
    defined, 13
    testing, 54
Flax, N., 411

Fleming, A., 327
Flom, M.C., 143, 146, 148, 157, 162,
    166, 171, 172, 173,
    186–187, 188–189, 192, 334,
    345, 406
Flom Swing technique, 334–347,
    344, 346–347
Flynn, J.T., 140
Fly stereopsis test, 58
Form fusion, 12–14
Four base-out prism test, 106
Fourth nerve (trochlear) palsy,
    235–236, 438, 442, 445
Foveal fixation, 297, 300
Foveal localization (fast pointing),
    303, 316
Foveal tag techniques, 300–305
    afterimage transfer training,
        300–301
    foveal tag training, 301–305
    basic central fixation training, 301
        foveal localization (fast point-
            ing), 303
        pursuits with tag, 303–304
        resolution practice with tag,
            304–305
        saccadic movements with tag,
            302
        steadiness of fixation training,
            301–302
    Haidinger brush training, 300
Framing and prisms, 426
Franois, J., 285
Franzbrau Coordinator, 295
Fresnel Press-on (TM) prisms, 376,
    377
Frisby test, 54
Frontal eye-field lesions, 246
Frontomesencephalic pathway le-
    sions, 29, 31
Fry, G.A., 56, 264
Fusional supplementary convergence
    (FSC), 51
Fusional vergence, 8, 46, 414–415
    deficiency, 367
    dysfunction, 50, 59
    at far, 47–49
    at near, 50
    testing, 46–49
Fusion field expansion, 442–443

G

Gamblin, G.T., 240
Garzia, R.P., 26, 284, 291, 307
Gay, A.J., 33
Gaze paretic nystagmus, 254
Gellman, M., 201
Generalized fibrosis syndrome,
    243–244

Getz, D.J., 354, 359
Glaser, J.S., 235
Global stereopsis, 56–57, 58
Goldberg, J.B., 465
Goldrich, S.G., 409
Goldrick, S.G., 430
Goodier, H.M., 191
Goss, D.A., 140–141
Graded occlusion method of Revell,
    326–327
Gradient method, 65–67, 128, 223
Graphical analysis, 92–93
Graves, R.J., 239
Graves' disease (dysthyroid eye dis-
    ease), 239–241, 458
    diplopia and, 240
    management of, 240–241
    systemic treatment of, 240
Greenwald, I., 326
Griffin, D.C., 21
Griffin, J.R., 27, 41, 42, 45, 52, 57,
    103, 195, 291, 454
Grisham, J.D., 42, 43, 48, 49, 83, 84,
    89, 213, 252, 336, 406, 432,
    485
Groffman's visual tracing patterns,
    295, 311
Gross convergence, 70, 344, 408,
    414, 416

H

Haddad, H.M., 485
Haidinger brush testing
    and amblyopia, 159–160, 300
    and ARC, 333, 339–341
    and macular integrity, 160
Hallden, U., 172
Hamsher, K.deS., 57
Hand mirror superimposition,
    359–360, 367
Haplopia, 9, 10
Harding, GFA., 154
Harmon distance, 37
Harmonious ARC (HARC), 164, 165,
    166, 181–182, 324, 339–340,
    343
Hart charts, 297–298, 316, 477
Haynes, H.M., 37
Head trauma, 245, 445
Head turn, 242, 243, 449
Heath, G., 334
Heinsen,, 30
Heinsen-Schrock system, 20–21
Helmholtz, 264
Helveston, E.M., 140, 200, 411
Hemenger, R., 464
Hering-Bielschowsky test, 338, 342
Hering's Law, 7, 8, 234, 236
Hess-Lancaster test, 118–119, 121, 128

Heteronymous (crossed) diplopia, 10, 11
Heterophoria, 54
    evaluation of, 129
    prognosis, 185, 195–196, 197, 199
    therapy, 353, 365, 367, 479
    see also Heterophoria case analysis
Heterophoria case analysis, 63–94
    bioengineering model, 92–94
    fixation disparity analysis, 73–81
        definition and features, 73–74
        measurement, 75–81
        prescribing prism, 81
    lens and prism prescription,
            71–73, 86–87
        clinical wisdom, 72
        Morgan, 71–72
        Percival, 73
        recommendations, 86–87
        Sheard, 72
    Morgan's normative analysis,
            70–71
    tonic convergence and AC/A,
            64–67
        calculated AC/A, 65
        gradient AC/A, 65–67
    validity of diagnostic criteria,
            81–86
    vergence anomalies, 87–88
        basic esophoria, 90–91
        basic exophoria, 89
        basic orthophoria with re-
            stricted zone, 91–92
        convergence excess, 91
        convergence insufficiency,
            88–92
        divergence excess, 89–90
        divergence insufficiency, 90
        normal zone with symptoms, 92
        zone of clear single binocular vi-
            sion, 67–70
    see also Heterophoria
Hiles, D.A., 407
Hirsch, M.J., 84
Hirschberg, J., 102–103
Hirschberg test, 45, 102–103, 414
Hoffman, L.G., 42, 45
Hofstetter, H.W., 36, 199, 264
Holopigian, K., 367
Home training, 351, 364, 366, 382,
            482–483
    instruments,394, 367
    versus office training, 270–271
    regression of skills and, 274–275,
            336
Homologous points, 54
Homonymous hemianopsia, 246
Homonymous (uncrossed) diplopia,
            10–11

Horopter
    in ARC, 166–170
    defined, 10
Horror fusionis, 171, 192, 266, 446
Howard-Dolman peg test, 55
H-S Scale, 30–31
Huber, A., 242
Hugonnier, R., 173, 198, 338, 343
Hurtt, J., 198
Hydrocephalus, 245, 247
Hyper-accommodation, 39
Hyper deviations, 228, 229
Hyperopia, 476
Hyperphoria, vision therapy, 479
Hyperthyroidism, 239–241
Hypertonic accommodation, 39
Hypnosis, 202
Hypnotherapy, 446, 447
Hypoplasia, 251

I

Identical visual direction (IVD)
        horopter, 10
Ill-sustained accommodation, 42–43
    testing, 42–43
    therapy, 43
Illumination gradient and flashing,
        358
Image degradation amblyopia, 141
Infantile esotropia, 173, 188,
        216–220, 230, 430
    amblyopia and, 217
    characteristics of, 101, 216–219
    management, 219–220
        optical treatment, 219
        surgery, 226
        vision training, 219–220
    nystagmus and, 218–219
Infantile noncomitant deviations,
        437–438
    diagnosis, 437–438
    management, 438
Infantile nystagmus. See Congenital
        nystagmus
Infant visual acuity assessment,
        152–154
Infections, 245
Infranuclear lesions, 31
Ingram, R.M., 216
Interferometry, 155–156, 157
Intermittent photopic stimulation,
        449–450
Intermittent stimuli, 353. See also
        Flashing
Internal ophthalmoplegia, 237
Internuclear and supranuclear disor-
        ders, 244–248
    internuclear ophthalmoplegia
        (INO), 245–246

supranuclear horizontal gaze
        palsy, 246
    brainstem lesions, 246
    frontal eye-field lesions, 246
    occipital and parietal cortical
        lesions, 246
supranuclear vertical gaze palsy,
        246
    parinaud syndrome, 247
    Parkinson's disease, 248
    progressive supranucler palsy,
        247–248
Internuclear ophthalmoplegia (INO),
        245–246
    features of, 245
Interpupillary distance (IPD), 45
Intractable diplopia, 171
    case example, 458
    causes of, 444
    diagnosis, 443–445
    management, 445–447
        hypnotherapy, 447
        occlusion strategies, 445–446
        prism displacement, 446–447
        surgery, 444
    risk of, 310, 323, 325, 343
Inverse prisms, 194
Irvine, S.R., 162
Ishikawa, S., 450
Isoametropic amblyopia, 141, 279
Isolated inferior oblique palsy, 237
Isolated inferior rectus palsy, 237
Isolated medial rectus palsy, 237,
        245
Isolated superior oblique palsy, 237
Isolated superior rectus palsy, 237
Isometric vergence training,
        269–270, 382–383, 414, 417

J

Jaanus, S.D., 201
Jacobson, M., 51
James, M., 285
Jampolsky, A., 115, 132, 198, 200,
        222, 343, 353, 408
Javal, L.E., 18, 261–263, 264, 265,
        349, 486
Johnson, L.V., 244
Jones, R., 103
Joubert, C., 80
Jump focus, 474, 477–478
Jump vergence training, 269, 424

K

Katz, S.L., 290
Kavner, R.S., 191
Kenyon, R.V., 50
Kerr, K.E., 172
Kestenbaum, A., 452

Keystone Colored Circles (lifesavers) Card, 422–423
Keystone Eccentric Circles, 394–395, 424, 479
Keystone Telebinocular, 380, 381
Keystone Test 1, 53
Kinesthetic stimulation, 354
Kinetic cover test, 480
King-Devick Test, 25–26, 28
Kirschen, D.G., 450
Kleinstein, R.N., 464
Knapp procedure, 238
Knapps Law, 462
Kohn, H., 202
Krimsky test, 103–104
Kutschke, P.J., 284

L

Lang, J., 226
Lang test, 55
Late acquired strabismus, 98, 188
Latent hyperopia, 39
Latent nystagmus, 256
  characteristics of, 253
Lateral adherence syndrome, 244
Lebow, K.A., 465
Leigh, R.J., 453
Lenses, 197
  adaptation to, 279
  CAMP, 35
Lens prescription, 71–73
  validity of diagnostic criteria, 81–86
  see also Prism prescription
Lens rock, 477
Levator muscle, 5
Levi, D.M., 139, 142–143, 153, 157
Leyman, I.A., 409, 411
Leyman, I.R., 285
Lid apraxia, 248
Lid retraction, 239
Lieberman, S., 25
Lighthouse (LH) symbol tests, 152, 153
Lite-Brite game, 468
Liu, J.S., 41
Lo, C., 251
Local stereopsis, 56–57, 58
London, R., 93, 445, 446
Low vision, 140
Ludlam, W.M., 187, 192, 328, 337–338
Ludlam's method, 328
Lyle, T.K., 263

M

MacDonald, A.L., 133
McNear, K.W., 202
Macular degeneration, 9

Macular evasion, 171
Macular Integrity Tester-Trainer (MITT), 159, 160, 300, 301
Macular massage, 331, 359
Maddox, E., 264
Maddox, W.D., 44, 63, 92, 93, 129, 486
Maddox rods, 125, 126, 463
  vector method, 441
Magnetic resonance image (MRI), 251–252
Magnetic resonance imagery (MRI), 453
Major amblyoscope
  and amblyopia therapy, 178–181
  and anomalous correspondence therapy, 328–347
  and antisuppression therapy, 358–359
Mallett, R.F.J., 449–450
Mallett Fixation Unit, 76, 78–79, 85
Manas, L., 195
Manley, D.R., 187, 201
Marsden ball, 294, 295, 316, 441, 472, 481
Matsuo, V., 453
Maumenee, A., 181
Mechanical restrictions of ocular movement, 241–244
  Brown (superior oblique tendon sheath) syndrome, 242–243
  Duane retraction syndrome, 241–242
  fibrosis of the extraocular muscles, 243–244
    adherence syndromes, 244
    orbital anomalies, 244
Medial longitudinal fasciculus (MLF), 245
Mein, J., 198
MEM retinoscopy
  to assess accommodative accuracy, 37–38
  to assess accommodative excess, 39
Mental effort, 262–263, 355, 358, 471
Meridional amblyopia, 141, 279
Metamorphopsia, 444, 446
Method-of-adjustment, research technique, 35
Metzger, E.L., 448
Mezawa, M., 450
Michaels, D.D., 29
Microesotropia. See Microtropia
Microstrabismus. See Microtropia
Microtropia, 226–228, 344
  case example, 402–403
  characteristics of, 226–227
  management, 227–228

primary and secondary, 226
prognosis, 228
testing, 227, 228
Milam, J.B., 289
Miotics, 201, 286
  accommodative esotropia, 213
  nonrefractive esotropia, 215
  side effects, 215–216
Mirror Stereoscope/Cheiroscope, 360
Misdirection syndrome, 236–237
Mobius syndrome, 235
Monocular estimate method (MEM). See MEM retinoscopy
Monocular fixation training, 292–299, 315–316
  eye-hand coordination techniques, 292–297
  fixation and ocular motility activities, 292–299
  resolution techniques, 297–299
Monocular telescope, 299
Monocular training, 266
Monocular vision, 9
Monofixation pattern. See Microtropia
Monovision, 465–466
Monovision occlusion, 446, 465
Morgan, M.W., 70–72, 83, 84, 88, 92, 171, 264, 334
Morgan's expected criterion, 71–72
Morgan's normative analysis, 70–71
Moser, J.E., 51
Mother Goose Vectogram, 388–389, 399, 418
Motor dominance, 129
Motor fusion, 53, 54
Motor fusion training. See Sensory and motor fusion training
Multiple sclerosis, 235, 245, 246, 445, 453
Muscle cone, 5
Muscle paretic nystagmus, 254
Myasthenia gravis, 238–239
  features of, 238–239
  treatment of, 239
Myogenic palsies, 238–241
  chronic progressive external ophthalmoplegia (CPEO), 241
  dysthyroid eye disease, 239–241
  myasthenia gravis, 238–239
Myopia, 39, 222, 406, 409
Myopic anisometropia, 406
Myotomy or myectomy, 198

N

Nawratzki, I., 289
Nearpoint of convergence, 44, 45
Negative disparity divergence. See Fusional vergence at far

Negative fusional convergence (NFC), 70. *See* Fusional vergence at far
Negative fusional vergence. *See* Fusional vergence at far
Negative relative convergence (NRC), 69
  measuring, 47, 49
Neural summation, 14, 15
Neurogenic palsies, 233–238
  diplopia and, 234
  fourth nerve (trochlar), 235–236
  general considerations, 233–235
  mobius syndrome, 235
  primary and secondary deviations, 233
  sixth nerve (abducens), 235
  third nerve (oculomotor), 236–238
Neutral density filters testing, 162
Night myopia, 39
Nixon, R.B., 216
Noncomitancy
  defined, 107, 108
  testing for, 109, 112
Noncomitant deviations
  acquired, 438–443
    diagnosis, 438
    management, 438–443
  infantile, 437–438
    diagnosis, 437–438
    management, 438
  recording, 115
Noncomitant intermittent hypertropia, case example, 456–457
Noncomitant strabismus, 13, 233–238, 438
Noncontoured stereoacuity tests, 187
Nonrefractive accommodative exotropia, 211, 214–216
Normal binocular vision, 3–15, 486
  anatomy of the extraocular muscles, 5–6
  motor components of, 3
  neurology of eye movements, 6–8
  sensory aspects of, 3, 9–15
  value of, 3–5
Normal retinal correspondence (NRC), 9, 178, 312, 327, 367
Normal zone with symptoms, 92
Nott dynamic retinoscopy, 37, 39
Nuclear lesions, 31
Nystagmus, 141, 248–256
  acquired, 453–454
  blockage syndrome, 252–256
  characteristics of, 249
  congenital, 250–252, 447–453, 458–459
  and infantile esotropia, 218–219
  latent, 256
  physiologic, 249
  rare types of, 254–255, 256, 453
  voluntary (flutter), 249–250
Nystagmus blockage syndrome, 252–256

O

Ober 2: Visagraph, 22, 23
Occipital and parietal cortical lesions, 246
Occipital lobe, 8
Occipitomesencephalic pathway lesions, 29, 31
Occluders
  alternate, 439
  binasal, 439–440
  central field, 446
  constant, 445
  contact lens, 284, 445
  graded, 350
  monovision, 446
  opaque, 280, 283
  partial, 440
  translucent, 280
  types of, 282–283
Occlusion, 191, 197
  in acquired noncomitant deviations, 438–440
  in amblyopia therapy, 279, 280–292, 414
    direct, 280–282
    efficacy of, 284–286
    inverse, 280
    motivation and patching management, 283–284
    patching progress, 284
    penalization, 286–290
    prism therapy and, 290
    red filter therapy and, 290
    short term, 291–292
    total or partial, 280
  in anomalous correspondence therapy, 325–327
    binasal, 326
    constant, total, 325–326
    graded method, 326–327
  in antisuppression therapy, 350
    graded method, 350
  classification of variables, 280
  in intractable diplopia, 445–446
  inverse versus direct, 305
  prevention of contractures, 439, 440
  prevention of diplopia, 438–440
  see also Occluders
Occlusion amblyopia, 282, 288
Ocular albinism, 251, 447, 459
Ocular calisthenics, 441
Ocular dominance, 15
Ocular motility, loss of, 241
Ocular myopathy of von Graefe, 241
Ocular torticollis of the head, 234
Oculogyric crisis, 248
Oculomotor disorders, 233–256
Oculomotor palsies
  etiological frequency of, 233–238
  features of, 236
Office training, versus home training, 270–271
Ogle, K.N., 73, 79, 80, 85, 264, 463
Oliver, M., 284
Open environment training, 337–338, 375, 376, 410
  versus instrument training, 271
Open space training, on amblyoscope, 323, 374
Ophthalmic artery, 5
Ophthalmography
  for saccades, 21–22
Ophthalmoscopy, 161
Optical anisometropia, induced, 57
Optic atrophy, 447
Optic foramen, 5
Optic nerve, 5
Optic nerve atrophy, 9
Optimum, 294
Opti-Mum Computer Vision Therapy, 396
Opti-Mum System, 273
Optokinetic nystagmus (OKN), 153–154, 155
Optometric Extension Program (OEP), 265
Optometric vision therapy, 262, 264–265
Optometrist, 265
Orbital anomalies, 244
Organic amblyopia, 140
Orthophoria, vision therapy, 480
Orthopic fusion training, 394–395
Orthoptics, 197, 261, 262
Orthotropia, 445
Oscillopsia, 249, 251, 450, 453

P

Pantano, F., 433
Panum, P.L., 9
Panum's areas, 9, 14
Papilledema, 247
Paracentral fixation lock, 161
Paradoxical ARC type one (PARC I), 165, 167, 324
Paradoxical ARC type two (PARC II), 165–166, 168, 324
Paralysis, 233
Paramedial pontine reticular formation (PPRF), 246

Parasympatholytic (anticholinergic)
    drugs, 35
Paresis, 108, 233
    true, 112
Paretic strabismus, 234
Parinaud syndrome, 247
    ocular signs of, 247
Parkinson's disease, 248
Parks, M.M., 112, 190
Patching. See Occluders; Occlusion
Pathological diplopia, 12
Pathological suppression, 132
Patient motivation, 410
    feedback and, 273–274
    mental effort, 262–263, 355, 358,
        471
    and patching management,
        283–284
    rapport with children, 272–273
    in vision training, 271–273
Payne, C.R., 84
Penalization, 286–290
    distance, 287
    efficacy of, 289–290
    management, 288–289
    methods, 286–288
    near, 286
    optical, 287–288
    total, 286, 287
    without spectacles, 286
Pencil pushups and pushaways,
        420–422
Penlight and filters, 359
Perceptuomotor pen, 295, 296, 354
Percival, A.S., 73, 81
Percival's criterion, 73, 86
Periodic alternating nystagmus
        (PAN), 254, 453
Peripheral fusion, 170
Peripheral fusion rings, 386, 415
Peripheral stereopsis, 13–14
Pernicious anemia, 245
Pharmacological treatment, 35,
        201–202
    side effects, 201
Philosophies of vision therapy,
        261–265
    English School, 263–264
    French School, 261–263
    optometric, 264–265
Phi phenomenon, 125
Phoria line, 67
Phorometry measurements, 264
Phospholine Iodine, 215
Photopic stimulation, 449–450
Physiological diplopia, 10–11
    training, 357, 362–363, 416–417
Physiological suppression, 10,
        131–132

Physiologic nystagmus, 249
    characteristics of, 250
Piaget, J., 272
Pickwell, L.D., 279
Picture cards, 149–152
Pierce, J.R., 51
Pierce Saccade Test, 24–25, 28
Pigassou, R., 290
Pilocarpine drops, 286
Pleoptics, 197, 305–309
    Bangerter's method, 305–306
    Cüppers' method, 306–307
    efficacy of, 307
    practical techniques in, 307–308
Pleoptophor, 305, 306
PL 20/20 Infant Vision Tester, 153
Plus-lens-acceptance training, 476
Plus-lens additions, 476–477
Point zero, 132, 133
Pola-Mirror, 365–366, 427
Polarizing filters, 55
Pope, R.S., 42
Positive fusional convergence (PFC),
        70
Positive relative convergence (PRC),
        69
    measuring, 48, 49
Postar, S.H., 199
Pratt-Johnson, J.A., 133
Preferential looking tests, 153
Presbyopic exophoria, 88–89, 432,
        476
Press, L.J., 127
Priestley, B.S., 309
Primary comitant esotropia (PCE),
        220–221
    characteristics, 221
    management, 221
Primary comitant exotropia (PCX),
        221–224
    characteristics, 222–223
    intermittency, 222, 226
    management, 223–224
Primary eye care, 487
Primary visual cortex, 9
Principles of vision therapy,
        265–270, 350
Prism adaptation, 44, 46, 47–48, 197,
        328
Prism adaptation test (PAT), 86, 87,
        198–199
Prism compensation, 440–441, 458
Prism confirmation procedure, 86, 87
Prism diopters and degrees, conver-
        sions of, 491
Prism displacement, 446–447
Prism overcorrection, 327–328
    case example, 344–345
Prism prescription, 71–73

associated phoria criterion, 77–78,
        86
    clinical wisdom criterion, 72, 86
    fixation disparity and, 81
    Morgan's expected criterion, 71–72
    Percival's criterion, 73, 86
    prism adaptation test, 86, 87
    prism confirmation procedure, 86,
        87
    recommendations for, 86–87
    Sheard's criterion, 72–73, 84, 86
    Sheedy's criterion, 86
    validity of diagnostic criteria,
        81–86
Prism-rack afterimage technique, 339
Prisms, 197
    compensating, 198–199
    inverse, 290–291
    yoked, 448, 457
Prognosis, 186
    case examples, 202–209
    heterophoria, 195–196
    strabismus, 186–195
        associated conditions, 191–192
        cosmetic cure, 186, 193–195
        Flom's criteria, 186–187,
            188–189
        functional cure, 186–193
        level of stereopsis, 187
        other factors, 192–193
        prognostic variables of the de-
            viation, 189–191
    see also Diagnosis; Vision therapy
Progressive supranuclear palsy,
        247–248
Proptosis, 239–240
Proximal convergence, 46, 93
Pseudo DE. See Simulated (psuedo) di-
        vergence excess
Pseudomyopia, 39, 476
Pseudostrabismus, 98
Psychic vergence, 46
Psychogenic amblyopia, 140
Psychometric analysis, 148
Psychometric charts (S-chart),
        148–149
Ptosis, 201243
Pursuit eye movements, 7–8, 18,
        29–33
    in amblyopia, 144
    characteristics of, 29
    defined, 29
    factors affecting performance of,
        29, 31
    functional training procedures
        and, 32
    inaccurate and jerky, 29, 31
    neurologic disease and, 31–32
    signs and symptoms, 31–32

Pursuit eye movements (*continued*)
  testing
    afterimages, 31
    direct observation, 30
    pursuit skills, 29–31
  tests
    Bernell Rotator Trainer, 31
    fixation, 32
    Heinsen-Schrock System, 30
    H-S Scale, 30–31
    Marsden Ball, 30
    recommended, 33
    SCCO, 30
  velocity of, 29
  vision training
    general approaches, 471–474
    specific techniques, 473
Pursuits, cogwheel, 246, 248
Pursuits with tag, 303–304

Q

Quoits slides, 481

R

Radiation therapy, 247
Rashbass, 49
Ray, J.M., 289
Reading bars, 366, 367, 391, 426
Reading Eye Camera, 22
Reading for resolution, 299
Reading problems, 485
Recognition acuity tasks, 152
Rectus muscles, 5
Red filter and red print, 311, 367
Red filter therapy, and occlusion, 290
Red lens test, 136
Referrals
  to other professionals, 59, 202, 438
  for vision therapy, 58
Reflex fusion stress test, 50–52
Reflex fusion test, 49–50
Refraction techniques
  in amblyopia, 160–161, 279
  in congenital nystagmus, 447–448
Refractive accommodative esotropia,
    211, 212–214
Refractive error, management of,
    278–280
Reindeer stereopsis test, 58
Relative accommodation
  poor negative (NRA), 36
  poor positive (PRA), 36
  ranking of, 36
Relative vergence, 47–49
Remy, 262
Remy Separator, 361–362, 393–394
Repka, M.X., 288, 289
Resectioning, of muscle or tendon, 198
Reserve vergence, 70

Resolution practice with tag, 304–305
Restricted zone, 91–92
Retinal correspondence, 9–10, 14
Retinal function testing, 162–163
Retinal image disparity detection, 14
Retinal receptive fields, 10
Retinal rivalry, 15, 132, 360
Retraction syndrome (Duane),
    241–242
Revell, M.J., 262, 327
Richman, J.E., 26
Rindziunski, E., 339
Rising eye syndrome, 237
Risley prisms, 47
Ron, A., 289
Ronne, G., 339
Root Rings target, 415
Rosner, J., 51
Rosner TVAS training, 468
Rouse, M.W., 42, 45, 313, 327, 336,
    397
Rubin, W., 290
Rush, J.A., 234
Rutstein, R.P., 343, 409

S

Saccades, 7
  fine and gross, 19
  types of, 7
Saccadic blindness, 18
Saccadic eye movements, 18–29
  in amblyopia, 144
  duration and velocity of, 18
  functional and dysfunctional prob-
    lems, 19
    symptoms of, 19
  neurology of, 18
  suppression, 18–19
  testing, 19–29
    for saccadic skills, 19–29
    standard scoring system, 27–28
    subjective, 24–27
    summary of, 28–29
  tests
    DEM Test, 26–27, 28
    five-dot, 21, 22
    Heinsen-Schrock system, 20–21
    King-Devick Test, 25–26, 28
    ophthalmography, 21–22
    Pierce Saccade Test, 24–25, 28
    recommended sequence of, 28
    SCCO system, 19–20
    sequential fixation, 22–24
  vision training, 19, 466–471, 484
    general approaches, 466–471
    specific techniques, 467–468,
      469–470
Saccadic Fixator, 467
Saccadic movements with tag, 302

Saladin, J., 84, 86, 93
SCCO system, 19–20
SCCO 4+ System, 33
Schapero, M., 87, 91, 92, 162
S-chart. *See* Psychometric chart
Schor, C.M., 46, 47, 74, 93
Schor, M.C., 143, 153
Schrock, R., 30
Sclera, 200
Scotoma, 161, 162
Scott, A.B., 202
Scott, S.H., 445
See saw nystagmus, 254, 453
Seizures, 357–358
Selenow, A., 139, 142–143, 156,
    157
Sensory and motor fusion training,
    356, 358, 366
  in acquired noncomitant devia-
    tions, 441–443
  in eso deviations, 373, 374–376
  in exo deviations, 374, 409–410
Sensory fusion, 9, 10, 52–59, 263
  classification, 53
  flat fusion, 54
  obstacles to, 15
  simultaneous perception, 53
  stereopsis, 54–58
  superimposition, 53–54
  suppression, 53, 54, 556
  testing
    at the centration point, 193
    recommendations from results,
      58–59
    summary of, 58
  theories of, 14–15
  therapy (*see* Sensory and motor fu-
    sion training)
  types of, 12–14
Sensory fusion disruption syndrome,
    445, 446
Sensory orthophoria, 338
Sensory strabismus, 230
Sequential fixation tests, 22–24
Sheard, C., 70, 72–73, 81, 84, 264
Sheard's criterion, 72–73, 84, 86
Sheedy, J.E., 4, 81, 84, 86
Shepard, C.F., 56
Sherrington's law, 7, 8
Shippman, S., 293
Sidkaro, Y., 230
Simulated (psuedo) divergence ex-
    cess, 89–90, 223
Simultaneous perception, 12–13, 53
  testing, 53
Singleness Horopter, 10
Single oblique mirror stereoscope
    (SOMS) Trainer, 360
SITE IRAS Interferometer, 156, 157

Sixth nerve (abducens) palsy, 235, 438, 439–440, 442
Skeffington, A.M., 265
Sliding vergence training, 268, 375
Smith, D.R., 223
Snellen, H., 146
Snellen charts, 4, 146–147
Solomons, H., 18
Spasm of accommodation, 39
Spasmus nutans, 252
Spatial localization testing, 115–116
Spiral of Tillaux, 5, 6
Spirangle Vectogram, 389, 480
Split field perception, 170
Stanworth mirrors, 334, 358
Static cover test, 480
Steadiness of fixation training, 301–302
Steele-Richardson syndrome, 247
Step vergence training, 268–269, 382–383, 389, 391, 417–418, 426, 479
Stereoacuity
    calculations, 492
    see also Stereopsis
Stereograms, 382, 383, 384
Stereopsis, 3, 4–5, 9, 54–58, 375
    central, 13, 14
    defined, 133
    fixation disparity and, 74
    and level of induced anisometropia, 57
    local versus global, 56–57, 58
    norms for stereoacuity, 58
    percentage of, 56
    peripheral, 13–14
    screening for binocular problems with, 56
    testing
        Howard-Dolman peg test, 55
        Lang test, 55
        percentage of stereopsis, 56
        ranking results of, 59
        screening for binocular problems with stereopsis, 56–58
        vectographic methods, 55, 480–482
    vision therapy, 480–482
Stereopsis Fly tests, 187
Stereoscopes. *See* Brewster stereoscope; Wheatstone stereoscope
Strabismic amblyopia, 9, 140, 143, 191, 284, 286, 319
    case example, 319–321
Strabismic deviation. *See* Strabismus testing
Strabismus, 5, 12, 54, 56
    A and V patterns, 224–226

accommodative esotropia, 188, 211–216
    acquired, 98, 188
    amblyopia, 319–321
    case examples, 202–209
    cause of, 99, 263
    congenital, 98
    consecutive, 230–231
    convergence excess esotropia, 214
    cyclovertical deviations, 228–230
    developmental, 211–231
    diagnosis and prognosis, 185–209
    early acquired, 98, 188
    essential infantile, 98, 173
    infantile esotropia, 98, 216–220
    intermittent, 367, 98, 121–123, 130
    late acquired, 98, 188
    microtropia, 226–228
    nonaccommodative acquired, 188
    noncomitant, 13, 233–238, 438
    paretic, 234
    primary comitant esotropia, 220–224
    primary comitant exotropia, 221–224
    pseudostrabismus, 98
    psychogenic, 188
    sensory, 230
    sensory adaptations to (*see* Strabismus, sensory adaptations to)
    testing (*see* Strabismus testing)
    types of, 211–231
    vision therapy (*see also* Vision therapy), 261–275
Strabismus, sensory adaptations to
    amblyopia, 138–163
        as a developmental disorder, 142
        case history, 145
        classification, 139–141
        eye disease evaluation, 161
        fixation evaluation, 156–163
        visual acuity testing, 145–156
    anomalous correspondence, 163–183
        characteristics, 166–173
        classification, 163–166
        testing, 173–183
    suppression, 131–137
        characteristics, 132–135
        testing, 135–137
    see also Strabismus; Strabismus testing
Strabismus fixus, 243
Strabismus testing
    AC/A, 128
    comitancy, 107–121
        causes, 107–108

criteria and terminology, 108–109
        ductions, 111–112
        primary and secondary deviations, 109–111
        recording noncomitant deviations, 115
        signs and symptoms, 116–117
        spatial localization testing, 115–116
        subjective testing, 117–118
        three-step method, 112–115
        versions, 112
    cosmesis and, 127, 130
    detection and measurement, 101–107
    detection and measurement of
        alternate cover test, 104–106, 124
        angle kappa, 102
        Brückner test, 107
        direct observation, 101
        four base-out prism test, 106–107
        Hirschberg test, 102–103
        Krimsky test, 103–104
        strabismus, 101
        unilateral cover test, 104
    deviation
        direction of, 123–125, 189
        frequency of, 98, 121–123, 135, 189
        magnitude of, 99, 103, 125–128, 129–130, 135, 189–190, 194–195
        variability of, 129–130, 190
    examination record, 494–495
    eye dominancy, 129, 190–191
    eye laterality, 128–129, 135, 190
    history, 97–101
    see also Strabismus; Strabismus, sensory adaptations to
Streff syndrome, 59
Stroke, 246
Subnormal binocular vision. *See* Microtropia
Suchoff, I.B., 191
Superimposition, 53–54
    testing, 13, 53–54
Superior adherence syndrome, 244
Superior oblique muscle, 5, 6
Suppliers and equipment, 496–497
Suppression, 131–137
    with amblyopia, 310
    characteristics of, 132–135, 367
    classification, 133
    defined, 131, 349
    end-point, 358–359
    and exotropia, 407, 409

Suppression (*continued*)
  intensity of, 133–135, 136
  pathological, 132
  physiological, 10, 131–132
  prognosis and, 191
  in sensory fusion, 53, 54, 56
  testing for, 24, 135–137
    amblyoscope workup, 137
    history, 135–136
    red lens test, 136
    Worth dot test, 136–137
  therapy for (*see* Antisuppression
    therapy)
Suppression zone, 133, 134
Supranuclear disorders. *See* Internu-
    clear and supranuclear disor-
    ders
Supranuclear horizontal gaze palsy,
    31, 246
  brainstem lesions, 246
  frontal eye-field lesions, 246
  occipital and parietal cortical le-
    sions, 246
Supranuclear vertical gaze palsy,
    246–248
  parinaud syndrome, 247
  Parkinson's disease, 248
  progressive supranuclear palsy,
    247–248
  review of pathways, 246–247
Surgery
  and A and V patterns, 225
  and accommodative esotropia, 213
  and acquired noncomitant strabis-
    mus, 443
  ARC and, 341–343
  complications, 200–201
    overcorrections, 230–231
  and congenital nystagmus, 452
  and esotropia, 376–377
  and exotropia, 411
  and Graves disease, 240, 241
  and infantile esotropia, 220
  and nonrefractive esotropia, 216
  see also Extraocular muscle surgery
Swann split field effect, 170
Swinging ball training, 294
Sylvian aqueduct syndrome, 247
Sympathomimetic (adrenergic)
    drugs, 35
Synoptophore, 137, 138, 178, 180,
    181, 329, 333, 351, 449

T

Tachistoscopic training, 299
Tactile stimulation, 354
Tanlamai, T., 140–141
Task performance, 4
Taylor, D.M., 187–188, 220

Television trainers, 364–365, 426
Tenectomy, 198, 243
Test anxiety, 29, 31
Third nerve (oculomotor) palsy,
    236–238, 457–458
  case example, 457–458
3-dot card, 416–417
Three-step method, 112–115
Throwing and hitting games, 293
Thyroid eye disease, 239–241
Tired eyes, 5
Tittarelli, H., 172
Tonic vergence, 46, 64–67
Toulouse, J.G., 290
Tracing and drawing, 293
Tracking with auditory feedback, 295
Tranaglyphs, 351, 386–390, 397,
    418, 479, 480
Translid Binocular Interaction (TBI)
    method, 310, 356–358, 367
Trimble, R., 198
Tromboning, accommodative, 477
Tromboning vergence training, 269,
    383–384, 418
Tropical illnesses, 35
True divergence excess, 223
Tucking, 198
Tumbling E cards, 149–152
Tumors, 245
Turned eye, 230

U

Unharmonious ARC (UNHARC), 164,
    181–182
Unilateral cover test, 104
Unilateral neutralization test, 227, 228
Upbeat nystagmus, 254

V

Vaegan, 269
Vascular lesions, 245
Vectograms, 386–390, 397, 418,
    480–481
Vectogram stereopsis enhancement,
    480–482
Vectographic slides, 13, 77, 78, 386,
    390, 419
Vectographic tests, for stereopsis, 55
Vergence, 18, 44–52
  absolute convergence, 44–46
    developmental considerations,
      46
    functions and norms for, 45–46
    testing techniques, 44–45
  accommodative, 195
  anomalies (*see* Vergence anomalies)
  demand, methods for changing,
    375
  excessive convergence, 195–196

  facility, 49–52
    studies on, 51
    testing of, 50–51, 52
  fusional, 195
  Maddox classification of, 44, 63
  neurology of, 8, 44
  relative convergence, 46–49
    fusional vergences at far, 47–49
    fusional vergences at near, 49
    testing and norms, 46–49
  sensory fusion, 52–59
  stamina, 52
  terminology of, 46
  testing, 44–52
    reflex fusion stress test, 50–52
    reflex fusion test, 49–50
    summary of, 52
  vision training, 479–480
    methods, 267–270, 433–434,
      478, 479–481
  see also Vergence anomalies
Vergence anomalies, 87–92
  basic esophoria, 90–91
  basic exophoria, 89
  basic orthophoria with restricted
    zone, 91–92
  convergence excess, 91
  convergence insufficiency (CI),
    88–92, 420–422, 431–435
  divergence excess, 89–90
  divergence insufficiency, 90
  normal zone with symptoms, 92
Vergence rock techniques (flipper
    prisms), 391, 397, 425–427
Vergence stamina, 52
Versions, 112
Vertical displacement of targets, 331
Vestibular nystagmus, 256, 453
  characteristics of, 253
Vestibular ocular eye movements, 7
Vestibular ocular reflexes (VOR), 7, 18
Video display terminal (VDT), 4, 5
Video game tracking, 293–294
Viral encephalitis, 35
Visagraph, 18, 22
Vision efficiency analysis, 92–93
Vision efficiency skills, 17–59
  accommodation, 34–44
    therapy for, 474–479
  aniseikonia, 462–465
  case examples of, 482–484
  emphasis on efficiency, 18, 265,
    462, 486
  evaluation testing outline, 493
  fixation, 33–34
  monovision, 465–466
  pursuit eye movements, 29–33
    therapy for, 471–474
  saccadic eye movements, 18–19

therapy for, 466–471
sensory fusion, 52–59
stereopsis, 480–481
therapy, 461–487
    finishing concepts, 478
    future directions in, 462,
       485–487
    for visual comfort and perform-
       ance, 462
    vergences, 44–52
    therapy for, 478–480
Vision loss
    postoperative, 200
    sensory strabismus and, 230
Vision therapy, 196–202, 261–275
    botulinum injections, 202
    computerized programs, 395–396
    for eso deviations (*see* Eso devia-
       tions, vision therapy)
    for exo deviations (*see* Exo devia-
       tions, vision therapy)
    extraocular muscle surgery,
       198–201
       general approach, 198–200
       prior to training, 187–188
       surgical considerations, 2
         00–201
    fusion training, 263
    home training
       office training versus, 270–271
       retainer, 274–275
    lenses, 197
    modes of, 196–202
    monitoring progress, 273–274
    occlusion, 197
    office versus home training,
       270–271
    open environment versus instru-
       ment training, 271
    other approaches, 202
    patient motivation, 271–273
    pharmacological treatment,
       201–202
    philosophies of, 261–265
       Javal and the French School,
         261–263
       optometric, 264–265

Worth and the English School,
    263–264
    principles of, 265–270, 350
    prisms, 197
    referral for, 58
    sequence of, 265–267
    strabismus, 261–275
    vergence training, 267–270
    vision training, 193, 197
    see also Prognosis
Vision training, 193, 197
    accommodative esotropia, 213
    computer-based, 273
    and congenital nystagmus,
       448–452
    and infantile esotropia, 219–220
    and nonrefractive esotropia, 215
    orthoptics, 197
    pleoptics, 197
    visual perception therapy, 197
Visual acuity, 4
    and visual efficiency, calculations,
       491
Visual acuity testing, and amblyopia
    Bailey-Lovie chart, 147
    infant assessment, 152–154
    interferometry, 155–156
    psychometric charts, 148–149
    Snellen charts, 146–147
    tumbling E and picture cards,
       149–152
    visually evoked potential, 154–155
Visual cortex, 9, 10
Visual field testing, in amblyopia,
    161–162
Visually evoked cortical potential
    (VECP), 154
Visually evoked potential (VEP),
    154–155, 156
    transient, 154–155
Visual perception training, 197
Visual tracing, 295
Visual tracking, 294, 311, 367
Visuoscopy, evaluating fixation,
    158–159
Vodnoy, B.E., 265, 308, 361, 374, 386
Vodnoy afterimage technique, 308

Vodnoy Aperture-Rule Trainer (ART),
    391–393, 419–420
Voluntary convergence, 413–414
Voluntary nystagmus, 249–250
    characteristics, 250
von Noorden, G.K., 127, 132, 162,
       172, 181, 198, 220, 223,
       228, 230, 236, 243, 244,
       288, 289, 290, 396, 397,
       445, 452

W

Wayne Perceptuomotor Pen, 295,
    296, 354
Wayne Saccadic Fixator, 467
Weige-Lussen,L., 199
Wesson, M., 149
Wesson Fixation Disparity Card, 76,
    79, 85
Westheimer, 49
Wheatstone stereoscope, 361, 379
White, C.T., 154
Wick, B., 46, 80, 93, 301, 309, 343,
       345, 376, 407, 429, 432, 443
Winter, J., 191
Wittenberg, S., 480
Wong, S.Y., 452
Worrell, B.E., 84, 86
Worth, C., 13, 53, 142, 263–264,
       328, 445, 486
Worth dot test, 136–137
Wybar, K., 190

X

X patterns, 224

Y

Yaniglos, S.S., 453
Yekta, A.A., 85
Younge, B.R., 234

Z

Zone of clear single binocular vision
    (ZCSBV), 67–70, 264
    relevant features of, 69–70
    useful characteristics of, 68–69
Zone of comfort, 73